Managed Care, Outcom[illegible]
and Quality:
A Practical Guide

Managed Care, Outcomes, and Quality: A Practical Guide

Edited by

Steven F. Isenberg, M.D.

With Forewords by
Uwe Reinhardt, Ph.D
and
Nancy Snyderman, M.D.

MAR 2 1999

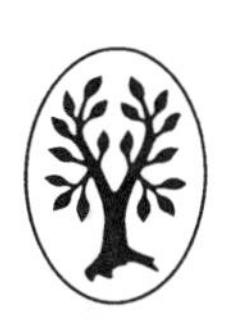

1998
Thieme
New York • Stuttgart

W
130
M31.5
1998

Thieme New York
381 Park Avenue South
New York, NY 10016

Managed Care, Outcomes, and Quality: A Practical Guide
Steven F. Isenberg, M.D.

Library of Congress Cataloging-in-Publication Data

Managed care, outcomes, and quality : a practical guide / edited by
Steven F. Isenberg ; with forewords by Uwe Reinhardt and Nancy
Snyderman.
p. cm.
Includes bibliographical references and index.
ISBN 0-86577-687-3 (TNY).— ISBN 3-13-109941-0 (GTV)
1. Managed care plans (Medical care) 2. Outcome assessment
(Medical care) I. Isenberg, Steven F.
[DNLM: 1. Managed Care Programs—United States. 2. Physician's
Practice Patterns—United States. 3. Practice Management, Medical—
United States. 4. Quality of Health Care—United States.
5. Outcome and Process Assessment (Health Care) W 130 AA1 M19
1997]
RA413.M266 1997
362.1'04258—dc21
DNLM/DLC 97-17252
for Library of Congress CIP

Copyright© 1998 by Thieme Medical Publishers, Inc. This book, including all parts thereof, is legally protected by copyright. Any use, exploitation or commercialization outside the narrow limits set by copyright legislation, without the publisher's consent, is illegal and liable to prosecution. This applies in particular to photostat reproduction, copying, mimeographing or duplication of any kind, translating, preparation of microfilms, and electronic data processing and storage.

Important note: Medical knowledge is ever-changing. As new research and clinical experience broaden our knowledge, changes in treatment and drug therapy may be required. The authors and editors of the material herein have consulted sources believed to be reliable in their efforts to provide information that is complete and in accord with the standards accepted at the time of publication. However, in view of the possibility of human error by the authors, editors, or publisher of the work herein, or changes in medical knowledge, neither the authors, editors, publisher, nor any other party who has been involved in the preparation of this work, warrants that the information contained herein is in every aspect accurate or complete. Readers are encouraged to confirm the information contained herein with other sources. For example, readers are advised to check the product information sheet included in the package of each drug they plan to administer to be certain that the information contained in this publication is accurate and that changes have not been made in the recommended dose or in the contraindications for administration. This recommendation is of particular importance in connection with new or infrequently used drugs.

Some of the product names, patents, and registered designs referred to in this book are in fact registered trademarks or proprietary names even though specific reference to this fact is not always made in the text. Therefore, the appearance of a name without designation is proprietary is not to be construed as a representation by the publisher that it is in the public domain.

Printed in the United States of America

5 4 3 2 1

TNY ISBN 0-86577-687-3
GTV ISBN 3-13-109941-0

This book is dedicated to all my patients.

Contents

STEVEN F. ISENBERG

Preface xi

Foreword xiii
Nancy Snyderman

Foreword xv
Uwe Reinhardt

Acknowledgements xix

Contributors xxi

I. The Essentials of Managed Care and Capitation

1. Capitation 3
Art Wilmes

2. Reimbursement Systems and Managed Care 11
Cheryl Toth, with an addendum by Lee Eisenberg

3. Referral Guidelines 23
Michael S. Benninger

4. Negotiating Managed Care Contracts 31
T. Forcht Dagi

5. The Legal Issues of Managed Care Contracts 51
Tom Neal

6. Understanding Profiling 67
Susan Bellile

7. Ethical Challenges of Managed Care 73
Carl A. Patow and Ruth D. Gaare

II. Utilizing Outcomes in a Managed Care Environment

8. Outcomes Research: Where We Have Been, Where We Need to Go 85
Michael G. Stewart

9. Meaningful Outcomes Research 99
Richard M. Rosenfeld

10. Improving Health Care: Measuring Outcomes and Implementing Change . 117
Eugene C. Nelson, Julie J. Mohr, Paul B. Batalden, Stephen K. Plume, and Christine C. Mahoney

11. Project Solo/Physicians' Information Exchange: Organizing Physicians Around Quality 167
Steven F. Isenberg

III. Quality in the Front and the Back Office

12. Improving Office Efficiency in a Managed Care Environment 185
Cheryl Toth

13. Staffing Requirements in Managed Care 193
Cheryl Toth

14. Surviving and Thriving as an Independent Practitioner: The Search for Continuous Quality Improvement 203
Steven F. Isenberg

15. Information Management in Managed Care and Capitation 233
Vinson J. Hudson

16. Malpractice Issues 239
Thomas M. Kidder

IV. The Physician's Response to Managed Care

17. Network Mergers and IPAs: The Legal Issues 249
Matthew L. Howard

18. Physician Organizations 257
James Unland

19. Single-Specialty Networks: The Mature Network 277
Gary Stone

20. Single-Specialty Networks: Initial Stages 289
Michael D. Weiss

21. Mergers and Acquisitions 295
T. Forcht Dagi and Jay Mayes

22. Evolving a Single Specialty Into a Multispecialty Network 315
Ramie A. Tritt

23. Will Doctors Take Back Health Care? 325
Uwe E. Reinhardt

Index 333

Preface

This book is for medical and surgical practitioners—those physicians who actually examine and treat patients. You know who you are. You're the physicians who could be on call at 3:00 AM on Christmas Day; the physicians who face an office full of patients or a complicated surgical case after a long, stressful, sleepless night of caring for a critically ill patient; the physicians who must fit diagnoses, treatment plans, and reimbursement into America's milieu of ICD-9s, CPTs, HMOs, PPOs, Medicare, Medicaid, malpractice, and the Hippocratic oath. You are the physicians who now must add the financial vulnerability of your practice to the standard patient care questions that precipitate your insomnia. I am one of you, and this book is for us. From one who walks the talk, let me invite you to read about the important practice management and socioeconomic issues that face today's medical and surgical practitioners.

Let me also invite those readers—nurses, administrators, business people, third party payers, and patients—who are interested in the physicians' response to the recent changes in America's healthcare. Laura Archer Pulfer of the *Cincinnati Enquirer* read an editorial on National Public Radio, August 2, 1996. Reportedly, there was a huge response from listeners for copies of the transcript. In her editorial, she questioned physicians: "Isn't it about time you rescue medicine from the questionable mercies of business and politics? Why aren't you running this show? Are you really prepared to become just another employee?"[1] This book was also written to answer the questions asked by Ms. Pulfer. It was written by physicians, for both physicians and all of us who currently are, have been, or will be patients.

I've divided this book into four sections. In the first section, Art Wilmes will lead us through the complicated and risky business of capitation. Cheryl Toth will then examine reimbursement in a managed care environment. Lee Eisenberg, a member of the AMA CPT Editorial Panel, writes an addendum to Cheryl's chapter and will highlight some important CPT issues in a managed care environment. The idiosyncrasies of managed care contracts will be detailed by Tom Neal. T. Forcht Dagi, acknowledged expert in negotiations, will assist us in learning how to negotiate with managed care companies. Susan Bellile will focus on practice profiling and Michael Benninger will present his expertise on referral guidelines. Referral guidelines have proven to be useful for primary care physicians, specialists, and patients. In Section I's final chapter, Carl Patow and Ruth Gaare explore the ethical issues of managed care.

In Section II, Michael Stewart and Richard Rosenfeld describe outcomes research. Both are ENTs, but their chapters apply to all physicians. Dr. Rosenfeld then provides useful information to permit practitioners to implement outcomes research in community-based office practices. This wonderful introduction to outcomes is complemented by the tetralogy of Eugene Nelson, Paul Batalden, Stephen Plume, Julie J. Mohr, and Christine C. Mahoney from Dartmouth. Outcomes research permits us to know where we are, but we then need to know how to implement change to improve quality. The four-part series authored by this nationally acknowledged and award-winning physician-focused team from Dartmouth will provide the reader with the tools that we require to provide healthcare for our patients in the next century. My chapter on organizing physicians around quality concludes Section II.

Section III section provides some nuts and bolts. Cheryl Toth begins with her chapters on improving office efficiency and managing staff in a managed care environment. Vinson Hudson then leads us through the important and complicated software selection process for the individual practitioner's needs. With my eighteen years of experience as a private practitioner, I offer my insight into managing a medical practice in the next chapter. Thomas Kidder completes this section with some helpful pointers to avoid malpractice claims.

Section IV provides the physicians' response to managed care. In this section, Matthew Howard discusses the legal issues of mergers and networks. Several practicing physicians from different geographic areas outline their personal experiences in the rapidly changing world of physician network development. James Unland, a national expert in physician organizations, details the idiosyncrasies of organizing physicians. Michael Weiss, a nationally recognized speaker on physician networks, outlines his experience with the frugal development of a network in Maryland. Gary Stone, from Florida, provides detailed information on his mature network. T. Forcht Dagi and Jay Mayes provide an in-depth review of mergers and acquisitions. Both physicians are Wharton graduates, and their expertise is extremely valuable in this complicated area. Ramie Tritt, from Atlanta, another expert in specialty network development, outlines the development of a multispecialty network and sophisticated practice management for a large group in a major metropolitan area. In the book's final chapter, Uwe Reinhardt, Princeton economist, leaves us with his expertise on how physicians can take back healthcare. Dr. Reinhardt's innovative thoughts on this matter are widely quoted.

Across America, physicians are organizing—into single and multispecialty networks and physician-owned practice management and insurance companies, for example—to regain control of healthcare. We were caught off guard by organized third-party payers, but by focusing attention on the patient–physician relationship, quality, and our combined abilities to control cost, physicians can "rescue medicine from the questionable mercies of business and politics." The future of this movement appears to rely on, as Uwe Reinhardt writes, whether independently minded physicians (eagles) will fly in formation.

Drs. Reinhardt and Snyderman follow this Preface with Forewords. Dr. Reinhardt warns of the danger that lurks amidst the opportunities that are available to physicians. Dr. Snyderman, physician–surgeon, author, radio talk show host, and ABC national reporter, describes the relationship between the media and medicine. These two outstanding authorities will help the reader understand the physician's role in the future of healthcare.

To "cut the Gordian Knot" is to solve a seemingly insoluble problem with a brilliant stroke. Gordius, the mythologic founder of Phrygia, tied a knot in a chariot thong that could be unraveled only by someone proclaimed by the oracle to become the ruler of Asia. All who had come to that place failed in the attempt, but Alexander the Great simply cut the Gordian knot with one blow of his sword. Sometimes America's healthcare problems can seem insoluble. Physicians, under the aegis of peer-directed solutions, are in the best position to cut the Gordian knot of healthcare in America.

REFERENCES

1. Pulfer L A. National Public Radio; 1996, August 2.

Foreword

NANCY SNYDERMAN

Drop in on any M.B.A. class these days and you might be surprised to find physicians in various stages of their careers. This isn't some midlife lark, but a real need, some say, to understand what so many in the business world have been saying for years—that American medicine may be the best in the world, but it is too expensive and there is no real data to support that high cost necessarily affords the best care. That is not to say that this premise and the transition to managed care have been easy. They have not. And while there were certainly abuses and excesses in the old days of fee for service, we have watched the pendulum swing so far the other way, it is unconscionable to most of us when CEOs of HMOs walk away with multimillion dollar paychecks. We are straddling a widening gulf of the haves and have-nots and our patients are the losers.

The sanctity of the traditional doctor–patient relationship is meant to ensure that we will always support what is in the best interest of our patient—with all financial incentives out of the equation. It is idealistic, should be practical, and is certainly naive. And now we are paying a price—literally and figuratively—in the United States. Medicine as we knew it of several decades ago is dead and I do not think it will be coming back. We may remember it as innocent because we loved the autonomy. We made decisions, charged fees, and the insurance companies wrote the checks. When the occasional patient fell on hard times or appeared at the front desk without coverage it was OK because the greater pool allowed us to cover it.

We have always coveted our autonomy and have bristled at bureaucracy. And yet the independence so many of us grew up with also allowed some to abuse a good system. We were lured by temptation and some overoperated, overcharged, and failed to realize the backlash that was waiting for us. Who would have foreseen the day when financial incentives would be to withhold care rather than provide it? We scream with outrage. But we should not be shocked.

I have worked for ABC News since 1986. As a correspondent for *Good Morning America* and *Prime Time Live,* I have traveled the country talking to physicians and interviewing patients with all sorts of stories to tell. During this time I have been witness to this change in medicine from the inside as a doctor and from the outside as a reporter. I have come to believe that while the doctor–patient relationship has been eroded and HMOs have made access to specialists more difficult, the press has become the patient's advocate.

Consider this scenario that took place in 1996. Kaiser-Permanente announced that women undergoing uncomplicated vaginal deliveries would be discharged from the hospital within 8 hours of delivery. A female OB-GYN was trotted out during the press conference and contended that women want to be home with their families because they were more comfortable there. There was no mention made of the fact that women would not be allowed to stay even if they wanted to or of the struggles with exhaustion, mastering breast feeding, and potential lack of support at home. It was meant to be a simple event and instead turned into a public relations nightmare. Why? Because the press dubbed this new policy "drive-through deliveries" and women and doctors across the country cried foul and blasted this decision. Next thing you know, the governor of New Jersey, Christine Todd Whitman, saw the ripple effect of one HMO starting policy changes for others and put her foot down. Legislation was enacted in New Jersey that required all insurers to allow a woman to stay up to 48 hours in the hospital if she so desired. Her move prompted other states to introduce the same policy and finally legislation was pushed through the U.S. Congress. The good news is that the press acted as the patient's advocate in this case and good policy was set. The downside is that this is one small slice of the pie and the press can't be there for every inequity nor can we count on legislation to take care of every one of our ills.

In fact, most of the time, the patient is left to struggle as an individual. Who fights for them? We try, but are one very small piece of the puzzle. We threaten and the faceless bureaucracy laughs. Don't like the rules? Leave. But play the fight out on national television and suddenly water cooler conversation turns into legislation.

These changes are not relegated to the private community. Every medical center is feeling the pinch and I believe the changes will change our teaching centers for a long time to come. The day of courting high-priced senior professors is over. There will be no need for "stars." They come with too high a price tag. Instead the system will cultivate worker bees, good physicians who come cheap. It's an easy equation to follow. Well-trained, young doctors can offer high quality health care without the salary demands. It's one step that many companies and universities see as essential.

Through all of this it is important that we keep our eyes on one of our most important roles—that as patient advocate. We must fight to provide each American with the best health care available and face the bureaucracy when need be. These are uncertain times. But there is no reason to give up. We will adapt and turn our attention to studying the correlation between cost, quality, and outcomes research. The business community wants this information as much as we do.

The pendulum will swing back. It may not be tomorrow. But we are not going to be shoved out of the picture. We are needed and we must make our voices heard. Our patients are counting on it.

FOREWORD

UWE REINHARDT

A while ago, as I was desperately racking my brain for a snappy title to an upcoming keynote address, my Chinese wife calmly wrote down the following characters:

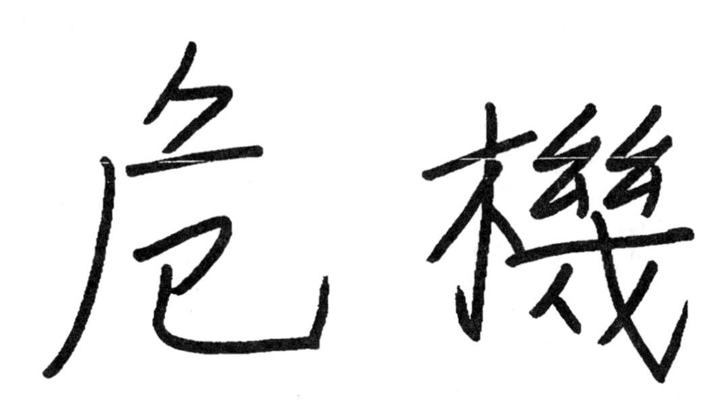

"Talk about that," she said. "It fits American healthcare to a tee." To my dumbfounded look she responded: "It's the Chinese word for 'crisis.' The character on the left side, you see, means 'danger.' The character on the right side means 'opportunity.' That's what 'crisis' spells for the Chinese people."

It is what the word "crisis" spells for the American physicians as well. There is no question that the current revolution in American healthcare carries with it great danger for the individual physician and for the profession as a whole; but it also offers enormous opportunities—opportunities to practice truly the best medicine in the world and in history; opportunities to regain, once more, clinical and also administrative control of American healthcare. It is also an opportunity to strike it truly rich, if that is the goal.

The crisis into which the American medical community has tumbled has partly been of the profession's own making although, under the circumstances, it could have happened to any profession. For reasons that will long puzzle historians, Americans decided sometime in the mid-1960s to simply set aside the normal laws of demand and supply for health care and to replace that system of checks and balances with one of unilateral and unquestioned trust in its medical profession and in other providers of health care. "Do to and for us, as patients, as you think best," we told our physicians. "Enlist in your treatment plan whomever you wish, and somehow we, our insurance carrier, or our government will politely pay you and your allies, usually without question or reservation, for whatever you write down on your bill." It was an arrangement such as the world had never seen before and surely will never see again. And it begat a health system that represents, not surprisingly, both the very best and the very worst to be found in the industrialized world. In many ways, the system is splendid beyond belief, and also expensive. In other ways, it is shoddy, haphazard, and cruel. People the world over may come to our medical schools and health care facilities to study medicine or to seek clinically advanced care. But people the world over also hold up our health system—which includes the manner in which we pay for health care and protect individuals from the fiscal inroads of ill health—as the bogeyman of health policy, as an example of where they may end up if they do not get their own act together. Americans may boast that theirs is the best health system in the world. The rest of the world thinks of that system as asocial.

Basking in the deep trust offered up by the American people and in the economic good fortune that rode on that trust, American physicians took too much for granted for too long. Sometime during the 1980s, the erstwhile trust gave way to suspicion as both public and private third-party payers saw their healthcare budgets run out of control and as physicians and other providers of healthcare found themselves unable to defend either the enormous regional and even intraregional variations in the prices for seemingly identical services or the equally stunning geographic practice variations in the per capita use of health services by seemingly similar populations. These geographic variations, in particular, led to the thought that the medical profession could not be counted on to observe proper economy in the use of scarce resources. Gone was the trust that had ruled American medicine in happier days, and in came the concept of "managed care."

At its core, "managed care" may be described as the continuous, external monitoring of the ongoing doctor–patient relationship and, if deemed necessary, the external micromanaging of that relationship, with the goal responding to given medical condition with appropriate medical interventions that are procured at the lowest attainable cost to those who pay for those interventions. In a broader sense, "managed care" can be brought to include the structure of selective contracting between those who pay for healthcare and those who provide the care. In principle, selective contracting permits those who pay for healthcare effectively to fire particular providers of health care found wanting either because their prices are too high, or because their treatment regimens are needlessly intensive, or both. Selective contracting allows payers to extract price discounts from providers and to impose on them the supervision and clinical control implied in the term "managed care."

Selective contracting basically takes two distinct forms, with many hybrids in between. At one extreme there is the "savvy purchase" model. Under that model, insurance carriers who collect insurance premiums either from patients, from employers, or from government (e.g. under Medicaid managed care) can try to control the providers of health care with the ancient principle of divide et impera. That system works best if providers of healthcare are compensated on a fee-for-service basis, albeit at steeply discounted fees, and controlled clinically through externally imposed practice guidelines (typically, by means of an 800 number staffed by nurses and physicians thousands of miles away). It is the model of selective contracting that has driven physicians to despondency. It also remains the dominant form of "managed care."

The alternative extreme to the "savvy purchaser" model is the "incentive alignment" or "risk delegation model." Under that model, the insurance carriers who collect the premium from employers, government, or patients channel a certain percent of it through to integrated networks of providers in the form of a flat capitation, shifting with it the full financial risk for the insured's ill health onto the shoulders of the providers of care. The insurance carrier effectively functions as a mere broker of insured lives who lives off the (typically huge) difference between the premium collected from insured clients and the capitation paid the providers.

In between are a myriad of hybrids with partial capitation of providers, carve-outs for special diseases or special components of medical treatments that are placed under capitation, and models in which insurers and providers truly act as one unit.

Although from the physician's perspective, full capitation for comprehensive healthcare may seem harsh and risky, it actually constitutes the only effective escape from the yoke of externally "managed care." With the shouldering of financial risk, physicians regain control over their clinical work, for it is they who must manage their own colleagues' care so that actual costs remain at or below the capitation. Therein lies the opportunity inherent in the crisis currently besetting the profession.

But the capitation model also carries with it certain dangers of which physicians must be ever mindful.

First, if recklessly exploited by the providers of care—especially physicians—capitation may breed deep suspicion and anger among patients. For better or worse, patients are likely countenance profiteering by insurance carriers with much greater equanimity that they will profiteering by physicians, especially if anecdotal evidence can be construed as support for the latent thesis that physicians might withhold need healthcare for the sake of money. Maintaining the patients' trust under full capitation will challenge American physicians as they have never been challenged before.

Second, full capitation for comprehensive healthcare necessarily requires extensive, multifaceted delivery systems that must be either physically or virtually integrated. At the moment, physically integrated health systems are a bit out of favor; the nouvelle vague among the management gurus is virtual integration. Virtually integrated systems, however, are figments of someone's imagination held together temporarily by networks of computers. It is my guess—although I have been wrong before—that they will never be able to kindle the kind of brand-name loyalty that comes with more visible and more permanent integration. In any event, physicians must take great care that they do not disgrace themselves in the eyes of patients through a never-ending, opportunistic game of musical chairs among virtual systems.

Third, physicians must search for the optimal degree of hierarchy for the integrated, capitated health systems they might seek of establish. Here, too, one can think of extremes. One extreme would be a purely capitalistic mode, founded and managed by people with M.D. degrees, with tradable ownership certificates. Even if such a model initially seeks to retain a majority stake in the hands of participating physicians, it is unlikely to be stable over a long period of time and may well be sold to outsiders sooner or later, when the riches top management might reap from such a sale prove irresistible. At the other extreme is the purely collegiate model that is run by the professionals, but that does not endow the latter with tradable or cashable ownership certificates. The Mayo Clinic is such a model, as is any private university (for professors).

There is great speculation at this time which form of "managed care"—the one driven chiefly by commercial insurance carriers or the one driven by physicians and hospitals—will carry the day in American healthcare. In the near future, much will depend upon the fate of the federal Medicare program. In principle, both the Clinton administration and the Republican Congress appear willing to turn over the task of controlling cost and quality for the Medicare program to private "regulators" (HMOs or provider service networks [PSN's]) as much as possible. Meanwhile, private employers so far have shown little taste for contracting directly with providers, as they always have. Therein, ironically, lies a major opportunity for American physicians to regain control over their own destiny. In the end, the much-loathed public sector may yet turn out to be medicine's best friend.

Acknowledgments

I am deeply grateful for my supportive family and my dedicated staff. My sincere thanks to the contributing authors, the members of Project Solo/Physicians Information Exchange, my peers and mentors, and Thieme New York.

I am most grateful to the higher power that guides me every day.

Contributors

Paul B. Batalden, M.D.
Director, Healthcare Improvement
Leadership Development
Center for Evaluative Clinical Sciences
Dartmouth-Hitchcock Medical Center
Lebanon, New Hampshire

Susan Bellile, M.A., M.B.A.
Founder and President
Q3, Inc.
Westchester, Illinois

Michael S. Benninger, M.D.
Department of Otolaryngology—Head and Neck Surgery
Henry Ford Hospital
Detroit, Michigan

T. Forcht Dagi, M.D., M.P.H., M.B.A.
Clinical Professor of Surgery
The Medical College of Georgia
Atlanta, Georgia

Lee Eisenberg, M.D.
Clinical Associate Professor of Otolaryngology
Columbia University College of Physicians and Surgeons
New York, New York
and
Private Practice
Englewood, New Jersey

Ruth D. Gaare, J.D., M.P.H.
Program Director
Johns Hopkins University Bioethics Institute
Baltimore, Maryland

Matthew L. Howard, M.D., J.D.
Kaiser Permanente Medical Center
Santa Rosa, California and
Private Practice
Ukiah, California

Vinson J. Hudson, M.S.E.E.
President/POMIS Industry Analyst
Jewson Enterprises
Menlo Park, California

Steven F. Isenberg, M.D.
Director and Founder
Project Solo, Physicians Information Exchange
and
Private Practice
Indianapolis, Indiana

Thomas M. Kidder, M.D.
Assistant Professor or Surgery
Medical College of Wisconsin
Milwaukee, Wisconsin

Christine C. Mahoney, R.N., M.S.N.
Clinical Nurse Specialist
Surgical Specialties Unit
Dartmouth-Hitchcock Medical Center
Lebanon, New Hampshire

Jay Mayes, M.D., M.B.A.
Vice President for Medical Affairs
Health Partners Health Plans
Health Partners of Arizona
Phoenix, Arizona

Julie J. Mohr, M.S.P.H.
Research Associate
Director, Healthcare Improvement
Leadership Development
Center for Evaluative Clinical Sciences
Dartmouth-Hitchcock Medical Center
Lebanon, New Hampshire

Tom Neal, J.D.
Kreig Devault, Alexander, and Capeheart
Indianapolis, Indiana

Eugene C. Nelson, DSc. M.P.H.
Director, Quality Education, Measurement, and Research
for the Office of the President
Lahey Hitchcock Clinic
Dartmouth-Hitchcock Medical Center
Lebanon, New Hampshire

Carl A. Patow, M.D., M.P.H.
Associate Professor of Otolaryngology—Head and
Neck Surgery
The Johns Hopkins University School of Medicine
Baltimore, Maryland

Stephen K. Plume, M.D.
President, Lahey Hitchcock Clinic
Dartmouth-Hitchcock Medical Center
Lebanon, New Hampshire

Uwe E. Reinhardt, Ph.D.
Professor of Economics
Princeton University
Woodrow Wilson School of Public and
International Affairs
Princeton, New Jersey

Richard M. Rosenfeld, M.D., M.P.H.
Associate Professor of Otolaryngology
State University of New York Health Science Center
and
Director of Pediatric Otolaryngology
Long Island College Hospital
Brooklyn, New York

Michael G. Stewart, M.D., M.P.H.
Department of Otolaryngology and
Communicative Sciences
Baylor College of Medicine
Houston, Texas

Gary Stone, M.D.
Medical Networks Enterprises
Miami, Florida

Cheryl Toth, Ph.D., M.B.A.
Karen Zupko and Associates
Chicago, Illinois

Ramie A. Tritt, M.D.
President and Chairman of the Board
Physicians Specialty Corporation
and
Private Practice
Atlanta, Georgia

James Unland, M.B.A.
President, The Health Capital Group
Chicago, Illinois

Michael D. Weiss, M.D.
Private Practice
Owings Mills, Maryland

Art Wilmes, F.S.A., M.A.A.A.
Consulting Actuary
Milliman & Robertson, Inc.
Indianapolis, Indiana

■ SECTION ONE ■

The Essentials of Managed Care and Capitation

1

Capitation

ART WILMES

Connecting the Disconnect

The dynamics of the delivery and financing of healthcare are changing. Although extensive federal government reform initiatives have either subsided or died, the reform efforts of the health insurance market continue and will likely result in the models that will be used in the near future.

One discussion of what is wrong with healthcare, by physicians and nonphysicians alike, is the disconnect that occurs between the delivery of healthcare and the financing of healthcare. This discussion is at the root of some managed care initiatives and has resulted in more risk being assumed by the individuals and organizations that provide healthcare services. Capitation and other risk-sharing arrangements represent methods intended to connect the disconnect.

Full-risk assumption occurs under capitation. Under capitation, a healthcare provider is responsible for providing medical services that are specified in a contract. The healthcare provider becomes a manager of care. The provider is paid for managing a patient's needs as opposed to being reimbursed for providing services.

Why Capitation?

Healthcare costs, as measured by the Consumer Price Index (CPI), have historically increased by an annual rate that is 4 to 6% higher than the Urban CPI, which is a measure of the rate of increase in all segments of the economy. (See Figure 1–1.) The rate of increase became more pronounced during the late 1970s and early 1980s, as the federal government sought to control increases in Medicare and Medicaid. Revenue reductions from government programs were initially passed on to the commercial insurance market. These additional costs leveraged commercial insurance costs, as Medicare and Medicaid deficiencies were passed through to the commercial market on top of their own cost increases.

The commercial insurance market was unable to sustain these leveraged costs for an unlimited amount of time. Lower-cost health insurance options were needed as employer health insurance costs incurred double-digit trends. The introduction of managed care organizations led to different healthcare management methods, such as precertification, preadmission testing, increased use of ambulatory surgery, and concurrent inpatient review. These management methods had a significant initial impact, but failed to have the necessary long-term impact on costs. Additional financial control methods were introduced to lower costs. These controls included discounted fees, physician withholds, case rates, and capitation.

Capitation Defined

Capitation is a payment method used to finance the cost of healthcare benefits. The American College of Physicians (ACP) formally defines *capitation* as:

> A way of reimbursing physicians that transfers the financial risk of care to physicians and away from the health plan or the patients. Capitation also refers to the per capita payment for providing specific health services to a defined population over a set period of time. Typically, the provider receives in advance a negotiated monthly payment from the HMO, usually

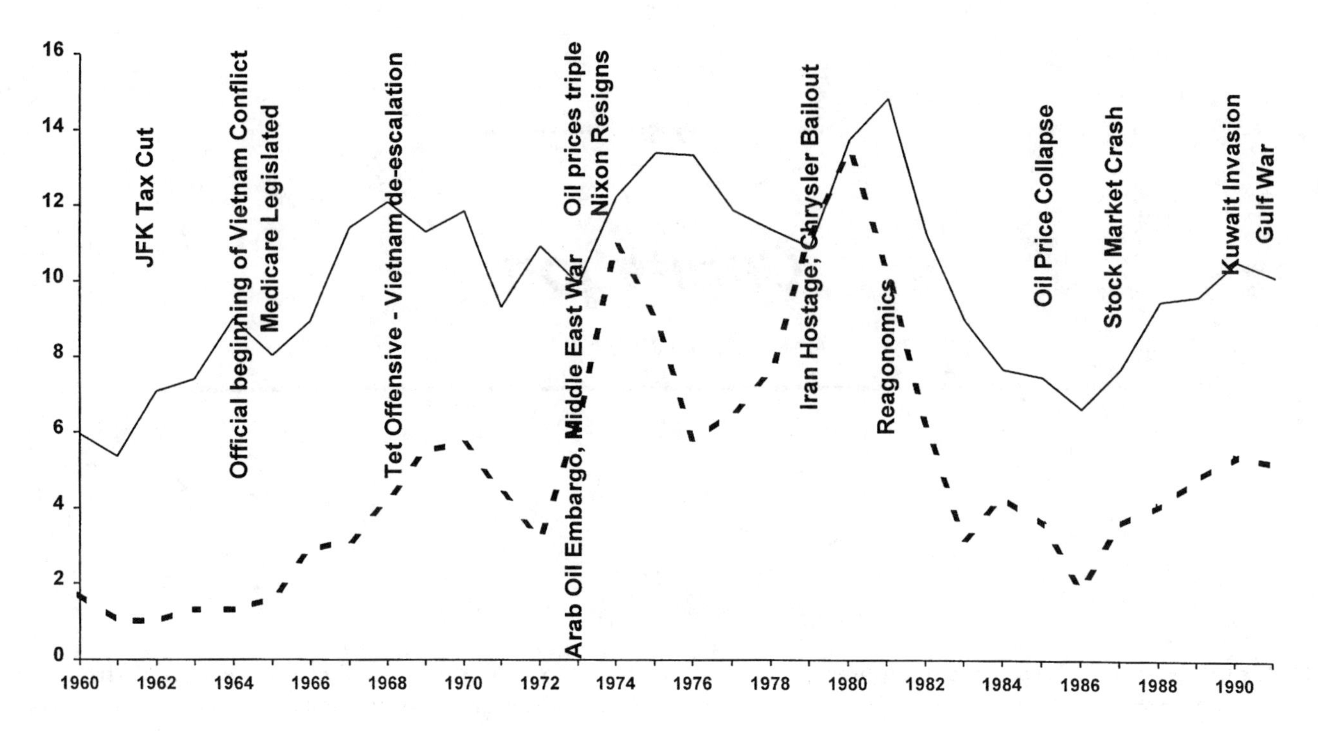

FIGURE 1–1. National health expenditures (annual trend).

referred to in terms of a "per-member-per-*month*" *(pmpm) payment. This payment stays the same no matter how much service the physician or group actually provides.*[1]

The ACP presents its definition of capitation from the perspective of the physician. The reality of capitation is that it is a method used to finance healthcare for physicians, hospitals, and other healthcare providers that supply their services in a commercially insured or government-provided health insurance program.

Capitation has evolved over time and, along the way, has accumulated its share of proponents and critics. It has been promoted as the Hippocratic version of the Emancipation Proclamation, whereby physicians are finally free and as a result are unencumbered by the shackles of third-party payers. At another extreme, capitation has been ridiculed as a method that works great in theory . . . just like communism.

In practice, capitation shares characteristics of both these extremes. Physicians do tend to have more freedom under capitation. One purpose for transferring risk to physicians is to provide them with incentives to make cost-effective treatment choices. Treatments do not necessarily need to be externally qualified. The physician is free to be innovative in treatment approaches. Prevention programs can also be introduced. The provider bears the cost of innovations with the incentive for reduced expenditures flowing to the bottom line.

The top three reasons for consumer purchases have often been defined as Price, Price, and Price. Current capitation approaches have generally followed this marketing axiom. Third-party payers tend to concentrate on evaluating a provider's price proposal first and assuming that the quality of care is a commodity shared uniformly by all providers. This results in a perverse incentive for providers to conserve the services they provide to patients in order to limit withdrawals from a fixed capitation pool. Market forces are theoretically available to create competition and to raise the level of quality. Patients can re-enroll with different providers or formally register grievances with health plans through patient appeal committees. These remedies do not always work as planned. Consumers lack the sophistication to distinguish quality differences among healthcare providers, and third-party payers continue to focus on financial issues before quality issues.

The greatest challenge for capitation is to create an environment where the patients must depend upon the physician to take the correct course even when it is against their economic self interest.[2]

■ Types of Capitation

Capitation rates vary as to the services that are covered. The most familiar types of capitation are those paid to individual physicians. The physicians receiving the payment are directly responsible for providing the services covered under the capitation. The most common is the primary care capitation, which covers the services provided by primary care physicians. Subspecialty capitations are the capitations made to various subspecialty physicians, such as orthopedic surgeons, otolaryngologists, obstetricians, or general surgeons.

Full physician capitation refers to all physician services and covers all the services provided by primary care physicians and subspecialty physicians. This type of capitation is generally paid to multispecialty physician groups which represent the full spectrum of physician services. When this is done, the full capitation payment is generally allocated to the various physicians by means of a formula, percentage allocation, or combination of methods intended to equitably distribute the revenue to the physicians. The full physician capitation may also be paid to a primary care group. The primary care group is responsible for ensuring that all physician services are available when needed, which means that it will need to arrange for subspecialty services.

Full-risk capitation refers to all medical benefit services and covers all the services provided by primary care physicians, subspecialty physicians, hospital services, prescription drugs, and other related ancillary medical services. This type of capitation is generally paid to a physician-hospital organization (PHO). Like a full physician capitation, the capitation payment is generally allocated among the physician specialties and the hospital. This type of capitation has also been accepted by multispecialty physician groups and primary care physician groups. This results in insurance regulatory questions as to whether these types of provider groups, which are not licensed as insurance or prepaid health plan organizations, can accept what amounts to full insurance risk. Insurance regulators are receiving a lot of pressure from health maintenance organizations and insurance companies to regulate the unlicensed acceptance of insurance risk. Allowing unlicensed acceptance of risk places licensed groups at a competitive disadvantage because they must maintain minimum levels of capital, collect premium taxes, and comply with the myriad regulatory provisions that do not currently apply to unlicensed groups.

What Is the Right Capitation Rate?

Physician capitation rates can be estimated by means of two primary methods: actuarial cost method and physician productivity method. Both methods rely upon actuarial estimates of medical services, but vary with respect to the way in which they determine physician compensation.

Actuarial Cost Method

The actuarial cost method relies upon a prospective estimate of the services to be delivered to an insured population. This estimate is combined with a fee to be charged for the services in order to determine the final capitation value.

The basic capitation formula for the actuarial cost method is shown in the following equation. This formula relies upon various parameters, which are described as follows:

$$\text{Capitation PMPM} = \frac{\text{Utilization Rate} \times \text{Cost Per Service}}{12}$$

Covered Services

The level of the capitation payment depends upon the number of services required by the capitation agreement. With the actuarial cost method, a prospective estimate of the PMPM is made for each CPT-4 procedure code. Therefore, it is very important that the capitation contract explicitly list the CPT-4 procedure codes that are to be provided by the contracting physician. Services can be defined as either exclusive services or general services. An exclusive service is a service that will be exclusively provided by the contracted physician. An example of an exclusive service would be a pediatrician or other primary care physician that is solely responsible for providing all well-baby exams denoted by CPT-4 procedure codes 99831/99832, 99391/99392, and 99432.[3] No other physician would be responsible for providing these services. Other physicians' capitation payments would not make a provision for well-baby exams.

A general service is a service that is provided by more than one physician. An example of a general service is physician office visits denoted by CPT-4 procedure codes 99201–99205, 99211–99215, 99354/99359, and 99361–99376.[3] Under a capitation contract, all physicians are responsible for providing the office visits necessary for the normal conduct of their specialty practice.

Although covered services are generally defined by CPT-4 procedure codes, some services may be defined by ICD-9 codes. ICD-9 codes are often used to identify high-risk patients who may be reimbursed outside of the capitation contract.

Annual Utilization Rates

The prospective estimate of the services to be provided under the capitation contract are defined in terms of utilization rates per covered member. A covered member is an insured individual who is eligible for services. Because utilization rates tend to be small, they are generally expressed as a rate per 1000 covered members.

Utilization rates are defined differently depending upon the provider of the service. Hospital inpatient services are defined as the number of hospital days needed for 1000 covered members. Inpatient services are sometimes further split into rates of admission per 1000 covered members and the average length of stay per admission. Utilization rates for hospital outpatient services are generally defined as the number of encounters per 1000 covered members. Utilization rates for physician services are defined as the number of CPT-4 procedure codes per 1000 covered members.

Utilization rate estimates generally are made by actuaries who monitor fee-for-service and managed care claims experience.

Demographic Factors

The morbidity of individuals is affected by various health status indicators, such as age, sex, height, physical build, smoking, genetic traits, chronic disease, or personal habits. In a commercial insurance market, age and sex are the standard methods by which capitation payments will vary. In the long term care Medicaid market and other risk pools primarily composed of chronically ill patients, factors such as disease state are also used to adjust capitation payments.

Utilization is centrally impacted by age and sex. In addition to utilization, age and sex may also affect the intensity of healthcare services. Population class will also affect utilization and service intensity. Population class can be defined of a class of insured lives for which a community premium rate PMPM is established. Examples of population classes include commercial insurance, Medicare, and Medicaid. Medicare and Medicaid classes can also be further divided into subclasses based upon health status. For example, Medicare may have separate PMPM values for aged and institutionalized individuals. Medicaid may have separate PMPM values for AFDC and long-term care individuals.

Table 1–1 illustrates sample age and sex adjustment factors associated with total physician services. The source of these factors is the *1996 M&R Health Cost Guidelines.*[4]

Age and sex factors are generally used to adjust capitation rates where there is substantial risk of age and sex fluctuations. Contracts for which physician groups accept a large number of patients (e.g., 100,000 or more) may not adjust for age and sex. Any adjustments, if made, occur in increments. Under such contracts, the actual age and sex mix of the group is monitored. If the composite age and sex index varies by ± 5%, a prospective adjustment is made. The age and sex index is calculated as the weighted average age and sex factor for the group.

Average Cost per Service

Utilization rates are the prospective estimates of services that are to be provided under a capitation contract. Value is ascribed to the PMPM by assigning an average cost to each service estimated to be provided. The average costs will vary by individual CPT-4 procedure code.

Average cost per service may be based upon the charges that a physician normally bills patients in a fee-for-service setting. Unfortunately, capitation contracts anticipate that fees will be discounted for reasons such as guaranteed cash flow, exclusivity, market share, or elimination of bad debt concerns. As such, the average costs usually reflect a discount to the physician's usual fees.

Fees may also be tied to a relative value basis. The most common relative value bases are Medicare's Resource-Based Relative Value Scale (RBRVS) and McGraw-Hill Relative Value Units. These two bases have their own unique characteristics. One very important point regarding them is that they value services differently. The scales used by each basis also differ. As such, the conversion factors that convert the relative value units to fees will also differ.

Putting it all Together

Table 1–2 provides a sample actuarial cost model for otolaryngology services. The model has been developed for a commercial insurance contract.

The model has been summarized and grouped into physician service categories in order to limit some of the detail. Underlying the summary model in Table 1–2 is a detailed model that has specific utilization and average charge estimates for each covered CPT-4 procedure code. The primary services in the Evaluation/Management category are office visits with CPT-4 procedure code 99213[3] being the most prevalent. The primary services in the Medicine category are testing services, with tympanometry (CPT-4 procedure code 92567)[3] being the most prevalent. The primary services in the Surgery category are respiratory, auditory, and other surgeries with tympanostomy, laryngoscopy, and nasal Endoscopy (CPT-4 procedure codes 69436, 31575, and 31231)[3] being the most prevalent.

Copayment Income

The actuarial cost model in Table 1–2 ignores the effect of copayments. Copayments are the fees that patients pay when certain services are received. It is the responsibility of the individual physician to determine the copayment status of each patient and collect the copayment at the time that a service is rendered.

Capitation contracts generally represent a blend of copayments. Managed care organizations tend to offer a variety of general service contracts which result in a variety

TABLE 1–1. Sample Age and Sex Adjustment Factors Total Physician Services

Age Cell	*Male*	*Female*
≤ 22	0.431	0.431
25–34	0.515	1.336
35–44	0.730	1.506
45–54	1.132	1.710
55 +	2.269	2.299

Source: Milliman & Robertson[3] For illustration purposes only.

TABLE 1–2. Sample Actuarial Cost Model for Otolaryngology Services Capitation, Commercial Insurance

Service	*Utilization Rate/1,000*	*Average Charge*	*PMPM*
Evaluation/Management	66.102 visits	$40.00	$0.220
Other Medicine	3.948 services	35.00	0.012
Surgery	19.371 services	500.00	0.807
Pathology	1.329 tests	30.00	0.003
			$1.042

Sample insured population: Commercial Lives
Source: Milliman & Robertson, Inc.[4] For illustration purposes only.

TABLE 1–3. Effect of Copayment Income: Sample PMPM Values for $5, $10, and $15 Copayments; Copayment Applies to Office Visits Only; Commercial Insurance

		Co-Payment Level		
		$5	*$10*	*$15*
	Utilization per 1,000	56.19	56.19	56.19
(times)	Copayment	×$5	×$10	×$15
(divided by)	12,000 Member Months	÷ 12,000	÷ 12,000	÷ 12,000
(equals)	Value of Copayment	$0.023	$0.047	$0.070

Sample insured population: Commercial Lives
Source: Milliman & Robertson, Inc.[4] For illustration purposes only.

of copayment terms. It is difficult for these organizations to track copayment levels and adjust for actual copayment provisions. Physicians, however, should be provided with information to determine a member's copayment based upon an identification card that will either contain the copayment amount or a plan number that can be cross-referenced to a master list of copayments.

Copayments are generally assessed to office visits. An actuarial cost model is also used to estimate the PMPM value for copayments. Since copayments are income paid directly by patients to physicians, a capitation contract will discount the PMPM amount to reflect the value of copayments. Table 1–3 provides sample PMPM values for office visit copayments of $5, $10, and $15. The utilization estimate is a portion of the total Evaluation/Management utilization value shown in Table 1–2.

Coordination of Benefits

Capitation contracts place the obligation of coordination of benefits (COB) upon the physician. COB is an insurance clause generally contained in managed care organizations' general service contracts. It allows for the subrogation of benefit payments for services that are provided to a patient where the patient is covered by other insurance. Subrogation can be made if the managed care coverage has secondary payment status to the other insurance coverage. Treatment related to an industrial injury or illness would result in a COB opportunity if Workers Compensation is primary. Automobile insurance may also create COB opportunities.

The level of COB collections will vary by type of physician. For example, Orthopedists may increase their capitation income by 3 to 5% due to COB collections. Other physicians may have negligible collections. The actual value of COB collections will be dependent upon educating staff with respect to COB detection (e.g., reviewing patient claims for cause) and collection methods.

Physician Productivity Method

The physician productivity Method relies partly upon a prospective estimate of the services to be delivered to an insured population. This is its only similarity to the actuarial cost method. The process underlying the method is summarized in Table 1–4.

Estimated Physician Productivity—Physician Office Visits

This section of Table 1–4 estimates the capacity of an individual physician. The estimates in this section are based upon the physician group's target for productivity per physician. The example in Table 1–4 defines productivity as 82.5 patients seen per week. Not all patients evaluated by a physician in the office are reimbursed. Some patients

TABLE 1–4. Illustration of Physician Productivity Method: Commercial Insurance Model; Otolaryngology Example

Estimated Physician Productivity—Physician Office Visits	
Hours per Week Spent on Target Services:	27.5 hours
× Patients Seen per Hour:	× 3 patients
Patients Seen per Week:	82.5 patients
− Estimated Patients Covered by Global Fees (30%):	− 25.0 patients
Net Patients—Nonglobal:	57.5 patients
× Weeks Worked per Year:	× 47.0 weeks
Estimated Physician Productivity per Year:	2,702.5 patients
Actuarial Estimate of Target Services	
Annual Utilization of Office Visits:	56.187 visits/1,000
Estimated Member Capacity per Physician	
Estimated Physician Productivity per Year:	2,702.5 patients
÷ Annual Utilization of Office Visits:	÷ 56.187 visits/1,000
× 1,000 members	× 1,000 members
Estimated Members per Physician	48,000 members
Estimated Commercial Insurance PMPM	
Target Gross Revenue per Physician:	$500,000
÷ Estimated Members per Physician:	÷ 48,000 members
÷ 12 months	÷ 12 months
Target PMPM	$0.868 PMPM

represent presurgical and postsurgical encounters. Compensation for these patients is generally covered under the global fee paid for the surgical service. The example has reduced the per-physician productivity to reflect that not all visits result in a collected fee. The net weekly productivity is multiplied by the target number of weeks worked per year in order to arrive at a final estimate of physician productivity. Other methods could be used to arrive at this estimate. Irrespective of the method, the estimate should be an achievable target for the average physician working within a group.

Actuarial Estimate of Target Services

This section of Table 1–4 summarizes the actuarial estimate of physician office visits. It represents the number of reimbursable office visits per year estimated for an insured commercial group of 1000 members. Since the actuarial estimate is based upon reimbursable visits, it is on the same basis as the target physician productivity per year.

Estimated Member Capacity per Physician

This section of Table 1–4 estimates the number of members per physician. This estimate is calculated by dividing the annual physician productivity by the actuarial estimate of office visits per year. This example estimates a ratio of 48,000 members per otolaryngologist. This differs from some published values that tend to estimate between 35,000 and 40,000 members per otolaryngologist. The difference results because the estimate in Table 1–4 is based upon a commercial insurance model that has fewer expected office visits per 1000 members. Published estimates are based on a blend of commercial and Medicare insurance, which would result in a higher number of expected office visits per 1000 members.

Estimated Commercial Insurance PMPM

An estimate of the commercial insurance PMPM can be made once the number of members per physician is calculated. The PMPM is calculated by dividing the target risk revenue per physician by the estimated number of members per physician per month. In the example in Table 1–4 the $500,000 target revenue is spread over 48,000 members and results in a monthly PMPM estimate of $0.868.

■ Other Issues

Primary Care Guidelines

Before signing a capitation agreement, ask for and review the primary care guidelines that apply to medicine. These guidelines, if developed properly, will clearly define the responsibilities of the primary care physician. Complementary to that, the guidelines will also clearly define the responsibilities of the subspeciality physician.

Imaging guidelines may also be in place. These guidelines will be important if radiology services are part of the capitation agreement. MCOs see duplicate imaging as an area of inefficiency. As such, imaging guidelines may place restrictions on the views that may be desired by the physician. Review the guidelines to determine the imaging restrictions and the effect they may have upon your standard of practice.

Primary care guidelines can be your enemy if you misunderstand their purposes, which are to (1) clearly define what a well trained primary care physician should do and (2) clearly define the procedures and grounds for a specialty referral. The effect of the guidelines will be to eliminate unnecessary referrals and concentrate the otolaryngologist's skills on high level, specialty services.

Benchmarking

Medical care managers should develop utilization guidelines to monitor the patterns of ambulatory physician services. The appropriate level of delivery efficiency for a particular system will be dependent upon the medical needs of the system's patients. Factors that impact utilization will include age, sex, health status, and other factors.

The measurement of outcomes is necessary to assess the efficacy of treatment guidelines and the benchmarking of actual utilization results against management targets. In addition to detailed benchmarking, "high altitude" general rules can be used to assess results and prompt additional review. Examples of such general rules[3] include:

1. The number of visits per member should be no more than four visits per member per year.
2. Seventy to 80% of members will be seen by a physician during a given year.
3. The visits per member seen should be no more than five visits per member seen per year.
4. Primary care physician visits should comprise 70 to 80% of the total visits. This percentage will be higher for pediatric patients and lower for adults under the care of family practitioners or internists.
5. Referrals to specialists should be no greater than 0.5 per member per year.
6. Ambulatory visits by specialists should average no more than 2.5 visits per referred patient per year. This average will include mental health services with as many as six visits per member seen per year.
7. Ancillary services should average less than one ancillary service per visit when there has been a large number of visits.
8. The services per encounter should be no more than 2.0 services per encounter.
9. The total number of office visits, including primary care visits, specialist consultations, outpatient mental health care, and periodic health appraisals, as well as new patient visits, should exceed the number of ancillary services, including laboratory testing, radiology testing, other miscellaneous medicine services, immunizations, injections and physical therapy visits.

A detailed benchmarking system should be developed. Compare the utilization results with two endpoints of healthcare management: (1) unmanaged care and (2) optimally managed care. *Unmanaged care* is defined as utilization for a relatively unmanaged delivery system. It represents the projected utilization for an insured population that reflects very little healthcare management other than hospital preadmission authorization.

Optimally managed care is defined as utilization for a very well-managed delivery system. It represents the projected utilization for an insured population that reflects very comprehensive healthcare management. Examples of comprehensive management include, but are not limited to, preadmission authorization and concurrent patient management, comprehensive patient treatment guidelines (inpatient, ambulatory, and phone triage), and the existence of a compensation system that provides incentives for efficient performance.

Reinsurance—Physician Aggregate Coverage

This reinsurance provides coverage for physician charges that exceed a specified aggregate retention level. This coverage protects a physician against excessive utilization from a group of insured members. The retention level is generally established as a multiple (e.g., 110%) of a target PMPM. The charges for this reinsurance will vary by physician specialty and local market. Underlying the reinsurance premium will be estimates of utilization and average charges. As with all reinsurance products, the reinsurer will increase its expected cost by a risk margin. Such risk margins may be up to or exceed 100% of the expected cost.

Reinsurance—Physician-Specific Coverage

This reinsurance provides coverage for physician charges that exceed a specified retention level per individual claim. This coverage protects a physician against an outlier patient by setting a maximum exposure level. The retention level is generally established at fixed dollar levels, such as $5000, $10,000, or $15,000. Measurement of charges are generally based upon a contractual fee schedule. Similar to aggregate coverage, the reinsurer will increase its expected cost by a risk margin.

Reinsurance—Benefit Carve-outs

Some reinsurers have developed reinsurance products for organizations that only want to reinsure specific types of risk. Examples include organ transplants, prescription drugs, substance abuse, and psychiatric disorders. These reinsurance products are called benefit carve-outs. These contracts operate like a subcapitation. A PMPM is charged and the reinsurer is totally responsible for the cost of the benefits subject to the carve-out.

■ Epilogue

Capitation represents a significant challenge to physicians. It is not clear how physicians will ultimately embrace capitation, or, as has often been stated, how capitation will embrace physicians. It is also not clear whether capitation is a long-term solution or a passing fad that will subsequently be replaced by the next generation of reimbursements.

The ultimate reimbursement methodology, whether it be capitation or the next generation, will need to embrace two important issues in order to be truly effective. It must not influence individual physician decisions, and it must encourage integration and innovation in the delivery of healthcare services. Capitation compromises the first of these two issues. It does, however, appear to be an initial step in the evolution of empowering the physician.

REFERENCES

1. What capitation really means. *ACP Observer,* 1996.
2. Payment by capitation and the quality of care. *New England Journal of Medicine.* 1996; 335:1227–1231.
3. CPT codes, descriptions and two digit numeric modifiers only are copyright 1995 American Medical Association. AU rights reserved.
4. *Health Cost Guidelines.* Seattle, Washington: Milliman and Robertson, 1996.

Art Wilmes is a consulting actuary in the Indianapolis office of Milliman & Robertson, Inc. He is a principal of M&R and has been with the firm since 1980.

His major area of expertise is individual and group health insurance and disability income, including strategic planning, new product development, financial projections, mergers and acquisitions, and benefit plan design and funding. Art's continuing client base includes healthcare providers (hospitals and physicians), prepaid health plans, insurance companies, ancillary medical service providers, and self-funded insurance plans.

Art has developed an expertise in the recent trends affecting the delivery and financing of healthcare. This expertise is evidenced by his continuing service to over 35 hospitals and health maintenance organizations. In addition, Art is a consultant for two large pharmaceutical companies and one medical device company in the areas of disease management and capitation. He is currently a faculty member for a series of educational seminars sponsored by The American Academy of Otolaryngology, The American Academy of Dermatology, and The American Association of Neurological Surgeons. He also delivered a series of capitation lectures at the 1995 annual meeting of the American Academy of Orthopedic Surgeons.

Art is a fellow in the Society of Actuaries and a member of the American Academy of Actuaries. An honors graduate of Ball State University, he is an active speaker and participant in various regional and national professional meetings.

2

Reimbursement Systems and Managed Care

CHERYL TOTH, WITH AN ADDENDUM BY LEE EISENBERG

It's no surprise that managed care has changed the reimbursement playing field considerably for physicians. But although reduced reimbursement is probably talked about the most, changes in plan billing rules and guidelines, stipulations on filing limitations and payment remittance, also affect a practice's reimbursement systems. Take this short quiz to see if your internal operation is ready for the managed care reimbursement revolution.

Are You Ready For Reimbursement Change?		
	Yes	No
1. Our fee schedule is based on either RBRVS or McGraw-Hill and we've done a comparative analysis with our top managed care plans to determine how each of them affects our business.		
2. The billing team analyzes explanation of benefits (EOBs) forms in detail and shares significant findings with physicians—who take an interest and develop action steps toward solutions.		
3. The billing team posts payments on a line item basis; plans are called if EOBs are not received with this detail.		
4. We've developed our computer file architecture so we can review reimbursement and accounts receivable by plan, and adjustments in great detail.		
5. We verify benefits prior to surgery, and our scheduler collects presurgical deposits.		
6. Physicians code operative reports using CPT and ICD-9-CM codes; the information is submitted to the reimbursement team within 48 hours of the procedure.		
7. Our practice preregisters all new patients; insurance eligibility is verified, and patients are informed of their deductible and copay prior to their visit.		
8. The partners review individual physician coding choices for office visits and consultations by running a CPT code frequency report.		

What's your score? If you got all eight correct, good for you—this chapter will be a refresher. But if you could answer fewer than seven with "Yes," you're missing significant reimbursement opportunities. Read on to discover ways of maximizing reimbursement in your practice.

■ Understand the Domino Effect

It's critical for physicians to realize that they are the first "domino" in the complex process that ends with a claim getting paid. Think about it. If you don't code your cases for weeks, staff cannot post the charges, get a claim out the door, or collect money in a timely way. If you see non-emergency patients in the office without a referral for a consultation—or you go ahead and treat the patient when the referral is for "consultation only"—staff can't collect on the claim. If you don't understand the key details of the plans you've signed, you may instruct the surgery scheduler to "*Schedule Mrs. Jones for Friday,*" when it takes at least a week to obtain preauthorization for the procedure. Physicians must take responsibility for their part in the reimbursement process or the process won't work—leaving physicians frustrated, and legitimate dollars on the table.

A physician's biggest contribution to the reimbursement process is supplying the CPT and ICD-9-CM codes to staff. Reimbursement staff do not have "M.D." at the end of their name, and they aren't in the OR or exam room with you and the patient. Don't expect them to read your dictation and accurately code the case or visit. And since your future with managed care is dependent on the clinical outcomes payers now collect, it's more important than ever for physicians to be sure CPT codes are correct, and that all diagnoses are present and coded to the highest level of specificity.

Attend a coding and reimbursement course *annually.* Not only will you learn all the new coding rules, you'll hear how other physicians have been successful at incorporating the coding process into their operational and reimbursement systems and developing coding "cheat sheets." Lee Eisenberg addresses the importance of CPT coding in a managed care environment in the Addendum at the end of this chapter.

■ Be Sure Staff Are Brilliant on the Basics

Once the physicians realize their role in the reimbursement "play," it's time to focus on the role played by staff. Let's start at the beginning. If your staff doesn't understand the building blocks of how to bill, follow up, and monitor payments, you've got a problem. Could this be true in your practice? Maybe. Here's how to diagnose the level of severity.

1. Do you hire people who understand the basics of reimbursement—or warm bodies to fill positions? A key biller, with you for five years, decides to have a child and not return to work. Your manager has a difficult time finding qualified candidates, and finally "settles" for someone who worked in the hospital billing department. Warning! If this individual does not have the technical skills for managing *physician* reimbursement, it's better to wait for someone who does instead of hiring because you need someone quickly. Managed care reimbursement requires specialized training and expertise. Smart practices give "technical assessments" to candidates to determine if they understand the basics of CPT and managed care, and can successfully solve reimbursement scenarios.

2. Does the billing process make sense—can you easily flowchart the process? There's something to be said about simplicity. If staff complete twenty steps before sending out a claim, it's likely they've only added managed care rules to the process they've followed since fee-for-service days. Solution? Take a step back and determine which of the steps are necessary in a today's medical practice, and which are not. You may be surprised to find how many manual systems are still in place, even though you have a computer system. (For more information about process improvement techniques, read Chapter 12, "Improving Office Efficiency In a Managed Care Environment.")

3. Do all staff—and your manager—understand the front-end elements of the reimbursement system? The front-end of the system includes preregistering new patients so staff can verify eligibility and benefits prior to the patient's arrival in the office. It also includes the reception staff making sure the patient has a proper referral for the visit, and updating all insurance and demographic information for *every patient* at *every visit.* If staff are not properly trained about how their performance affects the practice's ability to be reimbursed, the practice is missing out on legitimate reimbursement. (Read Chapter 12, "Improving Office Efficiency In a Managed Care Environment," for more information about how to set up effective front-end operations in your practice.)

4. Are unpaid claims diligently followed up at 45 days? Are rejected claims followed up within 24 hours of receiving the rejection? Problems can quickly occur if staff do not keep after claims at a "young age." Your manager must monitor staff workloads to be sure unpaid claims are a priority—the longer staff wait, the less of a chance there is of collecting on the account. Remember, managed care plans clearly state their filing limitations in the contract—you don't have an unlimited amount of time to question the plan's rejection or lack of payment.

5. Do staff understand how to follow up? It's amazing how many staff do not pick up the phone and call a plan about a rejection or claim that has not been paid. Good follow-up skills don't fall down from the sky; your staff must be properly trained. For example, sending "tracers" on unpaid claims, or letters on rejected claims that state, "Please reconsider this claim" are *passive,* ineffective collection attempts. Staff should prepare to call a plan with several claims at a time (each managed care plan has a different limit on how many claims they'll address per phone call), determine the problem, fix it, and *then* resubmit.

Use the Account Follow Up Form (Fig. 2–1) as a training tool for staff, and instruct them to submit ten large, outstanding surgical balances for the physicians to review monthly.

6. Are payments from managed care plans scrutinized? If your practice did not request complete payment schedules from each plan prior to signing the contract, reimbursement is being missed. Your staff must be equipped with payment schedules to be sure the plan pays what was agreed on in your contract negotiation. Better yet, enter the payment schedules in the computer system so that staff are alerted automatically when the payment being posted by line item is incorrect. (Line item posting means that each payment is applied toward a specific CPT code—not the total account balance.)

A Chicago physician with a talent for reading EOBs became very interested when he noticed a pattern of fraudulent discounts taken by carriers. Simply put, if the plan

<table>
<tr><td>Patient Name:</td><td>Account Balance:</td><td>Primary Surgeon:</td></tr>
<tr><td>Primary Insurance:
Secondary Insurance:</td><td>Phone Number of . . .
Primary Ins.:
Secondary ins.:</td><td>I Spoke With . . .
His/her position:</td></tr>
<tr><td>Date of Service(s):</td><td>Date Claim Filed:</td><td>Date of Last Activity on Account:</td></tr>
<tr><td>Did Payer Receive Claim?
Yes No
If yes, on what date was it received?</td><td>Where Can We Fax Claim to Speed Payment?
Name:
Fax Number:</td><td>Internal Problem? Contractual Adjustment Not Taken, Unbundling/Coding?
Yes No
Explain:</td></tr>
<tr><td colspan="3">Services or Procedures Denied/Not Paid (List actual CPT code and name of procedure):</td></tr>
<tr><td colspan="3">Why Was Claim Not Paid or Is Not Being Paid? What is the Reason for the Denial?</td></tr>
<tr><td colspan="3">Action Taken To Get Paid (What You Did):</td></tr>
<tr><td colspan="3">Comments:</td></tr>
<tr><td>When Can We Expect Payment:</td><td>Date I Will Follow Up if Claim Not Paid:</td><td>Staff Name or Initials:</td></tr>
</table>

Today's Date: ____________________

FIGURE 2–1. Account Follow-Up Form

had agreed to pay $80, random checks would come in for, say, $73.75. Realistically, staff in most physician practices don't go after the remaining $6.25—but this physician did, and was automatically paid the full amount. "*This happens with enough different payers that I'm convinced it's a deliberate strategy. You have to look up the fee schedule you agreed to, and then check the math . . . they'll nickel and dime you any way they can,*" says John McMahan, MD.[1]

■ Develop the Right Tools

It's impossible for anyone in the practice—physicians, manager, or staff—to have every step in the reimbursement system committed to memory. And, although miracles have been known to happen, the miracle of staff knowing details about reimbursement policies or managed care rules without anyone telling them probably won't occur in your practice anytime soon. In lieu of a miracle, develop sound tools that assist both physicians and staff in the quest for proper reimbursement.

1. **Create *written* reimbursement policies.** Have physicians sat down to discuss and agree to policies *as a group?* Staff should have written protocols about the physicians' philosophy for:
   - **Nonurgent vs. urgent appointment and surgery scheduling.** Depending on the managed care plan's definition of "urgent," you may be able to see the patient or perform surgery without a referral or authorization and get paid. But if the "urgent" criteria is not met, you will not get paid.
   - **Precertification versus preauthorization.** Precertification means, "*Yes, you can do the surgery, according to the diagnosis,*" but preauthorization means "*We'll pay you for doing the surgery.*" Big difference!
   - **"Accept assignment."** Overall, a bad idea. First, professional courtesy via the "accept assignment" method is fraudulent. Second, if you are offering professional courtesy this way, understand that many physicians—and others to whom you extend this courtesy—have deductibles of $1000, $5000, or more. Chances are, the charges on the claim submitted go toward the deductible—leaving you with no reimbursement.
   - **Posting managed care payments and withholds.** Clearly state how payments are to be posted, adjustments taken, and withholds tracked. If the plan's reimbursement is correct, staff should allocate the contractual adjustment to a specific adjustment category for the plan, and the withhold amount to a specific withhold category for the plan. Remember, the withhold is a *potential receivable.* In the event the plan does its math wrong (yes, it's possible), you've got accurate information to use when you contest.
   - **Collection policies.** What can be collected at the time of service? (Copays, deductibles, and past due balances should be the answer.) Are staff authorized to set up budget plans? What is collected presurgically? When are accounts turned to outside collection—how is this done?
2. **Be sure the encounter form is updated for a managed care environment.** An old familiar friend, the encounter form (aka charge slip, route slip, Superbill) is your best internal control tool for reimbursement. In addition to being sure all the appropriate CPT and ICD-9-CM codes are listed on the form, be sure managed care information is on there too. Most computer systems can print plan names, copay amounts, and insurance/patient balances—all excellent pieces of information to use as collection tools. If your encounter form still has 90060 listed, or if you haven't updated this essential tool in the last year, use Does Your Encounter Form Need Re-Tooling? (Fig. 2–2) It is provided as a guide for improving the practice's internal reimbursement process.

   The back of the encounter form can serve as an ICD-9-CM cheat sheet for physicians. Create a list of the most commonly used diagnosis codes to be sure physicians can easily select the correct diagnoses.
3. **Create a matrix and reference manual that contains plan guidelines.** We've said it before, and we'll say it again: if you and staff don't know which managed care plans you've signed, what their copay and noncovered services are, which plans require referrals and/or preauthorization for procedures, and the lab and hospital the plan has contracted with, your practice is losing out on reimbursement opportunities. Do we understand that collecting and organizing this information takes time? Yes. But let's think about priorities here—do you want to delegate this project or continue to miss out on money that should be yours?

   A step-by-step guide to organizing a matrix and reference manual is contained in Chapter 12, "Improving Office Efficiency In a Managed Care Environment." Delegate it, and make sure it gets done!
4. **Develop an effective tool to capture hospital consultation and ER charges.** With reimbursement on the decline, it's more important than ever for physicians to capture and bill for every charge they can. To do so effectively, these charges must be submitted to the reimbursement team in a format that is *useful* for proper billing and collecting. Does that mean cocktail napkins, pieces of scratch paper, and matchbook covers are "out" as reimbursement tools? Absolutely. But a coding card is "in"; and, better yet, it's sure to get you paid.

	Yes	No
1. Has it been *updated* to reflect current E/M and in-office procedure codes?		
2. Are *all* necessary codes listed? All 5 codes in each series of E/M, 99024 (post op follow up), in-office procedures, etc.		
3. Are all codes listed necessary? The encounter form is an internal document. Hospital services and operative codes should not be listed.		
4. Are supplies itemized using HCPCS II and III? (As opposed to 99070.)		
5. Is there a simple way for physicians to correlate CPT and ICD-9-CM codes?		
6. Are there fields for the patient's name, address, and *complete* plan name to print?		
7. Is there a way for physicians to communicate to staff the need for prior authorization?		
8. Is there a field for date of injury or first symptom?		
9. Does the patient's copay amount print? How about the names of the hospital, testing center, and lab approved by the patient's plan?		
10. Does the patient's account balance print—aged, with insurance balance separated from patient balance?		
11. Does it have computer-generated, sequential numbers for proper audit control?		

Coding Card

Patient Name:______________________ Date of Service:______________

Hospital:______________________ Physician:______________

Diagnoses (see reverse side): ______________________

____

____

____

Initial Hospital Visit	Subsequent Hospital Visit	Initial Hospital Consultations	Follow Up Consultations
99221 Detailed/Straightforward-Low	99231 Prob/Straightforward-Low	99251 Prob./Straightforward	99261 Add CPT
99222 Comprehensive/Moderate	99232 Exp. Prob./Moderate	99252 Exp. Prob./Straightforward	99262 language
99223 Comprehensive/High	99233 Detailed/High	99253 Detailed/Low	99263 here
	99238 Discharge	99254 Comprehensive/Moderate	
		99255 Comprehensive/High	

How to Use the Coding Card

- Print on pocket-sized, hard stock paper.
- Circle the code you've used, and supply staff with the ICD-9-CM codes in order of primary, secondary, etc. (Have common ICD-9-CM codes printed on the back.)
- Submit to billing staff *daily*, along with the hospital face sheet if the patient has never been seen in your office before (they need this information to send a claim).
- Instruct staff to file the cards; conduct periodic spot checks to see if everything physicians submit is actually billed.

FIGURE 2–2. Does Your Encounter Form Need Retooling?

Date ______________________ Physician ______________________

Patient Name ______________________

Street Address ______________________

City/State/Zip ______________________

Home Phone ______________________ Work Phone ______________________

Subscriber Name ______________________

Employer ______________________ Phone ______________________

I.D. Number ______________________ Group Number ______________________

Plan ______________________ Phone Number ______________________

Representative ______________________ Ext. # ______________________

Office Visit Copay ______________ Deductible ______________ Met? ______________

Surgical Deductible: Inpatient ______________________ Outpatient ______________________

Out of Pocket Maximum ______________________ Met? ______________________

Reimbursement Rate: Insurance % ______________________ Patient % ______________________

Any Pre-Existing Conditions? ______________________

Where Do We Mail Claim? ______________________

Staff Initials ______________________

FIGURE 2–3. Verification of Eligibility and Benefits Form

5. **Create a Verification of Eligibility and Benefits form for use with all new patients.** Each patient should be asked a number of key questions prior to coming into the office. Under managed care, this information is critical to getting reimbursed. If your practice has not yet developed a complete verification of eligibility and benefits form, use Figure 2–3 as a guide. It can mean the difference between getting paid or not.

   More and more software vendors are offering electronic verification of eligibility. Instead of calling a managed care plan and being put on hold for 15 minutes, staff can either log on to the plan's computer system or swipe the benefit card and dial up the carrier for an eligibility check. Ask your vendor about the status of this efficient process in your area.

■ Go Electronic for (Nearly) All Claims

If you're like many physicians, you submit claims electronically to Medicare, Medicaid, and Blue Cross. Good for you. But do you realize the amount of additional claims that could be submitted electronically? Submitting managed care and commercial claims through an electronic clearinghouse saves significant staff time—and means quicker reimbursement turnaround. Some clearinghouses inform the practice within 72 hours that the claim will be either paid or rejected. If your staff only had to wait four days before following up on a rejected claim, just think how your cash flow would improve!

If your practice doesn't send managed care and commercial claims through a clearinghouse, contact your computer vendor and find out how you can. These days, the per claim charge costs less than a stamp.

Electronic *payment remittance* is here to stay. No, we're not talking about electronically depositing money in your bank account—although that too is available. *Electronic payment remittance* is a modem transfer of payment information directly into your computer system—by line item! Ask your vendor if payment remittance is available in your area. Remittance for Medicare, Medicaid, and Blue Cross is common and managed care and commercial claims remittance is on the way. Talk about saving significant staff time—no more posting EOBs. (Ultimately, this will lower staff costs all together, since fewer people will be needed on the reimbursement team.)

■ Monitor Reimbursement Symptoms Before They Become Acute

Your manager and staff could implement the reimbursement systems in this chapter, but if physicians do not pay attention to whether they work, it will have been all for naught. Physicians must take an interest in their business. *"But I'm a busy doctor, and I don't have time to look at numbers,"* you say. All the more reason for you to be clear with your manager about the specific reimbursement information you need to review. Best advice? Stick to the essentials.

Before you can even get to reviewing essentials, however, you need to be sure the data you're looking for is meaningful. Garbage in, garbage out, right? If your information system has not been properly set up to track reimbursement information in the detail you need, the file architecture of the database will need to be modified. Don't worry—this is a common issue with physicians new (and even not so new) to managed care. The key is to make the changes now, so the practice has meaningful, clean data for the future. Figure 2–4 clearly outlines the specific category alignment necessary to track good data in a managed care environment. Use it as a guide to determine if your database has been set up with good categorization or whether it needs improvement.

"If we determine our database isn't the best it could be, does that mean we don't have any information to review?" No, it simply means you realize that the data isn't perfect—but practically speaking, use what you have. Here's what to review:

1. **Managed care plan "quick hits."** There are three key things to review, for each plan you've signed:
   - **Payor mix.** This is the percentage of your total business, for each plan. It's typically measured in charges, although you could calculate the percentages for payments too. To determine last year's payer mix, for example, take the annual charges for PruCare, and divide them by the practice's annual charges. Do this for each payer and/or each payer type. For instance, you may wish to know what percentage of the practice is HMO. To do this, take the annual charges for all HMO plans and divide them by the practice's annual charges.
   - **Days in receivable.** In essence, this is the payer's turnaround time. The plan's contract always states within how many days they promise to pay—you need to be sure the plan delivers on this promise. To determine the days in receivable for each plan, use the following equation:

$$\frac{\text{Total Accounts Receivable for Aetna Choice PPO}}{\text{Annual Charges for Aetna Choice PPO/365}}$$

   - **Percentage payment on your fee.** Physicians should monitor, by plan, the "cents on the charge dollar" reimbursement for each contracted plan. This way, you can glean information about your poor payers, and gather useful data about reimbursement in your market. (It's helpful to have this documentation in future plan negotiations.) To determine this percentage, simply divide the total payments for MetLife by the total charges for MetLife, for a quick summary. If you really want to get specific, include the frequency of each code used in the calculation to get a weighted average. In other words, take the frequency of 99243—let's say it's 250—and multiply it by both the payments for 99243 and the charges for 99243. Do this for all codes, and sum both the payments and the charges. Then divide the payments by the charges for the weighted average calculation.

     If you find that plans consistently reimburse at a low percentage of your fee, it may mean your fee schedule needs review. Use a relative value scale such as RBRVS or McGraw-Hill, as well as plan payments and the EOBs of commercial carriers, to round out the analysis.
2. **Review EOBs at Least Quarterly.** Your manager should do most of the legwork, then bring examples of problem EOBs to physician meetings. What are you supposed to look for? The following EOB information is commonly seen. Suggestions about what to do if you find the information appearing on your practice's EOBs are provided.
   - **Multiple procedure discount is taken improperly by carrier.** Call the carrier and advise them of the rules, then appeal.
   - **Physician selected the correct modifier, but the plan doesn't recognize it as valid.** Many plans have poor information systems, with incorrect information. Call the carrier and determine why they don't recognize the modifier; refile.
   - **The practice tries to bill for things such as an assistant surgeon, but the plan doesn't reimburse for an assistant surgeon for that procedure.** Assistant Surgeon is one of the many things managed care plans have stopped paying for. Be sure physicians know the rules, and staff determine what's reimbursable during preauthorization.
   - **"Procedure is included in another procedure."** This is unbundling of a code. Too much of this can be a red flag to carriers that there is a coding problem in the practice; it gives them cause to investigate your claims and charts. Just one more reason physicians need to have a firm grasp on the principles of CPT coding.
   - **Plans consistently pay several dollars less than what they contracted to pay you.** Appeal the

Basic Account Type/Status	Made Up Of Insurance Carriers . . .
Medicare	Medicare
Medicaid	Medicaid
Medicare/Medicaid	Medicare/Medicaid
Worker's Compensation	Traveller's Union
	Metropolitan
	Steel Worker's Union
	Etc.
Commercial Insurance	Prudential Indemnity
	Aetna Life & Casualty
	Connecticut General
	John Hancock
	Guardian
PPO	Physicians Health Plan
	Pru Plus
	Aetna Health Plans
POS	Patient Choice
	WeCare Plans
	Cigna Choice Option
IPA/Medical Group (i.e., SPA)	MetraHealth
	Aetna Choice
	PruCare
Senior HMO	Secure Horizons
	Prudential Gold
	Seniors Plus
Patient Balance After Insurance	Category shows what patients owe after insurance pays
Uninsured without insurance coverage	Category shows balances of patients without insurance coverage
Litigation	Category shows accounts that have litigation pending

FIGURE 2–4. Track Data Right!

Contractual Adjustment Categories
Medicare Contractual Adjustment
Medicaid Contractual Adjustment
Medicare/Medicaid Contractual Adjustment
HMO #1 Contractual Adjustment
HMO #2 Contractual Adjustment (etc.)
PPO #1 Contractual Adjustment
PPO #2 Contractual Adjustment (etc.)
Worker's Compensation Plan #1 Contractual Adjustment
Worker's Compensation Plan #2 Contractual Adjustment (etc.)
Other Write Off Categories
Multiple Procedure Write-Off
Deceased Patient Write Off
Bad Debt Write Off
Collection Agency Write Off (if you use two agencies, there should be one Write Off for each)
Professional Courtesy Write Off*
Employee Courtesy Write Off
Charity Care Write Off
Small Balance Write Off
Pre-authorization Not Obtained Write Off
Patient Not Eligible on DOS Write Off
No Referral
Withhold Categories
Withhold: Plan #1
Withhold: Plan #2 (etc.)

***Important!** Plans have recently won court battles against physicians for writing off the patient's financial obligation after a commercial insurance pays its share. DO NOT use this as a professional courtesy policy. The only legal way to offer professional courtesy is to write off the entire charge. These totals should be tracked by physician.

Remember there is no need for a "commercial adjustment," because you are able to balance bill the patient up to your fee-regardless if the payor states you are "above usual and customary."

FIGURE 2–4. Track Data Right!
continued

claim. Alert! If this is habitual for some plans, call the state governing board that oversees them. For example, HMOs are governed by the State Board of Corporations.

- **The plan is reimbursing you less for a supply than you paid for the supply.** Write a script.
- **The plan won't accept 99070, the general supply code—it requires the HCPCS code.** Refile with HCPCS code.
- **Claim rejection: "Not a covered service."** Bill patient. How do you avoid this? Develop a matrix and insurance manual for plan rules, and be sure staff collect from patients at the time of service.
- **Claim rejection: "Patient not eligible on date of service."** Bill patient—good luck collecting. No one called to verify eligibility. How do you avoid this? Hold your manager accountable for being sure staff verify eligibility in the future.
- **Claim rejection: "No referral authorization."** You'll probably have to write this off; most plans don't allow for retroactive referrals anymore. This could be a physician problem; physicians want to see the patient even if he or she presents without a referral. How do you avoid this? These patients should be rescheduled, and recalcitrant physicians informed that this must not continue.

3. **Review the frequency of CPT usage by physician.** Generate a frequency report at least quarterly to review each physician's selection of CPT codes—specifically E/M codes. Many payers have computer systems that are set to identify dissimilar group coding patterns or "bell curve" distribution that favors high level codes. To keep the fraud squad off your doorstep, be sure the physicians in the group have similar coding habits, and if high-level codes are used, the physician's documentation clearly supports them, according to the principles of CPT.
4. **Review cumulative withhold totals quarterly.** Since withholds are a potential receivable, physicians should be aware of just how much money is in the withhold accounts. You also need to be sure that when the plan does pay, the payment is accurate.

REFERENCES

1. McMahon, J., How Low Can Fees Go? *Med Economics,* April 7, 1997.

■ Addendum by Lee Eisenberg

In today's marketplace, the physician must be more aware of coding then ever before. In the fast disappearing world of indemnity insurance, one billed the patient and was not primarily concerned with proper coding. The patient was responsible for payment. The contract or coverage was between the carrier and the patient. This has obviously changed in recent years, and may reach a point in which the patient has no concerns about physician reimbursement. Physicians now contract with the payers. If not coded appropriately, we are at risk for even less payment than has been agreed by contract. In many circumstances, there are now individuals in your practice whose primary responsibility is assuring accurate coding.

This addendum will only discuss matters of contract issues as they pertain to coding. One should remember that the contracts you sign become the basis for your reimbursement. I cannot overemphasize the importance of reading the contract and having legal assistance before signing.

If you code correctly, it will help with reimbursement but does not guarantee payment. There are the issues of non covered and medically unnecessary services. The contract often spells out how or if you can bill the patient for these two types of activities. In many instances, the contract prohibits the physician to bill for non covered and medically unnecessary procedures. This of course raises the larger issue of liability in the circumstance where the physician feels the service is warranted and the MCO doesn't, yet you are prohibited from charging the patient. How one deals with this begins with your original contract. Afterwards it may be too late, and you are in the position of giving away your services.

Coding has two components: ICD-9C-M and CPT. The ICD provides the diagnosis, while CPT gives the service. The two should always correlate. One needs to use the most detailed ICD code available. There are instances in which no ICD code exists. This is especially true for recurrent illness. In this situation, the closest possible match should be sought. Most payers are not as exacting as HCFA in their request for ICD codes, but is best to follow their convention. The ICD system can be quite daunting. Only with review of the book's introduction, frequent use of the ICD, and refresher courses, will you become more familiar with its usage.

Understanding CPT, which is somewhat easier, is of greater importance. A number of conventions need to be followed, and we will offer only a brief outline. The introduction in the AMA CPT book goes into greater detail.

One of the most important concepts is knowing what activities are contained in a specific CPT code. As an example, when coding for a tympanoplasty (69631), obtaining the graft is considered part of the procedure. Using a separate code would be considered inappropriate. In other instances, the graft may be coded separately. (30620—septal of other intranasal dermatoplasty—does not include obtaining the graft.) Many such examples occur throughout the CPT, and a careful reading of the codes is essential.

Another area of confusion is an indented code. When a code is indented it voids writing out the entire code for subsets of a family of codes. As an example

31020—Sinusotomy, maxillary (antrotomy); intranasal
31030— radical (Caldwell Luc) without removal of antrochoanal polyps.

In this instance, 31020 has a general description of the family before the semicolon (;) (Sinusotomy . . .) and a specific procedure (intranasal) following. The descriptor for 31030 is indented (radical . . .) and therefore includes a sinusotomy as part of the procedure.

When the term "Separate procedure" appears in the descriptor of a CPT code, it indicates that this specific code is a component of another procedure. It may only be used when done in isolation. For example:

31231—nasal endoscopy, diagnostic, unilateral or bilateral (separate procedure).

This indicates 31231 can only be coded separately if it is the only endoscopic procedure accomplished at the time of the service. One could not use this code in addition to any of the other endoscopic sinus surgery codes.

Another example is 69210—removal impacted cerumen (separate procedure), one or both ears.

There is also a significant amount of confusion regarding the use of modifiers. Each of the payers may or may not require any or all of these. Medicare is very stringent in requiring appropriate modifiers. Others ask for only a limited number. This inconsistency in modifier request often complicates the coding process. Additionally, many payers' software cannot recognize the use of two modifiers with the same CPT code and some have difficulty with even a single modifier. The one major exception is Medicare, which requires two modifiers to be used if indicated. For example, if you were performing a septoplasty (30520) and bilateral submucous resection of the turbinates, partial or complete (30140) the coding for Medicare would be:

30520
30140–50,–51

For other carriers it might vary and look as follows:

30520
30140
30140–50,–51

As you review the explanation of benefits (EOBs) from the different carriers, you will be able to determine their specific use of modifiers. Some commonly used modifiers include:

–25 Significant, separately identifiable management evaluation and management service
–50 Bilateral procedure
–51 Multiple procedures
–57 Decision for surgery
–62 Two surgeons

The following is an example of how each of these should be used.

When seeing a patient in the office and a procedure is accomplished at the same visit the –25 modifier as appended to the E&M (evaluation and management) code.

99243–25
92511 Nasopharyngoscopy
indicates that you performed a procedure at the same visit as the separately identifiable E&M service.

69436
69436–50
indicates that bilateral tympanostomy tubes were performed. An alternative would be: 69436–50. The first method is preferred, but may not be acceptable for all payers.

31201
30520–50
indicates that a septoplasty was done at the same time of an intranasal total ethmoidectomy.

99243–57
31600
indicates that a decision to perform a tracheostomy was made at the time of the E&M service.

61548–62
indicates that two separate surgeons performed a distinct portion of the transphenoidal removal of a pituitary tumor. Each surgeon would code identically.

As previously mentioned, these are a few of the more common modifiers used. New modifiers are occasionally added by CPT. A complete description of the modifiers and their use is available in the CPT book. It is important to reiterate that there is great variability among the carriers about modifier usage. In dealing with each of the different managed care entities, you must pay specific attention to coding correctly. Remember that just because you code for a procedure, it does not mean it will be paid as a covered service.

Incidental or "Component" Procedures

One of the most common difficulties encountered with HMOs is the statement that procedure A is considered either a component of or incidental to Procedure B. Unfortunately, there is wide interpretation by the managed care organizations (MCOs) regarding which code will be paid. The fee is set contractually as is the amount of discounting for multiple procedures. In some instances the submitted codes are improper. This would be the case in coding for obtaining a graft as an additional code when performing a tympanoplasty. You must be sure that you code for only distinctly identifiable procedures and not for each component. This avoids unbundling.

In the circumstance where the MCO denies payment for incidental or included reasons, referral to the CPT descriptor is important. You might ask why coding for obtaining a graft during tympanoplasty is not acceptable when it is not in the descriptor. In this case it is considered an integral part of the procedure. One cannot do a tympanoplasty without obtaining a graft. In the case of denial as "incidental," the argument is made that either procedure can be performed separately, and this is often done in combination to improve the results.

To deal with the "component" procedure, it is important to refer to the CPT book for a technical descriptor of the code. If the denied procedure is neither indented nor identified as a separate procedure, separate coding is appropriate. Often referencing a standard surgical text with detailed description of the procedure is helpful. One of the most common areas where this occurs is when performing turbinate surgery with a septoplasty. In many cases, the MCO often will deny payment for the turbinate surgery as either incidental or a component of the septoplasty. In response, you should use the arguments described above. The turbinate surgery is done to enhance the results, and is a distinct procedure. This is evidenced by lack of indentation of the code and the absence of the separate procedure descriptor. In fact, in CPT, there is a separate reference where to find the codes for turbinate surgery. Although success is not guaranteed, a reasoned response with request for physician review often resolves the problem. With any and all of the problems you encounter, direct contact with the medical director may be necessary.

Accurate CPT coding is essential for accurate reimbursement in a managed care environment. It remains important in capitation to track the fiduciary stability of your cap rate. Physicians must attend CPT coding courses frequently and actively code with your staff. Your CPT coding can often determine your reimbursement, and your practice's coding is only accurate if the physician assumes the responsibility.

Cheryl Toth brings to her consulting assignments a strong business background and extensive knowledge about accounts receivable management and other financial reporting issues. Her experience with staff training and proficiency on various computer software systems allows Ms. Toth to diagnose inefficiencies and implement practical business systems solutions.

Ms. Toth's consulting projects include on-site operational evaluations of surgical practices, operational re-engineering, and the redesign of organizational structure.

Ms. Toth has given presentations for the American Association for Neurological Surgeons, the American Society of Plastic and Reconstructive Surgeons, the American College of Osteopathic Surgeons, the Joint Council of Allergy and Immunology, and various pharmaceutical companies and hospitals. Topics included practice management issues, managed care, and financial management.

Ms. Toth has been quoted in *Medical Economics* and has also contributed to medical publications that focus on business management issues: the American College of Physicians *Observer, Journal of Practice Management, Medical Office Manager,* the American College of Osteopathic Surgeons "News," and "Hospital Practice." She developed and manages KZA's web site. She holds a master's of business administration degree in finance from Loyola University of Chicago, and a bachelor's degree from Western Michigan University in Kalamazoo.

Lee Eisenberg, M.D., F.A.C.S. is on the Editorial Review Board of the CPT Coding Panel for the American Medical Association. He practices Otolaryngology in Englewood, New Jersey, with a special emphasis on Pediatric Otolaryngology. Lee has served as the Coordinator for Practice Affairs, American Academy of Otolaryngology-Head & Neck Surgery. He is an Associate Professor of Otolaryngology, Columbia University College of Physicians and Surgeons. He has lectured extensively on practice management, coding and reimbursement, and managed care including capitation and cost accounting medical practices.

3

Referral Guidelines

MICHAEL S. BENNINGER

The past decade, particularly the last few years, has seen dramatic changes in health care in the United States. Although many of these changes have been the result of new clinical developments, technological advancements, and pharmacological interventions, the main thrust of health care changes have involved developments in care delivery patterns. Traditionally, health care in the United States has been led by speciality and subspeciality care supported by the primary care disciplines. Many patients received all of their care at the hands of specialists. Care delivery has been procedurally oriented, and technological and pharmacological advancements have been driven through these specialists. This paradigm of care has resulted in a rapid growth of subspeciality areas and training programs. Seventy percent of all practicing physicians were specialists or subspecialists and a growing number of training programs were created to support these specialities.[1] In some specialities, such as ophthalmology, nearly all doctors completing general ophthalmology residency training have gone on to subspeciality fellowships. Associated with this growth of subspecialization has been a parallel growth in subspeciality boards.

Health care economic realities have shifted the emphasis of speciality care delivery as the standard to a more primary care focus. Although it is generally felt that speciality care is a mechanism for delivering high quality care, there have been growing concerns related to escalating health care costs and some evidence that the speciality model is more costly than a more primary care pattern followed by speciality referral when needed.[1–6] Health care researchers and educators, the government, and purchasers of health care have supported a reverse of the 30% primary–70% specialty ratio.

This paradigm shift from a speciality care model to a primary care model will require changes in the patterns by which patients move between primary care providers (PCPs) and speciality care providers (SCPs). Furthermore, a better understanding of the mechanism of referrals and factors that influence the referral process needs to occur. Finally, refinement of the referral process is necessary to assure that patients are receiving the highest quality care in a cost effective and efficient manner. This chapter describes the current understanding of factors that are important to referral processes and those that influence referrals. It also presents the relationships of such processes to otolaryngology and discusses the experience of a study of the development and implementation of referral guidelines in the Henry Ford Medical Group and recommendations for a process for the creation of otolaryngology referral guidelines that are consistent with individual physician and community needs.

The Referral Process

Referrals appear to be a major component of health care delivery in the United States and the United Kingdom, with the percentage of patients being referred differing substantially between speciality groups. Generalists tend to have relatively few referrals (13%), while certain specialities have large percentages of their patients coming to them through referrals.[7] Seventy-six percent of patients seen by general surgeons are referred and this number is probably greater for certain specialities such as medical oncology and neurosurgery.[7] Overall, approximately 44% of all patients seeing a physician in the United States have been referred. Specialities who practice both primary or medically oriented care as well as specialized surgical or procedural care, like otolaryngology, would be expected to have referral rates somewhere between that of the generalists and general surgeons. With certain managed care delivery patters, particularly those who use PCP gatekeepers, referral rates would be expected to decrease because patients require referral to see the specialist.

Many factors play an important role in the referral process. The first major set of factors relates to the reason for referral. A referral could occur to make or confirm a diagnosis; for a special test, procedure, or operation; to assist in the care of a patient or assume the responsibility of care of that patient for that disorder or for all of the patient's care. Even within the context of these reasons, different patterns for referrals may occur. A confirmatory diagnosis may precipitate the need for additional testing or a procedure. Shared care could occur when the patient sees either the PCP or SCP interchangeably or begins with the PCP, followed by the SCP for a finite period of time or until the disorder reaches a certain status, and then receives the rest of the care with the PCP. In some internal medicine specialities, once a referral for a particular disorder is made, the SCP may assume the general care of the patient: that is, the endocrinologist or cardiologist who needs to see a patient frequently for diabetes or congestive heart failure may subsequently treat other chronic or acute conditions as they develop. This is often expedient to the patient or may be necessary because of the interaction of these other conditions with the principle endocrine or cardiac disorder. It appears that advice in treatment may be the most common reason to refer.[8]

Although research specific to the referral process is only developing, some patterns appear to be emerging and they have been identified through the referral process assessment that has been ongoing in the British medical system. The Royal College of Radiologists Working Party has developed guidelines to attempt to refine the referral process[9–11] and has shown that referral rates can decrease through the use of referral guidelines.[9–11] Such decreases may result, in part, from decreases in the variability of the referral process. Whatever the cause, there appears to be growing interest in developing a referral mechanism that maximizes the quality of care of patients while diminishing its total cost. Whether or not guidelines will ultimately accomplish both goals is yet to be seen. Recent work, however, would suggest that such tools can serve to refine the referral process to maximize efficiency of care.[12]

Referral rates have been shown to vary from between 1 and 11% of all primary care visits.[13] Research has identified significant variations in the practice of medicine[14–17] and variations have been identified in primary care to speciality care referral rates.[8,17,18,19,20,21,22] These differences do not appear to be explained by differences in case-mix alone.[23] In addition, decisions for referral also appear to vary, even within a given physician's practice by practice domain.[19,24]

Many factors can impact this rate of referral. Physicians with ready access to tertiary or speciality care centers and those in metropolitan areas tend to refer more frequently.[24,25] Referral decisions may be influenced by patient-related factors such as patient or family expectations, age, or insurance status.[18,26,27,28,29] Physicians who spend less time in clinical care and younger physicians tend to refer more commonly.[25] In some cases, greater familiarity with the disorder or field of speciality may be associated with more frequent referrals.[30,31] Referrals may be more common for acute, symptomatic disorders rather than chronic conditions for some disorders.[32] Access to the generalist may affect the desire to refer. As patient access becomes strained and wait times for a clinic appointment lengthen for PCP care, referrals appear to increase perhaps in an effort to decrease the backlog of patients or assure that patients receive care in a timely manner.[12]

It is clear that substantial variations in referral rates have been identified and that considerable clinical discretion is involved in the decision to refer.[26,33] Despite all these potential reasons for referrals, attempts to identify consistent, specific reasons for referral have found no dominant factor.[34] Furthermore, attempts to use referral rates as a means of judging quality have not been successful in evaluation of small numbers of physicians.[35] If this lack of association between referral rates and quality is born out in future evaluations, then the main reasons for developing referral guidelines should be predicated on improvements in efficiency, reduced costs, or increased patient satisfaction. Attempts to curtail referrals to specialists would therefore be appropriate only if existing referral rates reflected overutilization of referrals, if quality of care was poorer if delivered by the specialist, if patient preference and satisfaction were adversely effected by referral, or if the cost of care being delivered by the specialist was found to be greater (given equivalencies in quality and outcome). The latter has been suggested in some studies. For every one dollar generated by a family physician, two dollars are generated by the consultant. Furthermore, $5000 in combined professional and hospital charges are generated for every referral from a generalist to a university-based specialist.[36,37,38] Indications are that even after controlling for case-mix, specialists utilize more medical resources than PCPs, although little has been done to translate such utilization into differences in expenditures.[1,3,4,5,6] Some of this difference between the PCP and SCP charges may be related to the complexity of the disorder or contact. This, however, has not been clearly demonstrated when considering care delivered by the PCP compared with the SCP.[39,40] Balancing such studies are recent reports suggesting that for certain conditions, speciality care may actually be less expensive and more efficient than if it were delivered by the PCP, and that outcomes may be better if treated by the specialist.[40–43] Such decisions most likely will have to be individualized based on evaluations of cost and outcome. Many disorders can be competently treated by the PCP, but certain conditions will surely be identified where primary contact and treatment may be better accomplished by the SCP.

To determine whether overreferral or underreferral is present, the relationship of such consultations and referrals to quality and cost must be determined. One way to evaluate quality of care is to develop a panel model for creation of referral guidelines and then compare actual referrals with the guidelines to assess whether they are appropriate or inappropriate.[12] A similar model has been used to create guidelines for care through explicit criteria developed by an expert panel using the two-round Delphi model from the University of California Los Angeles and RAND.[44–48] These criteria have then been used to evaluate utilization rates and make recommendations regarding appropriateness of care.[49] Although this specific paneling methodology has been questioned, its application has grown. A more objective method for determining quality is to compare differences in the care delivered with the associated outcomes. One such study is the Medical Outcomes Study.[42] No difference was found in outcomes for patients with hypertension treated by PCPs and SCPs. However, outcomes for the management of foot ulcers were found to be better in those treated by endocrinologists than those treated by PCPs.[42] Overall, most studies have found no difference in the quality of care delivered by the SCP or PCP. Although some studies have shown quality of care to be better when delivered by the SCP[40,41,43] few have found improved quality from care delivered by the PCP compared with the SCP.[50]

■ Developing Primary Care Referral Guidelines

The decision to create guidelines for altering or improving the process of referral from the PCP to otolaryngology can be driven by a number of factors and each will influence not only whether or not to create the guidelines, but also what they are to accomplish. Each physician or group should clearly establish the purpose of the guidelines prior to the process of developing them because such purposes will dramatically impact their content. Guidelines can be created to improve access to otolaryngology or restrict such access. They can be developed to increase otolaryngology referrals or increase the autonomy of the PCP in managing otolaryngologic disorders. They can be used to educate PCPs in appropriate care and the preferred timing of referral or ensure that patients who require speciality care are referred in a timely fashion to prevent potential adverse outcomes or complications. They can be used to identify which disorders are best treated early or late by the otolaryngologist. Finally, they can be used to reduce expenditures or improve patient satisfaction. As we can see from these examples or the multiple other circumstances where guidelines are perceived to be needed, no universal set of guidelines will suit all of the potential purposes.

The first step in the creation of referral guidelines is to identify local and regional needs for such guidelines. Key factors are the potential benefits of guidelines to the patients, the community, and the individual otolaryngology practice. Do the PCPs desire or need such guidelines and would they be willing to assist in their development? The physician should assess purchaser/employer/payer requirements for referral guidelines and determine whether guidelines will be developed by or purchased for local payers. Identify what is expected to be accomplished by the guidelines. This will also be determined by community and practice needs. Possible goals for referral guidelines to otolaryngology from PCPs are noted in Table 3–1. If the physician is primarily practicing in a fee-for-service environment, guidelines may want to assure access of patients to the physician. In a discounted fee-for-service environment, the guidelines should maximize referrals that require high technical or procedural input because these will not only provide high quality care but may also positively impact revenues. In such an arrangement, low revenue care, which can be managed well by the PCPs, may want to be limited. Finally, in a capitated or at risk payment strategy, the physician may wish to create guidelines whereby patients would be referred only when they require speciality input for diagnosis, procedures, or specialized care. In mixed environments of reimbursement, it is important to make sure that the guidelines do not serve to put physicians in a position where they cannot support their practices or may adversely effect patient care.

Who will write the guidelines? Will it be the physician, PCP, or both? Under most cases the best arrangement is

TABLE 3–1. Goals of Primary Care Referral Guidelines

Facilitate early referral
Facilitate ease of referral
Aid the PCP in determining need for referral
Decrease the frequency of unnecessary referrals
Improve quality of care
Decrease costs or improve efficiency
Accomplish payer/employer desire to:
change referral patterns
limit referrals

to establish a collaborative venture with the PCPs. An open line of communication between the PCP and physician will foster a relationship that will ensure that the concerns and interests of both are well represented and therefore facilitate their implementation. Under some circumstances, such a collaborative venture is not possible, either because of practical difficulties or because one party does not wish to participate. It is in the best interest of the specialist to be an active participant, particularly in these times of a strong primary care focus. In general, the specialist can best address quality of care issues and perhaps the PCP is more familiar with general issues related to the patient, comorbidities, and other medical conditions. Furthermore, the PCP usually has an ongoing relationship with the patient and the patient's family that is best to preserve. If the guidelines are developed primarily by the physician, reviewing the guidelines with the PCPs prior to implementation will go a long way toward assuring their success.

The next step is to address the content of the guidelines. Much of this is predicated on the goals established above. Table 3–2 contains a list of possible types of disorders that can be placed in the guidelines. While writing guidelines, it is important to set standards or a mechanism for assuring that they meet quality of care standards. The most formal approach involves using the recommendations for guideline creation established by the American Health Care Policy and Research. (AHCPR).[51] Unfortunately, such efforts are often cumbersome, time-consuming, and expensive. They frequently require in excess of $500,000 as well as the input of multiple individuals and sources to develop just one guideline. Very few groups have such financial and information resources at their disposal.

Other methodologies are therefore usually required to establish guidelines. One reasonable way is to create consensus utilizing the experience of the clinicians who will be using the guidelines—that is, creating a local standard for referrals. This approach requires support from the peer-reviewed literature and community standards of care and traditional practice. The more regimented the methods and the more objective the composers, the more likely the guidelines will meet the goals and withstand adverse pressures.

TABLE 3–2. Disorders That May be Addressed in Referral Guidelines

Surgical indicators for those patients being referred for surgery
Disorders for which referrals are frequently made but are often unnecessary
Disorders where an impact can be made due to high frequency of referral
Disorders where early referral is needed or desired:
a. early referral will decrease costs
b. early referral will minimize risk of complications
c. early referral will enhance quality of care
Disorders where changes in referral patterns will enhance patient satisfaction
Disorders where referral guidelines will decrease costs
Disorders where referral guidelines will improve PCP care of their patients

One key area to consider early is the format of the guidelines since this may have a significant impact on their effectiveness. In general, the simpler the guidelines, the more they will be used. Some physicians feel very comfortable using written documents; others would prefer to have information readily available through computer or electronic media. It is important to assess the needs of the users up front and develop a format or formats (occasionally more than one will be needed) that will facilitate their utilization of the guidelines. In our referral guideline efforts at Henry Ford Hospital, we have used three separate mediums for implementation: a scripted, descriptive form that is on both hard paper copy and in our medical information system; a summary condensed version consisting of laminated sheets that are in a small looseleaf binder so that they can be changed when needed and combined with guidelines developed for other specialities; and algorithms to facilitate a quick review by the PCP. We found that these were all necessary because different PCPs had different experiences and global roll-out seemed preferable to focusing on an individual audience.

To create referral guidelines, we found it necessary to include some management information. If we were making recommendations to refer at a point in the care process, we needed to be sure that the PCP was familiar with the evaluation and treatment methods used to reach that point in care.

Perhaps one of the most important facets of implementing referral guidelines involves determining how to measure the success of accomplishing the goals of the guidelines that were established in the beginning. This measurement will also depend on style and format of the guidelines. Have there been detectable changes in referral patterns? Has quality of care been maintained? Are patients, primary care practitioners and physicians satisfied with the guidelines and their effects? Satisfaction should be expanded to purchasers, employers, or payers if they were instrumental in driving guideline formation.

The American Academy of Otolaryngology-Head and Neck Surgery (AAO-HNS) has attempted to develop a Referral Guideline Kit to assist all physicians in developing local referral guidelines.[52] These have focused on providing a format for guideline development and some examples that can serve as a format for the individual or group of physicians to create guidelines consistent with their goals and community standards. Because of concerns about expense in AHCPR level guidelines, and the wide variety of community and individual goals, it would be difficult to create guidelines applicable to all circumstances. Therefore, the AAO-HNS has not attempted to develop consensus guidelines at this time, although it is likely that these will be developed by the AAO-HNS and other primary care and speciality groups in the future.

■ Otolaryngology Referral Guidelines

As with all referral guidelines, the development of referral guidelines for otolaryngology will vary with the local needs of the patients and purchasers, the experience of both the PCP and the physician, and the specific characteristics of individual practices. The guidelines will be different if the primary purpose is to identify key disorders where early diagnosis and management are preferred, if a specific speciality carve out is desired, or if the main goal is to limit referrals to the otolaryngologist so that more care is delivered by the PCP.

In 1993, we initiated a pilot of otolaryngology referral guidelines in an attempt to improve the referral process and decrease waiting times for patients who see both the PCP and the otolaryngologist. Since most guidelines refer to a level of care when the referral process should be initiated, some mention of the management of the patient by the PCP prior to referral seemed necessary. We therefore elected to create guidelines that included summaries of appropriate management options and tests that should be able to be performed by the PCP prior to referral, the timing of referral, at what point a referral should be considered, and criteria that would be used to determine if surgery was indicated. Although the latter is most pertinent to the surgeon, it seemed reasonable to include this information in the referral guidelines so that the PCP who is referring for consideration of surgical treatment would know prior to referral whether or not the patient met the minimal criteria.

The pilot was initiated in the northeast region of the Henry Ford Medical Group (HFMG), which is a region of 6 ambulatory care sites serviced by 100 physicians with an equal mix of specialists and PCPs. Two otolaryngologists and two audiologists, all members of the Department of Otolaryngology-Head and Neck Surgery, serviced this region. The HFMG is a multispeciality group practice of 1000 physicians and scientists. Approximately 50% of the patients are members of a large mixed-model Health Maintenance Organization, while the other 50% participate in other payment plans including traditional indemnity insurances, Medicare, Medicaid, and some unreimbursed care.

Prior to guideline development, we identified key process variables that the region felt were important in improving the referral process. These included disorders with high prevalence where guidelines would have an impact, disorders with high levels of variance in referral recommendations by the different PCPs, those where the physicians perceived that many referrals were unnecessary, and disorders customarily treated by both PCPs and otolaryngologists. Using these key variables, members of the Department of Otolaryngology–Head and Neck Surgery identified 10 disorders for guideline development. These were: acute otitis media, otitis media with effusion, chronic sinusitis, acute sinusitis, globus sensation, tonsillitis, epistaxis, hearing loss, dizziness, and tinnitus. Following the pilot for evaluating the effectiveness of guidelines related to these disorders, we added additional disorders including epistaxis, external otitis, hoarseness, and nasal fracture. Supported by the peer-reviewed literature, recommendations for clinical indicators of the American Academy of Otolaryngology-Head and Neck Surgery, recommendations from the AHCPR, American Academy of Pediatrics, and the American College of Physicians, the physicians developed draft management and referral guidelines. These were reviewed by two physicians and a division head from general internal medicine, general pediatrics and family medicine, and the Managed Care Coordinator for the region. The guidelines were modified by the physicians based on these recommendations.

The guidelines were initially written in a text form with bulleted highlights. Each guideline included: (1) a description of the disorder, (2) the evaluation and methods used to make a diagnosis, (3) treatment options, (4) when to refer, and (5) surgical indications. In this format the PCPs could determine whether or not they felt they could manage the patient or if and when they should refer. In addition, the surgical indicators let them know when a patient had met the minimal criteria for surgery. Since the physicians would often receive consultations for surgical treatment, if the patient had not yet met these surgical indications, an unnecessary referral was averted.

Prior to implementing the guidelines, we obtained baseline data so that the impact could be measured. Accessibility to the physicians were assessed via 3 months of Lead Time Reports, which is a measure of the third available appointment for a new patient. Questionnaires were sent to all the regional PCPs to evaluate their comfort in treating these common disorders, ease of access to otolaryngology, and present referral patterns to otolaryngology. Questionnaires were also filled out by patients at the time of their ENT visit to assess patient satisfaction with the referral process, the length of time from referral until the time they were able to be seen by the physicians, and their perceptions of appropriate wait times. All new patients sent by the regional PCPs over a 3 week period were assessed as to whether or not they would have been referred if the PCP had used the criteria established in the guidelines. If they would have been, then the referral was considered appropriate; if not, then they were considered unnecessary. These same data points were reevaluated 6 months after implementing the guidelines and again 5 months later to assure that any changes that occurred were sustainable.

The guidelines were sent to all of the regional PCPs who were encouraged to call if they had any questions. The physicians attended the regional meetings of the various PCP groups and described the guidelines and answered any questions. In this way, all the PCPs were made aware of the purpose of the guidelines and any significant issues were addressed in advance of implementation. This open communication was encouraged throughout the implementation phase and carried forward for the subsequent 3 years. In practice, this open communication may be as critical as the content of the guidelines themselves. This is also the traditional approach to managing referrals that has been a part of medical practice in the United States for many years and may still be an important tool in some communities, particularly those where the PCPs and SCPs have frequent contact. Table 3–3 gives a summary of the impact of guideline implementation. Initially, 54% of the referrals were unnecessary. This dropped to 12% after implementation. Although this percentage increased to 20% 5 months later, it stayed at that level for the next 2 years. Therefore there was a 34% sustainable decrease in the unnecessary referral rate. Lead time reports did not show a change in wait times, but the total HMO patient volume/enrollment in the region dramatically increased and the amount of total ENT clinic coverage actually decreased, yet wait times remained constant. Furthermore, patient questionnaires showed a significant decrease in the time until their appointment. Overall patient satisfaction with the referral process improved.

Eighty-six percent of the PCPs used the guidelines and 82% used them at least one time per month and one-third used them 3 or more times per month. Many of the PCPs told us that the processing that was performed prior to guideline implementation was educational and obviated daily use of the guidelines. Rather, they would refer to them only if they could not remember the instructions or if the case was related to an area or disorder where they had less familiarity. Seventy-two percent felt that the guidelines improved their ability to manage these ENT disorders and 45% felt that the guidelines decreased the number of referrals to otolaryngology. Eighty-nine percent of the PCPs felt that they would continue to use the guidelines and 85% wished to expand referral guidelines to other speciality areas.

Initially, 63% of referrals were found to have disorders addressed in the guidelines. This decreased to 40% at 6 months and remained at this level 5 months later. This decrease in the number of patients seen who had disorders addressed in the guidelines allowed access to other patients who could not be managed as well by the PCP or those who had significant disorders that required otolaryngology input or surgery. Although quality of care is often difficult to measure, the physicians did not see any adverse results from the referrals nor any potential complications that were preventable by earlier referral. If written in a manner that recommends early referrals even for common disorders if there is a potential complication, these adverse results should be preventable.

This pilot study has clearly shown that primary care referral guidelines are effective in accomplishing the goals of the guidelines. Furthermore, roll-out of these guidelines throughout the entire medical group has been successful and can be expanded to other specialities. Different communities and different practices may have different goals for their guidelines, but thoughtful preparation and open communication between physicians should allow for these goals to be met.

REFERENCES

1. Eisenberg JM: Doctors *decisions and the cost of medical care. The reasons for doctors practice patterns and ways to change them.* Ann Arbor, MI: Health Administration Press, 1986.
2. Greenfield S, Nelson EC, Zubcoff M, et al: Variations in resource utilization among medical specialties and systems of care. Results from the medical outcomes study. *JAMA* 1992; 267:1624–1630.
3. Manu P, Schwartz SE: Patterns of diagnostic testing in the academic setting: The influence of medical attendings subspecialty training. *Soc Sci Med* 1983; 17:(18)1339–1342.
4. Greenwald HP, Peterson ML, Garrison LP: Interspecialty variation in office based care. *Med Care* 1984; 22:14–29.
5. Engel W, Freund DA, Stein JS, et al: The treatment of patients with asthma by specialists and generalists. *Med Care* 1989; 27:306–314.
6. Kravitz RL, Greenfield S, Rogers W, et al: Difference in the mix of patients among medical specialties and systems of care. Results from the medical outcomes study. *JAMA* 1992; 267:1617–1623.

TABLE 3–3. Referral Guidelines, Before and After Implementation

	Before	*6 Months After*	*11 Months After*
Appropriate visits	46%	88%	80%
Unnecessary visits	54%	12%	20%
Appropriate/unnecessary	32/29	52/7	23/10
Visits related to guideline	63%	40%	40%
Disorders related to guidelines (patients seen)	71/113	59/146	33/81

7. Gonzalez ML, Rizzo JA: Physician referrals and the medical market place. *Med Care* 1991; 29:1017–1027.
8. Coulter A, Naone A, Goldacre M: General practitioners referrals to specialist outpatient clinics. I. Why general practitioners refer patients to specialist outpatient clinics. *BMJ* 1989; 299:304–306.
9. Royal College of Radiologists Working Party: Influence of the Royal College of Radiologists guidelines on hospital practice: a multicenter study. *BMJ* 1992; 304:704–743.
10. Royal College of Radiologists guidelines on referral from general practice. *BMJ* 1993; 306:110–111.
11. Halpin SFS, Yeoman L, Duondas DD: Radiographic examination of the lumbar spine in a community hospital: An audit of current practice. *BMJ* 1991; 303:813–815.
12. Benninger MS, King F, Nichols RD: Management guidelines for improvement of otolaryngology referrals from primary care physicians. *Otolaryngol Head Neck Surg* 1995; 113:446–452.
13. Hart J, Kahan E, Derazne E, et al: Consultants perceptions of quality of referrals. *Isr J Med Sci* 1991; 27: 405–407.
14. Wennberg JE: Dealing with medical practice variations: A proposal for action. *Health Aff* 1984; 3:6–32.
15. Johnson RE, Freeborn DK, Mullooly JP: Physicians use of laboratory, radiology, and drugs in a prepaid group practice HMO. *Health Serv Res* 1985; 20:525–547.
16. Chassin MR, Brook Rh, Park RE, et al: Variations in the use of medical and surgical services by the medicare population. *N Engl J Med* 1986; 314:285–290.
17. Starfield BH, Powe NR, Weiner JR, et al: Cost vs quality in different types of primary care settings. *JAMA* 1994; 272:1903–1908.
18. Rothart ML, Rovner DR, Elstein AS, et al: Differences in medical referral decisions for obesity among family practitioners, general internists, and gynecologists. *Med Care* 1984; 22:42–55.
19. Calman NS, Bernstein HR, Licht W: Variability in consultation rates and practitioner level of diagnostic certainty. *J Fam Pract* 1992; 35:31–38.
20. Wilkin D, Smith AG: Explaining variation in general practitioner referrals to hospital. *Fam Pract* 1987; 4:160–169.
21. Wilkin D, Smith AG: Variation in general practitioners referral rates to consultants. *J R Coll Gen Pract* 1987; 37:350–353.
22. Moore AT, Roland MO: How much variation in referral rates among general practitioners is due to chance? *BMJ* 1989; 298:500–502.
23. Salem-Schatz S, Moore G, Rucker M, et al: The case for casemix adjustment in practice profiling. When good apples look bad. *JAMA* 1994; 272:871–874.
24. Blancquaert IR, Zvagulis I, Gray-Donald K: Referral patterns for children with chronic diseases. *Pediatrics* 1992; 90:71–74.
25. Sobal J, Muncie HL, Valente CM, et al: Self-reported referral patterns in practices of family/general practitioners, internists and obstetricians/gynecologists. *J Community Health* 1988; 13:171–83.
26. Langley GR, MacLellan AM, Sutherland HL, et al: Effect of nonmedical factors on family physicians decisions about referral for consultation. *Can Med Assoc J* 1992; 147:659–666.
27. Penchansky R, Rox D: Frequency of referral and patient characteristics in group practice. *Med Care* 1970; 9:368–385.
28. Ludke RL: An examination of the factors that influence patient referral decisions. *Med Care* 1982; 20:782–796.
29. Hurley RE, Freund DA, Gage BJ: Gatekeeper effects on patterns of physician use. *J Fam Pract* 1991; 32:167–1174.
30. Calman NS, Hyman RB, Licht W: Variability in consultation rates and practitioner level of diagnostic certainty. *J Fam Pract* 1992; 35:31–38.
31. Reynolds GA, Chitnis JG, Roland MO: General practitioner outpatient referrals: Do good doctors refer more patients to hospital? *BMJ* 1991; 302:1250–1252.
32. Ettinger ER, Schwartz, Kalet AL: Referral patterns of primary care physicians for eye care. *J Am Optom Assoc* 1993; 64:468–70.
33. Lawler FH, Purvis JR, Glen JK, et al: Physician referrals from a rural family practice residency clinic: A pilot study. *Fam Pract Res J* 1990;10:19–26.
34. Lawler FH, Hosokawa MC: The relationship between utilization and referral for family physicians. *Fam Pract Res J* 1987; 7:22–28.
35. Knottnems JA, Joaster J, Dams J: Comparing the quality of referals of general practitioners with high and average referral rates: An independent panel review. *Br J Gen Pract* 1990; 40:178–181.
36. Glenn JK, Lawler FH, Hoerl MS: Physician referrals in a competitive environment. An estimate of the economic impact of a referral. *JAMA* 1987; 258:1920–1923.
37. Schneeweiss R, Ellsbury K, Hart LG, et al: The economic impact and multiplier effect of a family practice clinic on an academic medical center. *JAMA* 1989; 262: 370–375.
38. Kues JR, Sacks JG, Davis LJ: The value of a new family practice center patient to the academic medical center. *J Fam Pract* 1991; 32:571–575.
39. Strauss MJ, Conrad D, LoGerfo JP, et al: Cost and outcome of care for patients with chronic obstructive lung disease: Analysis by physician specialty. *Med Care* 1986; 24:(10) 915–924.
40. Clark RA, Rietschel RL: The cost of initiating appropriate therapy for skin diseases: A comparison of dermatologists and family physicians. *J Am Acad Dermatol* 1983; 9:787–796.
41. Ward NO, Berry DW: Is there a role for primary care in the specialist's office? *Arch Otolaryngol Head Neck Surg* 1993; 119:721–722.
42. Greenfield S, Rogers W, Mangotich, et al: Outcomes of patients with hypertension and non-insulin-dependent diabetes mellitus treated by different systems and specialties. *JAMA* 1995;274:1436–1444.
43. Zeiger RS, Heller S, Mellon MH: Facilitated referral to asthma specialist reduces relapses in asthma emergency room visits. *J Allergy Clin Immunol* 1991; 87:1160–1168.
44. Bodner EE, Browning GG, Chalmers FT, et al: Can meta-analysis help uncertainty in surgery for otitis media in children. *J Larongol Otol* 1991; 105:812–819.
45. Brook RH, Chassin MR, Fink A, et al: A method for the detailed assessment of the appropriateness of medical technologies. *Int J Technol Assess Health Com* 1986:1; 53–63.
46. Gray D, Hampton JR, Bernstein SJ: Audit of coronary angiography and bypass surgery. *Lancet* 1990; 335: 1317–1320.
47. Merrick NJ, Fink A, Park RE, et al: Derivation of clinical indications for carotid endarterectomy by an expert panel. *Am J Public Health* 1987; 77:187–190.
48. Kosecoff J, Chassin MR, Fink A, et al: Obtaining clinical data on the appropriateness of medical care in community practice. *JAMA* 1987; 258:2538–2542.
49. Kleinman LC, Kosecoff J, Dubois RW, et al: The medical appropriateness of tympanostomy tubes proposed for children younger than 16 years in the United States. *JAMA* 1994; 271:1250–1255.
50. Weiner JP, Starfield BH: Measurement of the primary care roles of office based physicians. *Am J Public Health* 1983; 73:666–671.
51. Clancy CM, Lanier D, Grady ML: Research at the interface of primary and specialty care. US Dept Health and Human Services 1996; Pub No AHCPR 96-0034.
52. American Academy of Otolaryngology-Head and Neck Surgery. Referral Guideline Kit. Alexandria, VA, 1995.

Dr. Michael S. Benninger is an internationally recognized otolaryngologist, especially well known for his work with voice and nasal sinus disorders. He is Chairman of the Department of Otolaryngology–Head & Neck Surgery and Director of the Medical Center for Performing Artists in the Henry Ford Health System. HFHS is recognized as an innovator in health care delivery; it was one of the first organizations to develop a vertically integrated health care system and a national standard for combining managed care with academic and research pursuits. Dr. Benninger is very active within that organization and he and his department are innovators in otolaryngology care delivery, including management and referral guidelines, resource allocation, utilization management and cost effectiveness, and outcomes research.

Dr. Benninger has multiple local, regional, and national administrative responsibilities including Chair of the Board of Governors, Member of the Executive and Finance Committee, and Member of the Board of Directors of the American Academy of Otolaryngology-Head and Neck Surgery; President Elect and Program Director of the American Rhinologic Society; Chairman of the Scientific Advisory Board of the Voice Foundation and President of the Michigan Otolaryngological Society.

He is Editor-in-Chief of the one of the world's two completely on-line medical journals, the *Online Interactive Journal of Otolaryngology*, an Associate Editor for the *American Journal of Rhinology*, and an Editor for the *Journal of Voice* and *Phonoscope*. He has written multiple publications, book chapters, and two books and he is frequently interviewed for regional and national newspapers and magazines, as well as national radio and television regarding health care topics.

4

Negotiating Managed Care Contracts

T. FORCHT DAGI

There are dozens of books that promise to teach negotiating skills. All of us, they announce, are negotiators in the rough. We all negotiate every day of our lives. We don't get what we deserve, we get what we negotiate. Negotiating skills are easily learned, we are told, and these books purport to show us how to do it better.

It is true that negotiating skills *can* be learned, even if not quite as easily as the popular press would have us believe. It is also true that we negotiate daily, if often subliminally, and that most of us have a surprisingly well-developed instinctual sense of how the negotiating process works and what needs to be accomplished. This review of negotiating skills, tools, and strategies is intended as a guide to the methods and tactics applicable to negotiating the managed care environment.

■ The Concept of Negotiation

It is as difficult to find a simple and informative definition of the term "negotiation" as it is to speak of the subject in the absence of such a definition. In their widely cited book, *Getting to Yes,* Roger Fisher and William Ury simply assume we know the meaning of the term.[1] They construe negotiation in terms of a process or procedure. Edward de Bono, an English physician who has devoted his career to the study of problem resolution through creative thinking, suggests that negotiation is a process that resolves conflict by resolving competition.[2] This explanation captures some of the *mechanism* of negotiation, but still falls short of a definition. In one of the few writings to address the problem of negotiation in health care specifically, Leonard J. Marcus, director of the Program for Health Care Negotiation and Conflict Resolution at the Harvard School of Public Health, explains that negotiation is a "process to determine the exchange of tangibles and intangibles."[3] True, but incomplete. The stock and option markets arguably accomplish the same goal through the reconciliation of bids and sales and puts and calls, but these markets somehow do not involve negotiation in the way we commonly construe the process.

Negotiation is best defined as a process of communication among two or more parties in joint pursuit of an agreement or a relationship that will inure to their benefit. The term "communication" is used rather than "dialogue" or "discussion" because some forms of negotiation—like the Cuban missile crisis during the Kennedy administration—may initially involve forms of communication such as public threats and posturing rather than discussions or other more direct and efficient forms of interchange. The contemporary health care environment is also characterized by similar indirect and inefficient forms of communication.

Although negotiation is characterized by pursuit of benefits, these benefits do not necessarily work to the advantage of both sides equally, as some idealists would have us believe. Neither does each party to a negotiation necessarily care about *mutual* benefit. In *partisan* negotiations, each party works to benefit itself primarily and other parties' secondarily, if at all. In *integrated* negotiation, the process is optimized to benefit *all* parties at the table in more than a token fashion. Partisan negotiations are often referred to as *distributive bargaining* or *win–lose* negotiations. The pie to be divided is construed relatively narrowly. Each side perceives the pie as sufficient to benefit itself alone. Integrated negotiations are often framed as *cooperative* or *integrated* bargaining processes, whose purpose is mutual benefit, or a *win–win* model. In this model, the pie is *enlarged* by the negotiating process, and not constricted. It is reasonable to model negotiations as consisting of two parts: substance and relationship. Different types of negotiating strategy may emphasize one over the other, depending on the context in which the negotiation takes place.

Several models attempt to describe the character of the negotiation process while others explore what the negotiation process *ought* to be like. The culture of negotiation in the West draws heavily on the traditions of law, trade, and diplomacy. As a result, there has been a strong historical tendency to conceive of negotiations in terms of victory and defeat on the substantive issues, and to see each negotiation as isolated, independent events. An alternate view conceives of negotiations primarily in terms of relationships, and therefore as a potentially ongoing, or continuing series of events. The outcome of one negotiation in this model is linked to the outcome of the next. Still another model casts the negotiation process in terms of game theory and assumes that each party will act on the basis of radical self-interest.

The model used here draws heavily on a the idea of integrative bargaining. This model teaches the value of defining problems in terms of mutual interests and aspiring to elegant solutions of mutual benefit. It also emphasizes the importance of building relationships and developing a sense of efficiency in the negotiation process based on prior trust. This way of modeling the negotiation process is illustrated in Figure 4–1. Movement to the right is preferred. Movement involving substantive issues and relationship is generally linked.

Negotiation skills are of little value in the absence of the analytical basis for mounting a cogent argument. The types of information required can be divided into two categories: the first category pertains to the needs, interests, and abilities of all parties and stakeholders in the negotiation; the second pertains to the value system(s) that each party brings to the table. The integrative bargaining model relies on a full exploration of both categories.

President Jimmy Carter was a proponent of negotiation as the *morally* preferred way to resolve conflicts. It was and remains his view, that the process of negotiation is a good thing in and of itself, even if no agreement is attained. Carter emphasized relationship over substance. His reliance on negotiation as the major tool of foreign policy in the context of the crises confronting his administration was widely perceived as a sign of weakness, much as Chamberlain's negotiations with Hitler came ultimately to be judged. We prefer, however, to view negotiation as a tool by which to advance a particular strategy, without an immutable moral advantage. It may embody the moral high ground under certain circumstances, but certainly not all, nor does it necessarily represent the best way of advancing a specific end under all circumstances. Nevertheless, simply preparing for a possible negotiation may offer sub-

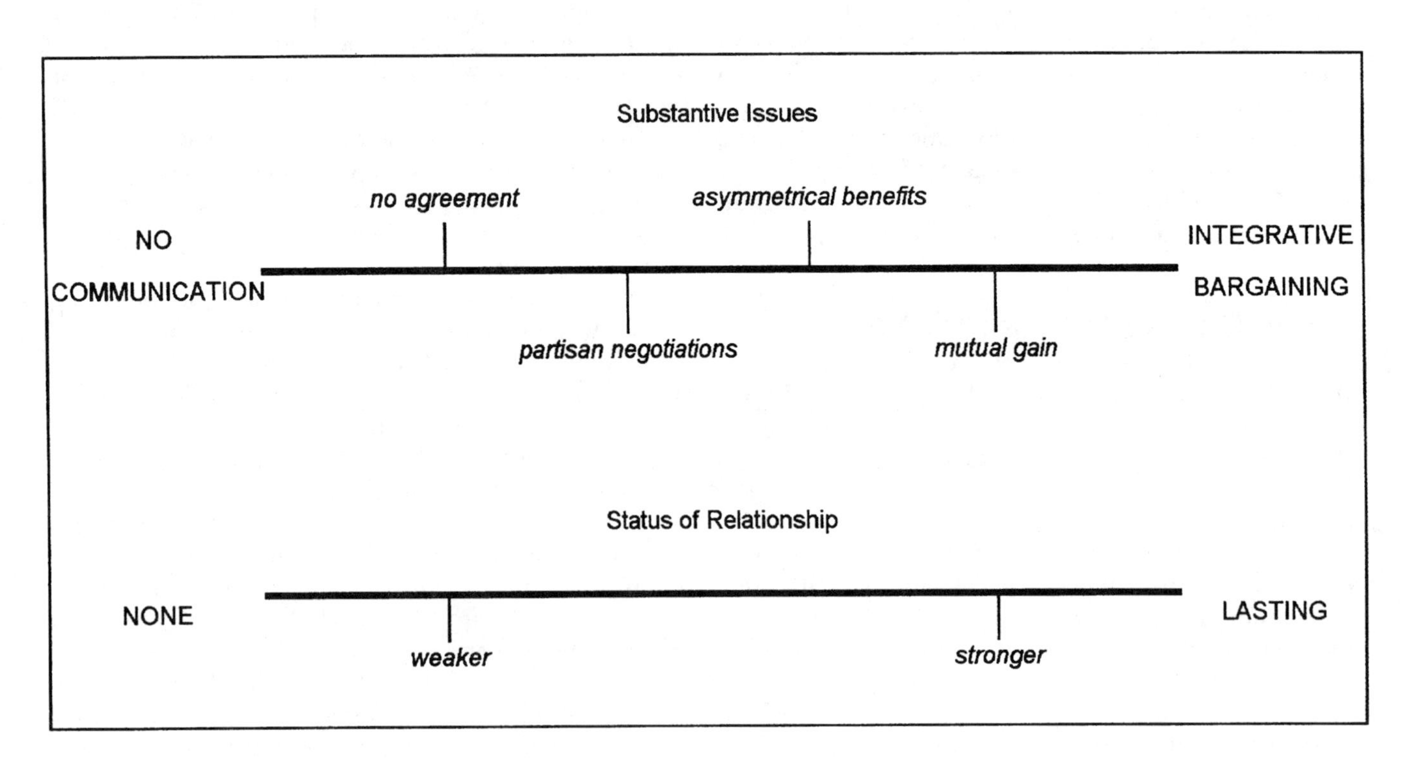

FIGURE 4–1. Modeling the negotiation process.

TABLE 4–1. Changing Parameters in the Management Care Environment

Parameter	*Traditional*	*New*
Patient flow	Based on professional relationships	Negotiated agreements
Management strategy	Jointly developed by patient and physician	Enforced protocol
Professional relationships	Based on personal and professional considerations	Dictated by payers without concern for preexisting relationships

stantial advantages to the parties concerned, whether or not they choose to proceed.

■ Managed Care and the Negotiating Mindset

The advent of managed care has changed not only the manner in which medicine is practiced, but also the skills necessary to be a "compleat" physician. From the physicians' perspective, the most salient changes fall into two categories: (1) those associated with patient referral patterns; (2) those associated with the way medical and surgical services are valued.

As a result of these changes, the skill set and knowledge required to be an excellent physician in the scientific, technical, and humanitarian sense no longer define the extent of the skill set required to develop and retain a competitive advantage in the medical marketplace. In addition, the process by which physicians develop a practice, and obtain and exercise the authority to treat and refer patients has also changed, as shown in Table 4–1.

Thus, patient flow no longer results from a network of professional relationships, but from negotiated agreements. Treatment no longer reflects an approach privately developed between physician and patient, but rather, in many cases, a protocol dictated by the payer. The practice of medicine has begun to evolve into a new kind of predefined, bounded encounters that differ in many significant respects from the types of relationships that were previously the norm.

The strategies for negotiating and ultimately moderating these shifts in authority and power require a change in attitude on the part of many physicians. These are some of the new skills that are required:

1. The ability to capture the costs of practice.
2. The ability to translate the costs of practice into terms commensurate with those by managed care organizations (MCOs).
3. The ability to reverse roles with payers and to view oneself and one's practice from the perspective of others.
4. The willingness to reexamine and possibly to modify deeply embedded practice patterns.
5. The willingness to reexamine the nature of the doctor–patient relationship.
6. The willingness to conceive of oneself as competing for patients on grounds other than the traditional triad of "ability, availability, and affability."
7. The willingness to examine one's practice milieu and recast it in terms of a "market."
8. The willingness to change in accordance with market demands.
9. The willingness to create new types of institutional alliances.
10. The willingness to learn new types of communication.

Practices aiming to succeed in the managed care environment must be prepared to accumulate and analyze information pertaining to issues of quality and capability as defined by others, and to learn how to present this analysis cogently, convincingly, and fairly to potential purchasers of the physician's services. This task is not easy for physicians. For as long as the profession has existed, quality and capability were defined internally, and the outside world accepted these definitions to a greater or lesser extent. It no longer does. To succeed, physicians must now at least acknowledge, if not actually accommodate, external benchmarks whose properties may stand at variance with the professional tradition.

■ Negotiating Skills

A number of rules have proven effective in improving the process of negotiation. In most instances, parties to a negotiation will begin by adopting a position that maximizes their benefit as they see it, and advocating staunchly for this position. The emphasis devolved is on substance rather than on relationship. The negotiation takes the form of two or more parties engaging in a contest of wills through which a compromise is forged. The compromise rarely satisfies all parties, and sometimes satisfies none. Fisher and Ury begin *Getting to Yes* with an admonition to bargain over interests rather than positions.[4] This advice is not universally applicable because it requires that all parties to the negotiation buy into this negotiating model and that a common idiom of interests can be developed. Nevertheless it is an ideal worth pursuing and constitutes

TABLE 4–2. Extremes of Bargaining*

	"Hard Bargaining"	*"Soft Bargaining"*
Context	Adversarial	Nonadversarial
Goal	Victory	Agreement
Concessions	A condition of the relationship	Intended to cultivate relationship
Method	Harshly demanding	Conciliatory
Trust	None	Presumption of trustworthiness
Attitude	Threaten, draw lines in the sand	Make offers
Honesty	Play games—disclose disinformation, incomplete information	Disclose bottom line, do not mislead
Strategy	Insist on one-sided gains (often as a condition to continuing negotiations)	Offer one-sided concessions to reach agreement
Type of Solution	Single answer acceptable to one side	Search for answer acceptable to other side
Focus	Increased power, prestige; protect your position	Amicable agreement: avoid contest of will
Use of Pressure	Apply as needed	Yield to pressure
Example	Soviet	Chamberlain

*The terms "hard" and "soft" bargaining draw on Fisher and Ury. Table adapted and modified from *Getting to Yes,* p. 13.

the basis for a number of important principles. Later we will discuss what to do when this approach is not workable. The following outline is organized around a series of principles to optimize the negotiating process and serves as the basis for our discussion. Principled negotiation is based on the idea that negotiation should center on *interests,* not positions.

Hard, Soft, and Principled Negotiations

"Hard" and "soft" negotiations are fundamentally different, as modeled in Table 4–2. In principled negotiations there are five basic rules:

1. Aim negotiations toward the solution of specific problems, ignoring such factors as pride, personality clashes, and, to whatever degree possible, previous history.
2. Move away from negotiating *positions* to negotiating *interests.*
3. Concentrate on inventing options to increase the ways in which a satisfactory solution can be crafted, satisfying needs on all sides.
4. Insist on establishing fair, objective, and verifiable criteria that all parties can agree to during the negotiations.
5. Break down large and seemingly insurmountable problems into small ones, if necessary, to which all parties can relate.

Principled negotiation differ from both "hard" and "soft" styles. The method of principled negotiation is summarized in the fourth column of Table 4–3, which also offers a comparison to "hard" and "soft" negotiating methods.

There are three stages to engaging in principled negotiations:

1. **Analysis:** gathering and processing information regarding the problem, as well as data to support one's arguments.
2. **Planning:** diagnosing the problem and developing creative solutions.
3. **Discussions:** the actual negotiating process in which parties communicate their interest and attempt to fashion a satisfactory agreement.

Although it may seem as though MCOs and physicians are far apart in their needs, they actually share more interests in common than many other negotiating partners. These interests make principled negotiating somewhat easier than in other venues. Many MCOs also train their people in negotiating strategies.

The method of principled negotiations has gained a large following. As a result, a physician who shows an appreciation for the choreography of principled negotiation is welcomed to a negotiating partnership more readily and quite differently than a physician whose accomplishments are purely clinical in nature.

■ Toward a Negotiating Method

A few good rules of thumb are terribly useful to the development of a disciplined and effective negotiating method. These rules are not intended to suppress the opportunity for personal expression and style, or the need to carefully balance issues of substance and relationship, whether for the short term or the long term. Negotiation strategy should be thought of not only in terms of outcome, but also in terms of efficiency—efficiency of effort, efficiency of time, and efficiency of communication.

A satisfactory *substantive* outcome may well be attainable *either* through positional bargaining or integrative

TABLE 4–3. Principled Negotiation

	"Hard Bargaining"	*"Soft Bargaining"*	*"Principled Bargaining"*
Context	Adversarial	Nonadversarial	Joint task force for problem solving
Goal	Victory	Agreement	Mutually satisfactory solution
Concessions	A condition of the relationship	Intended to cultivate relationship	Separate the problem from collateral issues
Method	Harshly demanding	Conciliatory	Cooperative but principled on the issues
Trust	None	Presumption of trustworthiness	Separate trust from the issues ("trust but verify")
Attitude	Threaten, draw lines in the sand	Make offers	Focus on interests, not positions
Honesty	Play games—disclose disinformation, incomplete information	Disclose bottom line, do not mislead	Disclose interests without intentional misinformation
Strategy	Insist on one-sided gains (often as a condition to continuing negotiations)	Offer one-sided concessions to reach agreement	Invent new options for the benefit of all parties
Type of solution	Single answer acceptable to one side	Search for answer acceptable to other side	Develop multiple options, decide later
Focus	Increased power, prestige; protect your position	Amicable agreement: avoid contest of will	Objective criteria by which to work
Use of Pressure	Apply as needed	Yield to pressure	Strive for consistency of principle, not pressure
Example	Soviet	Chamberlain	Trained mediators

bargaining techniques. Nevertheless, the likelihood of developing an efficient bargaining process for any *subsequent* negotiation involving the same party is much lower if the first agreement was achieved adversarially. In general, positional negotiating techniques degenerate into adversarial situations. One of the great advantages of integrative problem solving is that it encourages the establishment of lasting and useful relationships. Such relationships not only confer trust, but, if done well, also promote efficiency of communication and conflict resolution.[5]

There are very few instances of pure positional bargaining, integrative bargaining, "soft" bargaining, or adversarial bargaining. Most negotiations draw on, or require, multiple techniques. A clear preference for the model of integrative bargaining will be displayed in this discussion. Nonetheless, it is important to prepare to contend also with hard bargaining, adversarial negotiators, and unpleasant people. The conduct of negotiations under these circumstances is addressed at the chapter's end.

Determine and Agree on the Purpose of the Negotiation at the Outset

It is a good idea to begin every negotiating session by agreeing on the purpose of the negotiation. As a strategy, this step has two purposes: it establishes a goal to which the negotiations can move and it begins the negotiation on a point of agreement. The objectives of this initial step can often be satisfied implicitly. In a negotiation over the purchase of a car, for example, there is little need to belabor the obvious. Nonetheless, in situations of hostility, awkwardness, or wariness, or simply where no meaningful relationship exists and none is likely to evolve, the explicit articulation of a joint purpose often focuses the interaction very usefully, and serves as a point of reference should the negotiations become sidetracked for any reason. If the parties to a negotiation cannot agree about the purpose of the negotiation, it may be worth reconsidering altogether whether the negotiation should proceed. Negotiations in which the parties cannot agree on such a fundamental issue as purpose are usually doomed.

Differentiate between Substantive and Nonsubstantive Issues

Negotiations are generally conducted to resolve differences, real or perceived, that stand in the way of the aims and aspirations of one or more of the parties involved. The issues in question typically fall into two major categories.

- Issues of substance—the details of what one party wants another party to concede, permit, allow, or perform.
- Nonsubstantive issues—modes of interaction, personality match, ease and style of communication, respect, and other reflections of the nature and the tenor of the relationships between the parties and/or the negotiators.

The nonsubstantive issues tend to determine attitudes regarding the feasibility or the advisability of pursing negotiations in the first place. Even if they don't, at least one party to the negotiation will usually think they do. For ease of discussion, we will call the nonsubstantive issues relationship issues, even though there can be much more going on. In fact, it is worth remembering that while substantive issues and relationship are the two major *categories* of issues that come up during the negotiating process, the interests of the negotiating parties are unlikely to be quite so neatly parsed. Most negotiations, for example, usually involve both overt or manifest, and hidden or latent agendas.

■ Rule 1: Substantive Concessions Do Not Resolve Nonsubstantive Issues: "Separate the People from the Problem"

The famous aphorism, "Separate the people from the problem," is very widely cited in books and articles about negotiation, but not as widely understood. The aphorism refers to two points. First, it is important to avoid allowing negotiations to be sidetracked by unpleasant interactions or personality conflicts. Second, and much more broadly, it is important to distinguish substantive from nonsubstantive issues. They must be separated and negotiated separately. This section offers several brief observations on the problem of nonsubstantive issues interfering with the negotiating process.

Many nonsubstantive issues can be addressed through negotiation. Some cannot. If underlying nonsubstantive issues undermine the effectiveness of substantive negotiations, it may be advisable to reframe the negotiation. The nonsubstantive issues must take priority. They must be foremost on the list of issues to be resolved. If this strategy cannot be accomplished, it may be necessary to change negotiators or utilize third party mediation.

There is often a temptation to offer concessions on substantive issues to resolve nonsubstantive ones. This strategy rarely works. If it does, the agreement that ensues is very rarely stable. One must not expect substantive concessions to resolve nonsubstantive issues. Issues and negotiations must be matched.

The three most common sources of nonsubstantive problems are misperceptions, misunderstandings, and feelings of animosity. Misperceptions and misunderstandings go together. The problem of personal animosity is considered separately.

Managing Misperception and Misunderstanding

Perception refers to knowledge derived from the senses. Misperceptions are erroneously held beliefs, misidentifications, or mistaken ideas about reality. Misunderstandings are errors of meaning rather than perception. Things are identified correctly, but their significance is not wholly or correctly comprehended. Misunderstandings are equivalent to mistranslations of words. The distinction between misperception and misunderstanding is important. It allows a negotiator to focus on and manage the source of the problem. In the case of misperceptions, the parties to the negotiation must come to an agreement about fact—what constitutes a true belief and what does not. In the case of misunderstandings, the parties must come to an agreement about definitions and the meanings of language.

Because misperception is a function of erroneous *belief,* rather than erroneous *language,* it can only be overcome by changing belief systems. This task is rarely easy. Erroneous beliefs are no less strongly held for being wrong. It is necessary to understand the logic of a belief system before attempting to change it. The logic of belief systems reflects the ideas, the interests, and the opinions of the parties involved. The logic must be thoroughly understood as a preamble to renegotiating the misperceptions.

"Open and Frank Exchanges"

In diplomacy, parties to a negotiation may arrive at the realization that they have nothing in common. To avoid closing off communication altogether, they may engage in what in diplomatic parlance is known as an "open and frank exchange of views." On the one hand, this term is used as a euphemism to indicate that the parties involved could not agree on anything. On the other hand, it also suggests that the parties have undertaken the exercise of exchanging views and ideas, perhaps in the hope of a more satisfying interchange in the future. This exercise can become part of the foundation on which erroneous belief systems can be restructured on the one hand,[6] and an inherent part of the communication that anticipates the "real" or substantive business of negotiating on the other.

Even if parties hold differing view of reality, they might discover points of overlapping interest. These points may become the focus of negotiation. Here is a small example.

A managed care organization believes that its incentive structure will encourage physicians to become paid employees in the long term. This outcome would be in its interest. Consequently, the MCO woos surgical subspecialty practice groups with carrots and sticks directed at this goal. The physicians believe that neither managed care nor this MCO are likely to last because no physician in his or her right mind would voluntarily relinquish autonomy to be employed in such a setting. Irrespective of which projection proves correct, and even if neither party is wholly correct, the problem of providing care for a defined patient population is an issue that can be separated from the larger issues of the future of American medicine. The practical question here centers less on whether belief systems can be negotiated than whether problems at hand can be reframed or (in the British sense of the word) reconstructed independently of apparent misperceptions.

The process of undoing misperceptions is usually inseparable from the process of building trust. The reason these two processes are tightly linked is because reconciling belief systems involves the validation of external evidence contrary to internal belief. This process requires trust.

It is impossible to overstate the critical role of understanding the ideas and ideologies of other parties to the negotiation. They are central to the process of eliminating misperceptions. The renegotiation of misperceptions is facilitated by role reversal, but it is important to avoid the error of uncritical projection. For example, even the most successful role reversal does not *guarantee* that one can predict another party's intentions. Likewise, as Fisher and Ury have emphasized, it is unwise to "deduce . . . intentions from . . . fears."

Exchanges of ideas must include the needs, values, and concerns of all parties to the negotiation. Many of these ideas may not be specifically pertinent to the substantive negotiation at hand. Nonetheless, they may be critical to the nonsubstantive aspects, particularly to relationship building.

Blame

It is unwise to focus on assigning or transferring blame. Blame advances neither the process of reconciling substantive issues nor the process of healing rifts based on nonsubstantive issues. It is also very difficult and very time consuming to wade through past accusations that refer to past injuries and events. Although one cannot ignore the past altogether, it is useful to remind parties to a negotiation that past injuries are most likely to heal after more immediate concerns have been dealt with.[7]

Surprise

It never hurts to "surprise" opposing parties with unexpected gestures, nonsubstantive concessions, or even substantive concessions *when they do not conflict with one's interests.* Sadat did exactly that when he flew to Jerusalem to meet with Begin at the time of the Camp David agreements. Sometimes a small gift or a personal gesture is extremely effective *if the culture of the negotiating circumstance permits.* The gift or gesture must be one that could not be misinterpreted as an impropriety or an attempt to bribe or compromise the integrity of another party.

Avoiding Misperceptions

It is more efficient to avoid misperceptions than to resolve them. The key is communication and, where appropriate, exploration of both shared and alien ideas. In addition, it is very important to reflect on the process of negotiation even as it is pursued. One useful technique involves enlisting all stakeholders in framing problems and resolving them. It is important to include issues of *process* (how to decide) and *substance* (what to decide) in the discussion.

The Importance of Saving Face

Veteran negotiators learn the importance of face-saving opportunities, particularly where there is misperception or misunderstanding. Such opportunities inure to the benefit of all parties to the negotiation. It is very important not to make the other party appear stupid. Sometimes a misperception can be reframed as a *reasonable* or an *understandable* error. This gesture, however contrived, allows other parties to maintain their pride. It never hurts to let other parties to a negotiation be "right" if doing so neither derails the negotiation nor turns on something contrary to one's interests.

Animosity and Other Adverse Emotions

It is inevitable that the negotiator will encounter or even inspire various adverse emotions. These emotions are very powerful and cannot be suppressed. They will invariably come out. It is to the advantage of the negotiator to have them vented in as controlled a fashion as possible.

Personal and Principled Animosity

It is useful to distinguish between two types of animosity: personal animosity and principled or ideological animosity. Personal animosity is based on personal aspects of a relationship. Principled animosity is based on ideological objections. The personal identity and the personal beliefs of the negotiators may be entirely irrelevant to the ideological categories to which others assign them.

Acknowledging Emotions and Emotional Issues

Because animosity cannot be forever suppressed, negotiators skilled in eliciting the civil expression of emotions gain significant competitive advantage. It is insufficient, of course, to simply *solicit* emotion. The real trick is in creating a side negotiation to overcome the animosity or manage it in such a way that does not impair the effectiveness of the interchange. Negotiators who evolve strong interpersonal ties while remaining true to their agency role gain tremendously in effectiveness. There is much to be said for "off line" acknowledgment of emotional issues that might influence the negotiating process. One has to be careful not to allow personal involvements to become intrusive, however.

Nevertheless, it may be quite useful to acknowledge, preempt, and sometimes legitimize emotions and emotional reactions, particularly under two circumstances: when they are especially close to the surface, and when they can be discussed without violating privacy barriers. Privacy issues often mitigate *against* the free acknowledgment of emotional expression. Gestures of respect and concern, in contrast, are rarely rejected.

Avoiding Problems

Most problems can be avoided by communication. The problem is that some communications simply do not get through. It is worth developing a routine analogous to that used by modems when they communicate. In the computer world, this routine is called a "handshake." In negotiation, this process involves the following steps[8]:

a. Identification of data or information to be communicated, including, for example, the purpose of the communication.
b. Authentication of the negotiators—i.e., that the person(s) speaking possess(es) authority to speak as principal or agent on behalf of the party(ies) involved
c. Verification: things that are presented as fact are actually true.
d. Confidentiality: the privacy of the negotiation and the parties involves is secured.
e. Authorization: the negotiator(s) possess(es) the authority to negotiate on behalf of the party(ies) involved.[9]
f. Integrity: the communication is complete in its intended scope and purpose without corruption.
g. Availability: all the intended information has been conveyed and received.

Several other rules of thumb have proven effective.

1. It is critical to fathom the purpose of what is said and the implications of any ideas that are raised in other than a brainstorming session.
2. Personal relationships and organizational relationships should be linked when they are effective, but unlinked when they are not.
3. One ought to strive for working relationship, not a personal relationship, although there is no need to derail a personal relationship if one develops.
4. The focus of the negotiation should be on mutual problem solving, with an emphasis on the solution rather than the problem. This involves a commitment to a collective approach to discovering a solution.

■ Rule 2: Concentrate on Interests Rather Than Positions

Problems are generally definable and defined in terms of interests. Most opposing positions embody both compatible or shared, and incompatible or unshared positions. The goal of a successful negotiation is to unmask the shared positions and to reconcile conflicting interests. The idea is to convert conflicts of interest into complementarities of interest.

Tools for Finding Shared Interests

First, identify interests. They are to be articulated and reiterated. Next, it is useful to develop an understanding of the *basis* of an interest. This is accomplished through a series of "why" and "why not" questions. Finally, it is very helpful to enlarge the negotiation pie by addressing or readdressing specific needs and interests without regard to preconceived notions regarding solutions or agreements.

Never assume a single or monolithic interest or a full understanding of interests by any party. To the extent one can help clarify interests, one can help reframe positions advantageously.

It is also useful to try to mirror interests on each side of the table. There are some useful idioms and tools for discussing interests. These include:

1. Quantification and qualification of outcome: answers to questions about "how much," and "what kind."
2. The establishment of performance benchmarks and common denominators for discussion.
3. Invitations to openness: "I come with no preconceived ideas regarding solutions to the following problems. . . . "
4. Efforts to verify assumptions: "Correct me if I'm wrong."
5. Getting the other side(s) to see your point of view, articulate it, *and admit to it publicly.*
6. Getting the other side to acknowledge *your* interests as part of problem.

Advantages of Legitimizing Interests

Legitimization of interests goes a long way toward promoting agreement and understanding. The following suggestions may prove useful:

- Show you appreciate other side by reflecting on *their* problem as if it were yours and inviting criticism—"As I understand it, the following is the situation. Have I got it right?"
- Frame dialogues in terms of problems, not solutions—"we all agree you don't want your doctors to resent their working conditions."
- Do not concede on your own interests: advocate them—even though it may be necessary to concede on solutions.

Individuals and Institutions

Most negotiating textbooks focus on negotiations among individuals. Physicians, on the other hand, are more likely to negotiate with organizations than with individuals. The interests of individuals and the interests of organizations are comparable, as shown in

Table 4–4. Comparison of Interests

Individuals	*Organizations*
Security	Continuity, consistency, and company policy
Economic well-being	Profit
Sense of belonging	Company culture and, for the agent, respect for hierarchy
Recognition	Market share, market leadership, and other symbols of prestige
Control over one's life	Control over the economic milieu including links in the value chain and costs and sources of revenue

Table 4–4. Just as individuals are likely to resist any initiative that will threaten their basic interests and needs, so will organizations. This insight is worth keeping in mind as negotiations and solutions are structured. An organization is unlikely to agree to something that appears inconsistent, or that might become a unanticipated precedent for an change in company policy. The bottom of the negotiating range is inevitably defined by a profit factor over costs. No agent will chance agreeing to conditions that will flaunt an organizational hierarchy and threaten his position in the company culture. No company will willingly surrender market share or the quest for market leadership.

On the other hand, every organization will be favorably disposed toward solutions that respect its interests, including continuity, consistency, and company policy; that provide opportunities for profit; that conform to organizational culture; that promise a larger market share, a marketing opportunity, a public relations coup, or other prestige; and that offer control over costs and sources of revenue.

■ Rule 3: Enlarge the Pie by Inventing New and Elegant Options

Enlarging the pie in novel, elegant, and unexpected ways in one of the most powerful negotiation strategies. It serves to reconstruct the universe of possible solution, and, in that sense, reconstruct the problem under negotiation as well. Although it seems quite easy to invent new options, several obstacles need to be overcome.

Premature Judgment

It is important to avoid a rush to premature, and generally negative, judgment. There is a tendency to close down possibilities before they have been fully investigated. It is best not to shut down possibilities unless one intends to shut off negotiations.

Inventing and Adopting Options

A related issue is the confusion between *inventing options* and *deciding on them.* To come up with an idea does not mean one has to adopt it. This is a principle that industry has long understood, but physicians as a group have not fully grasped. Industry has adopted a system of "brainstorming" as a way of coming up with creative ideas. The system has a great deal to offer the negotiating team looking for unexpected solutions and novel options.

Brainstorming

Brainstorming involves the following steps:

- Deciding to set up brainstorming session.
- Defining the purpose of the brainstorming session.
- Enlisting the involvement of all participants.
- Controlling the milieu by
  - Keeping things informal
  - Keeping things private
  - Insisting on nonjudgmental communication without criticism of new ideas
  - Facilitating discussions during the brainstorming session by such contrivances as seating participants side by side rather than face to face to emphasize *jointness* of venture
- Clarifying the ground rules, for example:
  - Each participant must propose two ideas he does not espouse (believe in) together with each one advocated
  - All ideas are to be recorded
- After the session
  - Emphasize the most promising ideas.
  - Base further inventions on the most promising ideas.
  - Set up a specific time to evaluate and decide the next steps.

Keep Options Open by Choosing the Right Vocabulary

Certain words seem final and unconditional. Others are softer. Changing the vocabulary through which ideas are presented can be very important to the negotiating process. Words like *substantive, permanent, comprehensive, final, unconditional,* and *binding* are powerful and limiting. They close options. Words like *procedural, provisional, partial, in principle, contingent,* and *nonbinding* are less conclusive, and therefore keep options open.

Thus, one way of keeping a negotiation going is by discussing agreements *in principle,* or *contingent* on certain other events. The *procedural* aspects of a problem and *partial* solutions are much easier to negotiate than the *comprehensive* solution that *unconditionally binds* all the parties in a *permanent* relationship. This approach works for brainstorming sessions as well.

The Fallacy of Searching for Single Options

There is often a temptation to search for a single, comprehensive option in an attempt to reach a rapid, if not particularly novel or elegant solution. Rarely, however, is there only one workable solution, particularly in negotiating with MCOs. Tools like the four quadrant analysis help to match up problems and solutions. It is sometimes helpful to change the scope of the discussion altogether to create a new menu of options.

This is where thinking in terms of partial solutions becomes very helpful. For a writer, a partial solution might involve writing a chapter rather than a book. For the physician, it might involve carve outs instead of risk taking for an entire population. For the MCO, it might involve limiting capitation to certain specialties and paying others discounted fee for service. For the practice negotiator, it might involve accepting less than optimal fees "in exchange" for a computerized medical records installation or assistance in developing a medical informatics system that will catapult the practice to an enviable position with respect to other MCOs one or two years hence. Each of these solutions involve bundling two or more solutions corresponding to one or more interests. Brainstorming for creative and elegant options should not be restricted to a search for one option only.

The Four Quadrant Analysis

The four quadrant analysis shown in Table 4–5 offers a disciplined approach to analyzing issues under negotiation.[10] The outline of answers based on this analysis is used to develop a *negotiation memorandum* to serve as a template for the negotiator in conducting the negotiation. It also offers a disciplined approach to initial brainstorming by each side.

Another way to use this tool is to divide the negotiation into theoretical and practical issues. Agreement *in principle* is required for the theoretical issues. Substantive agreement is required for the practical issues. Agreement on theoretical aspects of the problem may be deferred or suspended so long as agreement can be reached on the practical side.

The contents of the quadrants are basically the same. Quadrant 3 is where the majority of the creative thinking occurs; quadrant 2 is next. From an administrative standpoint, agreement in quadrant 1 must preceded the negotiation. Agreement in quadrant 4 closes the negotiation (see Table 4–6).

Facilitating the Brainstorming Process

Once the brainstorming session has been set up and the analysis begun, success is still not guaranteed. The brainstorming process still needs to be facilitated. For example, it is worth emphasizing several times during the process that one should avoid, at all costs, assuming that the pie has been fixed *a priori*. There are a number of initiatives that help brainstorming sessions work. These are listed in Table 4–7.

Disjointed Interests

We have assumed thus far that all parties agree to pursue joint interests as a mechanism for establishing and concluding the negotiating process. But there are two circumstances in which this assumption may prove incorrect. First, one or more of the parties may not *wish*

TABLE 4–5. Four Quadrant Analysis

1. Define and frame the problem *Why are we here?* *Goals of the negotiation?*	3. Look for appropriate remedies *Strategize* *Creative brainstorming* *Enlarge set of options* *Nothing excluded a priori*
2. Describe, analyze, and diagnose *Underlying issues* *Categorize reasons and causes* *Why is the problem a problem?*	4. Action plan *What next?* *What do we agree upon?* *Steps and means to monitor?*

TABLE 4–6. Bringing Together Theory and Implementation

	What's Wrong	To Do
Theoretical Issues	Frame and define problem: *Quadrant I*	Look for appropriate remedies: *Quadrant III*
Implementation	Describe, analyze and diagnose:	Action steps:

TABLE 4–7. Facilitating the Brainstorming Process

Brainstorm with each party separately and with all parties together

Solicit "unofficial views"—off the record and not for attribution—from all parties

Look through eyes of, and solicit the views of various experts—lawyers, accountants, consultants, both inside and outside the negotiating process—for new ideas

Focus on finding shared interests—e.g.:

- Specialists can reduce their costs by co-ordering supplies in bulk with the MCO
- Specialists can increase their value be instructing PCPs or assisting in developing clinical pathways
- MCOs may have the ability to provide software and hardware for computerized medical records or for outcomes analysis
- Develop shared goals—reduction in length of stay, increased patient satisfaction, definitions of quality
- Dovetail differing interests—market surgical subspecialists together with the HMO

to conclude a negotiation. The unwillingness or inability to find joint interests then becomes a reflection of the underlying disengagement from the process. One cannot *force* a negotiation under these circumstances. All one can do is to point out the phenomenon and ask whether it is the intention of the recalcitrant parties to close off their options for negotiation. If so, the negotiation is ended. If not, one can discuss the negotiation process, including, at this point, the method of finding joint interests.

There is, however, a second possible scenario. Sometimes the parties to a negotiation have asymmetrical conflicting interests—more important to one side than the other—that eclipse those held in common. Until these interests are elucidated and articulated, they cannot be addressed. Table 4–8 lists some of the more common opposed, or conflicting interests.

These 10 points are not intended to form a comprehensive list. They do serve as a quick guide, however, to possible avenues through which negotiating impasses can be overcome. When an impasse is reached, it is important to look for:

- Different belief systems
- Different time values inviting
- Different future forecasts
- Different risk/value curves
- Asymmetries of values
- Cultural conflicts

Table 4–8. Commonly Conflicting Interests

Form	v	Substance
Economics	v	Politics
Internals	v	Externalities
Symbols	v	Practicalities
Short term	v	Long term
Results	v	Relationship
Progress	v	Tradition
Precedent	v	Ad hoc solution
Prestige	v	Outcome
Autonomy	v	Control

Different belief systems can generally be resolved only through arbitration. They may not ever be truly reconciled. Complete reconciliation is not necessary to reach an agreement. Shared belief is not required. To reach an agreement, it is necessary only to agree on mutually acceptable *behavior.*

Different values along a time scale can sometimes be negotiated by appeal to an installment plan. In an installment plan, one does not pay everything up front. Instead, one pays a premium for payment over time. The installment plan becomes, for all intents and purposes, a loan. One side has the use of an object or service. The other receives a premium for deferring repayment. If you believe something is more valuable today than it will be tomorrow, you will sell it today, assuming that maximization of cash is the rule by which you abide. By the same token, if you believe something will be more valuable tomorrow than it is today, you will buy it today if you are rational.

In managed care negotiations, one might negotiate a higher premium (by analogy) for patients seen at one time than another. The time factor adds or subtracts value. Thus, part of the negotiation may revolve not only *what* should be done (buy or sell) but also *when* it shall be done.

Another twist on the issue of time has to do with differing forecasts of what the future might bring. Different forecasts often entail different risks. An impasse based on different forecasts can sometimes be resolved by articulating the differences and insuring against them through a process of indemnification or other guarantees.[11] Thus, if the contract suggested by the MCO assumes a certain growth factor; if the future as forecast by the physician looks more like decreasing growth; and if the contract requires the physician to hire another specialist to service the population as envisioned by the MCO, it may be possible to negotiate a guarantee in which the MCO indemnifies the physician against the cost of the additional specialist if the anticipated growth does not materialize.

Sometimes, differences in forecast result in different risk assumptions. The MCO might say, in an instance opposite to the one above, that there will be no growth, whereas the physician fears that he will be overwhelmed by the patient volume he foresees. This type of problem can also be managed by an insurance scheme once the problem is articulated. The MCO can be held to either find another specialist or indemnify the physician for additional help on a *locum tenens* or a permanent hire basis if its forecast is surpassed by a certain amount.

Asymmetries of value and cultural conflicts are the most difficult to overcome and cannot be discussed here.

Steps to Take

The following practical steps may prove helpful. Begin by listing options for all parties in the negotiation. Ask for more options from every side. Ask for preferences. Above all, look for means to facilitate decisions so long as no significant barrier is broached. Try to find a series of ideas to which agreement is likely. A series of agreements is likely to break whatever ice is underfoot. This principle is sometimes captured by the admonishment to find "yesable" propositions. Substitute offers for threats, particularly offers to help the other side. Surprise works very nicely in this setting.

■ Rule 4: Objectify Criteria

Negotiating is best modeled not a process of bargaining in which agreement is reached through a series of compromises (*e.g.*, "splitting the difference" between offers) but as a process that appeals to objective criteria for a basis on which agreement is reached. The principle search, therefore, must be for objective criteria for whatever is under negotiation. Examples of objective criteria that are open to review by outside agencies—and therefore to verification—are listed in Table 4–9.

Objective standards are meant to be fair and independent. They are also meant to be externally verifiable. The use of standards pertains to valuation and procedure. Anything may be open to valuation, but there are advantages to defining, insisting on, and negotiating *both* fair standards and fair procedures.

TABLE 4–9. Examples of Objective Criteria

Market value	Count
Precedent	Fairness
Judgement	Equal treatment
Standards	Tradition
Costs	Reciprocity

How can this idea be converted into practice? Here are some examples:

- Frame issues in terms of joint searches for objective criteria.
- Discuss
  - Which standards are most appropriate.
  - How to apply them.
- Offer concessions on principle only.
- Articulate the principles on which concessions will be offered.
  - Ask for the theory on which a concession is demanded.
  - Articulate the principles derived from the theory.
  - Try to generalize the principles as part of the "externally verifiable" definition of good objective criteria for negotiation.
- If needed, utilize external experts to discuss *standards.*
- Refuse to bow to pressure tactics.
- Acknowledge and confront pressure tactics.

■ Rule 5: Develop the BATNA (Best Alternative to Negotiated Agreement)

One of the critical moments in any negotiation is the point at which one or more parties either *threatens* or *intends* to walk out. Assuming the parties to be rational and not self-destructive, and assuming that the reason for ending the negotiation is not based in personal or organizational frustration alone, it is safe to conclude that one or more of the parties believes it has better alternative than that promised by the negotiation process. The concept of the *Best Alternative to a Negotiated Agreement,* or BATNA, is critical to any negotiation process. The BATNA defines the very bottom of the negotiating range, the range below which there is no rational advantage in continuing the discussion.[12]

The phrase "no rational advantage in continuing the discussion" is purposely intended to be very strong. Invoking BATNA often means that communication shuts down. Relationships end. Further discussion is likely to become more difficult than it was before. On the other hand, it doesn't always have to be that way.

The way one concludes a negotiation is as important to one's future possibilities as the way one has conducted the negotiation, even though a negotiated agreement has not necessarily been concluded. Invoking the BATNA does not necessarily have to mean that the negotiation ends on a note of animosity, only that the interests of one or more parties to the negotiation are not as well served by continuing.

How to Use the Idea of a BATNA

If other side does not seem to be interested in a negotiated settlement:

- Assume that there is a cogent reason behind the position.
- Try to fathom or to strategize the reasons independently from the other parties.
- Invite criticism and explanation to opposition to your ideas.
- Ask questions—avoid hostility.
- Use a third party mediator.

It is critical to understand one's own as well as the other side's position. This requires that one develop a substantial understanding of the financial and contractual positions of one's own practice. It also helps to gain a substantial understanding of the details of the other side's position(s).

The BATNA is a double-edged sword. On the one hand, it can be used to define the range that the negotiation must adopt. On the other, it can be used to force an end to a negotiation. The BATNA is not a fixed milepost. Every negotiation has its BATNAs for each party, and the BATNA should be well understood and strategized before the negotiation is undertaken.

The BATNA is also the instrument for creditable threats. There is a major difference, for example, between a threat defined by a position, and a threat defined by interests. In the first instance, statements tend to take the form "I shall walk out if I do not get what I want." In the second instance, statements tend to take the form "There seems no point to negotiating if my interests are not protected to this point."

In many respects, the BATNA should be the first part of the negotiation that the negotiation team decides on.

■ Tools for Hard Bargainers

In the last section we discussed the problem of diagnosing and overcoming disjunctive interests. In this section we discuss the problem of hard bargainers—individuals or organizations who prefer positional negotiation to integrative negotiation, or who simply don't know any better.

Whatever type of negotiation goes on, it is necessary to understand the rules of the game.[13] The term "game" is used to describe the rationale that determines the moves, or choices, made by each party to the negotiation. The game model of negotiation assumes that negotiation, like any other game, has agreed on rules.

The existence of definable rules makes it possible to challenge, or at least to query, deviations and aberrations from those rules. Objectionable moves should be framed and conceptualized as deviations from the agreed on rules. They should not be framed or conceptualized as, for example, personal affronts or insults. The more general formulation of this rule stipulates that objectionable moves ought to be discussed in terms of agreed on rules, principles, or behavior, in an objective fashion rather than in personal or particular terms.

Deception

An excellent example is the problem of deception. To greet deception with indignation is neither effective nor, in the long run, satisfying. A better way of dealing with deception is to frame the move for what it is, and to ask, for example, "Why are incorrect facts being introduced?" "What are the intentions underlying this strategy?" "What benefits do you believe to achieve through less than full disclosure?" If no satisfactory answer is provided, the negotiation may not be possible, and the only reasons to continue would be the side benefits of communication and contact.

Psychological Warfare

Some negotiators like to engage in psychological warfare. Attacks on other negotiators often degenerate into *ad hominem* confrontations. In other instances, one party may adopt a "good cop–bad cop" strategy to confuse or frustrate their opponents into concessions. Still another strategy is brinkmanship, in which threats that cannot be discounted, but that are also slightly less than credible, are used to push the other parties in a certain direction. The Soviets were past masters at this type of negotiation, which often puts parties with a sensitive social conscience at tremendous disadvantage. This category of hard bargaining can only be negated by insisting that one negotiate only on the merits of the solutions under discussion, and not in response to threats. Thus, the query "Is it *really* in your interest to launch missiles against the United States, or would you rather conclude a trade agreement?" has more promise than a counterthreat of bigger and better missiles or breaking off the negotiation.

Positional Pressure Tactics

The threat of launching missiles has been made on numerous occasions, of course. Such threats have become classic metaphors for positional pressure tactics. Positional pressure tactics are typically employed when there is a perception by one or more parties to the negotiation that there are insurmountable asymmetries of power that accrue to the advantage of the party mounting the threat.

Positional pressure tactics always boil down to a "take it or leave it" approach, sometimes modified to a "take it or else," and sometimes to the proverbial "silver or lead," carrot and stick proposal.* The first point that must determined is whether the threat is credible and whether the asymmetry of power is really as stark as it is made out to be. If the threat *is* credible, and the asymmetry of power *is* stark, the threatened party may have no choice.

Assuming that the threatened party believes it has a choice, or at least that it is willing to chance the consequences of not conceding, two approaches can be tried. The first is to confront the confrontation. Do other parties want you to follow their lead? A threat is tantamount to a tactical refusal to bargain. Is this the intent of the other party(ies)? The second approach is to state that one does not know how to negotiate under the conditions that have been imposed, and then to inquire about the purpose of the move. Was this move intended to precipitate capitulation, for example? If so, is it the intention of the other parties to revert to a "take it or leave it" position? If so, there are only two options: to accept the proposed conditions (to capitulate) or to break off the negotiation. Take it or leave it. If that is not the intention of the other party, new ground rules for negotiation must be established.

Extreme Demands

The situation that we have just worked through is a classic example of an extreme demand. Extreme demands seldom result in satisfactory agreements. Even if concessions are made, the conceding party rarely walks away satisfied.

If no further contact between the parties is anticipated, the fact that one party feels cheated may not be particularly relevant. But if there is any thought of further negotiations once a contract lapses, or on other matters, one can be sure the previous animosity will come up again. In the political arena, changes in the balance of power may eliminate or reverse previous asymmetries. Renewed conflict is sure to arise.

In the best of all possible worlds, extreme or radically unrealistic demands would never be presented. Why, then, do otherwise capable negotiators do this? Sometimes, extreme demands are present as a show of power. Only a very powerful opponent, the reasoning goes, would dare make such an extreme demand. The move is intended to intimidate.

Another reason to make an extreme demand is to establish a bargaining range. The idea is to make an extreme demand with the expectation that a compromise will be reached. The mechanism of the compromise is thought to be sensitive to the original positions of the negotiators. Agreement, in other words, is implicitly associated with some arbitrary middle ground, achieved by somehow splitting the difference between the opening positions of each side. According to this theory, if a less extreme demand were offered unilaterally, the compromise would inevitably favor the other side. This reasoning often comes up in managed care negotiations with physicians.

It requires careful thought and strategy to contend with extreme demands. It is helpful to begin by assuming that the demand may be reasonable, whether or not it is. This assumption telegraphs respect to the other parties, and opens the door to the next step, which is to request objective and verifiable justification for the demand. As emphasized earlier, the idea is not to come up with an arbitrary compromise based on splitting the difference between the parties involved, but to conclude a contract based on mutually satisfactory standards. If other parties insist on splitting differences, the best tactic is to ask whether it is the understanding of the other parties that this mode of negotiation leads to objective standards on which subsequent negotiations can be based and, if so, how.

Negotiation with hard bargainers often requires the "enlightened" party to educate the other side. Negotiation is always easier when all sides are predisposed to speaking the same language and viewing the negotiation through the same lens. One useful technique is to invite role reversal. Role reversal often sensitizes each party to the thinking of the others. Role reversal fails in two ways. Other parties are either *unwilling* or *incapable.* Unwillingness often signals the imminent failure of the negotiation. Lack of capacity to reverse roles may mean that no relationship is likely to evolve through the negotiating process. It may also signal imminent failure, however. There are several other specific tactics that merit review.

Escalating Demands

Each time an agreement comes into view, a new demand is added or the conditions for fulfillment are escalated. This is frustrating and annoying, as well as deceptive. To contend with escalating demands, point out to the parties concerned the pattern of behavior. Try to recapitulate the negotiating process and inquire whether any important interests have been left out or have changed. Try to understand the underlying concerns without in any sense giving in. Determine, for example, whether there might be fear or opposition to a negotiated agreement. Finally, ask all negotiating partners to put *all* their interests on the table at once. In a totally fruitless and frustrating circumstance, it may be necessary to couch this last request in the form of an ultimatum that, if not accepted, will cause the negotiation to close.

*Silver or lead: If you do as I tell you, you will be rewarded. If not, you will be shot.

Lock-In

Another form of manipulation is the lock-in. This term is used to describe a situation in which opposing parties restrict the possible options or solutions in ways that accrue only to their individual advantage. The only response is to refuse to play, if at all possible. The lock-in is a form of the "take it or leave it" method. It does not allow true negotiation. For this reason, it becomes necessary to diagnose and articulate the pattern of behavior, and to challenge it, preferably while trying to understand why this pattern has arisen and addressing any underlying problems that are discovered.

Sometimes the lock-in position is expressed through a series of calculated delays, missed documents, unmet appointments, or unreturned communiqués. The question, once again, becomes one of conscious or unconscious action. Whatever the conclusion that is eventually reached, one might try to attack this problem as a sidebar negotiation. The object of the negotiation is threefold: (1) to determine the motivation behind the lock-in strategy; (2) to determine whether the strategy is purposeful, unmindful, insouciant, or simply rude; and (3) to try to establish rules for acceptable negotiating behavior. Should such rules be unattainable, either the negotiating team must change or the negotiation must be closed.

General Rules for Dealing with Hard Bargainers

Hard bargainers are called hard not because they are tough in an admirable sense, but because it is hard to achieve the goals that have presumably been established at the outset. It usually does not take long to realize that one is working with hard bargainers. Here are some general rules for making the process go as smoothly as possible.

- Define the process and the closure in terms of specific aims and goals from the outset of the negotiation.
- Craft a framework agreement that defines everything except for the final details: concentrate on the details.
- Prepare tentative drafts and working documents: restrict discussion to revisions of these drafts and documents.
- Pursue interests without preconceived rigid solutions.
- Stage the negotiation and the agreement, and insist on proofs of commitment along the way.
- Make sure test proofs of commitment are culturally consistent for all parties.

Positional Bargaining

Positional bargaining is not exactly the same as hard bargaining, though it is often pursued in the same way and has the same impact. Sometimes, parties to a negotiation engage in positional bargaining because they don't know any better. But assuming that the tactic of positional bargaining is both purposeful and conscious, one must determine once again whether the potential consequences of *not* negotiating are worse than the potential outcome of negotiating.

The short-term success of positional bargaining tactics rests on asymmetries in three domains: asymmetries of relationship—the relationship is more valuable to one party than another; asymmetries of substantive concerns—the substantive issues are more important to one party than another; and asymmetries of power. These asymmetries may be real or perceived. It is the *perception* of asymmetry that allows positional bargaining to go forward.

It is generally difficult to convince a party that perceives itself to have the upper hand that it does not. As a result, direct confrontation is rarely effective in positional bargaining. What sometimes works is to counter the perception of strength by obtaining the intelligence necessary to stand firm. This often requires that one insist on going second, not first, in any interchange. People often disclose more about themselves than they mean to. Look at past tactics, histories, and any other information that comes to hand. Build options. But unlike in other situations, here the option building and the strategizing should be conducted privately, not in the open. The process is no longer collaborative, nor should it be assumed to be carried out in good faith. Build defenses, ways out, asymmetric incentives for the other side, and verification strategies. Learn, but do not necessarily disclose, the weaknesses of all parties. Concentrate as much on weakness as on strength. Stay focused on both the primary mission and secondary and tertiary goals.

The frustration involved with positional bargaining can be intense. Nonetheless it is critical to suspend emotional reaction and concentrate on developing and pursuing objective standards. When accusations or *ad hominem* arguments are floated, it is important to counter accusations by demanding a statement of relevance, or a standard of validity for the association.

In principled negotiation, the negotiation range may not be overtly stated, but neither is purposefully hidden. In positional bargaining, only the high end of the negotiation range is disclosed. The rest should remain absolutely private.

Prepare a menu of wants and needs that are converted into requests. Contrive a menu in which what is desired becomes bundled indistinguishably with what may be conceded. Concede what is least desired. The low end of negotiating range is the BATNA. The BATNA can appear, or be made out to be a threat. The efficacy of this move with BATNA is directly proportionate to the degree it accurately reflects one's interests, and one's intent to quite the negotiation. The idea of BATNA works only if one is willing to accept there are some unacceptable concessions.

It is important to distinguish between strategy and posturing, and between perception and truth. As one formulates a list of interests, the interests should be stratified between those that are of high importance and those of low importance, those that are essential and those that are not. Be prepared to concede items of low importance and those that are unessential if the concession can be couched as a concession to principle, and try not to pressure.

It is tempting to respond to positional threats with other threats. Threats are useful *only* so long as they are credible, only so long as they can be implemented. A threat should not be left implicit. Threats are most effective when choices and consequences are explicitly outlined.

Conclusion

This chapter has developed the rudiments of one approach to negotiations. There are many possible approaches. The method of principled or integrative bargaining has the advantage of efficiency and simplicity once learned, and also the advantage of encouraging relationships, trust building, and follow-on opportunities in the long run. Because it qualifies as a "method," and is relatively widely known (at least in its rudiments), the integrative method serves as an Esperanto for negotiation, a universally recognized language.

Negotiating with Managed Care Organizations

There are no "universal specifics" for negotiating with MCOs. The general interests of such groups are not difficult to infer: access to care; cost containment; quality of care; patient satisfaction; rapid response to referral requests; parsimonious utilization; perhaps involvement by specialists in the education of PCPs. Neither are the interests of surgical subspecialists particularly arcane: for autonomy; adequate reimbursement; access to advances in technology; respect; and easy relations with MCOs, for example.

In any particular situation, however, these interests may be weighed one way or another, or supplemented by the needs of the moment. A managed care organization seeking to comply with certain specific licensing requirements may be willing to pay more for trauma care than for outpatient surgery. Another may be interested in capitating all services for administrative purposes even though discounted fee for service might cost less. One group of physicians may be willing to relinquish autonomy for higher fees. Another may structure its priorities differently.

Negotiations with MCOs should be approached as an exercise in defining one's BATNA, building relationships, inventing creative options, and finding opportunities to arbitrage, honestly and openly, asymmetries of interest. To the extent such asymmetries can be identified, they can be quite useful. For example, it may be very inexpensive and relatively straightforward for an MCO to provide a group of practitioners with the hardware and software to verify the eligibility of patients, maintain electronic records, and document outcomes. The cost to the group, which would have to install such a system sooner or later in any event, would be much higher. Part of the negotiation might involve bundling the provision and maintenance of such a system as part of the reimbursement package.

It is critical that physicians negotiate with principals of the MCO. Principals are individuals authorized to speak for the company and negotiate on its behalf. Managed care organizations unwilling to provide principals for liaison are unlikely to afford easy communication in the future. The way to assure that the representative is, in fact, a principal is to make this a condition of the negotiation. The representative must also verify that he or she bears this authority at the time of the negotiation.

Virtually anything can be negotiated. Physicians should think twice before routinely signing new managed care agreements. Can the contract be negotiated? One will not know without trying. A company unwilling to negotiate *before* an agreement is signed will have no greater incentive to build a relationship *after* it has been signed.

Twelve Commandments of Negotiation

I. Options are the tools of the negotiator.
II. Strategies are the rules for their use.
III. Think in terms of goodness of fit—will the agreement satisfy the interests of the parties involved?
IV. Aim for a low maintenance agreement.
V. Evaluate the relative importance of substance and relationship—try to build relationships as well as "winning" on substance.
VI. Hybrid creations work well—be innovative.
VII. Think in terms of value for others, costs for you.
VIII. Accept conflict and recognize the consequences—beware of unsubstantiated threats.
IX. Formalize the motives for every move—especially concessions.
X. Learn the other side.
XI. Enlarge the pie.
XII. Find the logic.

REFERENCES

1. Fisher R, Ury W: *Getting to yes. Negotiating agreement without giving in.* 2nd Ed. New York: Penguin Books, 1991. This book has been extremely successful in defining the genre of integrative bargaining ("win-win") as opposed to distributive bargaining ("win-lose"). Though widely cited, it has been criticized for being overly simplistic and unrealistic. It re-

flects the thinking at the Negotiation Project at the Harvard Law School, which the authors founded.

2. De Bono E: *Conflicts. A better way to resolve them.* New York: Penguin Books, 1986. See too, by the same author, *Practical thinking.* New York: Penguin Books, 1971; *Tactics: The art and science of success.* Boston: Little Brown & Co., 1984.
3. Marcus LJ, Dorn BC, Kritek PB, Miller VG, Wyatt JB: *Renegotiating health care. Resolving conflict to building collaboration.* San Francisco: Jossey-Bass Publishers, 1995, p. 417.
4. Fisher R, Ury W: *Getting to yes,* p. 13.
5. The rules that follow are adapted from several sources, including Fisher and Ury, Marcus and colleagues, the teachings of Professor Stuart Diamond at the Wharton School of the University of Pennsylvania, and personal experience.
6. The process of restructuring belief systems is in itself a negotiation, and should be regarded as such.
7. The present and future significance of interests based in objectionable yet irreversible events from the past is often underestimated. They not infrequently engender a wish for remediation or revenge that colors all subsequent substantive negotiations. In a sense, the negotiation is asked to become a *redemptive* event. Unless this hidden interest is uncovered, addressed, and brought into the negotiation, substantive differences will either become irreconcilable or, in the case that asymmetries of power or other circumstance dictate that they be superficially resolved, the agreement will sooner or later prove unstable. Substantive concessions *alone* are extremely unlikely to resolve latent, non-substantive issues. The other side of this coin, however, is that past injuries are most likely to heal only when more immediate concerns are also resolved, because the circumstances that allow the resolution of immediate concerns are the ones most likely to afford remediation of the past. It is not the substantive aspects of the negotiation that are redemptive, but rather the circumstances and other non-substantive aspects.
8. Jeffrey Kalwerisky, C.A., vice-president of consulting at Security First Technologies, initially brought this analogy to my attention. The four aspects of computer security he described were confidentiality, referring to who had the authority to see data; authorization, referring to who had the authority to change data; integrity, referring to the continuity and change of data; and availability of data. The extension of the metaphor is my own.
9. Authentication confirms that they are accredited spokesmen; authority confirms that they may initiate *changes* from initial negotiating positions.
10. This version of the table is borrowed, but modified, from Fisher and Ury.
11. The model of insurance is often used. Insurance reduces risk for a premium. One pays a certain amount to be secure in the knowledge that one is covered up to a certain dollar value for loss. The maximum loss is then given by the formula $L_{max} = V_L - V_P - P$ where L_{max} stands for the maximal loss, V_L for an agreed on value for the loss, V_P for the value of the reimbursement payment, and P for the value of the premium.
12. The idea of the BATNA is not new, but it was given this name by Fisher and Ury in *Getting to Yes,* with which it has subsequently been closely identified.
13. The term "game" is used in an economic, not a pejorative sense. For an economist's approach to the negotiating process based in elements of game theory, see Raiffa H: *The art and science of negotiation.* Cambridge: The Belknap Press, 1982. For a more general view of economics and social behavior, see Landsburgs E: *The armchair economist.* New York: The Free Press, 1993.

Appendices

Principles of Communication

Before the Negotiation

During the Negotiation

After the Negotiation

1. Focus on purpose of communication.
2. Relate to purpose of exchange.
3. Understand and communicate your own position.
4. Depersonalize conflict and isolate emotions.
5. Recognition and prestige are usually irrelevant to negotiation unless they constitute hidden agenda on one of the parties.
6. Understand how you are perceived.
7. Speak to the audience.
8. Query what you don't understand.
9. Unless communication relates to the negotiation at hand or to building relationships, it probably serves little purpose—avoid debates over the moral high ground.

Hosting a Negotiation: Implementation Checklist

Before the Negotiation

1. Determine degree and source of interest.
2. Set agenda.
3. Explore agency and authority.
4. Prepare:
   a. Interests
   b. Reserve Price
   c. Data
   d. Alternatives
   e. Role reversal
   f. Walkaway position
   g. Negotiation memorandum
5. Decide on venue.

During The Negotiation

1. *Strategies*
   a. Frame issues
      i. Recognize joint problem
      ii. Negotiate to solve problem
      iii. Agree that some solutions are better than none
      iv. Use as "prenegotiation"
   b. Establish standards

i. Establish
ii. Agree to use
c. Check on communication
i. Query
ii. Language
iii. Culture
iv. Signals
v. Perceptions
vi. Reflective summary
d. Agree on process
i. How and when decisions can be made
ii. How long
iii. Financial issues and their basis
iv. Changes
v. Reviews
2. *Negotiate issues*
a. Types of bargaining
b. Separate people from
c. long-term versus short-term relationship

Endgame—Closing the Negotiation

1. Offers
a. Commitments
i. Publicity
ii. Escrow money
b. Written memorandum
c. Time aspects—when agreement will start, how long will it run
d. Conditions and consultations
e. Default modes
2. Terms of agreement
a. Consult with outside groups or other parties
b. Establish relationship
c. Build relationship improving steps into agreement
d. Create/avoid dependency
e. Reality check vis à vis original strategy
f. Escalation clauses
g. Make unexpected concession
h. Require unexpected concession
3. Verification strategies
4. Alternatives
a. Mediation
b. Mutual walkaway
c. Cost of walkaway

Afterwards

1. Keep notes and impressions from the negotiation
2. Continue relationship building

■ Principles of Managed Care Negotiations

WHO: Authority, not title
WHAT: Service: time, level, duration, extent
Reimbursement: quantity, form
Contract: contents, duration, exclusivity, carve out, future
Relationship benefits: information and data, software packages, marketing
WHEN: Proactive and when existing contracts about to end (overcome inertia)
WHERE: Careful consideration
HOW: Negotiation skills, especially framing, standards, joint solutions; also consider mediator
WHY: Purpose and focus: *e.g.,* simple service contract, long-term relationship, networks, referral patterns, cash flow, exposure, control, other linkages

■ Checklist for Managed Care Negotiations

1. Know your costs.
2. Know your capacity.
3. Define your competitive advantages.
4. Ask the organization to help you define the market.
5. Consider a consultant to obtain data.
6. Develop an understanding of standards.
7. Formulate contracts in terms of defined levels of service, e.g.,:
a. Population size
b. Population mix
c. Service mix
d. Numbers of visits
e. Postoperative visits
f. Imaging studies
g. "Extra services"
8. Start amassing patient satisfaction data: demonstrate sensitivity to data, ability to change.
9. Learn the interests of the organization.
a. Costs
b. Capacities
c. Quality issues
d. Expansion plans
e. Network interests
10. Frame negotiations in terms of
a. Mutual gain
b. Mutual success
c. Relationship issues
d. Cost savings
e. Risk sharing

   f. Performance standards
   g. Shared profits (watch for legal pitfalls)
11. Be sure managed care negotiator has necessary authority for purposes of your negotiation.
   a. Learn organizational structure.
   b. Medical director will rarely negotiate, but is almost always accessible.
   c. Make the first approach with data in hand.
12. Establish precedent for renegotiating contracts when predetermined benchmarks are met.
13. Look for additional benefits ("What else could you give me") to enlarge the pie during negotiation.
14. Define and adhere to BATNA.

Dr. Dagi is a neurosurgeon as well as an expert in the areas of negotiation, practice mergers and acquisitions, and the management of early stage ventures. In addition to serving as Clinical Professor of Surgery at the Medical College of Georgia and maintaining a private practice of neurosurgery in Atlanta, Dr. Dagi is the managing general partner of Cordova Technology Partners, L.P., an early stage venture capital fund, and a principal in Cordova Advisors, a management consulting group. He has lectured widely on negotiating strategies, and has taught negotiation techniques and consulted on negotiation strategies to physician groups, government agencies, and private industry nationwide.

Dr. Dagi studied at the Julliard School and graduated from Columbia College, where he was named Italian Government Traveling Scholar. He received an MD and MPH from Johns Hopkins and an MBA with distinction in Finance and Strategic Planning from the Wharton School of the University of Pennsylvania. He completed his neurosurgical and neuroscience training at the Massachusetts General Hospital and Harvard Medical School in Boston, and at the Guy's, Maudsley, and King's College Hospitals in London. He was awarded the Mendeleyeff Travelly Fellowship, a Neuroresearch Foundation Fellowship, and appointment as the Joseph P. Kennedy, Jr. Fellow at Harvard University. Subsequently he served on the neurosurgical and law facilities of Georgetown University, and the medical faculties of the Uniformed Services University of the Health Sciences, and Brown University, where he was appointed to the Weyland Collegium. While a faculty member at Georgetown, Dr. Dagi became Special Assistant to the Assistant Secretary of the Administrative Conference of the United States. He is a Fellow of the American College of Surgeons and was recently elected to Fellowship in the College of Critical Care Medicine.

Dr. Dagi has written over 150 articles and edited three books. He sits of the boards of several privately held corporations.

Quadrant Analysis Revisited: Three Types of Negotiation

	QUADRANT I	***QUADRANT II***	***QUADRANT III***	***QUADRANT IV***
Negotiation Type	***Goals***	***Underlying Issues***	***Strategies***	***Implementation Steps***
Overt conflict resolution	Define and frame problem	Reasons and causes	Working on creative options and ideas without deciding a priori what will work. Problems vs positions.	What to do now? Steps and means to monitor.
Information gathering	Obtain specific data or general Information	Asymmetry of information	Share information to mutual advantage. Trade information. Data precondition to negotiation. Data part of agreement. Third party mediator. Further nondisclosure agreement.	Agree on domain of information. Define standards for disclosure. Third party monitors?
Contract	Mutually satisfactory agreement	Overlapping interests, differing needs.	Frame issues as joint problem. Share data, external standards of conformity and standards. Process. Trade-offs in time, reward, other factors. Relationships. Stepwise segmentation. Islands of commitment. Separate/collapse hide/disclose interests	Concessions for optimum contract length and quick decision. Achieve rapid mutual understanding of positions. Offline discussions.

5

The Legal Issues of Managed Care Contracts

TOM NEAL

Understanding MCOs and Types of Agreements Offered to a Provider

No Prior Knowledge on Contracting Is Common for Providers

The types of contracts presented to providers from MCOs in scope of compensation and management range from not quite sublime to very nearly ridiculous. Many types of questions and pressures are presented to providers in their decision-making process in evaluating contracting opportunities. Many physicians, historically and currently, have a view of their business marketplace skewed by their own narrow experience and lack of accurate information of the larger context in which their business is placed. Many individual providers have no information from an independent or authoritative source regarding the identity or management style of the MCO. It is still surprising, but common, that many physician decisions on contracts having long range economic consequences are based on very little knowledge of the subject matter and many unfounded assumptions.

Look for Advice

A number of organizations offer assistance to the physician in analyzing and negotiating a managed care contract. Some are medical societies or other professional organizations. Some are networks or semi-integrated organizations of providers that have the size and staff to offer analysis for these particular contracts. Often the most common source of advice to a practitioner is his or her colleagues, a business partner, a friend at the hospital, or a spouse. Sometimes this advice can be enlightened and insightful. More often, such advice is based on some small piece of information from a personal experience, without any knowledge of the larger market picture. This type of advice is not helpful. This chapter is designed to highlight a number of elements in the managed care contracting arena that should be brought to mind by the practitioner in evaluating whether to undertake negotiations or accept a particular business opportunity.

Types of MCOs Submitting Contracts

The range of possibilities varies in relation to the type and size of MCO presenting the contract. The contract may be proposed by a provider network broker, a local or national network offering discounted preferred provider services (PPO), a national health maintenance organization (HMO), a local HMO, a local hospital or hospital affiliate, a local or national employer, a national or local consortium of employers in a group-purchasing vehicle, an insurance-based health plan, or any combination of the above. These companies may have a significant market share in the service area of the provider or no business in the entire state. Some may have a large network of providers already. Some may not have signed up a single person. The provider needs to ask pointed questions regarding the size and scope of the MCO and its book of business in that service area. Ask for specifics about the names and locations of other network providers and the source of the number of the enrollees in the plans under contract.

Find Out About the MCO

The insurance department of every state keeps a record of companies licensed to engage in the business of insurance. In the field of health insurance, any contract under which a company charges a prepaid fee (premium) to pay for the cost of future health care services, becoming at risk for the amount of the utilization of the services, is considered the "business of insurance." HMOs fall into this general definition and are licensed by each state insurance department. MCOs selling such prepaid health coverage products need such a license or access to one. The information at the insurance department will list the number of covered lives or enrollees reported by the licensed companies, but this information is generally over a year old. Startup time is fairly lengthy for many HMOs, and they will not report many covered lives for several years.

If the provider is part of some larger contracting organization, such as an independent practice organization (IPA), a physician-hospital organization (PHO), or some hybrid of a group practice, the provider has some assistance through a contracting committee whose job is to find out the answers to some of these basic questions. Often the state or local medical association may have general information on the number and size of MCOs marketing in a particular area. Local hospitals will have information on many MCOs. Certainly if the local hospitals or other alliances in the area are marketing their own products, information about those can also be obtained from these sponsoring organizations.

Relationship of Parties

Relationship of the parties is measured in a business transaction by the amount of leverage one party has over another. The more equal the parties are in the negotiating session, the more equitable the contract provisions can be expected to be in the final product. The most extreme example of leverage entirely on one side is embodied in the concept of *adhesion contracts.* This term refers to the contrast of bargaining power between the parties being so severe that one party has the ability to force the other to "adhere" to the former party's will. An example of an *adhesion contract* in the traditional business sense would be a small proprietor or farmer being forced to deal with a larger conglomerate or (in the past, a trust) that controlled the marketplace for the commodity that either the farmer was trying to sell or the proprietor was trying to buy. The small businessperson had no choice but to deal with the large business on the large business's terms.

Many physicians in dealing with MCOs feel that they are in the same position as the farmer or store owner. They have signed managed care contracts exactly as presented to them as if they had no alternative but to submit to the "will" of the larger MCO. While it is true that a sole practitioner is only one voice in a much larger market of physician services, physicians need to be aware that they have a great ability to negotiate terms and even prices in managed care contracts if they will take the time to learn the elements and the range of possibilities.

It is important in considering a capitation contract to analyze the records of the current practice with regard to costs and payment structure. The number of managed care contracts in the office is also a factor to consider. For example, it is a good strategy not to be overly dependent on any one large managed care contract. If over 20% of the practice revenues come through one contract, there is a much decreased ability to resist contract amendments and other payment reductions from that payer. Leverage and negotiability are greatly reduced for the physician. On the other hand, a broadly diffuse and diverse payer mix will provide minimal amounts of patients to the total practice so that the physician has leverage to deal with each one. The consolidation of the payer community in certain states has decreased physicians, ability to resist major payer contracts. This has, in turn, caused the consolidation of the provider community. The combination of both of these elements distinctly reduces competition in the marketplace and reduces the patient's choice also. Neither one of these results is viewed by either the government or the public as necessarily good.

Contract Types by Payment Method

PPO

The most common managed care contract circulating outside the far West, Florida, parts of Texas, parts of Minnesota, Wisconsin, and New England is still a preferred provider organization type. This contract uses a discounted, fee for service payment, usually accompanied by mildly intrusive medical management procedures, whereby certain tests, treatments, or admissions must be approved in advance before the company will authorize payment. Historically, most physicians have executed these documents without much examination, believing that a 10% to 15% discount is something that can be absorbed and that the practice should never be in a position to be left out of these programs. Many practices have from 20 to 50 of these PPO contracts lying around the office, with varying elements of discounts and preapproval procedures. Many practices have no idea when these contracts expire, when they renew, or what type of termination notices are required.

Any Willing Provider

The PPO network may be subject to a number of state statutes referred to as "any willing provider" laws. These are generally found in state insurance codes and may only apply to PPOs operated by insurance companies or licensed health plans (HMOs). "Any willing provider" laws require such plans to contract with any provider who will accept their terms and payments, subject to various limitations as to geography, capacity, and credentialing requirements. If a PPO contract is offered by a group of providers or employers, it may not be subject to these requirements.

The PPO Network Broker Model

A broker model is a PPO network that is not in itself a payer or health plan, but arranges contracts between payers and a network of providers. This network can recruit providers to a PPO contract without having any business to offer the providers. It then markets the providers to the local payers at a discount. This enables the particular insurance company or network to reprice the market below current commercial rates, effectively using the PPO contracts of the local physicians to establish a lower price for their services for perhaps the same patients they have been seeing.

Traditionally most physicians have simply signed these contracts believing that they needed to be in every discount network plan or they would be denied access to a certain percentage of the local commercial patient population. **However, each contract presents challenges to the physician and should be evaluated for impact.** The effect of some is often repricing existing patients with discounted rates. These types of contracts should be identified and regarded differently in negotiation from the contracts that actually represent substantial numbers of patients who are new to the practice or are in the practice and could be redirected.

PPO—Medical Management

With most PPO-type products, the medical management imposed on the provider is not so much management as it is notice and approval for certain procedures. Review these contracts to spot the precertification procedures, the rules and protocols, and how the provider manuals operate. Many times this is not explained in the actual contract. The provider manual should be reviewed at the same time the contract is reviewed. Often the PPO models require approval from personnel not trained at the doctoral level. Review and appeal mechanisms need to be established in these MCOs to allow physicians quick access to an MCO physician for quick answers on treatment authorization.

HMO

The other basic type of managed care product offered to providers will be a type of plan shifting some or all of the risk of the costs of utilization to the provider(s). Because these programs first originated with HMOs, the products are often generally referred to as HMO contracts, although they can be offered by a number of different MCOs or employers. The payment model in the contract is characterized by an assumption of the risk of the cost of utilization by the entity providing the care and the method of prepayment of a single rate that is calculated to cover all care costs. The capitation model is the most common, but other hybrids have developed.

These contracts tend to separate providers, rather than treat them as colleagues in continuity of care, due to the tension created by the different payment schemes for the different categories of providers, primary care, speciality care, hospital services, and ancillaries. Each category is under pressure to obtain the highest compensation for its services. Under a capitated or global pricing system, one provider only increases payment at the expense of another. However, only through this total sharing of the risk do they also have incentives for reducing costs across the board.

One common feature of the first capitated risk contracts has been the gatekeeper duty of the PCP. The classic gatekeeper model builds economic incentives for the PCP for controlling "upstream" referrals. One method for rewarding the PCP is for him or her to share in the year-end surpluses of the speciality and hospital pools. Some of this has been cause for negative publicity, when patients discover that the payment methodology used to reward physicians in such systems is based on conserving the resources consumed by specialists referrals. This can be interpreted as payment for denying care or access to care. Consumers are generally uncomfortable with plans that limit their choices or decisions and appear to reward their managing physicians for being the agent of this limitation.

Direct Contracts with Employers

A third type of contract is from either single large employers or employer *consortia*. These group-purchasing organizations sometimes represent large employers on a regional basis, sometimes small employers. Employers are increasingly becoming more sophisticated in their design of benefit plans and their purchasing of health services for their employees. Major employers have traditionally granted broad health benefits, beginning in an era when their costs were more manageable than the costs of granting pure salary increases. Reducing these benefits is extremely difficult. Rather than reducing the benefits, employers are moving to control the costs of utilization of the benefits. They are also asking employees to share in these costs. They are attempting to negotiate risks and rewards in provider contracts to give providers incentives to control costs.

Further, employers have found that the administrative services needed to manage a self-insured benefits program need not come directly from an insurance plan or HMO. Many major employers and an increasing number of small employers banded together in groups are self insured for their health benefit plans, using third party administrators to process claims and collect data. Self-insured employers need not qualify for and obtain a state license as an HMO to take and share the risk of these plans, as they are managing their own resources. If they seek to shift the risk directly to providers, however, some states will require the providers to have or use an HMO license. State insurance departments vary with such matters, depending on the maturity of managed care in the state.

Employer Contracts Have a Major Impact

The local employer contract represents a known number of enrollees or patients. These covered lives are not a projected or hypothetical population. Employer contracts represent real people in a service area who have been the patients of local providers for years. The direct employer contract represents a more direct challenge to a local provider's practice. An employer product will cause an impact on a practice because it will control an immediate number of local patients. If the employer is the local employer of some prominence, as in many cities, these contracts can present somewhat of a "do or die" situation to local providers.

A corollary of having a known population is that the employer will have good information on its work force. Good demographic and experience data can be used to calculate meaningful capitation rates or other fixed prices that a provider can rely on with greater security. However, an experienced actuarial consulting firm still must be used to make sense from the employer's data.

Employer Contracts May Be More "User-Friendly" for Providers

The upside of the employer direct contract is that many local employers are more than willing to negotiate many terms and payment methodologies with local providers, rather than present a "take it or leave it" national adhesion contract. While national HMOs and insurance companies will have contracts and contract negotiating skills well honed on the fields of battle with providers in many states, their terms will often be fairly rigid, local employers may not be so willing to offend the entire medical community, and will not have been in the health plan business very long. They are really only seeking to conserve the local costs of health care, a goal that should not be dismissed by the local medical community. Often the medical management of such contracts is fairly open to negotiation and can be created in a unique setting in the local community that fits the practice parameters and idiosyncracies of the local market. Local employers should be open to suggestions to management techniques offered by local physicians. There are also many different varieties of payment methodologies in systems that can be crafted onto a self-insured plan if it fits the goals of the employer and practice needs of the providers. The initial direct contract with a major local employer is a good opportunity for local providers to educate this payer in medical management procedures that are effective and to gain acceptance of payment systems that are realistic.

■ Precontracting Issues to Consider

Business Objectives

All managed care contracts should lead the provider to assess the risks and benefits of the contract opportunity, just as a patient would assess risks and benefits of a proposed treatment or procedure. Consider the business goals and objectives of the two sides of the contract. Different companies have different cultures and management styles. The goals of the contract will reflect this culture. The business objective of one type of MCO may be simply to wring from the system all available cash. The motivation for this contract is the shift of wealth from the provider side to the payer side. While it is alarming to many that health care contracting is taking on such industrial qualities, the reality is that the real change in medicine has come from the increased size of the bargaining parties. With size come big numbers and much at stake. The consolidation of both payers and providers at great speed in some part of the country has caused these contracts to carry so much impact. The basic transaction is not that much different from any other business agreement. Physicians should prepare for negotiations with as much information as is available on the subject.

Business Plans

Consider the contract in the context of the business plan of the provider or the provider's organization. How much and what type of business does the contract represent? Sometimes the first question is, however, does the provider even have a business plan? Then consider what is the business plan of the MCO. Is the provider or his organization central and necessary to the success of the MCO's business plan? Is the MCO's book of business, in terms of the market share of enrollees, central and necessary to the success of the provider's business plan? To the extent that the parties need each other, they will find a point at which they can agree.

Provider Panic

The provider or the provider organization must avoid the "panic/stampede" syndrome, often seen in subtle ways in a medical community. Speakers to medical societies are often fond of quoting the phrase that organizing physicians is like "herding cats." However, experience has shown that those cats herd quite easily at the first rumble of a stampede in the valley from other physicians rushing to sign a contract that is thought to be essential to everyone's practice. No negotiation is then possible if the physician's fear of exclusion is readily apparent.

Provider Patience

One of the primary rules of negotiating such contracts is to master the art of patience. A time-honored tradition of negotiating tactics includes the art of exhausting the other side to the point where they simply throw up their hands in frustration and recognition that they do not have the will to outlive the other party. While these tactics are more commonly seen in industrial settings with management and organized labor, such protracted negotiations can be experienced in any business if the parties on each side feel that the contract is crucial to their well-being, but that the terms are unpalatable.

Where both sides have considerable strength in the marketplace, such negotiations can continue for many months. Physicians who have traditionally viewed themselves as independent professionals, unused to such frustrating tactics or turns of events, whether intentional or not, often need to acquire a sustained mental attitude necessary to participate in a contract negotiation that can extend beyond 12 months. Without the size to have strength in the marketplace, individual physicians will usually not be able to sustain such an effort. Size for these physicians would come in the form of membership in some contracting organization, such as an IPA or a PHO.

For an example of how these matters can drag on indefinitely, reflect on the negotiations between major hospital systems concerning alliances, mergers, and acquisitions. Yearlong negotiating efforts are not uncommon when major systems are attempting to deal with one another. Likewise, if a physician or provider organization or network is dealing with a major insurance payer or health plan in its local area, similarly protracted efforts may be realized when the parties are determined to achieve certain mutually exclusive economic or management goals. Generally, the result of such efforts is not just to see which person is the first one to blink, but which entity really has the strongest need for the other. In the end, the party with the greatest business need will generally agree to certain terms to implement the transaction.

Provider Size

In evaluating managed care contracting from a solo physician's perspective, one item to consider is whether the physician needs size or significant leverage on his or her side to level the playing field with the size of the MCO proposing the agreement. Size is often not necessary. Individual physicians with healthy practices in desirable areas will often be able to renegotiate many unreasonable terms with the largest HMO or PPO. If size is necessary, then the physicians have a variety of options open to them in that they may ultimately be negotiating with a payer. These options include several that do not require the provider to be an employee of a larger group or hospital system. Physicians do not need to sell their practices to gain size in contracting with MCOs. Rather, a variety of organizational means are being developed to offer the physician various contracting vehicles. These include the many forms of IPAs, PHOs, and nonintegrated collective efforts of networks. These more loosely organized efforts have many legal and regulatory hurdles between the member physicians and the executed contract, but they allow the physicians to achieve two otherwise contradictory goals: stay independent and achieve leverage of size in the market. Antitrust laws and tax regulations are the main hurdles to watch for in joining or forming these networks and nonintegrated associations, but they will not prohibit effective aggregation of local practices if done carefully in consultation with experienced advisers.

■ Contract Elements and Issues

An old expression continues to be just as valid in managed care as in any other business: "Whatever they're talking about, they're talking about money." The initial elements to review in contracts will be the economic ones.

What is good about the process of evaluation is that once the physician has invested the time and effort in becoming oriented to the terms and concepts used in the complex payment schemes, this education carries over into all other managed care contracts, MCO, integrated delivery systems, hospital alliances, provider networks, and so forth. All these managed care payment principals and terms are used throughout the entire reorganization of the marketplace. Understanding the economics of the contract opens the doors to understanding all of managed care.

Orientation to Terms

If the provider is completely "at sea" in dealing with these terms, he or she should seek assistance from a local provider-directed network, a professional association representing physicians, or experienced consultants. Many physicians, though, with a technical acumen of their own, find the movement into this field quite natural. Many of those most skilled in mastering the payment complexities in this field have medical degrees. This is the first step of what most of the literature in the field is coming to recognize—that physicians, once oriented and aroused to the issues presented, will become the masters of the field as their experience increases. This is often referred to by medical groups and societies as "taking back medicine" or "controlling our destiny." However expressed, it is generally agreed that physicians will be the decision-makers in health care, both with regard to payment methodologies and medical management of systems, once they are oriented to the new economic terms and issues in substantial numbers throughout the country. As managed care is slow to come to many different markets and localities, physicians have had no interest or necessity in spending the considerable capital in time, effort, and money to become skilled in these matters. Nevertheless, as managed care spreads across the country in some form, physicians will be called on to gain these skills to preserve the independence of their profession.

Contract terminology will often be subject to the MCO's definitions listed at the front of a contract. The following terms are key items often covered in a definition section: "covered services," "excluded services," "emergency services," "authorized services," "medically necessary," "disputes," "clean claims," "authorized communications," "utilization management," "in-network or out-of-network," "point-of-service," "balance billing," "eligible enrollees," and "timely payment." These terms vary with each MCO and its management style. Physicians often have the ability to renegotiate the definition and function associated with these elements to better fit local practice patterns and practical considerations. Most of these terms have economic consequences.

If these terms are not defined in the MCO agreement, a physician should insist on definitions and supply his or her own language, geared toward practicality and enhanced independence of medical decisions by the physician, as well as ease of claims processing and payment procedures.

Payment Rates and Schedules

The payment methodology and rates for contracts are usually found on a schedule attached to the contract. This schedule may not be available to the physician at the initial stages of the contract orientation. Payment schedules and compensation formula are generally attached as schedules because they are the items that are so often changed and are different in every market, while the standard managed care contract is made up of "boilerplate" clauses, which are uniform (or at least attempted) throughout the service area in which the MCO operates.

Discount Fee-For-Service Rates

If the compensation is based on a discount, it may be expressed in terms of a comparison to a well-known industry standard, such as Medicare. It may be expressed in terms of a numerical percentage below the physician's usual and customary rate. It may be expressed in a numerical percentage below some other payment barometer, such as a historical or fixed figure or an accepted average or standard in the community, by zip code, and so on.

Withholds and Incentive Pools in Discount Schedules

A discounted fee for service contract may have a withhold deducted from each claim paid, as an incentive payment mechanism for the physician to modify certain practice behaviors. The concept is to use this amount to heighten the physician's awareness of costs and efficiencies. Arguments vary as to the validity of this premise. This amount to be withheld from each claim paid will then be placed in some reserve fund, which is to be paid out at the end of the term to various recipients. The recipient may vary, depending on the experience of the entire health plan, the experience of that particular provider, the experience of that class of provider, or the experience of that particular health insurance product. The physician may receive his or her money or may share it with others. The physician's control over receipt of this money is directly proportional to the proximity of the conditions of payment to his or her own performance under the contract. Payment conditions based on total health plan experience are far beyond a single provider's control, easily manipulated by the health plan, and the payments are easily lost by the physician. Payment conditions dependent entirely on the physician's own activity, expenses, or outcomes are greater incentives for changed behavior and have greater likelihood of producing additional payments for the physician. Where the MCO is inexperienced in pricing its products in the particular service area or has insufficient experience in paying claims and dealing with a particular patient population, payment conditions should not be dependent on total health plan performance.

Fee Schedules

The discounted MCO contract can come in a variety of forms, apart from a simple percentage off of the physician's usual and customary charges. The health plan can have a predetermined fee schedule, which it presents in an attachment to the contract. This fee schedule, taken as a whole, may result in an overall or average discount in payment rates by a certain percentage below the physician's usual and customary rates.

However, within the fee schedule itself, there will be a variety of different reductions in payment on each CPT Code from modest to severe, used to achieve the overall discount. For example, if the fee schedule presented appears to have an average reduction in rate of 15% below the physician's usual and customary rates overall, this may be achieved by discounts ranging from 0 to 40% or more on individual service codes. The actual fee schedule itemized by code may not be available with the contract. The physician should obtain the actual fee schedule by service code. He should compare this to his own practice service codes of most common usage and current allowable rates offered by his current payers. Otherwise, the physician has no ability to project the effect of the new fee schedule on his own practice. He should also identify the number of codes that appear to be unrealistically low in reimbursement and use those in negotiation to obtain changes in the fee schedule. Health plans will usually negotiate on individual code payments.

Amending Fee Schedules

The ability of the MCO to amend this fee schedule with or without notice is important. The MCO may seek the ability to make significant changes by simply giving the provider a 30-day notice. If the provider does not object, the changes go into effect automatically. If the provider does object, the result may be that the MCO will terminate the contract entirely. Both alternatives are unacceptable. The physician needs to keep the benefit of her initial bargain. Better language for the provider is that the MCO must give notice of amendments, and if the provider objects to the change, the change does not go into effect for that provider's agreement until the expiration of the contract's current term.

Risk-Bearing or Risk-Shifting Payment Schemes

If the contract presents any payment methodology shifting the risk of the cost of utilization to the provider or a group of providers, its analysis is more complex. An entire industry has grown up in the last 10 years of consulting services and publications devoted exclusively to educating both the medical and legal professions in the labyrinth of capitation and other risk-shifting contract elements. Risk-shifting contracts are of three basic types. The most widely discussed is capitation, a prepaid amount given to the providers, calculated on a per-member per month basis, which is to cover all services excluding certain ancillaries or special services. Typically, pharmacy, laboratory, mental health, and dental services will be "carved out" of capitation or paid separately. The capitation system is widely discussed and analyzed, but is not common in its pure form outside mature managed care markets such as the West Coast. In capitated systems, primary care, speciality care, ancillaries, and hospital services are all separated and paid differently. The scheme of payment will vary according to local conditions and the scope and size of the payer and providers.

The second type is a discounted fee for service claims systems with substantial (20%) withholds reserved from claims to be paid from risk pools. The third type is a system whereby the health plan credits a percentage of the total premium sold for the benefit plan to a series of risk pools, from which all payments to providers are drawn.

Percentage of Premium Credited to Risk Pools

If the payment is drawn from a pool of funds expressed in the terms of a percentage of premium charged by the MCO to the payer, the risk for the provider is twofold. First, a concern is in the calculation of how much of the premium comes to his or her provider group. Second, a concern is what that premium price will be. Health plans may use payment methods whereby various subcategories of providers are gathered into risk pools for purposes of incentive payments and one group subsidizing another. The costs of primary care, specialty care, hospital care, and carve outs of various kinds may be taken from various pools of funds, the total of which is based in premium charged to the ultimate payer.

Contracts that are expressed in terms of premium percentages may be open ended, because the premium charge to the customer may be unknown at the time the contract is signed. The premium may vary depending on market conditions, the ability of the marketing department, and the skill of the underwriting department of the health plan. Any managed care contract with this risk that does not have a premium floor, below that the premium cannot fall, should be avoided. The physician should determine and negotiate a figure, below which the contract would convert to a fee-for-service mechanism. The MCO will not desire a floor for its premium, however, because this inhibits its marketing of its products. The provider needs considerable leverage in the negotiating session to establish a floor below which the premium will not control reimbursement.

Function and Flow of Risk Pools

Often the relationships of the risk pools will not be clear from an initial review of just the numbers that appear on a compensation schedule attached to a risk contract. A complete explanation of the relationship of primary to specialty to hospital to ancillary risk pools or carve-outs should be requested and received from the MCO. A pool of funds may be of two types. It may represent all the money available to pay claims or to prepay providers for contract services, or it may represent the reserved withholds to be paid at year's end as a supplement to the normal claims paid through the contract. The pools are subject to creation of deficits and surpluses depending on utilization. The provider needs to understand the source of the funds flowing to the pools as well as the source of support to make up for a deficit in the pool if service utilization exhausts the funds in the pool. For example, will the hospital pool be used to support a deficit in the specialty pool? Will the specialty pool be used to support deficits in the primary pool?

Will physicians share in surpluses from the hospital pool? How will physicians distribute surpluses from their own category pool or from other pools in which they may participate? The significance of the pools comes from the lower rates being paid to providers either per case or per member per month. The economic incentives are "aligned" in such a way that the only way providers can achieve a total compensation approaching historic levels will be from the distribution of the pool surpluses at the end of the term.

Sharing Among Risk Pools

There may be incentives in the flow of funds among the different providers to subsidize or support different segments of the provider network. Specialists may need to recruit primary care and therefore use some of their pool to raise the level or rates for primary care. Hospitals may do the same for either primary or specialty care. A great variety of percentages and spillover or pour over methods of sharing are available to design these systems. Physicians should participate in these decisions that help determine intraprofessional relationships as well as redistribute income. These sharing methods should be appropriate for local goals and delivery systems. "Cookie-cutter" plans from one region may make no sense for another local area.

Specialist Reimbursement Issues

The distribution of surpluses within a capitated system is more significant to specialists and subspecialists. Typically, primary care providers will realize a compensation level in a capitated system either equivalent to fee for service revenues or slightly higher. Risk systems are designed to squeeze money out of specialty services and hospital services. Where managed care contracts include a health system, hospital services, and primary care, tension exists among the providers. The specialist has to defend his or her reimbursement in dealing with the hospital, the MCO, and primary care. Each segment is trying to keep its rate up or justify an increase.

Specialists have an additional problem with the consolidation of all specialists and subspecialists into one risk pool. The ultimate internal distribution of surpluses within the risk pool becomes an internal contest among specialists. The MCO may have a scheduled design for this, or the providers may be able to design their own system. It is important to determine which specialist will be doing which kind of procedure. The payment system and incentives must match the local idiosyncracies of the care delivery system. A specific and finite number of physicians must be identified as participating in the specialty risk pool and authorized to perform certain services. The specialties may be subcapitated or they may be paid on claims a fee schedule. Subspecialty subcapitation requires large numbers of enrollees and sophisticated data analysis on population history and experience to set the subcapitation rate. Consulting firms are in order here. Many published subcapitation rates are available by subspecialty, but these are anecdotes gathered from the experience of different markets and health systems. They may not be analogous to the local market.

Another issue for specialists is dealing with the economic incentives of the PCPs. Primary care is often capitated, while network specialists are paid on a fee schedule, due to low numbers of enrollees and no good data on the enrollees. With the economic incentives realigned, PCPs may be drawn to refer cases to the specialists that they used to perform themselves. Referral protocols within the contract network will help to solve this problem. Nonreferral is also an area for problems for the provider network. If efficiency is a goal of the network, a quick and early referral to a knowledgeable specialist is more efficient than primary care's keeping the patient for multiple visits before referring what has become a real problem. The diagnostic skill of primary care in a network is a real issue in managing the total care through a capitated system, where primary care acts as a gatekeeper.

Data Necessary in Advance

Obviously, the best way to manage a particular population and price the services appropriately is to have considerable demographic and medical experience information on the patient population in question. Surprisingly, the health plan may have no data at the front end of the contract. Physicians with plan-based withholds are silent partners in this effort to roll the dice on the cost of utilization in that particular enrollee population. Experienced MCOs will have a distinct advantage over newcomers due to the need for data. The providers need the ability to revisit the payment mechanism to make adjustments or begin the contract with fee for service payments until some experience has been learned.

Unknown Patient Demographics

It is well known that statistically significant numbers must be present for the basic assumptions of the arithmetic to work in prepaid payment systems. Perilously low numbers of prepaid patients being enrolled in a particular area for a plan present an enormous danger to the provider. One or two severe illnesses may consume all the money set aside for all the rest of those patients in the contract year. A tool in negotiating on a risk-based product where the number of patients and demographics of the patients are completely unknown is the use of an initial method of fee for service until enrollment reaches a predetermined number.

Stop-Loss Insurance

The great unknown factors from future enrollment numbers and utilization are generally covered by reinsurance of MCO losses above a predetermined level, known as "stop-loss insurance." Reinsurance for all losses or claims over a certain level is necessary in any capitated or risk system. The trigger for the stop-loss should be known by the providers. The question of who bears the cost of the reinsurance and who has the obligation to procure it is important. Reinsurance is not inexpensive in managed care systems, because the risk of excessive claims is very real. Apart from the MCO, it may be worthwhile for the providers, if organized, to consider stop-loss insurance on their own. This would be contracted through their organization, such as an IPA or PHO.

Administrative Costs

The health plan or network operator generally keeps a certain percentage of a risk contract for administrative costs. The lean system will have an administrative cost of somewhere between 6 and 10%. Often 12 to 14% is common, and certain health plans may have an administrative cost approaching or exceeding 20%. Nonprofit and for profit MCOs have different approaches to this calculation. In understanding a managed care contract, this type of information is significant. The administrative costs in excess of 10% may contain a considerable profit margin. The components of the administrative cost should be questioned. The cost of reinsurance should be included in the administrative overhead, for example. Claims processing, marketing, accounting, and other costs should be itemized within the general amount claimed by the MCO for administration.

Even though physicians can be taught all the elements of complex reimbursement mechanisms, many contend that their interest is not in the economics of the contract. Most physicians, interests remain focused on the treatment of their patients and the procedures and protocols to be used in that regard. It is from this perspective that the second major element of the contract is identified as the tools, processes, protocols, and philosophy (or lack of any interest) in management of the medical decision-making process in a managed care system. Here the two extreme possibilities at either end of the level of MCO intrusion on the physician are both bad. If the health plan focuses only on payment, all the medical management for "new" efficiencies is up to the provider. The plan gives no guidelines or assistance, only punishment for being inefficient. On the other hand, if the health plan has extensive rules and procedures that interfere with the physicians, independent exercise of medical judgment, this can be just as bad as no rules at all.

Liability for Management Decisions

The law still holds the physician responsible for his or her medical judgment used in treatment of a particular patient, regardless of whether the managed care plan has agreed to pay for the service or not. To fulfill the physician's professional responsibilities with regard to this patient, the physician must provide care at a level equivalent to the community medical standards, and often national or regional standards implied for specialty care. The physician cannot allow an initial determination of "medically unnecessary" as a reason for nontreatment, if the physician believes that the treatment is clinically justified and appropriate under the prevailing standards. The matter must be taken up with the health plan through appeals to determine the best treatment plan.

Personnel working for an MCO who are on the front line of this type of approval and appeal may not have the training of the physician who is requesting the authorization. One element of the medical management of a contract should be a requirement that the reviewers of such matters, if not the initial personnel who determine such matters, should be physicians trained in the same background as the requesting physician. Any review and appeal of such matters must be done in a very quick time frame, so that the patient will not suffer the consequences of an inappropriate denial of care. While the details of this will not be in the contract document itself, the procedures themselves should be found in the manual.

Systems: Management to Measurement

The enormity of the administrative work in managing such a system currently threatens to overwhelm many providers. The administrative costs to a physician's office for caring for a patient base that is made up of many different contracts with many different rules is burdensome and currently uncompensated. In twenty-first-century health care, the winners will be those organizations that have devised systems that eliminate most, if not all, of the bureaucracy attendant to the management of the physician's decision. The future will belong to those systems that allow the physician his or her independent professional judgment for which he or she is trained, but pay not so much for services as for results. The measurement of the results will be the hard part. Physicians for the immediate future will be burdened with the necessity for constant communication with various degrees of trained personnel on behalf of the managed care organization in trying to arrive at a mutually approved treatment plan.

The level of intrusiveness of this approval requirement overlaid on the payment system is an important medical management component. Frustrations over the initial efforts in this type of management have lead to a national search for critical paths and treatment protocols developed by, for, and through physicians, so that the continuum of care can be designed from the beginning, guided by such a protocol. When the protocols have matured to the point where they have been used in practice and have earned the confidence of practitioners, they will provide an efficient and often better source of treatment decisions for the practicing physician. The physicians contracting through networks or IPAs of various kinds can participate in the development of local varieties of critical paths and protocols. Hospitals have begun to create such paths within their environments for their high cost procedures. Most of the specialty colleges have published similar protocols. Local communities, however, often have idiosyncratic patterns in referrals and treatment of different diseases that need to be taken into consideration. The enlightened approach is for local providers to take a very proactive role in determining the appropriate path or protocol for certain disease management within a managed care system.

Management Issues in a Short-term Contract

Part of the problem in the inability to develop paths and outcome measures is not only the lack of good information from automated systems, but the normal short term or life of a managed care contract. The success of these paths is measurable with information over a sustained period of time. Most of the paths and protocols are being developed initially for chronic disease management. It is difficult to ascertain the efficiency or efficacy of such a protocol over only a 12-month period. Thus there are conflicting pressures: (1) to keep the managed care contract short term for purposes of economic salvation, in case all the financial assumptions and calculations go awry, and (2) from a medical management perspective, to have the contract long term, so that the clinical results of effective critical paths and protocols, especially chronic conditions and high cost items, can be studied and evaluated. The resolution of these two conflicting needs is a challenge in each local market.

"Terminating" the Disruptive Patient

The ability of the physician to "terminate" a plan patients if the patient is unruly, disruptive, fails to follow orders, or is otherwise an incompatible match with the physician should be included in the contract. When health plans assign patients to the physician or the enrollees choose physicians from the health plan's network, the arrangement should not interfere with the normal professional relationship a physician traditionally has with the patient. The patient should have free choice of a physician, and the physician should have the ability to accept or not accept the patient. Most health plans will agree to this language if requested, but it often is not included in the standard health plan contract.

Provider Manual

The provider manual seldom accompanies the contract, unless it is requested. Obtain a copy of the provider manual in advance, if at all possible. Note the procedures for utilization review and medical management. Look for appeals and dispute resolution mechanisms. Look for times to submit claims, times for claims payment, times to request treatment authorization, how emergency services are handled, how noncovered services are handled, and so forth. The details of all these elements will be in the provider manual and only briefly referenced in the actual contract. Note in the contract how the provider manual is amended. Often it can be amended through the contract by simple issuance by the health plan of additional pages. The provider must then object to the amendments, but may be excluded from the network by virtue of his or her objection. Try to gain the ability through the contract for nonacceptance of amendments to the manual if they are materially different from the initial contract.

Credentialling

Most health plans make some reference to credentialling of the providers in their network and various accreditation standards for the network itself. If the network claims to adhere to standards from an accrediting organization, the physician should know which standards may cause some difficulty. Is an office survey by the health plan or an accrediting body required for membership in this network? Has the provider's office ever been subject to such a survey and what would be the elements of the survey, if conducted? Many of these surveys, just as in hospital surveys, require written policies for all office personnel and procedures, extensive documentation with regard to office records and medical records, and other paper-intensive review. Be aware of this before it is imposed on you by the contract. Will the accreditation or credentialling survey contact patients of the physician? Will it send them patient satisfaction surveys without the provider's knowledge? All of items need to be clarified in advance.

Records Requirements

Generally, health plans will require that medical records and other clinical statistics be kept and available to the health plan in a manner that fits their business practices. Usually this is not problem for physician's offices, unless the health plan has some highly unusual method for collecting data from its network physicians. The health plan will also want the ability to audit the medical records and the financial records in the physician's office. These audit requirements should be limited to the health plan's need to verify that the services were actually provided to the patient and match the billing from the physician. The financial inquiry should be limited to the billings on that health plan's enrollees only, and sufficient to verify that the billings in the physician office match those received by the health plan. Overly broad audit provisions authorize fishing expeditions. The physician should require confidentiality covenants from the health plan that provide that any information obtained through the physician's records will be kept confidential by the health plan and will not be shared with any third party. The physician owes this duty to the patient, with regard to clinical records, and the physician needs this coverage with regard to this financial records.

Closing the Practice to New Patients

The physician should have the ability to close his or her practice to new enrollees of the health plan if the physician cannot accept increased volume at a particular point in time. The health plan will need a notice in some time period before the physician's practice closure. The physician needs to have this notice period be as short as possible, such as 30 days.

A corollary to this is that some health plans or networks will require that the physician accept a predetermined number of enrollees in certain contracts. Sometimes this number is quite high per contract, and would amount to a staggering patient load coming to the practice if the managed care organization is successful in obtaining its target contracts. The impact of this obligation on the practice could be substantial, and the physician should weigh the likelihood of the arrival of these new patients and his or her ability to handle this additional volume, in addition to the impact of these discounted patients compared to those paying standard commercial rates. In capitated contracts, large numbers are desirable, but capacity of the practice is still an important consideration.

Key Procedural Sections

Balance Billing

The term "balance billing" refers to a physician's ability to collect the contract payment from the health plan and bill the patient for any balance that would raise the charge to the physician's usual and customary rate. All MCOs prohibit this practice. The patient has, of course, paid a premium to the health plan under the assurance that he or she will not be billed for items on covered services beyond what the health plan will pay. This is sometimes referred to as "holding harmless" the patient from the liability for the balance of the cost of the care. Balance billing will violate the contract between the patient and the health plan. If the patient authorizes treatment beyond what is covered, however, the physician should be able to bill customary charges.

Coordination of Benefits; Other Payments

The payment section will also discuss coordination of benefits (COB) and co payments and deductibles with regard to the physician's obligations for each one. "Coordination of benefits" refers to the process of identifying the layers of insurance coverage and payments from the multiple health plans or insurance companies that are associated with the care of a particular individual. For example, an individual may have coverage from a spouse or at his own employment, or some other arrangement such as workers, compensation. There may be different layers of coverage committed to the payment for one injury or illness. An injury may have been caused by the act of a third party. Managed care contracts impose varying degrees of responsibility on physicians for identifying such coverage and payments. Generally the physician will at least have the responsibility to gain all coverage information from the patient and supply this to the health plan. The health plan should seek payment from the separate layers on its own. Physicians should avoid being used as the health plan's collection agency.

Deductibles and copayments are portions of the cost of the care that are the responsibility of the patient to pay. Generally the physician is required to obtain these payments from the patient directly. Be sure that the physician is entitled to keep these payments once he or she has collected them.

The physician should also be entitled to direct compensation from the patient when the patient has specifically authorized in writing a particular type of treatment that is not covered by the health plan. The contract should state that once the physician has explained that a treatment is not covered, but the patient authorizes it anyway, the physician is free to provide such care, bill the patient directly, and collect the usual and customary fee for this service.

Ability to Amend or Renegotiate

The contract should provide for the ability of the parties to come back to the table, once the experience of the contract is known, to renegotiate elements of the payment system that were obvious errors or basedon bad assumptions. This does not mean that the entire contract needs to be renegotiated because someone lost money in a particular month, but if a particular CPT code is being paid at a large loss compared to other codes, it is often the case that the calculation for that was simply in error. Many MCOs do not spend the kind of time on these fee schedules and payment rates that the physicians would, simply because it is not in their interest to fine tune it. Physicians who are adversely affected by errors and omissions in the system, however, have an interest in fine tuning. The contract should provide that this fine tuning can go on, in good faith, over the course of the contract when items are presented for review and that the entire agreement need not be scrapped because of it.

Clean Claims

If a fee schedule and claims are part of the system, a mechanism should be established and referenced in the contract with regard to "clean claims" and claim payment periods. A "clean claim" is one that is coded properly and contains all items necessary for prompt payment, including all eligibility information regarding the patient. If a disputed claim is withheld from this process, what makes it a disputed claim? How will the disputes be resolved? Is the MCO's last word on the subject reviewable? What are the elements of a clean claim? Ideally, such matters should appear in a "definitions" or "payment" section of the contract. This may also be in the provider manual. Experienced HMOs and health plans have extensive rules and procedures in their provider manuals. These should be reviewed up front, if possible.

Termination Causes and Rights

The termination provisions of the contract are essential to the provider's ability to escape a disastrous payment system and enforce the obligations of the MCO. Some agreements are offered to physicians with many termination provisions in favor of the MCO, citing a series of events causing the physician to default, while silent with regard to causes for MCO default. The first task in negotiation is to "mutualize" all such provisions so that each party has relatively equal rights to leave the contract if certain things go wrong.

The MCO has an obvious interest in immediate termination rights if the physician loses his license to practice medicine, his professional liability insurance, his hospital privileges, or any number of other such predetermined credentials. The physician should likewise have the ability to terminate the agreement immediately if the MCO defaults in timely payment, compliance with various eligibility procedures, enrollment procedures, or information reports that support the physician. A default by either party should be cause enough for the other to terminate.

The physician should not be defaulted for the MCO's determination that he or she has "acted improperly," "acted against the best interests of the MCO," or otherwise communicated with his or her patient about the MCO, the plan benefits, or treatment coverage. Avoid vague and general wording as cause for termination, as well as the "gag orders" often seen that attempt to prevent candid communication between doctor and patient.

Contract Term

The actual term of the contract can be a negotiable item. If a good termination section is included for the physician, a longer initial term may be favorable. It allows more experience to collect and analyze data and avoids price renegotiation annually. Most managed care agreements are only of 1 year's duration. Many have automatic renewal clauses with different notice periods for a termination at the anniversary date. Every physician's office should have some sort of tickler system alerting the staff to the notice provision upcoming for the anniversary date of each managed care contract. If the physician has been dissatisfied with the experience under that health plan, a simple letter sent in a timely fashion will cancel the contract. Otherwise, termination usually will only be for cause. Many contract provisions have long termination notices prior to the anniversary date, such as 90 days. It is a good point to obtain the shortest possible notice period for anniversary termination in the initial stages of executing the managed care contract.

Dispute Resolution

Each managed care agreement should have some dispute resolution mechanism referenced for a simple way of arriving at a resolution without resorting to litigation. Often these contracts refer to arbitration. Generally, arbitration will be a much quicker resolution than litigation in court, but it can be just as expensive for both parties. Avoid dispute resolution mechanisms that ultimately refer to some employee or appointee of the MCO as the final arbitrator of these decisions. This is not an equitable method for resolving differences.

Continuing Care after Termination

One of the primary sources for complaints by physicians in HMO contracts is the requirement that the physician must continue to care for the enrollees under the health plan even after termination, if termination is during a contract term. This obligation varies in each contract, but is designed to allow the health plan ample time to transfer that patient to another provider. Most state insurance departments will require some variant of this requirement for all HMO-type contracts. This is a consumer-protection item, which is designed to protect an enrollee who had paid a premium to cover care for a period of time, should the MCO go bankrupt or otherwise be unable to function. The continuing care obligation extends to MCO insolvency as well as termination during a contract term. Avoid clauses requiring the physician to continue to care for the enrollees until the end of their enrollment period. These continuing care obligations should be limited to a distinct number of days or to the good faith efforts of the physician and the health plan to transfer the patient to another member in the network.

Exclusivity

Watch for exclusivity terms in the agreement. Most health plan agreements do not bind the physician to deal only with that health plan. However, some network agreements do have exclusivity clauses in them. Eventually, lines will be drawn in a given market, and one particular health plan or system will exclude physicians who are members of a rival health plan or system. Physicians should be aware of the impact on the practice if he or she signs with one MCO and cannot sign with its major competitor. Many times these consequences or conditions are not stated in the contract, but are more subtle matters. One health plan will simply not offer a contract or will terminate a contract with a physician if his or her membership in the other is learned.

Professional Liability Insurance; MCO Indemnification

Most health plans will require the physician to carry constant professional liability coverage in an amount acceptable in that particular state or jurisdiction. In states that have medical malpractice statutory plans where limitations are provided or state pools or funds are involved, the health plan should require that the physician participate in such state programs. Beyond this, the health plan may require coverage of general liability exposure for the office of the physician.

Indemnification provisions of the health plan by the physician are sometimes requested. The physician's general or professional liability carriers usually will not insure contractual indemnification of the MCO by a physician. The professional liability for a licensed practitioner's acts of negligence is the basis for the cost of the policy issued to the physician. Contractual indemnification covering the corporate liability that could be incurred by the MCO for some errors, omissions, or design of its management system is not included in the basic liability policy written for most physicians. Many carriers will either not write such a rider or charge an excessive premium for this additional coverage.

The physician should avoid underwriting the liability of a MCO in health care or patient treatment settings. The MCO should carry its own managed care liability insurance, which will cover it for exposure from utilization review and management decisions, under which it may have some impact on the access to and type of care its enrollees receive.

"Change in Law" Sections

Often a managed care contract will have a section called "change in law." In the volatile environment of the health care market currently, both regulatory agencies and state legislatures are constantly reviewing and modifying rules under which both managed care plans and providers must operate. Consequently, what has been viewed as standard operating procedure one month might become illegal or anti-competitive in the next. Thus, a change in law section really benefits both parties and enables them to terminate or otherwise modify a business relationship that might be condemned by governmental authorities or subject the parties in the transaction to some liability that was unknown at the time the contract was signed.

Amendment Provisions

The contract should have an amendment provision that specifies clearly how the contract may be amended. Avoid language that allows the managed care organization to simply issue an amendment. The provider may be forced to object to it and lose the contract or accept it. The contract should only be amended by mutually agreed written documents that are understood by both parties. Unilateral amendments, if objected to, should only be effective on a new or renewal term.

Which Law Governs

With the advent of many MCOs having a nationwide scope of operations, the provider may find that the contract presented is subject to and governed by the laws of a state other than the one in which he practices. The provider should request that the governing law for his business contracts be the law of the state in which he is located. In this way, even though there may be a dispute resolution mechanism that tries to avoid the courts of that state, the law of that state will be applied by any arbitration or other judicial review mechanism. Local lawyers and advisers for the physician will be knowledgeable in the local law, and he will be much more comfortable with complying with laws that have always governed his practice, rather than being surprised by the application of a law from a state with which he has no connection.

■ Special Capitation Elements and Issues

Analysis of Existing Practice

Physician office data can be categorized as history data, encounter data, and results data. The history data is made up of standard history and physical information on patients. The encounter data consists of the diagnosis, CPT code treatment data, pharmaceuticals, referrals, age, sex, payer determination, charges and allowable payments, and patient satisfaction. The results data tends to be the traditional outcome measurements of morbidity and mortality, symptom presence, cure, regression, activity levels, and other such measurements of treatment success.

Analysis of the data in your files will show where patients come from, current charges, collections, the percentages of patients from each health plan, the percentage of patients from each zip code, how dependent the practice is on certain payers and how patients and their payers relate to the practice with regard to positive or negative cash flow.

One method of analysis of practice data that is useful and recommended by many consultants in the field is the use of zip code grouping. The number of patients coming to you by zip code is easily obtained through the zip codes in your address and billing information on your office systems. As managed care contracts generally are contracted through employers, and employers generally have well-known areas of residence for their employees, zip code or geographically based data can be a useful tool for determining the probability of patient selection under a particular plan, as well as a replacement factor if current patients choose the new capitated plan.

Patients can be sorted by zip code and then subsorted by age, sex, charges, and allowable charges. Zip code patients can also be sorted by diagnosis, by CPT code, and other treatment-oriented categories. Patients can also be sorted by payer, and sub-sorted by charges billed, allowed, and collected.

Analysis of Practice Costs

The next step is to use this information to arrive at a cost per encounter or visit on a per member per month basis to understand what the impact of a capitated rate would produce if all of the existing patients were paid on a per member per month basis. Only in this way will you know if a proposed per member per month capitation rate is the equivalent of what you are currently receiving, higher, or lower. The proposed rate multiplied by the number of covered lives that could be expected from that plan, or the number of covered lives that would be removed from your current commercial population and covered under this plan, will begin to project the impact of the capitation rate on your practice.

This exercise is designed to arrive at the total expense of delivering a chargeable service, which would include the encounter experience, the materials and supplies used, and the administrative overhead that must be charged to each service unit. The average cost per service is used to determine the capitation rate.

The office visits on an annual basis are divided by 1000 and multiplied times the average cost for a visit, determined by the number of visits compared to the total expenses for the office. The cost of the office visit per member per year is the product of the average cost for office visits times the number of visits, or your annual figure divided by 1000. The cost of the visit per member per year is then divided by 12 for a per member per month figure. From this is deducted any copayments that are routinely obtained by the practice for that visit, and the result is a figure that is used as the cost of your office visit per member per month, against which any proposed capitation rate can be measured for positive or negative impact.

Calculate a Capitation Rate

To calculate a capitation rate for your practice by service code, based on your current patient population, list the services by CPT code that you would provide under the proposed capitated contract. Try to obtain from the plan or other sources an appropriate number for utilization for each CPT code in a recent year for the appropriate medical specialty or some reasonable estimate of utilization for the proposed enrollee population. Use a charge figure for each service according to your typical charges for indemnity coverage. The utilization for each service is multiplied by the charges for a total for all services. Divide the total dollar amount by the number of patients estimated for enrollment under this capitated contract. This is the equivalent of the capitation rate for prepaid care for this same population. This rate should be discounted by the practice's normal collection percentage. Compare this resulting number with the capitation rate being offered by the MCO. The variance in your rate versus the rate proposed by the managed care contract then presents a challenge in several respects. If the MCO's rate is favorable, the practice will likely do well under the contract. This probably also means that the MCO is attempting to initiate capitation in a market where it is relatively rare. If the capitation rate offered by the contract is less than the number arrived at, the rate will reduce your income unless a higher rate is negotiated or utilization and the costs of delivery of service are curtailed or controlled.

This type of analysis can be used to evaluate payment rates for much more specific data sets within your office, other than just gross patient visits. Depending on the information available, it is possible to analyze by CPT code for the charges, utilization, and per member per month rates for your current practice population, as well as the projected population coming through the proposed managed care contract. Divide your annual utilization numbers by 1000. Multiply those times the normal charges for that CPT code to get your annual figures. Adjust those figures for your usual collection rate. Divide those per year numbers by 12 to get a per member per month rate. This will give you the capitated rate per CPT Code. The cost per code would be determined by the same method, using expense figures, rather than revenue or charge figures.

Consulting firms and accountants who specialize in health care will be able to provide these evaluations for your practice. A fairly sophisticated office manager or administrator with good data from your system would also be able to do this.

Look Behind the Proposed Capitation Rate

The capitation rate proposed by the MCO should be an actuarially sound figure, but it may not be. You need to ask through your negotiations if this rate has been determined by an actuary and who that was. What assumptions are built into the rate? Is the rate adjusted for age and sex? What are the covered services to be provided under this rate? What are other revenues the provider should receive, such as co-payments or other fees? What are the utilization rates for this population built into this plan? The lack of data will make any comparative analysis difficult and raise credibility questions regarding the MCO.

Capitation Reports

One final point in capitation matters that is extremely important is the frequency and type of reports given by the MCO to the providers on a regular basis. The more frequent and more thorough these reports can be from a financial and statistical viewpoint, the better the providers are. It is very dangerous for a provider or a provider organization to continue down a path of ignorance of the consequences of practice patterns through 9 months of a 12-month capitation contract, only to find too late that the various risk pools or other sources of bonuses and surpluses have been exhausted, and that in fact there may be huge deficits that need to be repaid. The consequences of lack of control of utilization and of referral patterns need to be checked on a very frequent basis so that the behavior of the providers can correspond to the economic reports from the payer. If the provider is part of a large provider system or network, it is possible that this information can be collected and analyzed by the provider network itself. However, individual providers are dependent on the MCO for this information.

Localize the Contract

Most negotiated managed care contracts with capitation plans or percent of premium plans are tailored to each local community and provider network. To paraphrase a famous Speaker of the House of Representatives, all health care is local. The arrangements made in your community may not resemble the arrangements in a neighboring community. Care should be taken in negotiations to make sure that the proposal of a MCO new to your community fits the practice patterns and idiosyncracies of hospital and physician services in that locale. The MCO will want this fit to work, or everyone will lose money. Therefore, the MCO, while it will resist efforts to shift wealth from the insurer to the provider, nevertheless should welcome an ability to tailor the procedures to make sure that patients are well served and that providers remain reasonably satisfied with the compensation.

Capitation Requires Critical Paths for Predictability

Managed care organizations generally have very limited ability to develop or impose critical paths or treatment protocols for any type of disease management philosophy or plan of action without active support or even initiation by the providers. If the providers in the community have such measures developed or in mind, these can be quite successful in improving care, reducing inefficiencies, and cutting costs. The development of good treatment protocols in management systems will be similar to the development of software in the electronics industry. Therefore, the first group to create a better "program" will capture the business from both the payer and provider side. This challenge is not addressed in nearly as comprehensive a manner as the economic side of managed care contracts. However, it is in these systems, which will come through the outcomes side, that success or failure of the concept of managed care will ultimately be determined.

Thomas R. Neal's practice includes corporate, reimbursement, medical staff, organizational, and management issues for hospitals and physicians. Mr. Neal is a former Deputy Corporation Counsel for the City of Indianapolis and Deputy Attorney General of Indiana. Mr. Neal served as general counsel for hospitals, community mental health centers, organized hospital medical staffs, and a variety of physician practices, networks, and PHOs. He is a past chairman of the Healthcare and Medicine Section of the Indiana State Bar Association and a frequent speaker on physician practice reorganization and managed care for the Indiana State Medical Association. He is the author of numerous articles on law and medicine. He is listed in the 1993–98 editions of *The Best Lawyers in America,* published by Woodward White, Inc. Mr. Neal graduate from Indiana University and its School of Law. He is a partner in the Indianapolis firm of Kreig DeVault, Alexander, & Capehart.

6

Understanding Profiling

SUSAN BELLILE

The Importance of "Outcome" Data to Physicians

In the current managed care environment, physician groups will only be successful to the extent that they can document and deliver high quality, cost effective care.

Data captured through the process of handling claims is being used by health plans to compare, evaluate, and even select providers for participation. Some plans are beginning to require the submission of additional "outcome" data from participating providers. Although these efforts have progressed more quickly in certain geographic areas and among certain specialties (e.g., cardiac surgery), the trends are clear. Physicians are competing with other physicians for patients and for health plan contracts. Physicians are being challenged to prove that their practice is "the best."

Changes in the way health care is managed and reimbursed are also creating new requirements for internal practice management information. Reports showing *billed charges versus payments* by physician are meaningless under capitated agreements. As physicians are added to existing groups or networks are formed for contracting purposes, participants need to know that the care provided by *all* members is consistently high quality and cost efficient. Financial results will be increasingly dependent on a group's ability to monitor and manage care for a given population of patients. Information is the key to success in this new environment.

Three Approaches to Outcome Measurement

Current approaches to measuring health care outcomes can be categorized as follows:

1. **Outcome research** is usually sponsored by academic institutions and/or professional societies. These studies generally focus on outcomes for specific procedures or diagnoses, such as total hip replacement, asthma, and so on. Some studies include patient reported, functional status, and long-term outcome measures. Results are based only on patients and providers who participate in the study. For the most part, these initiatives are designed to compare outcomes for different treatment regimens or patient types, not to compare the practices of specific providers.
2. **Hospital based** analysis compares costs and outcomes for inpatient stays, by DRG, diagnosis, or procedure, often with adjustments for patient severity. The reports are based on hospital financial data, not including all physician fees. They typically compare the length of stay and charges for Surgeon A's cases to the length of stay and charges for similar patients treated by other physicians or treated at other hospitals.
3. **Insurer/managed care** "report cards" or profiles are based on billing data. As bills are submitted and paid, managed care plans capture the claims data from all physicians and facilities for each member of their plan. They then use analytic software to

generate reports on the number or cost of services "per thousand patients" or "per member per month".

Unlike quality measures, utilization and charge data are available and already reported in a somewhat standard format (see the discussion of source data).

▪ The Managed Care Perspective

The remainder of this chapter focuses on managed care profile reports. Before examining the content of these reports in more detail, it is helpful to consider the perspective of the organizations that are producing and using them. The business of insurers and managed care plans is to take in premium dollars from employers and individuals and pay out claims to providers for services rendered to the population that is insured. It should not be surprising that the focus of their analysis is utilization (number of services provided) and cost (amount paid for claims).

Health plans are receiving increasing pressure from employers and consumers to also collect and report data on the quality of care they provide. Two well-known initiatives are the National Committee for Quality Assurance (NCQA) *Health Plan Employer Data and Information Set* (HEDIS 3.0) and the Foundation for Accountability (FACCT). Both organizations are developing standard methods for health plans to report quality indicators (in addition to member satisfaction and financial and enrollee data).

As health plans are increasingly evaluated on such "quality" indicators, they will likely incorporate similar measures in their evaluation of individual providers. However, at the current time, most insurers are still profiling physicians on the basis of activity and dollar figures.

▪ Source Data

The information that a physician's office staff puts on each insurance claim form is used to determine payment. That same information is accumulated to "profile" the services provided by specific physicians and compare their practice to that of other physicians in the same specialty. Although insurers have been analyzing this claims data for some time, most have only recently begun to share the analysis reports with physicians.

Although coding is not a specific focus of this chapter, *the importance of accurate coding cannot be overemphasized.* The choice of diagnosis and procedure codes reported on claim forms now not only affects revenue—it also affects the way a practice is viewed by external organizations. For example, omitting secondary diagnoses may cause cases that actually *are* complex to be compared with cases that *are not* complex (which can cause the incorrectly coded cases to appear higher cost for no apparent reason).

Profile Reporting for Specialists

Managed care profile reports for specialists such as otolaryngologists typically analyze how services or charges per patient treated compare to the average for all otolaryngologists who treated patients in the plan. Figure 6–1 is an excerpt from an actual report received by an

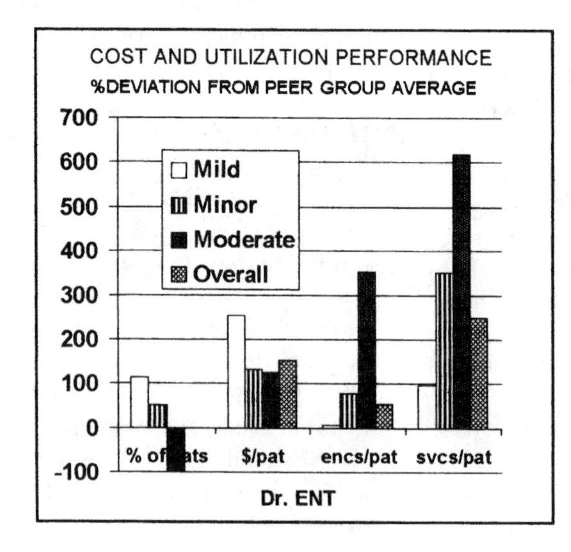

"Shows percentage deviation from the peer group average for each complexity level"

Physician's Actual average paid per patient	$1000
Physician's Expected average paid per patient	$450

FIGURE 6–1. Physician profile report

"ENT" physician. The shading of the bars represents different levels of patient "complexity." In other words, patients were categorized as mild, minor, or moderate based on the combination of diagnosis and procedure codes reported in the insurer's database. The first set of bars shows how the complexity level of this physician's cases compared to that for all ENTs (this physician had more mild and minor patients, fewer moderate). For each complexity level and overall, Dr. ENT is compared by

- **$/pat.** The total amount of claim dollars per patient treated.
- **encs/pat.** The number of encounters per patient treated. An encounter includes all services related to one course of treatment (e.g., it includes related lab testing with an office visit).
- **svcs/pat.** The number of services per patient treated (counting each individual CPT code charged for).

In this example, Dr. ENT is far above his peers on all three measures. The "actual average paid per patient" to Dr. ENT was $1000; the plan "expected" to pay out an average of $450 per patient. The expected number is based on the average for all ENTs, adjusted for patient complexity.

Formats for reporting profile data vary considerably from one plan to another. However, most include essentially the same information as in this example. The data may be presented in a table, rates per 100 patients may be shown (instead of % deviation), or numbers that vary significantly may be "flagged." Physicians should be particularly cautious with reports that show only percents and rates (and do not include actual numbers). Particularly for certain procedures, a given physician may only have treated a few patients. For those low volume procedures, percents and rates can be very misleading.

Profile Reports for Gatekeepers

Reports produced by managed care plans for PCPs are different from the specialist reports just described. Members of managed care plans are typically assigned in some way to a PCP. The PCP's profile analyzes all services provided to the assigned plan members—services provided directly by the PCP as well as services provided by specialists. Utilization on these reports is generally calculated as a rate "per 1000 members." Total expenditures are reported as a dollar figure "per member per month."

Primary care reports are also of interest to specialists because of their focus on the number and cost of referrals. Figure 6–2 is an excerpt from a PCP's profile. It suggests that the patients managed by Dr. Primary Care cost more than expected and were *referred to specialists* more often than expected. Dr. Primary Care learned from this report how many bonus pool dollars were *not* received based on this data.

Primary care physicians whose patients utilize more nasal endoscopies per 1000 or have higher specialist expenditures per member per month will be forced to change their referral practices. It is in the PCP's as well as the specialist's best interest to establish and use guidelines for appropriate referrals. Physicians do not benefit from seeing inappropriate patients; those who are capitated will be penalized for such unnecessary visits.

PHYSICIAN PROFILE		
Dr. Primary Care		This report was created and distributed by a health plan, using paid claims data.
Actual ACP	$1970	ACP = "actual annualized average cost per patient". Expected is "based on the mean cost of the peer group for a like population".
Expected ACP	$1120	
Actual referrals	230	Rate per thousand of referrals to a specialty
Norm referrals	93	
Overall Z-Score	1.2	"The Z-score is the difference between the actual and expected ACP, using a weighted average...represents the standard deviation from the norm."

The report concludes with an explanation of how the Z-score is used to distribute the bonus pool

FIGURE 6–2. Primary care profile report

Limitations of Managed Care Reports

One of the major limitations of managed care reports is the source data itself, as discussed earlier. Inconsistent or inaccurate coding by providers submitting claims, timing gaps in claims processing, and the exchanges of data from claims submission through processing/payment and entry into the profile reporting system all offer opportunities for error.

Even when collected, coded, and transmitted accurately, very little *information* is found on a typical claim form: patient identifiers; procedure dates, codes, and charges; and one or two diagnosis codes. Although statistical techniques such as risk adjustment improve the ability of managed care plans to make appropriate comparisons, the only numbers available to compare are utilization (e.g., procedures per 100 patients) and charges (usually the amount paid by the insurer, not the amount billed).

A related limitation is the fact that it is often difficult—if not impossible—to identify the factors underlying any differences identified. That is, if Dr. Jones's report suggests that she utilizes a procedure more often or that her average charges per patient are higher, there is no way to determine *why* that may be the case. If a listing of patients is included, the physician can do her own investigation, but not all profile reports include patient specific detail.

Because reports are created by individual plans and most physicians treat patients from many different payers, any profile report will only reflect a small percentage of a physician's practice. Different plans use different analysis and reporting methods, making it difficult to compare data from one report to another.

One final challenge to using profile reports has been poor report design and confusing (or missing) explanations of the information reported. There have been instances where physicians received in the mail a fuzzy photocopy of a page swimming with tiny numbers, without so much as a cover letter. Using profile data is new to managed care plans as well as physicians. Most plans are continuing to review and improve their analysis methodology, report format, and communication process and are open to provider feedback.

When and How to Respond

Given these limitations, it may be tempting to simply ignore or "roundfile" any profile reports sent by managed care plans. Remember, however, that other organizations—*other organizations that pay your claims*—are looking at this data. While the information may not prove to be particularly helpful or enlightening, it is important for physicians to obtain, review, and understand all available profile data.

First, does the report seem reasonable? Given the definition of each data field or column and your knowledge of your practice and the patients in this plan, are there any numbers that seem completely out of line—for example, numbers of cases or charges for a particular procedure? If so, ask the report provider for an explanation. Next, focus on the areas where you have a significant volume of cases. Ignore data that averages across only a few cases. For the high volume areas, do your numbers compare favorably to the peer group norms provided?

Given the normal distribution of data, 90% of physicians will find that their results are not statistically significantly different from the norm. If that is the case, no further follow-up may be needed. If, however, your numbers compare unfavorably or the report shows "flags" or "outliers" (again, for procedures with a significant volume), further investigation is warranted. Start by identifying the specific cases that were analyzed. Check office data/records to confirm the numbers and begin to identify issues that may be driving the differences.

Particularly since specialist reports use "patients treated" as the denominator for calculating utilization rates, a fairly common occurrence is that a physician will be "flagged" for procedure codes that represent his or her individual speciality focus. In other words, a physician who sees a unique population and/or receives referrals for complex cases may be "flagged" for a higher than average utilization of the unique and complex procedure codes.

When the explanation is "Of course, Dr. Smith uses those codes more often—that's the type of practice he has!," some documentation and a communication to the payer may be useful. Additional documentation to consider is (1) if the hospital or ambulatory surgery center tracks procedure indications (specific criteria demonstrating the necessity of a procedure) or (2) the practice has data on the insurer's own "precertification" criteria and the number of times that proposed services or payments have been denied. Such information would support the fact that Dr. Smith is not overutilizing these procedures.

Case Study

A major insurer distributed a profile report to otolaryngologists that was organized by procedure group. For cases in each procedure group (e.g., tonsillectomy/adenoidectomy), "episodes" of treatment were analyzed. The report showed, for the individual physician and for all cases (for that insurer) in the state, the number of episodes, the average surgeon charges, and the average hospital charges.

It is interesting to note that the *physician* profiles included *hospital* charges. Surgeons practicing at high cost hospitals had higher overall "episode" charges than their peers.

The profile of one otolaryngologist with a large number of patients in this plan showed high costs relative to the statewide average. With the assistance of an expert data analyst, this physician went back to the individual patient detail to determine what might be driving these cost differences. He enlisted the hospital's assistance in evaluating hospital charges and costs for common case types. One critical issue turned out to be the way that procedure groupings had been defined for the profile reports. For example, the report labeled "Septoplasty" included cases in which only a septoplasty had been performed *as well as* complex sinus surgeries that included septoplasty. Using office data, this physician's consultant was able to demonstrate very different outcomes when patients were grouped in more similar and logical categories. In this case, the insurer was receptive, appreciated the input, and plans to modify its future reporting.

■ Profiling Is Here to Stay

There is no question that all activities and all participants in the health care system will be scrutinized more closely in the future. Managed care plans are playing an increasingly important role in physician practices. For better or worse, the data they have, the analysis they do, and the incentives (or disincentives) they provide have a significant impact on physicians.

Understanding and proactively addressing managed care profile reports is an important first step. However, as illustrated in this chapter (and appreciated by most physicians), managed care profile data does not provide a complete picture of any physician's practice. Individually and collectively, physicians need to take the lead in defining more meaningful quality and efficiency measures, collecting and analyzing data, and using it to continuously improve patient care.

Susan K. Bellile specializes in using data to help physicians measure—and *improve*—their effectiveness. Her practical approach finds answers to physicians' key questions: "What are the critical areas of our practice? How well are we performing? How can we do better?"

Ms. Bellile is founder and president of Q3, Inc., a firm that supports physicians in managing clinical information—rather than being managed by it. She recognizes that in today's health care environment, data is best used *not* as a weapon to control physician practice, but as a tool to support the management of patient care.

Ms. Bellile has more than 15 years' experience in health care data analysis and information systems consulting. She has held top management positions at Iameter, MediQual Systems, Baxter International, and Healthcare Knowledge Resources (now a division of HCIA).

She is known for her talent in sorting through volumes of data to find meaningful and useful information. Ms. Bellile has been instrumental in developing several cutting-edge process improvement approaches, including MediQual Systems' "Clinical Benchmarking" program and Baxter International's "Value Improvement Program." Ms. Bellile realizes a medical practice's future depends on how well it manages the care it provides. She uses her years of experience in data analysis to help physicians develop an information plan specifically for their practice. Her guidance lets physicians negotiate from a position of strength, able to demonstrate their practices' quality and cost effectiveness. Ms. Bellile holds a master's degree in management from Northwestern University, a master's degree from Loyola University of Chicago, and a bachelor's degree from Valparaiso University.

7

Ethical Challenges of Managed Care

CARL A. PATOW AND RUTH D. GAARE

I wish to begin by making a public confession: In the spring of 1987, as a physician, I caused the death of a man.

No person or group has held me accountable for this—for this was a half-million dollar savings to my employer. In fact, this act secured my reputation as a good company doctor and insured my advancement in the health care industry—in little more than a year I went from making a few hundred dollars a week to an annual six-figure income.

In all my work, I had one primary duty: to use my medical expertise for the financial benefit of the organization. According to the managed care industry, it is not an ethical issue to sacrifice a human being for savings. I was told repeatedly that I was not denying care, I was only denying payment.

I am not an ethicist whose opinions have come just from books. For me, the ethical issues were born in the trenches, fed by the pain I know I have caused. . . .

Testimony by Linda Peeno, MD, a former medical director for three managed care organizations, before the U.S. House of Representatives Subcommittee on Health and the Environment in May 1996.[1]

This compelling testimony gives voice to the fears of many health care providers and patients about the potential dangers and abuses in the health care system as it undergoes a rapid and dramatic transformation to managed care. More important, however, these words speak to the need for an equally dramatic paradigm shift in the ethics of the health care profession—a shift in focus that goes beyond the traditional emphasis on the provider–patient relationship to a broader consideration of the health care organization and the effects of the complex management systems under which care is now delivered. Just as the managed care organization considers not only the care of an individual patient but also the health of its entire population, so too medical ethics must now examine the ethics of patient care from a systems perspective. This organizational approach to medical ethics is needed to address the new conflicts of interest; the new complex relationships among provider, patient, payer, and managed care organization; and the new ethical issues born in the trenches of a managed care system that uses such management tools as clinical practice guidelines, physician incentives, utilization review, physician gatekeepers, and networks.

The delivery of health care services in the era of managed care, which depends heavily on quantitative assessments of costs, benefits, and quality, presents great challenges as well as great opportunities. One challenge is to preserve and reinterpret the cornerstones of medical ethics: the traditional provider–]patient relationship that is built on a covenant of trust, and physician and patient autonomy. The opportunities include better coordination of patient care by a primary care physician; an improvement in the quality of care through the use of clinical guidelines based on outcomes research; and equality of access for all members of the managed care organization.

An organizational approach to medical ethics will draw attention to the ethical dimensions of these challenges and opportunities through ethical analysis of the measurement tools and the management and implementation policies within an organization. For instance, the organization will carefully examine the benefits and burdens of a particular policy for both its patient population as a whole and for individual patients and will attempt to balance the benefits and burdens in a consistent way; it will be sensitive to the underlying values implicit in its decisions about what to measure as part of costs and quality; it will question whether policies or determinations about coverage disproportionately impact one subset of its patients and therefore raise questions of distributive justice. This focus on ethical reflection within an organization can ensure that the time-honored values of beneficence, respect for patient and provider autonomy, and justice will endure by becoming embedded in an organization s corporate mission and structure. It also will highlight the critical role of organizational ethics in fostering a culture that encourages ethical relationships and nurtures responsibility and ethical behavior by both professionals and patients.

The field of medical ethics provides a rich storehouse of reflection dating from the days of Hippocrates,[2] and a significant revival in medical ethics during the last 30 years has helped the medical profession and society manage dramatic scientific and technological advancements. Ethical analysis similarly can illuminate the moral dimensions and challenges brought about by the managed care transformation by fostering the following:

1. An acknowledgment and careful exploration of the effects of financial and other contractual constraints on patient and provider autonomy, and of other potential conflicts under managed care that challenge the provider–patient relationship. Examples include conflicts between the provider's role as advocate for an individual patient and the provider's responsibility for the interests of other patients and the MCO's population as a whole; between the goals of cost containment and the quality care; between respect for the integrity of the provider as clinical decision maker and contractual limitations on treatment as well as clinical guidelines and utilization review.
2. The development of guidelines on ethics and the establishment of assessment strategies like ethics report cards that include criteria for measuring provider and organizational behavior on ethical issues.
3. The promulgation of an organizational medical ethic that is built on such values as honesty, disclosure and accountability, as well as on such time-honored values as beneficence, justice, and respect for the patient.

Effects of Managed Care on Physician and Patient Autonomy

A careful exploration of the effects of managed care on physician and patient autonomy begins with acknowledgment that medical decision making now involves three parties. The ethical principle of autonomy is compromised in managed care by the interjection of the MCO into the doctor–patient relationship.

The presence of a third party in health care relationships, however, is not new. One hundred and seventy-eight million people in the United States have some form of private health insurance coverage; coverage for 150 million of them is employment related.[3] Historically, this coverage was provided by employers purchasing a group contract under which an insurance carrier offered indemnity coverage by employers for employees—that is, the insurance company paid all usual, customary, and reasonable charges incurred by an employee for medical care, subject in some cases to an annual deductible and a percentage of covered expenses, co-paid by the employee for each service.[4] Increasingly, however, indemnity carriers have sought to control costs by assessing appropriateness through utilization review, including preauthorization for admissions, precertification for surgical procedures, and retrospective denial of payment. In addition, many employers, seeking opportunities to cut medical expenditures, have become self-insured for medical costs, often using a third party to administer the claim payment process. At present, pure indemnity insurance is relatively rare, and in nearly every health care transaction, except self pay and no pay , there is a third party interest in the cost and quality of the patient–physician interaction. In the United States, patient autonomy has been reduced, to varying degrees, by all health insurance plans, as efforts are made to bring the rate of health care expenditures closer to the growth rate of the rest of the economy.

Managed care relies on the assumption that the doctor–patient relationship will be preserved as fiduciary and trusting, despite the fact that it may be contractually based. Patients expect that physicians will act on their behalf, even if financially disadvantageous for the physician. For example, patients expect that physicians will appeal medically inappropriate administrative care management determinations made by the MCO. The patient expects that by selecting managed care the physician will work within the system to provide for the patient's best interests.[5]

The most often cited potential for ethical compromise of the fiduciary relationship in managed care is the payment of physicians by capitation. Not all managed care physicians are reimbursed by this arrangement. However, where physicians receive a set monthly amount for care of a given patient population, there is the potential for an inverse incentive to inappropriately limit services and access to specialists. The uncertainty of patients as to whether they are receiving all appropriate and necessary services has the potential of undermining trust in the medical profession.

In addition, managed care may introduce other restrictions and controls that can potentially interfere with the doctor–patient relationship. Both the doctor and the patient may feel that autonomy has been compromised.

For the patient, managed care's emphasis on the health of the population of plan members is contrary to the historic fee-for-service concentration on individual health needs and desires. Determination of medical necessity, virtually unheard of in the free market atmosphere of fee-for-service medicine, is central to assuring equity of care under managed care. Patients may also have concerns about their physician's incentives to provide optimal care, regardless of cost. Patient's perceptions about physician reimbursement and incentives in managed care may raise significant issues of trust, even when contractually unjustified. In addition, the opportunity to independently select form a full range of providers, restricted only by the limits of insurance coverage, is lost.

Physicians autonomy is also threatened by managed care. The care management paradigm inherent in managed care challenges physicians to integrate complex administrative directives with medical practice. The degree to which administrative controls and directives are introduced into the patient–physicians relationship varies widely. Common mechanisms include clinical practice guidelines, restricted formularies, provider networks, and restricted referrals.

Clinical practice guidelines are commonly used by managed care to decrease variation in the process of providing care, and thereby more tightly control resource utilization. Guidelines vary by organization, in purpose and content.[6] There is no uniformity in the method of creation of guidelines or in their application. Guidelines can be used as simply a tool for better understanding of possible treatment options or as an unalterable dictum for rationing resources. As tools for making decisions, guidelines incorporate patient preferences, encourage self-determination based on informed decision making, and remain flexible in choices of options for care. As strict instruments of rationing, guidelines focus on total population resource utilization, at the expense of self-determination. The treatment outcomes of guidelines are not standardized. Outcomes may reflect cost, health and disease measures, or functional outcomes. The beneficiary of the guideline's efficiency may depend on the target outcome, and may be the patient, the provider, or the MCO.

The purpose, means of creation, contained assumptions, and intended outcome all have an impact on whether a guideline affects the autonomy of the patient and provider. A comprehensive guideline constructed to enhance patient awareness of risks, complications, and alternatives of scientifically validated treatment options may increase, rather than decrease patient autonomy. On the other hand, a rigid guideline that stifles clinical interaction, created to serve only managed care cost effectiveness, impairs both physician and patient ability to freely make care decisions.

The means of creation of guidelines have particular significance when considering their eventual use.[7] Havighusrt describes two dominant models for the development of guidelines. The Traditional Professional Model assumes that guidelines should be promulgated or validated by authoritative professional groups, especially the recognized specialty societies, and that these guidelines should not be hard and fast prescriptions, but parameters accommodating multiple approaches and accepting diverse opinions. Under this model, the guidelines are not seen as binding. The Traditional Professional Model, although founded on scientific scrutiny of the literature, suffers from the perception that specialty physicians may craft guidelines in their own interests over those of the patient.

The alternative model, the Political Model, explicitly includes nonmedical interests in guideline development, including consumer advocates. The Political Model has been used in federal legislation that mandates creation of guidelines.[8] The Political Model introduces nonscientific data into the formulation of guidelines, such as cost considerations. An important feature of this model is the apparent objectivity of this process and its political legitimacy. Guidelines developed under the Political Model are more likely to be considered as standards of care against which physician behavior is measured. While this approach may be advantageous for policy makers in government programs such as Medicaid and Medicare, individual physicians may find the guidelines threatening.

An argument has been made that if guidelines are constructed to include value choices of patients, then inherent loss of autonomy may be justified.[6] Advantages potentially include elimination of practices that deliver little value to the patient. Practice guidelines may be used as minimal standards for practitioners, possibly for licensing, disciplinary bodies, and credentialling by health care institutions. Network physician selection by MCOs might be facilitated by identification of high quality and low cost physicians who adhere to guidelines. Redman argues that a public policy that develops and uses practice guidelines judiciously and in ways known to benefit patients would be justified in limiting autonomy. Unfortunately, local development of clinical practice guidelines in physician practice associations may not consider patient values, and may be developed primarily by physicians using the Traditional Professional Model.

In many cases the guidelines developed only codify local accepted practice, without a rigorous scientific or economic analysis or consumer representation.[9] Little effort may be expended in evaluating the effects of the guidelines on costs or patient functional outcomes. Given the difference between hypothesized requirements for use of ideal clinical practice guidelines in policy and regulatory matters, and the lack of standardization of use, evaluation and improvement of guidelines in actual deployment, a justification for the loss of autonomy that is based on the merits of clinical practice guidelines should be carefully considered.

Restricted formularies also subvert the autonomy of the individual physician and patient by creating a centrally determined preapproved list of pharmaceuticals. Prescribing nonformulary medications usually involves a lengthy bureaucratic appeal. The list may be determined solely by a pharmacy administrator, without input from the physicians in the MCO. Furthermore, the pharmacy provider may be owned or controlled by a pharmaceutical manufacturer. Inclusion of a medication on the formulary may have more to do with its origin or the contract under which it is procured than its clinical effectiveness. Many MCOs, include physicians in creating the formulary, especially when the medications are included in mutually developed clinical practice guidelines. Patient preference, however, is often superseded in the effort to contain pharmacy costs.

Physicians are frequently asked by patients to prescribe brand-name medications, based on the patients subjective fear of generic medications or anecdotes regarding brand-name effectiveness. The physician is confronted with pleasing the patient and authorizing the brand name medication without scientific justification, or instructing the patient that the generic substitution is as effective despite the patient's bias. There are, of course, medications for which generic substitutes are known not to have equal potency (e.g., certain seizure medications). But for many routine prescriptions the generic may be as satisfactory. From the standpoint of the MCO, a prescription for brand name only due to allergies to all generic medications quickly raises the question of ethical compromise of the physician.

Provider networks are central for managed care, and are essential in assuring access to a broad geographical area under a single managed care system. Provider networks are often created by contractually obligating groups of physicians to participate in the care of managed care patients. In return, the MCO provides access to patients and a contractual basis for remuneration. Depending on the plan design, patients may or may not have options for access of care outside the network. In strict HMOs with closed networks, care obtained from providers not listed in the physician directory is not a covered benefit. More contemporary plan designs offer care options outside the network, but with higher copays and coinsurance. Patients who do not have the option to seek care outside the network without insurmountable personal cost may find themselves limited in care options, particularly if the network is small and the pathology in question is rare or complicated. With limited numbers of advanced specialists, patients can find themselves without a compatible physician.

Physicians also may find that exclusion from the managed care network has unacceptable consequences. In areas where the penetration of managed care is high, inability to access patients in managed care plans may mean financial hardship to physicians not participating as network providers. In an effort to assure access to all patients, physician groups in many states have petitioned legislatures to pass any willing provider laws that permit independent physician access to managed care patients, if the physicians agree to the financial terms accepted by network physicians. These laws may provide access to patients for nonparticipating physicians, but for MCOs any willing provider laws undermine efforts to manage quality through credentialling, education, and care management.

Definition of a network of providers has distinct advantages for providing care to a large population. Geographic distribution can be assured. Physician qualities, such as board certification, can be examined and unsuitable providers can be screened. Costs can be controlled through contractual obligations of participating physicians, and cost effective medicine can be incentivized. Education of physicians and office staff in providing effective, timely, quality care can be focused on a designated physician population. Monitoring of preventive medicine interventions, and reporting results of these analyses, can ideally lead to positive changes in community health.

Monitoring of physician utilization data can also lead to economic credentialling: the practice of termination of physician contracts for excessive utilization or for network oversupply of physicians in certain specialties. Fear of termination of contracts produces considerable pressure on physicians to avoid hospitalizations and overutilization of resources that would swell the MCOs' cost of care. The pressure to restrict hospitalizations becomes increasingly severe as the proportion of a physician's patient population is derived from a single managed care source. Loss of access to a large number of patients is a catastrophe to a medical practice relying on those patients for a steady income stream. For patients, however, the risk in economic credentialling of physicians is twofold. The physician may make treatment decisions based on fiscal pressures and delay admission until the outcome is adversely affected. And, second, the termination of the physician from the managed care plan my end the patient–physician relationship abruptly and at no fault of the patient. Multiple states have passed laws protecting physicians from termination without just cause.[10]

Contracts with physicians have specifically forbidden physicians to discuss certain issues with members, including disclosing treatments for which the MCO will not approve payment, and disclosing bonuses offered to physicians for restricting access to services.[11] These gag rules have received considerable political attention, and by March 1997 eighteen states had passed legislation prohibiting gag rules.[10]

While autonomy is threatened under managed care, both patients and physicians may benefit under managed care arrangements. Case management, by reducing health care costs, may decrease the rate of rise of community and personal health expenditures. In addition, cost containment arises from contractual sources, through assurance of suppliers of volume, and by competitive bidding. This type of leverage is not available to the individual patient. Quality monitoring by MCOs is performed to demonstrate that services provided to members and health outcomes are satisfactory. While the measurements are reported for populations of patients, no such monitoring is available under fee-for-service arrangements. The MCO also has a responsibility to assure the quality of providers through its credentialling process, a role that the patient must otherwise assume in screening potential personal providers. Unnecessary procedures and redundant testing is discouraged, decreasing patient inconvenience and possible complications.

For physicians, MCOs can provide advantages of scale not otherwise readily available, including immediate access to large patient populations and predictable income. Staff model HMOs may provide regular practice hours and minimal practice financial and administrative responsibilities. Financial incentives encourage cost-effective care.

Recent legislative attempts to regulate the behavior of MCOs arise in part from concerns that managed care executives have not acted ethically and responsibly in assuring good health care for members. The ethical principle of beneficence, promoting the welfare of others, has been described as having four elements: avoiding the infliction of harm, preventing harm, removing existing harm, and the affirmative promotion of good.[12] The application of beneficence to medical care is: the alleviation of disease, disability, and injury if there is a reasonable hope of cure or improvement. The harms to be prevented, removed, or minimized are the pain, suffering, and disability of injury or disease. In addition, the health professional is enjoined from doing harm, such as when interventions inflict unnecessary pain and suffering.

In testimony before the House of Representatives Subcommittee on Health and the Environment, a former managed care medical director detailed many egregious lapses of medical and business ethics used to deny care to beneficiaries.(see testimony at the beginning of the chapter).[1] Care frequently was denied on the basis of definitions of medical necessity, including classifications of treatment as being experimental, previously existing, or cosmetic. By defining services as not medically necessary, they become excluded from coverage. Health plans and insurers specify what is and what is not covered as medically necessary care in the insurance contract. However, the clarity of the definition, especially regarding experimental therapies, may allow for considerable latitude in making case-by-case determinations.[13] Relying on health plans to make coverage decisions while at the same time reducing costs is problematic. Health plans have an incentive to minimize the scope of benefits, to reduce expenditures, and maximize returns on available revenues.

Defining medically necessary care is difficult. There are conditions for which clear diagnostic criteria do not exist, and conditions that may not exist as distinct entities—for example, the Gulf War Syndrome. Medical treatment of other conditions may seem warranted to restore normal function, but what should we use as the definition of normality? Should average human experience be used as the measure, or an ideal standard of human capacity? Cosmetic procedures are usually not included in benefits packages, but should a patient be denied treatment of a giant congenital facial vascular nevus because it does not impair function? Should infertility and transsexual surgery may be excluded from benefit packages, as they often are? These questions illustrate that many managed care determinations about patient care and benefits are based as much on values and cultural preferences as on scientific data.

By first acknowledging and then examining the ethical dimensions of managed care in an open and fair forum, providers, patients, and health care organizations can mediate the tensions that grow out of their different roles and responsibilities. With ethical reflection, they will be better able to create a system that respects the autonomy of patients and providers.

■ Guidelines on Ethics and Provider Accountability

Guidelines on Ethics

Professional reports and guidelines on ethics have begun to address the inherent ethical conflicts that arise because of the managed care plan's responsibility to provide cost-effective medical care for a population and the traditional physician's role to advocate for each patient. Although still evolving, guidelines generally are emphasizing the central role of honesty, disclosure, and professional trust.

The American Medical Association's Council on Ethical and Judicial Affairs issued a report titled *Ethical Issues in Managed Care*[14] that includes guidelines for physicians, patients, and MCOs (an edited version follows):

> Patient advocacy is a fundamental element of the physician–patient relationship and physicians must continue to place the interests of their patients first.
>
> Broad allocation guidelines of a managed care plan that go beyond the cost-benefit judgments made routinely by physicians should be established at policymaking level so that individual physicians are not asked to engage in ad hoc bedside rationing.
>
> Regardless of allocation guidelines or gatekeeper directives, physicians must advocate for the medical care they believe will materially benefit their patients.
>
> Physicians should be given an active role in contributing their expertise to any allocation process and should advocate for guidelines that are sensitive to differences among patients.
>
> In some cases in which a physician believes that medical care that would materially benefit the patient has been denied, the physician's duty is to challenge the denial and argue for the provision of treatment in the specific case. When a physician believes that a health plan has an allocation guideline that is generally unfair in its operation, the physician's duty is to advocate at the health plan's policymaking level to seek an elimination or modification of the guideline.
>
> Physicians should promote full disclosure to patients enrolled in managed care plans and are obligated to inform patients of all treatment options, even those not covered under the terms of the plan. Patients should also be fully informed on enrollment in plans and at least annually thereafter of any incentives to limit care.
>
> Financial incentives for physicians should be limited and calculations encouraged on the basis of the performance of a sizable group of physicians rather than on an individual basis.

The AMA Report also addresses patient responsibilities: Patients have an individual responsibility to be aware of the benefits and limitations of their health care coverage. Patients should exercise their autonomy by public participation in the formulation of benefits packages and by prudent selection of health care coverage that best suits their needs.[14]

In adhering to the requirements of informed consent, managed care plans must inform potential subscribers of limitations or restrictions on the benefits package when they are considering entering the plan and must provide adequate appellate mechanisms for both patients and physicians to address disputes regarding medically necessary care, according to the AMA Report.[14]

Another report, *Ethical Considerations in the Business Aspects of Health Care,* issued by the Woodstock Theological Center, similarly argues strongly for the primacy of the physician–patient relationship. The Report proposes an aggressive role for health care professionals when rules conflict with their professional judgment:

1. The health care professional should not falsify requests or reports to carry out a preferred plan of treatment for a patient.
2. In the face of financial constraints, it is now professionally and ethically incumbent on health care providers to be knowledgeable about various alternative ways of arranging services to respond to the total health care needs of patients. Physicians, especially, should recognize the expertise of other health care professionals, and the health benefits that can result from their involvement in patient care, and they could be prepared to refer patients to them when appropriate.
3. The referring physician must be sufficiently informed about the competence and qualifications of these alternative health care providers to have confidence that the alternative provider can competently attend to the needs of the patient.
4. If a third party refuses funding for a course of treatment deemed by the provider to be indispensable for the health or survival of a patient, it is ethically proper for the health care provider to express strong disagreement, carry out the treatment, and strive to justify this decision after the event to secure funding. Failing successful resolution, the health care provider on the health care institution may have to absorb the cost, if it is entirely beyond the means of the patient. If this becomes a frequent or recurrent pattern, then, in the interest of patients, a health care professional and/or institution has an obligation to try to reform the system to rectify the offending resource constraint guidelines.[15]

Accountability and Report Cards

Another approach to assuring ethical behavior of physicians and organizations involves ethics report cards or accountability measurements that list criteria and methods for measuring professional and organizational behavior. Accountability involves the procedures and process by which one party justifies and takes responsibility for its activities.[16] Any organization or group, from a professional society to a small physician practice to a MCO or state Medicaid program, could develop a report card with criteria with which to measure and hold professionals accountable on ethical standards. Linda Emanuel, MD, PhD, writing for the Working Group on Accountability, has identified eight widely endorsed content areas and specific criteria for monitoring accountability in ethical conduct. The eight areas were developed from traditional codes, from recent statements by medical bodies and from consensus among the members of the Working Group on Accountability. The eight categories, including some of the specific assessable items listed under them, for use in physician, group, and institutional report cards are:

1. Medical decision making
   Decisions on life-sustaining intervention
   Decisions on participation in research
2. Confidentiality
   Physician knowledge and standards in confidentiality
   Precautions taken to preserve confidentiality
3. Fiduciary obligations
   Disclosure of conflict of interest policy
   Limits on conflicting incentives
4. Responsibilities arising from patient vulnerability
   Patient representatives or ombudsperson
   Human subjects research policies
5. Practitioner's personal standards
   Disclosure of training level
6. Equity
   Service to the under- and uninsured
   Allocation of resources decisions
7. Cultural representation
   Training in cultural representation
   Translation services
8. Procedures for resolving dilemmas
   Consultations in ethics
   Ethics committees
   Patient access to the above-mentioned and related resources
   Patient representative[17]

Although the Working Group notes the need for improved assessment measures, it identifies some methods for assessing conduct on the basis of the above categories, such as surveys among all involved parties, the testing methods used for accreditation, and limited audits. The authors endorse a two-step use of composite assessments on ethical practice: (1) as feedback information for internal adjustments within an organization, and (2) for consumer information.

Professional guidelines, like the AMA and Woodstock Reports, ensure that traditional medical values inform the new professional roles and responses to the ethical challenges of managed care. Report cards and measurable standards for accountability on ethics, developed through careful ethical reflection and analysis, ensure that the moral dimensions of health care delivery are recognized and part of the criteria used to measure quality care. Once criteria like the eight listed above have been adopted by an organization or professional group, then the process of refinement can proceed with surveys, discussion forums, and feedback and adjustment mechanisms.[17] As Arnold Relman, MD, then editor of *The New England Journal of Medicine* noted in 1988, The Era of Assessment and Accountability is dawning at last; it is the third and latest—but probably not the last—phase of our efforts to achieve an equitable health care system, of satisfactory quality, at a price we can afford."[18] Assessment and accountability on ethical values and behavior are critical for achieving these goals.

Organizational Medical Ethics

An organizational approach to ethics is based on the recognition that organizations and institutions "have ethical lives and characters just as their individual members do, and that (I)ndividual decision makers increasingly are being supplanted by the rules, standards, traditions, and collective decision process of organizations."[19] The focus is on the the role of the organization itself in fostering humaneness in the relationships and environment of the workplace.[19] The Joint Commission on the Accreditation of Healthcare Organizations (JCAHO) recognized the impact of an organization's behavior and business practices with the inclusion of a section on organizational ethics standards in the *1996 Comprehensive Accreditation Manual for Hospitals*.[20]

An organizational ethic begins with the formulation of an organization's or group's core values and mission statement. In the past, organizational mission statements were often not taken seriously, but ethicist Laurence O Connell, PhD, president and CEO of the Park Ridge Center for the Study of Faith and Ethics, has observed that in the current unsettled moral climate and with the great upheaval in the health care industry, health care organizations are now developing these ethical guidelines as much for themselves as the marketplace. It's an exercise in self-understanding.[21]

A six-year research project at the Stanford University Graduate School of Business suggests that it is this self-understanding and the articulation of core values and a core purpose that distinguishes companies and organizations with enduring success from others. "The dynamic of preserving the core while stimulating progress is the reason that companies . . . became elite institutions able to renew themselves and achieve superior longer-term performance," as James C. Collins and Jerry I. Porras note.[22]

Their research points to the critical importance of identifying an organization's core values (usually between three and five), which must stand the test of time, and its core purpose, which is a statement of its reason for being. Identifying an organization's shared core values is a process that works from the individual to the organization. People involved in articulating core values need to answer several questions: What core values do you personally bring to your work? These should be so fundamental that you would hold them regardless of whether or not they were rewarded. What would you tell your children are the core values that you hold at work and that you hope they will hold when they become working adults?[22]

For a health care organization, additional questions might identify values particular to organizations that deliver care to patients. Two of the values pertinent to health care organizations described by bioethicist Stanley Reiser are humaneness, a sense of benevolence to people in general and compassion for people in need, and trust, confidence in the integrity and reliability of individuals.[19]

Once formulated, values statements or missions must be incorporated into the day-to-day interactions within the institution. In addition to educational programs and leadership training, Reiser proposes administrative case rounds, similar to the medical case round model used in medical schools, in which cases featuring organizational issues about patient care or business-related issues such as marketing, patient billing, or computerized patient data are addressed from an organization's value-based perspective. Cases illuminating the relationships and actions of organizations can be used to test how effectively the values in institutional statements of purpose are applied in practice, to formulate and critique policies and goals, to analyze troublesome problems, and to create an institutional memory to guide future policies, explains Reiser.[19] He cites the need for research to explore other ways to connect values and actions within an organization.

In addition to internal ethical issues, organizational issues arising under managed care also include the MCO's responsibility to conduct research that can be shared with the larger medical community, and the organization's responsibility to the geographical community where it exists, particularly for traditional public health services.

■ Conclusion

The transition to managed care represents a profound change for the practice of medicine and presents significant ethical challenges. Medical ethics must broaden its focus to the health care organization and to new ethical obligations of providers to the health care plan, to the other patients in the plan, and to society at large, as well as to new obligations of providers to their individual patients about disclosure and financial aspects of care.

The emphasis in current ethical guidelines on managed care is on honesty, disclosure, and accountability. With teams of professionals in an MCO involved in patient care, future guidelines on ethics must give greater attention to principled organizational management and the processes of collective decision making to ensure sensitivity to the ethical dimensions of measurement tools, clinical practice guidelines, and complex professional relationships. The development of assessment tools on ethical behavior of organizations and professionals is important for accountability.

Achieving managed care's goals of equality of access, responsible cost-containment, and effective quality assurance will require honesty and fidelity—the same virtues embodied in the doctor–patient relationship.[23]

We shall not cease from exploration
And the end of all our exploring
Will be to arrive where we started
And know the place for the first time.

T. S. Eliot, *Four Quartets*[22]

REFERENCES

1. Peeno L. The dirty work of managed care. *AAO-HNS Bulletin* 1996(Oct):32–33.
2. Beauchamp T, Childress J. *Principles of biomedical ethics* 1994. New York: Oxford University Press.
3. Health Insurance Association of America. *Sourcebook of Health Insurance Data,* 1993. Washington, DC:HIAA, 1994, pp. 13–14.
4. Parker C. Practice guidelines and private insurers. *J Law Medic Ethics* 1995;13:57–61.
5. Puma JL, Schiedermayer D. Ethical issues in managed care and managed competition: Problems and promises. In Nash DB, The physician's guide to managed care. 1994. Gaithersburg, MD: Aspen Publishers, Inc., pp. 31–62.
6. Redman BK. Clinical practice guidelines as tools of public policy: Conflicts of purpose, issues of autonomy and justice. *J Clin Ethics* 1994;5(4):303–309.
7. Havighurst CC. Practice guidelines for medical care: The policy rationale. *Saint Louis Univ Law J* 1990;34:777–819.
8. Omnibus Budget Reconciliation Act of 1989. Pub. L. No. 101-239, 6103, 103 Stat. 2189 (1989).
9. Fang, E, Mittman BS, Weingarten S. Use of clinical practice guidelines in managed care physician groups. *Arch Fam Med* 1996;5:328–331.
10. Page L. State legislators spent busy year trying to manage managed care. *Am Med News.* September 9, 1996:6–8.
11. Bodenheimer T. The HMO backlash—righteous or reactionary? *N Engl J Med* 1996;335(21):1601–1604.
12. Faden R, Geller G, Powers M, eds. *AIDS, women and the next generation.* 1991. New York: Oxford University Press, p. 15.
13. Mariner WK. Patient's rights after health care reform: Who decides what is medically necessary? *Am J Public Health* 1994;84(9):1515–1520.
14. Council on Ethical and Judicial Affairs, American Medical Association. Ethical issues in managed care. *JAMA* 1995; 273(4): 330, 334.
15. Woodstock Theological Center. Ethical considerations in the business aspects of health care 1995. Washington, DC: Georgetown University Press, 21.
16. Emanuel E, Emanuel L: What is accountability in health care? *Ann Intern Med.* 1996 (Jan 15); 124:229.
17. Emanuel L. for the Working Group on Accountability. A professional response to demands for accountability: Practical recommendations regarding ethical aspects of patient care. *Ann Intern Med.* 1996 (Jan. 15); 124:243, 244.

18. Relman A. Assessment and accountability. *N Engl J Med* 1988; 11; 319:1220.
19. Reiser S. The ethical life of health care organizations. Hastings Center Report 24, no. 6(1994); 28, 31, 34.
20. Joint Commission for Accreditation of Healthcare Organizations. Patient Rights and Organization Ethics. *1996 Comprehensive Accreditation Manual for Hospitals,* 1996.
21. Appleby C. True values. *Hospitals and Health Networks,* July 5, 1995, 20, 22.
22. Collins J, Porras J: Building your company's vision. *Harvard Bus Rev,* September–October 1996; 65, 68.
23. Nash D., p. 54.

Carl A. Patow, M.D., M.P.H., F.A.C.S. is Associate Professor of Otolaryngology-Head and Neck Surgery at the Johns Hopkins University School of Medicine and Medical Director of an MCO, the Johns Hopkins HealthCare Employee Health Plan. He has served as a senior evaluator for the Malcolm Baldrige National Quality Award of the U.S. Department of Commerce. He also serves on the Ear, Nose and Throat Devices Advisory Panel of the Food and Drug Administration. From 1991 to 1993, he was the founding director of the Continuous Quality Improvement Council at Walter Reed Army Medical Center where he served as Assistant Chief of the Department of Otolaryngology. He has written and lectured extensively on quality measurement and ethics in medicine and surgery. As a practicing surgeon, an expert in quality assessment, and medical director of a regional MCO, he brings a unique perspective to the discussion of ethics in managed care.

Ruth D. Gaare, J.D., M.P.H., is program director of the Johns Hopkins University Bioethics Institute and the Greenwall Fellowship Program in Bioethics and Health Policy and teaches in the area of ethics, law, and health care business and management. She is member of the Johns Hopkins Hospital Ethics Committee and co-chair of its Subcommittee on Managed Care, and a member of the Johns Hopkins Health Care Advisory Committee and the School of Public Health's Committee on Managed Care. Ms. Gaare, who serves as a consultant to numerous organizations on ethical and organizational issues in managed care, is currently working with the State of Maryland to develop an ombudsmen program for its Medicaid Managed Care Program. She is also involved in a number of research projects on managed care and public health, and on patient care at the end of life.

Ms. Gaare has been coeditor with James Childress of *BioLaw,* a publication on law, ethics, and health care, since 1985 and an adjunct professor in philosophy at Loyola College, where she teaches undergraduate and professional development courses. For more than ten years Ms. Gaare has worked with hospitals and health care organizations to train health care professionals, ethics committees, and ethics consultants. Her education includes a law degree from the University of Virginia, a Master's of Public Health degree from Johns Hopkins, and certificates in mediation and conflict resolution from Boston University and Harvard University School of Public Health.

■ SECTION TWO ■

Utilizing Outcomes in a Managed Care Environment

8

Outcomes Research: Where We Have Been, Where We Need to Go

MICHAEL G. STEWART

■ Overview of Outcomes Research

In the field of health services research, the delivery of health care has been divided into three stages: structure, process, and outcome.[1] *Structure* refers to the "inputs" into the system, such as patients and providers, *process* refers to what is done to the patient, and *outcome* refers to the consequences to the health and well-being of the patient. Although initial efforts in health services research focused on the process of health care, outcomes assessment has become increasingly important. Outcomes include classical clinical endpoints—such as morbidity and mortality, pure-tone hearing threshold, respiratory disturbance index, and so on—or *expanded* measures of clinical outcome, including quality of life, functional or performance status, and patient satisfaction.

Quality of Life

Quality of life implies more than just the absence of disease or illness. Although there is no standard definition for quality of life (QOL), most researchers agree that QOL is both *subjective* and *multidimensional*.[2] In other words, QOL cannot be assessed without directly asking the patient for their perspective (e.g., subjective). In addition, a patient's QOL depends on several underlying domains or constructs, such as physical, emotional, mental, and social well-being (e.g., multidimensional).

Functional Status

Functional status, also known as "performance status," refers to the patient's ability to perform typical daily activities, such as physical activity, eating, and so on.[3] Although some investigators have used the terminology "quality of life" interchangeably with functional status, quality of life is a more global concept and should not be confused with functional status.[4] Many researchers refer to "disease-specific" functional status when describing the functional deficits caused by a particular disease process, such as visual loss or hearing loss.[5,6]

Comorbidity

The term "comorbidity" was coined by Dr. Alvan Feinstein to describe the presence of an additional disease process—other than the disease of interest—that may affect prognosis and/or treatment.[7,8] For instance, severe coronary heart disease would be an important comorbid factor affecting potential treatment options for conductive hearing loss, and immunodeficiency would be an important comorbid factor affecting treatment prognosis for chronic sinusitis.

Outcomes Assessment

A key theme in outcomes research is that QOL and performance status should be measured from the *patient's perspective.* This is typically accomplished through the use of *instruments,* or surveys, which are collections of individual *items,* or questions. The use of family members or health care providers as proxies to complete instruments in place of the patient is generally discouraged since bias may be introduced.[9] The assessment of health status in pediatrics is an obvious exception, since proxies are often necessary. Instruments to assess QOL and performance status must be both *valid* and *reliable.* Validity refers to an instrument's ability to measure what it purports to measure, and reliability refers to the dependability of an instrument. High levels of systematic error in assessment lead to low validity, and high levels of random error lead to low reliability. In other words, if an instrument is designed to measure disease-specific functional status in chronic sinusitis, then scores should (1) correlate with the severity of sinusitis (e.g., validity), and (2) not change when the severity of sinusitis does not change (e.g., reliability).

Disease-specific versus Global Instruments

There is evidence that disease-specific instruments are more sensitive to functional handicaps caused by a given disease—and to changes in functional status after treatment—than are global (or "generic") instruments.[5,10] Global instruments, however, have the advantage of being comparable across disease states so they can be used to "benchmark" for the relative impact or effect of a disease state on functional status or QOL. Since both generic and disease-specific instruments have distinct advantages, some authors recommend using both disease-specific *and* generic instruments when assessing clinical outcomes.[5,6,10] Other techniques include using only specific items from a generic instrument that are applicable to a given disease, or rewording generic items to apply to specific diseases (e.g., "*because of my hearing loss . . .* ?").[6]

Quality of Life Instruments

Interest in quality of life assessment has increased dramatically in recent years. A recent bibliography listed well over 1000 reported QOL instruments in the cumulative index, with more than 160 new instruments reported in 1993 alone.[11] The Medical Outcomes Trust (Boston), a nonprofit organization with worldwide membership, has developed an instrument review process utilizing a Scientific Advisory Committee of noted experts in outcomes research. Using strict criteria for instrument content, reliability, validity, responsiveness, interpretability, and respondent burden, the Trust has released a list of "approved" instruments (Table 8–1). The criteria used for instrument evaluation have also been published.[12]

Among the approved instruments is the SF-36 ("short form—36 items"), which is also one of the most widely used global QOL instruments in the United States. The SF-36 was developed to survey health-related QOL for the Medical Outcomes Study, a large multicenter prospective study designed to study variations in physician's practice patterns.[13] The SF-36 is divided into eight multi-item subscales: (1) physical functioning, (2) social functioning, (3) general health, (4) mental health, (5) role functioning due to physical problems, (6) role functioning due to emotional problems, (7) vitality, and (8) bodily pain. The SF-36 was designed for self-administration, telephone administration, or administration with a personal interview. The SF-36 is reliable and valid for comparisons of *group* data rather than individual patient data, and its responsiveness to change in clinical status is adequate. There is no overall sum-total score for the SF-36; instead, each subscale is scored individually. In addition, the SF-36 is relatively easy for patients to complete. The SF-36 has been used to assess the QOL of patients with several chronic medical conditions as well as otolaryngologic conditions,[14,15] and baseline data exists for multiple disease processes. In fact, much of the appeal of the SF-36 lies in the availability of comparison data and its widespread use and acceptance.

TABLE 8–1. Quality of Life Instruments approved by the Medical Outcomes Trust

- Quality of Well-Being Scale
- SF-36 Health Survey United States (English)
- Sickness Impact Profile
- SF-12 Health Survey
- London Handicap Scale
- SF-36 Health Survey United Kingdom (English)
- SF-36 Health Survey Germany (German)
- SF-36 Health Survey Sweden (Swedish)

One important caveat in the use of all QOL instruments—including the SF-36—is that a patient's self-assessment of quality of life is always made against some subjective "internal baseline." In other words, an elderly wheelchair-bound subject will likely have a different baseline perception of acceptable QOL than a healthy middle-aged marathon runner. Therefore an identical illness, such as acute sinusitis, may yield quite different decrements in QOL by our two hypothetical subjects. In addition to subjective differences in baseline QOL, the presence of comorbid diseases will certainly effect self-assessed QOL, so care should be taken when interpreting the "impact" of a given illness on QOL.

Types of Outcomes Research

The history of outcomes research and the methodologic requirements for conducting different types of outcomes research were very well delineated by Piccirillo[8] who identified four methodologic requirements for conducting outcomes research: establishment of diagnostic criteria for a given disease, creation of a clinical severity index, identification of prognostically important comorbid factors, and development of outcome measures that include clinical endpoints, functional status, and QOL. With these requirements in mind, we can classify the outcomes studies that have been performed to date in otolaryngology.

Other types of health services research related to outcomes research include studies of geographic variation in health care utilization and "appropriateness studies." The technique used in appropriateness studies involves development of a group of appropriate indications for a given intervention by a consensus panel of experts, followed by chart or large database review with ranking of the appropriateness of utilization by a review board—using the indications and criteria defined by the expert panel. Since patient satisfaction is also an outcome of medical care, studies that assess patient satisfaction can be considered outcomes research.

■ Outcomes Research: Where We Have Been

Geographic Variation

Dr. John Wennberg is considered one of the fathers of outcomes research because of his seminal investigations into geographic differences in health care utilization as well as his later work on the impact of benign prostatic hypertrophy on QOL. Using epidemiological techniques to compare small neighboring communities in Maine, Wennberg noted that the rate of tonsillectomies performed per eligible population varied widely: tonsillectomies were performed in the "highest rate" area almost *three times* more frequently than in the "lowest rate" area.[16] Incidentally, Wennberg has noted similar rates of variation between other surgical procedures with subjective indications, such as hysterectomy, prostatectomy, and hemorrhoidectomy.[17] Wennberg noted further that despite seeming agreement among specialists on appropriate indications for surgery, these differences persisted. Dr. David Wennberg performed a recent update of the analysis of tonsillectomy rates in Maine, and also noted significant differences in rates between metropolitan areas.[18]

Appropriateness Studies

The first major appropriateness study undertaken in otolaryngology generated significant controversy. Kleinman and colleagues used an established technique (described earlier) to assess the appropriateness of tympanostomy tubes in children less than 16 years of age in the United States.[19] The authors concluded that 42% of tympanostomies proposed were appropriate, 35% were equivocal, and 23% were inappropriate—based on a review algorithm and appropriateness criteria developed by a multidisciplinary expert panel. The authors did not have data on whether or not the children actually underwent tube surgery; these were procedures proposed to third party payors for precertification.

This article generated a tremendous amount of controversy, including no fewer than 11 published letters to the editor in JAMA and an editorial by the editor-in-chief of the *Archives of Otolaryngology—Head & Neck Surgery*. Several criticisms were raised. First, the initial step in the review process was a telephone interview concerning indications for surgery with "a member of the physician's office staff," who had the patient's office chart available for review. This was felt by many to be an inadequate method for assessing the full clinical history in children with protracted otologic problems. Second, there was significant disagreement among members of the expert panel on several appropriateness criteria, and the technique of assigning a "median appropriateness rating" was felt to be somewhat arbitrary. Further, two members of the expert panel felt that the contemporary clinical literature had not been considered strongly enough during appropriateness rating. Despite this disagreement among noted experts on indications for surgery, the authors reported their findings as exact percentages with narrow 95% confidence intervals, implying a high degree of precision—which was actually not present in the process. Third, the best possible appropriateness rating for children with recurrent acute otitis media was "equivocal," and this was in children with a high frequency of infections, and breakthrough otitis media while on antibiotic prophylaxis. In addition, a significant conflict-of-interest point was raised because the review was developed and performed by a for-profit utilization review corporation; potentially, such a company might have a primary motivation of finding care inappropriate and therefore reducing costs for a contracting third party payer. In summary, although the findings of this article generated much worthwhile discussion, the reviewers were probably unable to obtain all the relevant clinical information needed on which to base a decision on medical appropriateness. Although it is likely that some proportion of tympanostomy tubes proposed by physicians may be for equivocal or inappropriate indications, this is likely overstated by the article.

A similar study, using the same techniques for appropriateness rating, was performed in patients proposed for sinus surgery at one institution.[20] The authors found that 44% of cases were rated appropriate, 40% uncertain, and 16% inappropriate; surgery for chronic sinusitis was more likely to be found appropriate than surgery for recurrent acute sinusitis. The authors noted that office chart documentation was often incomplete, which led to an "uncertain" rating for appropriateness on several occasions. The authors noted that the decision algorithm developed for sinus surgery seemed easy to use and clinically appropriate.

Clinical Severity Staging System

Clinical staging of disease severity for prognostication has been an important part of the clinician's armamentarium for many years. The APGAR score for newborn babies, the Glasgow coma scale, the American Society of Anesthesiologists (ASA) preanesthesia risk score, and the TNM tumor stage are examples of some of the best known staging systems. Significant work has been accomplished in this area.

A recent literature review by Piccirillo of existing outcomes research studies in otolaryngology between 1992 and 1995 yielded 68 articles related to clinical severity staging.[21] The majority of these articles (54 of 68) were related to head and neck cancer, and the vast majority of those used mortality and local control as the outcomes of interest. In other words, most research efforts were directed toward stratification of patients to predict cancer control and mortality—rather than using QOL or functional status as outcomes of interest. In addition, most oncologic staging systems are based only on the *anatomic* extent of tumor, and no other clinical variables (such as weight loss, tumor growth rate, etc.) are considered.

An important contribution to clinical severity staging in head and neck cancer was made by Piccirillo et al. who added pertinent clinical variables to the TNM system in patients with laryngeal cancer.[22] Using their improved staging system, the authors were able to increase the accuracy of prognostic stratification for laryngeal cancer patients over the TNM stage alone. Similarly, Piccirillo included comorbidity data with anatomic tumor data for patients with laryngeal cancer and was able to improve prognostication over the TNM system alone.[23] In fact, using Piccirillo's system, patients with Stage I cancer and the presence of comorbidity had worse 5-year survival than patients with Stage IV cancer and no comorbidity.

Using similar techniques and data collected from a multicenter, prospective observational outcomes protocol for obstructive sleep apnea syndrome (OSAS), which was supported by the American Academy of Otolaryngology-Head & Neck Surgery, Piccirillo and colleagues were able to develop a clinical severity staging system for OSAS.[24] The authors used a sophisticated statistical technique called conjunctive consolidation (a type of multivariable analysis) to combine physical examination variables, sleep study variables, and the Epworth Sleepiness Scale score to create a clinical severity index that appears to have better prognostic accuracy than either sleep study data alone or clinician rating of severity. Further data analysis is still in process on this large database at the time of this writing (J. Piccirillo, MD, written communication, June 1996).

Meta-analysis

The concept behind meta-analysis is to combine the data from multiple clinical trials and use the statistical power of the large sample from combined studies to answer clinical questions that may be difficult or controversial with smaller sample sizes. Although this may not sound difficult, meta-analysis is actually a very sophisticated type of clinical epidemiology that requires significant statistical expertise. The technique of meta-analysis has been used several times in otolaryngology.

Rosenfeld and Post analyzed the efficacy of antibiotics in otitis media with effusion (OME) and found that antibiotics had a clinically and statistically significant impact on the resolution of OME.[25] Rosenfeld et al. also studied the use of systemic steroids for OME in children.[26] The authors found that the pooled reported studies favored the use of steroids, but the small number of studies in the literature raised the possibility of publication bias (e.g., studies without significant results—null results—are likely not published and therefore the data is not available for analysis), and suggested that additional study was warranted.

Garcia et al. analyzed topical antibiotic prophylaxis for post-tympanostomy otorrhea,[27] and found that the pooled studies favored the use of topical drops to reduce the prevalence of otorrhea. Williams et al. studied antibiotics used to (1) prevent recurrent acute otitis media and (2) treat otitis media with effusion.[28] The authors found small but significant beneficial effects of antibiotics in both cases. The authors also noted that most studies failed to identify potential confounding variables, and that most studies were unable to predict which groups of patients were most likely to benefit from antibiotic therapy.

Snyderman and D'Amico analyzed the use of carotid artery resection for malignant disease[29] and found no difference in survival curves between patients with advanced neck disease treated with carotid resection and patients treated with irradiation. Seventeen percent of patients who underwent carotid resection had a major neurological complication.

Sher et al. analyzed the results of surgical treatment of obstructive sleep apnea syndrome.[30] The authors found that uvulopalatopharyngoplasty was effective at treating less than 50% of patients with obstructive sleep apnea, although patients with less severe apnea had a higher probability of significant improvement.

Disease-Specific Instruments

As discussed earlier, disease-specific instruments are often necessary in otolaryngology to adequately assess the effects of treatment on disease-specific functional status. Fortunately, several validated instruments are available in otolaryngology, which are listed in Table 8–2. Although

TABLE 8–2. Selection of Validated Disease-specific Instruments Applicable to Otolaryngology

Name	*Application*	*Primary Author*
Hearing Status		
Hearing Handicap Inventory for the Elderly (HHIE)	Hearing loss—elderly	Ventry[67]
Hearing Handicap Inventory for Adults (HHIA)	Hearing loss	Newman[68]
Abbreviated Profile of Hearing Aid Benefit (APHAB)	Hearing aid satisfaction	Cox[69]
Hearing Aid Performance Inventory (HAPI)	Hearing aid satisfaction	Walden[70]
Hearing Satisfaction Scale (HSS)	Hearing loss	Stewart[71]
Hearing Evaluation and Auditory Rehabilitation (HEAR-14)	Hearing loss	Piccirillo[72]
Dizziness/vertigo		
Dizziness Handicap Inventory (DHI)	Dizziness	Jacobson[73]
Tinnitus		
Tinnitus Handicap Questionnaire	Tinnitus	Kuk[74]
Rhinosinusitis		
Chronic Sinusitis Survey (CSS)	Chronic sinusitis	Gliklich[15]
Rhinosinusitis Outcome Measure (RSOM-31)	Rhinosinusitis	Piccirillo[75]
Rhinoconjunctivitis Quality of Life Questionnaire (RQLQ)	Rhinitis/conjunctivitis	Juniper[76]
Head & Neck Cancer		
Functional Assessment of Cancer Therapy with Head & Neck module (FACT-HN)	H & N cancer	Cella[77]
University of Washington Quality of Life Questionnaire (UW QOL)	H & N cancer	Hassan & Weymuller[78]
Performance Status Scale-Head & Neck (PSS-HN)	H & N cancer	List[79]
European Organization for Research on the Treatment of Cancer (EORTC)	H & N cancer	Bjordal[80]
Head and Neck Radiotherapy Questionnaire	H & N radiotherapy	Browman[81]
Comprehensive Head and Neck Questionnaire	H & N cancer	Morton[82]
Voice		
Voice Handicap Inventory	Voice	Jacobson[83]
Treatment Benefit		
Glasgow Benefit Inventory	General benefit	Robinson[84]

all instruments included in the figure have been validated at least partially, the reader is encouraged to carefully review the reference article to ensure that a given instrument is appropriate for its intended use.

Retrospective, Cross-sectional and Prospective Studies

Several studies in otolaryngology have assessed QOL, functional status, or both. Many different techniques for data collection have been utilized, including retrospective, cross-sectional, and prospective designs, both with and without controls, or some combination of techniques. Instead of grouping studies by methodology, they are grouped together loosely by disease process in the following section.

Hearing Aid Benefit

In a study designed to measure the association between QOL and sensory impairment in elderly individuals living at home in Italy, single sensory impairments (either visual loss or hearing loss) were significantly and independently associated with increased risk for depression and decreased self-sufficiency in activities of daily living.[31] A more extensive study ($n = 1192$) of a similar group of elderly subjects in Italy demonstrated that patients with hearing loss who did *not* wear a hearing aid had significantly lower scores on a QOL instrument than subjects with hearing loss who *did* wear an aid.[32] In a study of elderly veterans in San Antonio, hearing loss was associated with significant emotional, social, and communication dysfunction.[33] Disease-specific instruments were more sensitive at detecting these changes than generic QOL instruments.

The same authors then performed another study: they randomly assigned patients with hearing loss to either receive a hearing aid or be placed on a waiting list.[34] A battery of disease-specific and generic instruments was administered at baseline, 6 weeks and 4 months. At baseline the two groups did not differ in demographic characteristics, disease-specific functional status, or generic QOL. The authors found significant improvements at 4 months in social and emotional function, communication and cognitive function, and depression in the group given a hearing aid when compared to the group on the waiting list.

Cochlear Implant Benefit

Harris et al. studied 9 adult patients who underwent cochlear implantation by administering a QOL instrument (the Quality of Well-being Scale) and instruments to assess depression and satisfaction with life, and measuring audiologic function and personal income from pretreatment to 3 years posttreatment.[35] The authors found that scores on the global QOL instrument and depression scale improved significantly and that personal income also increased during the postoperative period. A cost-benefit analysis performed by the authors found that the cost of the cochlear implant per well-year was $31,711, which compared favorably to other procedures that also improve QOL, such as total hip replacement and 2-vessel coronary artery bypass.

Dizziness/Vertigo

Grimby and Rosenhall studied elderly subjects living at home in Sweden using a disease-specific questionnaire to assess symptoms and severity of dizziness, and the Nottingham Health Profile (NHP) to assess global QOL.[36] The authors found that subjects who reported dizziness had lower scores on virtually all QOL dimensions than subjects who did not. Of note, subjects with dizziness also had a higher prevalence of comorbid illnesses. Fielder et al. used the Dizziness Handicap Inventory and the SF-36 to assess disease-specific functional status and global QOL in a group of British patients referred to a specialist for dizziness.[37] The authors found that three subscale mean scores on the SF-36 (role functioning-physical, vitality, and pain) were lower in the dizzy patients than normative population means. In addition, the DHI score correlated significantly with all 8 SF-36 subscale scores. The authors did not address the presence of comorbid conditions.

Chronic Sinusitis

Several noted rhinologists have reported subjective patient-based outcomes after the treatment of chronic sinusitis with endoscopic sinus surgery.[38,39] Most of these reports have used retrospective surveys that asked some variant of the following question: "Compared to how you felt before surgery, would you say you are . . . much improved, somewhat improved, etc?" Most authors have found that the majority of patients reported that they were improved after surgery, with very few reporting that they were worse.

The first attempt to prospectively assess outcomes in chronic sinusitis using a disease-specific health status instrument was performed by Hoffman et al. before and after endoscopic sinus surgery.[40] The authors noted significant improvement in patients' symptoms after sinus surgery. Unfortunately, however, although the instrument used was designed by a panel of noted experts, no data on validity or test-retest reliability were available, making the results difficult to interpret.

Gliklich and Metson have systematically assessed outcomes after endoscopic sinus surgery. They first assessed baseline generic QOL, using the SF-36, in a group of patients with proven chronic sinusitis.[41] The same authors then developed and validated a disease-specific instrument for chronic sinusitis: the Chronic Sinusitis Survey.[15] Subsequently, they used the Chronic Sinusitis Survey and the SF-36 to longitudinally assess changes in disease-specific health status and global QOL in a group of patients undergoing endoscopic sinus surgery.[42] The authors found that disease-specific scale scores increased significantly after surgery; SF-36 scores also improved, but did not return to the values seen in disease-free subjects.

In addition, Metson and Gliklich have studied computed tomography staging systems used in chronic sinusitis.[43] Using multiple readers on two separate occasions, the authors were able to assess the sensitivity, comprehensiveness, and both intra- and inter-rater reliability of several staging systems. The authors concluded that the Harvard and Lund systems were the most reliable, but the Harvard system was somewhat easier to use.

Rosenfeld performed a pilot longitudinal outcomes study in pediatric chronic sinusitis using a "stepped" treatment approach.[44] The primary outcome measure was an oral survey of disease-specific symptoms and overall QOL. The author noted that caregiver expectations of symptom and QOL improvement were exceeded more frequently in children who underwent endoscopic sinus surgery than in those who underwent medical therapy and/or adenoidectomy only. In his discussion, the author pointed out some potential limitations of the study, including the lack of psychometric validation of the instrument used, relatively small sample size, and potential treatment and investigator biases. Despite these limitations, however, this was an important study because the author was able to (1) achieve a 100% follow-up rate, and (2) incorporate outcomes assessment into routine clinical practice. It was also significant because the "stepped" protocol more closely resembles the actual practice of medicine than a randomized trial.

Head and Neck Cancer

One of the first studies to address QOL in laryngeal cancer was the so-called "fireman" study by McNeil et al.[45] The authors interviewed 37 healthy volunteers (12 firefighters and 25 executives) and asked for their preferences on survival and voice preservation using the time-tradeoff technique of utility analysis. Basically, this technique attempts to capture the importance of a given health state by asking the subject questions similar to the following: "If your life expectancy was 25 years, and you were going to have a laryngectomy and artificial speech, how many years of survival would you give up to maintain your normal voice?" Subjects were also asked questions to determine how *risk-aversive* they were. For example, if they had a choice of normal life for X number of years versus a coin flip that would determine either full-life expectancy or death within a few months, subjects who were risk averse would choose to give up a few years of survival to avoid the risk of the coin flip. Using known probabilities of survival for T3 laryngeal cancer, and subjects' attitudes about overall survival and voice preservation, the authors constructed utility curves for survival with normal and artificial speech. In their group of subjects, the authors calculated that the utility of 10 years of survival with normal speech was equivalent to seven years of survival with artificial speech. Furthermore, the authors estimated that 20 percent of subjects would choose a treatment to preserve their larynx, even if it meant potentially shorter survival.

This landmark article played an important role in raising the consciousness of physicians toward QOL issues in treatment selection by patients with laryngeal cancer. However, some important weaknesses of the study deserve discussion. First, the subjects were played tapes of patients using esophageal speech as a way of educating them on the relative quality of artificial speech after laryngectomy; subjects were not educated on use of the electrolarynx or the tracheo-esophageal puncture as techniques for alaryngeal speech. Further, patients who were treated with full-course radiation therapy were assumed to have "normal" voices after treatment, and clinical experience suggests that many patients experience some decrement in voice quality after radiation therapy.

In addition, because the authors studied healthy, active subjects, an important philosophical point should be considered. Many authors agree that the expected value—or utility—of a given health state may be considered quite differently by healthy subjects and subjects with disease, or by patients before and after a disease is diagnosed. Consider the following example. A healthy person is asked a series of questions to estimate the change in QOL that would be caused by chronic hemodialysis. Next, a patient with renal failure who is on chronic dialysis is asked a series of questions to estimate the change in QOL caused by the dialysis. The two values (utilities) would likely be different, since the patient with renal failure perceives the dialysis—however unpleasant—as a treatment which is keeping the person alive. This phenomenon has been studied explicitly by cognitive psychologists and is termed the "framing of decisions" by Tversky.[46] Tversky noted that the value-utility plots for gains and losses are actually not straight lines but curves, which are sloped differently depending on the frame of reference of the subject. For instance, subjects faced with a potential loss would exaggerate the negative effects of a *certain* loss compared to a probable loss. Which perspective is *more* important—that of a group of healthy people or a group of patients with disease—is an extremely important question to be grappled with by ethicists and policymakers. From an outcomes research standpoint, the important issue is that the perspectives are, in fact, different.

In addition, the way questions are phrased has a significant impact on the decisions made by healthy subjects. For instance, if identical probabilities are proposed to subjects but asked in two different ways (chance of *survival* and chance of *death*) subjects will make different decisions even though the probabilities are identical.[47] These complicated and emotional issues surrounding medical decision making, cognitive psychology, and loss of such a personal characteristic as the voice, make the results of the "fireman" study difficult to interpret conclusively. Nevertheless, this article has served an important role in defining the importance of QOL assessment in the treatment of laryngeal cancer.

Mohide et al. compared the relative importance of QOL dimensions as ranked by post-laryngectomy patients and health care professionals.[48] The authors found that the relative importance of dimensions differed significantly between the two groups. Health care professionals ranked communication impairment and self-image/self-esteem as the two most important dimensions, but patients identified communication as only the third most important dimension and self-image/self-esteem as the seventh most important. Post-laryngectomy patients ranked physical consequences and interference with social activities as the two most important QOL dimensions.

Plante et al. used the technique of decision analysis to assess treatment options in pyriform sinus carcinoma.[49] The authors used available data for morbidity rates and length of survival, but were forced to use estimates for decrement in QOL after various treatment interventions. After sensitivity analysis—changing the values of variables to assess the effects on quality-adjusted survival—the authors concluded that QOL issues were important variables for consideration when planning treatment.

Several authors have performed cross-sectional assessments of QOL after treatment of head and neck cancer. Jones et al. used the EORTC to assess QOL in a diverse group of head and neck cancer patients from Great Britain.[50] Ackerstaff et al. assessed communication, functional disorders, and lifestyle changes after total laryngectomy in a group of laryngectomees from the Netherlands.[51] Bjordal et al. used the EORTC to assess QOL[52] as well as psychological distress[53] in Norwegian patients who were cured of head and neck cancer 7 to 11 years after treatment. DeSanto et al. assessed QOL after laryngectomy in a group of patients from the United States who had undergone both total and near-total laryngectomy.[54] Harrison et al. used the PSS-HN to assess the performance status of patients who had undergone either primary surgery or primary radiation therapy at Memorial Sloan Kettering Cancer Center for base of tongue cancer.[55] Of course, these studies only assessed survivors, and there is always the possibility of nonresponse bias (e.g., extremely satisfied or dissatisfied patients, or those with recurrent or metastatic disease, may not respond to the questionnaires).

Several authors have also prospectively studied changes in QOL after treatment of head and neck cancer. Languis et al. studied QOL and functional status before and after treatment of oral cavity and pharyngeal cancer in a group of Swedish patients.[56] The authors found very large individual differences in self-assessed functional status, as well as a high study drop-out rate, which made interpretation of group data difficult. Morton prospectively studied the general life satisfaction of a group of patients in New Zealand with head and neck cancer.[57] The author noted poor follow-up compliance, but of the patients who were followed through to study completion (24 months after treatment) the group mean life satisfaction score had improved. In addition, high levels of pretreatment life satisfaction predicted higher levels of posttreatment life satisfaction. List et al. prospectively studied performance status and QOL using several instruments (the PSS-HN, the Karnofsky scale, and the FACT-HN) in a group of laryngeal cancer patients from the United States.[58] The authors found that performance status scores generally showed significant improvement after treatment. Although the QOL scores trended toward improvement, statistical significance was not achieved. The authors also found that both ability to speak and ability to eat were *not* correlated with overall QOL.

Cost-effectiveness Research

Wyatt et al. used a decision analysis model to assess the cost effectiveness of cochlear implantation in postlingually deaf adults.[59] The authors calculated the cost per quality-adjusted life-year (QALY), which is a widely used technique for assessing the cost effectiveness of medical interventions. Basically, since any given intervention has a cost, potential risks (each with its own cost), and potential benefits (increased survival or increased QOL during the remaining lifespan), the average cost per QALY can be calculated. A lower cost per QALY is preferable. The authors found that the cost per QALY for cochlear implantation was $15,600, which compared favorably with other interventions such as repair of symptomatic intracranial aneurysm ($18,500) and cardiac transplantation ($39,000).

Gates addressed the same issues when comparing surgical and medical therapy for otitis media.[60] The author had to use many assumptions—based on available data—in his analysis, but estimated the direct and indirect cost for adenoidectomy and tympanostomy tubes in children with chronic otitis media with effusion to be $2000 per QALY. This obviously compares very favorably with other common medical interventions. In addition, Gates noted that if surgery is used only in patients who fail medical therapy, the total costs of medical therapy for otitis media would represent two-thirds of the total societal costs of otitis media, even though surgical treatment is more expensive on a per-case basis.

Patient Satisfaction

Patient satisfaction is increasingly becoming recognized as an important outcome of the health care process. Patient satisfaction after outpatient office visits in multiple practice settings has been reported as part of the Medical Outcomes Study.[61] Project Solo, a organization of solo and independent medical practitioners headed by Steven Isenberg, M.D., employed a novel approach to the assessment of patient satisfaction.[62] Each physician was assigned a confidential bar code and given satisfaction surveys with only the bar code as an identifier to distribute to their patients. Completed surveys were sent from the patients back to Project Solo, where data was entered and analyzed. The return rate of completed questionnaires was adequate, and results from over 1800 surveys from 35 physician's offices indicated that patient satisfaction in private otolaryngologist's offices was as high as (or higher than) patient satisfaction in any practice setting identified by the Medical Outcomes Study.

Piccirillo studied patient satisfaction in an academic department using the same satisfaction instrument.[63] The return rate was adequate, and out of 482 returned surveys 79% rated the visit as excellent or very good. Both Isenberg and Piccirillo have gone a step further and are using patient satisfaction data as a way to monitor continuous quality improvement.[64]

Community-based Outcomes Research

Hoffman et al. articulated the importance of the collection of outcomes data by clinicians and described a methodology through which outcomes data could be gathered in a community-based setting.[65] The authors discussed the use of disease-specific and global health status instruments, and described a protocol for prospective data collection. The article reported that the methodology could be applied to several centers for additional data collection.

Isenberg, using Project Solo, attempted to do exactly that: organize and conduct a prospective, observational, multicenter outcomes trial to study external otitis. Twenty-nine otolaryngologists were enrolled in the study, but ultimately only five otolaryngologists returned data on nine patients. Isenberg and Rosenfeld subsequently identified several problems and pitfalls with the multicenter community-based approach.[66] Discussion with participants and a post-study mail-out survey indicated that factors impeding participation were: overly long and complex survey forms, multiple points of data collection, poor ongoing communication, and lack of enthusiasm for the project. The authors proposed several solutions to these problems, including starting with cross-sectional (rather than longitudinal) studies, using brief, easy to complete instruments, and identifying motivated "site coordinators" at offices to enhance patient accrual.

■ Outcomes Research in Otolaryngology: Where We Need to Go

Recommendations of 1995 Outcomes Research in Otolaryngology-Head & Neck Surgery Conference

The first annual conference on outcomes research in otolaryngology-head and neck surgery was held in Bethesda, Maryland, in 1995. As part of this conference, participants divided into four subgroups: ear and hearing, nose and sinus, larynx and airway, and head and neck cancer. Each subgroup discussed the important issues and future directions of outcomes research in the field. The leaders of each subgroup then synthesized the group discussion into a set of conclusions and recommendations, discussed below.

Ear and Hearing

The ear and hearing subgroup, led by George Gates, M.D., recommended the study of children with severe recurrent otitis media with effusion, and study of Meniere's disease, both early and late. The group recommended a randomized controlled trial for children with otitis, a stepped protocol for patients with early Meniere's disease, and a prospective, observational study for patients with late Meniere's.

Head and Neck Cancer

The head and neck cancer subgroup, led by Ernest Weymuller, M.D., recommended a cross-sectional cohort study of patient-based outcomes of surviving patients from the Veterans Administration Cooperative Study for laryngeal preservation. The study would test the hypothesis that QOL, performance status, and satisfaction with care do not differ between surviving patients in different treatment arms (e.g., laryngeal preservation, laryngectomy, and salvage surgery).

Nose and Sinus

The nose and sinus subgroup, led by Richard Rosenfeld, M.D., M.P.H., recommended study of chronic sinusitis in adults treated medically and surgically; they also recommended the development and validation of a disease-specific instrument for pediatric sinusitis. The group recommended a long-term prospective, observational protocol for the study of chronic sinusitis in adults.

Larynx and Airway

The larynx subgroup, led by Jay Piccirillo, M.D., recommended three studies as particularly important. The first was a cost-effectiveness evaluation of the diagnostic evaluation for patients with suspected obstructive sleep apnea syndrome. Second, the group recommended the systematic description and classification of patients with reflux-type symptoms, and third, the group recommended study of the management of benign laryngeal diseases.

Head and Neck Cancer

Laryngeal Cancer

Evidence is increasing that, in certain patients with laryngeal cancer, survival is unchanged whether patients are treated with laryngectomy or neoadjuvant chemotherapy and radiation therapy. While many have assumed that survival with an intact larynx is preferable to survival without a larynx, this has not been explicitly studied. In addition, there is good evidence that laryngectomees do not consider ability to communicate as the most important aspect of their QOL. Perhaps differences in QOL outcomes will ultimately be the deciding factor between surgical and nonsurgical treatment of laryngeal cancer when both options are possible. Of course, decision analysis has demonstrated that QOL issues are important even when clear survival differences exist between treatment types.

Other Head and Neck Sites

There is good evidence that, for many nonlaryngeal head and neck tumors, radiation treatment and surgical treatment may offer similar survival and morbidity rates. Systematic, prospective study of changes in QOL after different treatment modalities is needed to help guide treatment decisions in these patients.

QOL in Clinical Trials

If QOL and functional status data were routinely collected during clinical trials, changes in QOL and functional status could be used as statistical outcome variables, similar to the way local control and mortality are currently used. Statistical analysis could then be directed toward identifying factors that predict good QOL and functional status outcomes, as well as factors that predict improved survival. The identification of pretreatment factors that predict, say, poor functional communication status would be an important step toward improving both treatment selection and overall QOL and functional status after treatment. As discussed previously, QOL is multidimensional, and other factors such as a comorbid illness could significantly affect temporal changes in QOL during longitudinal trials.

Head and Neck Reconstruction

It is clear that microvascular free tissue transfer is an effective technique for head and neck reconstruction. Most centers report high success rates, low complication rates, and increasing utilization as the efficacy of the technique becomes apparent. Since we know that the technique is effective, the obvious next question is: Is it cost effective? It is probably more expensive to use a free flap than a local flap, but this initial incremental increased cost may easily be outweighed by long-term cost savings from, for instance, fewer fistulas and flap failures, better functional status, or improved QOL (e.g., cost per quality-adjusted life-year). QOL and functional status changes after free flap reconstruction should be assessed systematically, and the techniques of decision analysis and cost-effectiveness research should be applied to the use of the microvascular free tissue transfer.

Pediatric Otolaryngology

Measuring QOL and functional status outcomes in the pediatric population can be difficult because the patient typically does not have the language skills necessary to complete health status and QOL instruments. Therefore, in pediatric studies, the parent or primary caretaker is typically used as a proxy for data collection. Probably for that and other reasons, the field of outcomes assessment in pediatrics is less developed in general than in the adult population. In most otolaryngology practices, pediatrics constitutes a significant portion of the patient population and a significant portion of the otolaryngologic health care expenditure, so pediatric outcomes assessment is extremely important.

Recurrent Acute Otitis Media

As outlined by Gates, cost-effectiveness studies should be performed to compare medical prophylaxis and tympanostomy tube placement in recurrent acute otitis media.[60] To complete such an analysis and estimate the "utility" associated with various disease states, the QOL changes caused by acute otitis media, otitis media with effusion, and hearing loss must to be quantified. The American Academy of Pediatrics, with multidisciplinary involvement from specialist organizations, is currently developing a disease-specific health status measure for otitis media that may be used to help answer some of these questions.

Otitis Media with Effusion

Although the efficacy of adenoidectomy with tympanostomy tube placement for otitis media with effusion has been established in a randomized clinical trial, that trial included only patients from ages 4 to 8. Since *efficacy* has been established, the next step is to assess the *effectiveness* of treatment under "real-life" circumstances, and involving a wider age range of patients. Again, development of a disease-specific instrument is a necessary step for this research.

Tonsillectomy and Adenoidectomy

The efficacy of tonsillectomy for severe recurrent tonsillitis has been established in a controlled study. The efficacy of tonsillectomy for other indications (e.g., less severe recurrent infections, viral or culture-negative pharyngitis, hypertrophy, or sleep hypopnea/apnea) is more controversial. In addition, unexplained large geographic variations in tonsillectomy rates still exist. Therefore, a longitudinal study is needed to assess (1) functional status and QOL changes caused by tonsil and adenoid disease, (2) effects of medical treatment on functional status and QOL, (3) effects of surgical therapy on functional status and QOL, and (4) effects of "watchful waiting" on functional status and QOL. This research would require the development and validation of a disease-specific instrument for tonsil and adenoid disease.

Chronic Sinusitis

Many authors have demonstrated that short-term parental satisfaction after sinus surgery for chronic sinusitis is high. There is controversy, however, about the role of prolonged medical therapy, the role of limited versus extensive surgery, and the long-term effects of sinus surgery. In addition, comorbid factors (e.g., asthma, immunoglobulin deficiency, adenoid hypertrophy) may have a particularly large impact on outcomes in pediatric sinusitis. A longitudinal outcomes study is needed comparing different therapies, with appropriate stratification and adjustment for comorbidity.

Infant Hearing Screening

Although the importance of infant hearing screening is well established, the scope of screening (universal versus high risk), location of screening (in nursery versus first well-baby check), and technique for screening (auditory brainstem response versus otoacoustic emissions) are all controversial. The techniques of cost-benefit analysis could be used to address some of these issues in infant hearing screening. However, this is a potentially difficult area to study because the long-term effects (e.g., what is the "cost," or decrease in utility, of missed hearing loss) could be very difficult to quantify.

Otology

Conductive hearing loss

Although conductive hearing loss is usually well treated with otologic surgery, a hearing aid is often an equally effective and less expensive treatment. A prevailing presumption is that an otologic procedure that restores hearing to near normal is usually preferable to lifelong use of a hearing aid, although this has never been formally studied. A longitudinal study is needed comparing hearing-specific performance status and QOL in patients treated with hearing aids and surgery.

Chronic Suppurative Otitis Media

Similarly, a longitudinal study comparing outcomes between prolonged medical therapy and surgery for chronic suppurative otitis media is needed. Since the desired outcome is elimination of infection (in addition to improvement in hearing threshold), a disease-specific instrument would be necessary to assess treatment outcome. As in any other longitudinal outcomes study, assessment of prognostically important comorbid factors (such as eustachian tube dysfunction, duration of otorrhea, or systemic immunosuppression) would be important.

Vertigo

Typically the diagnostic evaluation of patients with vertigo or dizziness consists of a battery of tests (the content of the battery depending on the training and personal preference of the physician, as well as the availability of equipment and expertise). Even after this relatively costly group of tests is completed, results may be conflicting or equivocal and the diagnosis may be "multifactorial" dizziness. The techniques of cost-benefit analysis should be used to assess the cost effectiveness of the diagnostic evaluation of vertigo. Potentially, the ultimate goals of this research could be: (1) to describe a cost-effective battery of tests for vertigo, (2) to identify key factors in the patient's history or physical exam that may help direct the diagnostic workup, and (3) if feasible, to develop a screening-type algorithm to avoid utilizing every test in every patient.

Other

There are several other important issues in otolaryngology for which the tools of outcomes research could be applied. Although the effectiveness of endoscopic sinus surgery for *chronic sinusitis in adults* has been demonstrated, the long-term effects have not been well studied. In addition, direct comparison of the outcomes of surgical versus medical therapy has also not been performed. Further, identification of prognostically important comorbid factors and development of a comprehensive severity staging system are needed. Much important groundwork has already been accomplished in this area, making this an attractive field for further study.

Similarly, longitudinal outcomes assessment of patients with *obstructive sleep apnea syndrome,* including comparisons of available therapies (including laser-assisted or cold uvulopalatoplasty) is needed. The tools of outcomes research should also be applied to speech and voice disorders, measuring the effects of speech therapy, phonosurgery, vocal cord medialization procedures, and so on.

REFERENCES

1. Donabedian, A: The definition of quality and approaches to its assessment. In: Explorations in quality assessment and monitoring, Volume I, pp. 79–85. Ann Arbor, MI: Health Administration Press, 1980.
2. Cella DF, Bonomi AE: Measuring quality of life: 1995 update. *Oncology* 1995; 9(11 Suppl): 47–60.
3. D'Antonio LL, Zimmerman GJ, Cella DF, et al: Quality of life and functional status measures in patients with head and neck cancer. *Arch Otolaryngol Head Neck Surg* 1996; 122: 482–487.
4. Gill TM, Feinstein AR: A critical appraisal of the quality of quality-of-life measurements. *J Am Med Assoc* 1994; 272: 619–626.
5. Damiano AM, Steinberg EP, Cassard SD, et al: Comparison of generic versus disease-specific measures of functional impairment in patients with cataract. *Med Care* 1995; 33: AS120–AS130.
6. Patrick DL, Deyo RA: Generic and disease-specific measures in assessing health status and quality of life. *Med Care* 1989; 27:S217–S232.
7. Feinstein AR: The pre-therapeutic classification of comorbidity in chronic disease. *J Chron Dis* 1970; 23:455–468.
8. Piccirillo JF: Outcomes research and otolaryngology. *Otolaryngol Head Neck Surg* 1994; 111:764–769.
9. Epstein AM, Hall JA, Tognetti et al: Using proxies to evaluate quality of life. *Med Care* 1989; 27:S91–S98.
10. Gliklich RE, Hilinski JM: Longitudinal sensitivity of generic and specific health measures in chronic sinusitis. *Qual Life Res* 1995; 4: 27–32.
11. Berzon RA, Simeon GP, Simpson RL, et al: Quality of life bibliography and indexes: 1993 update. *Qual Life Res* 1995; 4:53–74.
12. Perrin EB: SAC instrument review process. *Medical Outcomes Trust Bulletin* 1995; 3(4):I–IV.
13. Ware JE, Sherbourne CD: The MOS 36-item short-form health survey (SF-36). *Med Care* 1992; 30:473–483.
14. Stewart AL, Greenfield S, Hays RD: Functional status and well-being of patients with chronic conditions: results from the Medical Outcomes Study. *J Am Med Assoc* 1989; 262: 907–913.
15. Gliklich RE, Metson R: Techniques for outcomes research in chronic sinusitis. *Laryngoscope* 1995; 105:387–390.
16. Wennberg JE, Barnes BA, Zubkoff M: Professional uncertainty and the problem of supplier-induced demand. *Soc Sci Med* 1982; 16:811–824.
17. Wennberg JE, Bunker JP, Barnes B: The need for assessing the outcome of common medical practices. *Ann Rev Public Health* 1980; 1:277–295.
18. Wennberg D: From variations to effectiveness studies: Physicians, patients and medical outcomes research. Presented at the Outcomes Research in Otolaryngology-Head & Neck Surgery Conference; October 1995; Bethesda, MD.
19. Kleinman LC, Kosecoff J, Dubois RW, et al: The medical appropriateness of tympanostomy tubes proposed for children younger than 16 years in the United States. *J Am Med Assoc* 1994; 271:1250–1255.
20. Piccirillo JF, Thawley SE, Haiduk A, et al: Indications for sinus surgery: How appropriate are the guidelines? Presented at the Annual Meeting of the Triologic Society; May 1996; Orlando, FL.
21. Piccirillo J: Literature review: Existing OR studies in ORL-HNS. In: Proceedings of the 1995 Outcomes Research in Otolaryngology-Head and Neck Surgery Conference; October 20–22, 1995; Bethesda, MD.
22. Piccirillo JF, Wells CK, Sasaki CT, et al: New clinical severity staging system for cancer of the larynx. *Ann Otol Rhinol Laryngol* 1994; 103: 83–92.
23. Piccirillo JF: Inclusion of comorbidity in a staging system for head and neck cancer. *Oncology* 1995; 9: 831–836.
24. Piccirillo JF, Schechtman KB, White DL: The development of the clinical severity staging system for obstructive sleep apnea. Presented at the Annual Meeting of the American Academy of Otolaryngology-Head & Neck Surgery; September 1995; New Orleans, LA.
25. Rosenfeld RM, Post JC: Meta-analysis of antibiotics for the treatment of otitis media with effusion. *Otolaryngol Head Neck Surg* 1992; 106:378–386.
26. Rosenfeld RM, Mandel EM, Bluestone CD: Systemic steroids for otitis media with effusion in children. *Arch Otolaryngol Head Neck Surg* 1991; 117:984–989.
27. Garcia P, Gates GA, Schechtman KB: Does topical antibiotic prophylaxis reduce post-tympanostomy tube otorrhea? *Ann Otol Rhinol Laryngol* 1994; 103:54–58.
28. Williams RL, Chalmers TC, Stange KC, et al: Use of antibiotics in preventing recurrent acute otitis media and in treating otitis media with effusion. *J Am Med Assoc* 1993; 270: 1344–1351.
29. Snyderman CH, D'Amico F: Outcome of carotid artery resection for neoplastic disease: A meta-analysis. *Am J Otolaryngol* 1992; 13:373–380.
30. Sher AE, Schechtman KB, Piccirillo JF: The efficacy of surgical modifications of the upper airway in adults with obstructive sleep apnea syndrome. *Sleep* 1996; 19(2): 156–177.
31. Carabellese C, Appollonio I, Rozzini R, et al: Sensory impairment and quality of life in a community elderly population. *J Am Geriatr Soc* 1993; 41:401–407.
32. Appollonio I, Carabellese C, Frattola L, et al: Effects of sensory aids on the quality of life and mortality of elderly people: a multivariate analysis. *Age and Ageing* 1996; 25:89–96.
33. Mulrow CD, Aguilar C, Endicott JE, et al: Association between hearing impairment and the quality of life of elderly individuals. *J Am Geriatr Soc* 1990; 38:45–50.
34. Mulrow CD, Aguilar C, Endicott LE, et al: Quality-of-life changes and hearing impairment: A randomized trial. *Ann Int Med* 1990; 113:188–194.
35. Harris JP, Anderson JP, Novak R: An outcomes study of cochlear implants in deaf patients. *Arch Otolaryngol Head Neck Surg* 1995; 121:398–404.
36. Grimby A, Rosenhall U: Health-related quality of life and dizziness in old age. *Gerontology* 1995; 41: 286–298.
37. Fielder H, Denholm SW, Lyons RA, et al: Measurement of health status in patients with vertigo. *Clin Otolaryngol* 1996; 21:124–126.
38. Lund VJ, MacKay IS: Outcome assessment of endoscopic sinus surgery. *J Roy Soc Med* 1994; 87:70–72.
39. Kennedy DW: Prognostic factors, outcomes and staging in ethmoid sinus surgery. *Laryngoscope* 1992; 102(12 Pt 2): 1–18.
40. Hoffman SR, Mahoney MC, Chmiel JF, et al: Symptom relief after endoscopic sinus surgery: An outcomes-based study. *ENT Journal* 1993; 72:413,414,419,420.

41. Gliklich RE, Metson R: The health impact of chronic sinusitis in patients seeking otolaryngologic care. *Otolaryngol Head Neck Surg* 1995; 113:104–109.
42. Gliklich RE, Metson R: The effect of sinus surgery on quality of life, *Otolaryngol Head Neck Surg,* in press.
43. Metson R, Gliklich RE, Stankiewicz JA, et al: A comparison of sinus computed tomography staging systems. Presented at the Annual Meeting of the American Academy of Otolaryngology-Head & Neck Surgery; September 1995; New Orleans, Louisiana.
44. Rosenfeld RM: Pilot study of outcomes in pediatric rhinosinusitis. *Arch Otolaryngol Head Neck Surg* 1995; 121:729–736.
45. McNeil BJ, Weichselbaum R, Pauker SG: Speech and survival: tradeoffs between quality and quantity of life in laryngeal cancer. *N Engl J Med* 1981; 305:982–987.
46. Tversky A, Kahneman D: The framing of decisions and the psychology of choice. *Science* 1981; 211(30):453–458.
47. McNeil BJ, Pauker SG, Sox HC, et al: On the elicitation of preferences for alternative therapies. *N Engl J Med* 1982; 306: 1259–1262.
48. Mohide EA, Archibald SD, Tew M, et al: Postlaryngectomy quality-of-life dimensions identified by patients and health care professionals. *Am J Surg* 1992; 164:619–622.
49. Plante DA, Piccirillo JF, Sofferman RA: Decision analysis of treatment options in pyriform sinus carcinoma. *Med Decis Making* 1987; 7:74–83.
50. Jones E, Lund VJ, Howard DJ: Quality of life of patients treated surgically for head and neck cancer. *J Laryngol Otol* 1992; 106:238–242.
51. Ackerstaff AH, Hilgers FJM, Aaronson NK, et al: Communication, functional disorders and lifestyle changes after total laryngectomy. *Clin Otolaryngol* 1994; 19:295–300.
52. Bjordal K, Kaasa S, Mastekaasa A: Quality of life in patients treated for head and neck cancer: A follow-up study 7 to 11 years after radiotherapy. *Int J Radiation Oncol Biol Phys* 1994; 28:847–856.
53. Bjordal K, Kaasa S: Psychological distress in head and neck cancer patients 7–11 years after curative treatment. *Br J Cancer* 1995; 71:592–597.
54. DeSanto LW, Olsen KD, Perry WC, et al: Quality of life after surgical treatment of cancer of the larynx. *Ann Otol Rhinol Laryngol* 1995; 104:763–769.
55. Harrison LB, Zelefsky MJ, Armstrong JG, et al: Performance status after treatment for squamous cell cancer of the base of tongue—a comparison of primary radiation therapy versus primary surgery. *Int J Rad Oncol Biol Phys* 1994; 30: 953–957.
56. Languis A, Bjorvell H, Lind M: Functional status and coping in patients with oral and pharyngeal cancer before and after surgery. *Head Neck* 1994;16:559–568.
57. Morton RP, Witterick IJ: Rationale and development of a quality-of-life instrument for head-and-neck cancer patients. *Am J Otolaryngol* 1995; 16:284–293.
58. List MA, Ritter-Sterr C, Lansky SB: A performance status scale for head and neck cancer patients. *Cancer* 1990; 66: 564–569.
59. Wyatt JR, Niparko JK, Rothman ML, de Lissovoy G: Cost effectiveness of the multichannel cochlear implant. *Am J Otol* 1995; 16:52–62.
60. Gates GA: Cost-effectiveness considerations in otitis media treatment. *Otolaryngol Head Neck Surg* 1996; 114: 525–530.
61. Rubin HR, Gandek B, Rogers WH: Patients' ratings of outpatient visits in different practice settings. *J Am Med Assoc* 1993; 270:835–840.
62. Isenberg SF, Davis C, Keaton S: Project Solo: an independent practitioner's initiative for confidential self-assessment of quality. *Am J Medical Quality,* in press.
63. Piccirillo JF: Patients' ratings of visits to an academic otolaryngology office. Presentation at the American Academy of Otolaryngology-Head & Neck Surgery; September 1995; New Orleans, LA.
64. Piccirillo JF, et al: The use of patient satisfaction data to assess the impact of continuous quality improvement efforts in an academic otolaryngology office. *Arch Otolaryngol Head Neck Surg,* in press.
65. Hoffman SR, Mahoney MC, Chmiel JF, et al: Conducting outcomes research in a community-based practice setting. *Am J Rhinol* 1994; 8:193–200.
66. Isenberg SF, Rosenfeld RM: Problems and pitfalls in community-based outcomes research. *Otolaryngol Head Neck Surg,* 1997; 662–665.
67. Ventry IM, Weinstein BE: The hearing handicap inventory for the elderly: A new tool. *Ear Hear* 1982; 3: 128–134.
68. CW, Weinstein BE, Jacobson GP, Hug GA: The hearing handicap for adults: Psychometric adequacy and audiometric correlates. *Ear Hear* 1990; 11:430–433.
69. Cox R, Alexander GC: The abbreviated profile of hearing aid benefit. *Ear Hear* 1995; 16:176–186.
70. Walden BE, Demorest ME, Hepler EL: Self-report approach to assessing benefit derived from amplification. *J Speech Hear Res* 1984; 27:49–56.
71. Stewart MG, Jenkins HA, Coker NJ, et al: Development of a new outcomes instrument for conductive hearing loss. *Am J Otol* (submitted, June, 1996).
72. Piccirillo JF, Valente M, Haiduk AM: The development of a new patient-specific hearing loss health status and quality of life measure (HEAR-14). Presented at the Association for Research in Otolaryngology; February 1996; St. Petersburg, FL.
73. Jacobson GP, Newman CW: The development of the dizziness handicap inventory. *Arch Otolaryngol Head Neck Surg* 1990; 116:424–427.
74. Kuk FK, Tyler RS, Russell D, et al: The psychometric properties of a tinnitus handicap questionnaire. *Ear Hear* 1990; 11:434–445.
75. Piccirillo JF, Edwards D, Haiduk A, et al: Psychometric and clinimetric validity of the 31-item rhinosinusitis outcome measure (RSOM-31). *Am J Rhinol* 1995; 9:297–306.
76. Juniper EF, Guyatt GH: Development and testing of a new measure of health status for clinical trials in rhinoconjunctivitis. *Clin Exper Allergy* 1991; 21:77–83.
77. Cella DF: Manual for the Functional Assessment of Cancer Therapy (FACT) Scales and the Functional Assessment of HIV (FAHI) Scale. Chicago: Rush-Presbyterian-St. Luke's Medical Center, 1994.
78. Hassan SJ, Weymuller EA: Assessment of quality of life in head and neck cancer patients. *Head & Neck* 1993; 15: 485–496.
79. List MA, Ritter-Sterr CA, Baker TM: Longitudinal assessment of quality of life in laryngeal cancer patients. *Head Neck* 1996; 18: 1–10.
80. Bjordal K, Kassa S: Psychometric validation of the EORTC Core Quality of Life questionnaire, 30-item version and a diagnosis-specific module for head and neck cancer patients. *Acta Oncologica* 1992; 31:311–321.
81. Browman GP, Levine MN, Hodson DI, et al: The Head and Neck Radiotherapy Questionnaire: A morbidity/quality-of-life instrument for clinical trials of radiation therapy in locally advanced head and neck cancer. *J Clin Oncol* 1993; 11: 863–872.
82. Morton RP: Life-satisfaction in patients with head and neck cancer. *Clin Otolaryngol* 1995; 20:499–503.

83. Jacobson BH, Johnson A, Grywalski C, et al: The voice handicap index (VHI)—development and validation. *Am J Speech Lang Pathol,* in press, 1996.
84. Robinson K, Gatehouse S, Browning GG: Measuring patient benefit from otorhinolaryngological surgery and therapy. *Ann Otol Rhinol Laryngol* 1996; 105: 415–422.

Michael Stewart, M.D., M.P.H., is the Chairman of the Continuous Quality Improvement Committee at Ben Taub General Hospital in Houston, Texas. Mike obtained his Master's in Public Health from the University of Texas School of Public Health with a special interest in outcomes research. He is a graduate of Johns Hopkins Medical School, and the recipient of the J. Charles Dickson Award for outstanding Clinical Research as a resident at Baylor College of Medicine. Dr. Stewart is the author of several scientific papers, poster presentations, and book chapters. A faculty member at Baylor College of Medicine, Dr. Stewart is actively involved in outcomes research.

9

Meaningful Outcomes Research

RICHARD M. ROSENFELD

Perhaps the best way to begin a chapter on meaningful outcomes research is with an example of the more prevalent meaningless variety. Dr. Hi Cost uses Quantum-Activated Computerized Kinesthetic (QuACK) surgery to cure refractory sinusitis. Based on the years of blood, sweat, and tears that went into developing the procedure, Dr. Cost feels justified in charging twice the rate of other, less qualified, sinus surgeons. Unfortunately, the local managed care companies beg to differ. Dr. Cost is certain, however, that some timely outcomes data will prove otherwise.

A chart review turns up 100 QuACK-treated patients, of which 20 complete an outcomes survey. Superb symptom relief and satisfaction are reported by 95% of respondents. But what if the 80 nonresponders were so inclined because their malpractice attorneys deemed it inadvisable to speak with Dr. Cost? Further, without an untreated comparison group we do not know if the improvement reflects a favorable natural history (independent of QuACK exposure) or a placebo effect from the perceived impressiveness of the device. Does the satisfaction reflect real clinical improvement, or is it perhaps secondary to the care, concern, and pampering offered by the amiable Dr. Cost and his compassionate staff? Finally, the 95% satisfaction rate is uninterpretable because outcomes surveys of unknown validity and reliability rarely yield "success" rates less than 90%.

Dr. Hi Cost's QuACK surgery may warrant a premium price, but he'll need more convincing data to prove it. In the words of Voltaire, "The art of medicine consists in amusing the patient while nature cures the disease." Insurers and consumers favor frugal amusement, unless meaningful outcomes data suggest otherwise. This chapter will acquaint physicians with the prerequisites for meaningful outcomes research and offer suggestions on how to perform simple office-based studies in a managed care environment. Also included are a brief overview of outcomes research, examples of clinical outcomes studies, and suggestions on using quality of life and satisfaction surveys.

■ What Is Outcomes Research?

The definition of outcomes research remains unclear, because the answer depends on exactly who is asking the question: patient, payer, or physician. The outcomes "movement" is as much political as scientific, based on the premise that health care outcomes have not received sufficient attention and that physicians know too little about what produces desired health effects. Understanding what each of the key players—patients, payers, and physicians—hope to gain from the outcomes movement is an essential precursor to any meaningful research effort.

Outcomes research deals with all identified changes in health status and quality of life arising as a consequence of how a health problem is handled. *Health status* is the degree to which a person is able to function physically, emotionally, and socially, with or without aid from the health care system. In contrast, *quality of life* is the degree to which persons *perceive* themselves as able to function. Both health status and quality of life extend far beyond the usual disease-specific treatment endpoints used to determine success or failure in clinical trials. A clinical trial may be interested in the hearing improvement achieved with tympanostomy tubes for otitis media, but an outcomes study would measure the actual and perceived benefits of improved hearing on the child's physical, emotional, and social function.

A Technology of Patient Experience

"We are drowning in information but starved for knowledge," noted the American business writer John Naisbitt. Similarly, Paul Ellwood noted in 1988 that our inability to measure and understand health care outcomes resulted in uninformed patients, skeptical payers, frustrated physicians, and besieged health care executives.[1] In response, he proposed a technology for collaborative action called "outcomes management:"

> Outcomes management is a technology of patient experience designed to help patients, payers, and providers make rational medical care—related choices based on better insight into the effect of these choices on the patient's life. Outcomes management consists of a common patient-understood language of health outcomes; a national data base containing information and analysis on clinical, financial, and health outcomes that estimates as best as we can the relation between medical interventions and health outcomes, as well as the relation between health outcomes and money; and an opportunity for each decision-maker to have access to the analyses that are relevant to the choices they must make.

To achieve these goals, Ellwood proposed (1) systematic measurement of the functioning and well-being of patients, along with disease-specific clinical outcomes, at appropriate time intervals, (2) pooling of clinical and outcome data on a massive scale, (3) analysis and dissemination of results from the segment of the database most appropriate to the concerns of each decision-maker, and (4) greater reliance on practice guidelines by physicians when selecting appropriate interventions.

Health Care Stakeholders

The number of individuals and organizations involved in outcomes research has grown rapidly over the past decade. Greater insight into the outcomes movement can be obtained by understanding what each of the stakeholders hopes to gain from the process.[2]

Pubic and private payers seeking to reduce health care costs may use effectiveness results to ration health care or establish national guidelines. Reimbursement and purchasing decisions could eventually be linked to quality assessment reflecting desirable or undesirable health outcomes. For hospitals and other health care organizations, effectiveness results would establish local treatment guidelines, identify opportunities for improvement, and be used for marketing purposes. Patients, the public, and individual providers could use effectiveness data to make informed treatment decisions, particularly when the preferred treatment for an individual patient is not obvious and the patient or caregiver is willing to participate in the decision-making process.

Medical Treatment Effectiveness Program

Since 1989, the Agency for Health Care Policy and Research (AHCPR) has funded special projects known as Patient Outcomes Research Teams (PORTs).[3] These large and complex 5-year undertakings, with average annual budgets of one million dollars, represent the leading edge of outcomes research methodology. Emphasis is placed on outcomes that patients understand and care about, such as quality of life, functional capacity, symptom relief, and cost (in contrast to physiological measures and parameters that focus more on organs than their owners). Questions of cost effectiveness and appropriateness are additional basic themes in this research.

Each of the PORTs follows a standard research model, which consists of (1) systematic literature review (meta-analysis), (2) analysis of variations in practice patterns and patient outcomes (primary data), (3) analysis of cost and claims data (secondary data), (4) decision analysis to define the optimal path to the desired outcome, and (5) strategies for effective dissemination and assimilation of research findings. Despite the grandiose goals of the PORTs, the methodology remains embryonic and has not yet been applied to clinical problems confronting the practicing physician.

AAO-HNS Outcomes Research Grant

When the American Academy of Otolaryngology–Head & Neck Surgery Foundation introduced its Outcomes Research Small Project Grant in 1996, the purpose was to foster research that would improve the effectiveness and appropriateness of medical practice. Projects supported under the program would develop and disseminate scientific information on the effects of otolaryngology services and procedures on patients' survival, health status, functional capacity, and quality of life. Three main categories of outcomes research were identified: patient-based studies, record-based studies, and process assessment (Table 9–1).

An ideal patient-based outcomes study would incorporate principles outlined above for the AHCPR PORTs. No effort of this magnitude is yet underway in otolaryngology, but smaller efforts are ongoing to develop and validate measures of comorbidity, disease severity, and disease-specific quality of life. Records-based outcomes studies have been more popular because they are easier, faster, and less expensive to design and conduct. Process assessment includes anything that happens between two evaluation points that might affect health. Although not

TABLE 9–1. Overview of Outcomes Research

Patient-Based Outcomes Research
- Creation and validation of health-related quality of life measures
- Creation and validation of disease-specific clinical severity scales
- Observational studies of treatment effectiveness

Record-Based Outcomes Research
- Analysis of administrative and financial data bases
- Regional variations in practice patterns and outcomes
- Meta-analysis, decision analysis, or cost-effectiveness studies
- Analysis of national data sets or population-based surveys

Process Assessment
- Continuous quality improvement
- Patient satisfaction with health care services
- Development of clinical practice guidelines
- Editorial peer review process

directly related to patient care, the editorial review process is included in this definition (Table 9–1) to acknowledge the importance of peer-reviewed publications as a foundation for evidence-based medicine.

Outcomes and the Practicing Physician

What impact will the outcomes movement ultimately have on practicing physicians? "The art of prophecy is very difficult, especially with respect to the future," observed Mark Twain. What is clear, however, is that the outcomes movement contains two separate, but related, agendas. *Outcomes management* by payers and hospitals tries to cut costs by controlling physician and patient access to health care resources. *Outcomes research* by physicians tries to identify management options that result in the highest overall and disease-specific quality of life for patients.

Lest they fall victim to the control paradigm of outcomes management, practicing physicians must participate in—or at least understand the fundamental principles of—outcomes research. Participation must be proactive and include both community physicians as well as university academicians. Howard Ruff, an American business consultant, noted astutely, "It wasn't raining when Noah built the ark." The remainder of this chapter introduces clinicians to the principles and practice of ark building.

How to Avoid Meaningless Outcomes Research

An uncanny aspect of outcomes research is the ease with which meaningless data arise. This occurs because outcomes studies are a type of observational research, in contrast to the experimental method that underlies randomized controlled trials (RCTs).[4] From an evolutionary perspective, outcomes research is a giant step backward from RCTs. Nonetheless, lousy RCTs are as feasible as lousy outcomes studies. The latter, however, are much easier to produce.

How can clinicians avoid the problems and pitfalls that accompany the seductive simplicity of outcomes research? By realizing that outcomes studies are subject to the same laws of statistical and epidemiological gravity that govern all other meaningful research endeavors. When asked how he invented the incandescent light bulb, Thomas Edison replied that after 10,000 failures he finally ran out of things that didn't work. The crash courses in epidemiology and statistics that follow are offered as an alternative to 10,000 failed attempts at meaningful outcomes research.

Crash Course in Epidemiology

Over the past 50 years, the definition of epidemiology has broadened from concern with communicable disease epidemics to encompass all phenomena related to health in populations. Epidemiology brings method to the madness of planning and conducting research studies, including outcomes research.

Epidemiologists are obsessed with avoiding bias and proving causality. *Bias* refers to any trend in the collection, analysis, or interpretation of data that leads to conclusions systematically different from the truth.[5] *Causality* is the ability to relate causes to the effects they produce. The fruit of these obsessions is the RCT, which since World War II has epitomized successful application of the scientific method to clinical medicine. As noted above, outcomes research is a giant evolutionary step backward from the RCT because of increased bias and reduced ability to demonstrate causality. Comparing these two types of research (Table 9–2) is a useful exercise in basic epidemiology.[6]

The virtues of RCTs are stated in the name itself: control groups and randomization. The presence or absence of a *control group* has a profound influence on data interpretation. An uncontrolled study—no matter how elegant—is purely descriptive.[7] Nonetheless, authors of case series or cohort studies—or uncontrolled outcomes studies—often delight in unjustified musings on efficacy, effectiveness, association, and causality. Without a control or comparison group, it is often impossible to distinguish natural history from treatment effects (Table 9–3)

The placebo and halo effects (Table 9–3) may account for on average 70% of good to excellent outcomes in uncontrolled studies.[8] The potential for these effects is proportional to the novelty or impressiveness of the treatment given and the setting in which it is administered. Coincidentally, surgical subspecialists often administer novel treatments in impressive settings (Dr. Hi Cost take notice!). Further, patients with chronic disease typically have fluctuating symptoms and seek medical care (and enroll in research studies) when symptoms are at

TABLE 9–2. Comparison of Randomized Controlled Trials and Outcomes Studies

Characteristic	*Randomized Controlled Trial*	*Outcomes Study*
Goal	Establish cause and effect	Demonstrate relationships
Level of investigator control	Experimental	Observational
Treatment allocation	Random assignment	Routine clinical care
Patient selection criteria	Restrictive	Broad
Typical setting	Hospital or university based	Community based
Endpoint definitions	Objective health status	Subjective quality of life
Endpoint assessment	Blinded	Unblinded
Time frame	Short or intermediate	Long
Statistical analysis	Paired or independent groups	Multivariate regression
Potential for bias	Low	Very high

their worst. Thus, the next change is likely to be an improvement (independent of therapy), a phenomenon called regression to the mean.

Studies with control or comparisons groups may be performed with or without randomization. In an RCT, the investigator randomly assigns patients to treatment or control groups. An RCT is an *experimental* study because conditions are controlled by the investigator for the express purpose of increasing medical knowledge, not for providing clinical care. In contrast, an outcomes study is a form of *observational* research. Treatment decisions occur as part of routine clinical care, without intervention from the investigator other than to record, classify, and analyze. This lack of control predisposes observational studies to numerous hidden biases, only some of which are overcome by using a control group (Table 9–3).

A major source of bias in outcomes studies are the individual judgments and other selective decisions that influence clinical management in the absence of randomized assignment.[9] Randomization balances baseline prognostic factors—known and unknown—among groups, including severity of illness and the presence of co-morbid conditions (e.g., asthma in a sinusitis trial). Because these factors also influence a clinician's decision to offer treatment, nonrandomized studies are prone to *allocation (susceptibility) bias* (Table 9–3) and false-positive results.[10] A typical example occurs when the survival of surgically treated cancer patients is compared with nonsurgical controls (e.g., radiation or chemotherapy). Without randomization, the surgical group will generally have a more favorable prognosis—independent of therapy—because the customary criteria for operability (special anatomic conditions and no major co-morbidity) also predispose to favorable results.

RCTs prevent two other biases that plague observational research: detection bias and transfer bias (Table 9–3). *Detection bias* occurs when unequal methods of surveillance and identification are applied to treatment and control patients, because observers are affected by their knowledge and prior expectations concerning therapy. Experimental studies can prevent this by double blinding patients and physicians to treatment status, but comparable measures would be unethical in observational research. *Transfer bias* arises from inequalities in accounting for all patients initially entered in the study. For example, if we limit our analysis to only those patients who survived surgery or were highly compliant with medication use our success rates would be falsely elevated. RCTs avoid this by analyzing according to intention to treat, rather than completion of treatment. Although not impossible, intention to treat analysis can be difficult in observational studies.

If RCTs lie at the top of the epidemiologic food chain, why bother at all with observational studies such as outcomes research? Because as they shed bias and donned the gown of causality, RCTs became increasingly divorced from the realities of everyday medical practice. In other words, the price of scientific purity was low generalizability to real world situations. Results of RCTs are limited by constraints of selective admission criteria, rigorous therapeutic protocols with measures to ensure compliance, and narrowly defined outcome measures. The treatment endpoints in RCTs are chosen for their objectivity, and are not necessarily important to patients (or physicians). RCTs are expensive and not always ethical, particularly for surgical therapies. Finally, randomized trials can become outdated quickly and often do not address issues of effectiveness and dissemination.

The outcomes movement has been fueled, in part, by the aforementioned inadequacies of using RCTs to guide medical therapy. Nonetheless, observational (outcomes) treatment comparisons may contain all the biases randomized trials are intended to prevent or reduce. The prognosis and choice of treatment can be affected by baseline co-morbidity, the pattern of symptoms, the severity of symptoms, and the pattern of disease progression. When these crucial clinical factors, called *covariates,* are suitably identified and classified, they can be used for adjustments that remove or reduce bias when observational data are used for therapeutic comparisons.

TABLE 9–3. Explanations for Favorable Results in Outcomes Studies

Explanation	*Definition*	*Solution*
Bias	Systematic variation of measurements from their true values; may be intentional or unintentional	Accurate, protocol-driven data collection
Chance	Random variation without apparent relation to other measurements or variables; e.g., getting lucky	Control or comparison group
Natural history	Course of a disease from onset to resolution; may include relapse, remission, and spontaneous recovery	Control or comparison group
Regression to the mean	Return to baseline state after exacerbation of a chronic illness, independent of other interventions	Control or comparison group
Placebo effect	Beneficial effect caused by the expectation that the regimen will have an effect; e.g., power of suggestion	Control or comparison group with placebo
Halo effect	Beneficial effect caused by the manner, attention, and caring of a provider during a medical encounter	Control or comparison group treated similarly
Confounding	Distortion of an effect by other prognostic factors or variables for which adjustments have not been made	Randomization or multivariate analysis
Allocation (susceptibility) bias	Beneficial effect caused by allocating subjects with less severe disease or better prognosis to treatment group	Randomization or comorbidity analysis
Ascertainment (detection) bias	Favoring the treatment group during outcome analysis; e.g., rounding up for treated subjects, down for controls	Blinded outcome assessment
Transfer bias	Inequalities in accounting for all initial patients; e.g., omitting postoperative deaths from survival rates	Intention to treat analysis

Unfortunately, appropriate covariates have not been adequately defined for most diseases. A major part of outcomes research, therefore, is to identify and classify these disease-specific covariates.

Crash Course in Statistics

"Every sensible person promptly associates the term 'statistics' with the thought: 'This is a bunch of lies'," observed August Bier, surgeon and philosopher. If you agree, you might as well skip this section. Regrettably, you will remain half in the dark when it comes to understanding outcomes research, because epidemiology is to statistics as leadership is to management: the epidemiologist (leader) makes sure that the right data are analyzed, but the statistician (manager) make sure that the data are analyzed right. Great data analyzed poorly are worth as much as poor data analyzed greatly. So please bear with me for the remainder of this section.

Accepting *uncertainty* is the key to understanding outcomes data. Uncertainty is present in all data, because of the inherent variability in biologic systems and in our ability to assess them in a reproducible fashion. Nearly 2000 years ago, Pliny the Elder reported with certainty, "The only certainty is that nothing is certain." For example, if you measure disease-specific quality of life in 20 children with stable disease on 5 days, how likely would it be to get the same mean result each time? Very unlikely, because of random and unpredictable fluctuations in response. Similarly, if you measured quality of life in 5 groups of 20 children, how likely would it be to get the same results in each group? Again unlikely, because of variations between individuals. We would get a range of similar results, but rarely the exact same result on repetitive trials.

Uncertainty must be dealt with when interpreting data, unless the results are meant to apply only to the particular group of patients in which the observations were initially made. Statisticians consider all clinical measurements to be *estimates* of some "true" value that can never be known, because some degree of unavoidable error is always present. Measurements made on a finite sample of observations are called *point estimates* because the values obtained in other samples are unlikely to be exactly the same. In medicine, however, we seek to pass from observations to generalizations, from point estimates to estimates about other populations. When this process occurs with calculated degrees of uncertainty, we call it *inference.*

Here's a brief example of clinical inference. After treating 5 patients with vitamin C for intractable vertigo, you remark to a colleague that 4 had excellent improvement in health status. She asks, "How confident are you of your results?" "Quite confident," you reply, "there were 5 patients, 4 improved, and that's 80%." "Maybe I wasn't clear," she interjects. "How confident are you that 80% of vertiginous patients *in general,* whether in your practice or mine, will respond favorably to vitamin C?" "In other words," she continues, "can you *infer* anything about the real effect of vitamin C on vertigo from only 5 patients?"

Hesitatingly you retort, "Maybe I'll have to see a few more patients to be sure."

The real issue, of course, is that a sample of only 5 patients offers low *precision*. How likely is it that the same results would be found if 5 new patients were studied? Actually, we can state with 95% confidence that 4 out of 5 successes in a single trial is consistent with a range of results from 28% to 99% in future trials. This *95% confidence interval* may be calculated manually or with a statistical program,[11–13] and tells us the *range of results consistent with the observed data.* Thus, if this trial were repeated we could obtain a success rate as low as 28%—not very encouraging compared with the original point estimate of 80%. A broad 95% confidence interval indicates a large amount of uncertainty, whereas a narrow interval indicates much greater precision. All main results in an outcomes study should be accompanied by a 95% confidence interval to aid interpretation.

The uncertainty plot thickens when comparing *two or more groups,* because errors in inference are inevitable. If we conclude that the groups are different, they may actually be equivalent (type I statistical error or false-positive). If we conclude that they are the same, we may have missed a true difference (type II statistical error or false-negative). All *statistical tests* (t-tests, chi-squared, etc) are simply a means of estimating the likelihood of a type I error. The *P values* produced by such tests indicate the likelihood that the purported association or relationship under study is really a false-positive finding. For example, if we find an association between passive smoking and otitis media at $P = .03$, there is only a 3% chance that this represents a fortuitous (false-positive) finding.

Outcomes studies use *multivariate analysis* to determine the independent effect of multiple predictor variables on an outcome. Predictors may be disease-specific (tumor stage, treatment administered, etc.) or general (age, sex, socioeconomic status, co-morbidity, etc.). Examples of multivariate analysis include logistic and proportional hazards (Cox) regression. Each produces a statistical model that predicts outcomes based on combinations of individual variables. The adequacy of the model as a whole is determined by R^2 (1.0 indicates perfect fit) and its associated P value. Each predictor variable has an associated coefficient and P value, which reflect the magnitude and significance of any effect on outcome adjusted for all the other variables in the model. Proportional hazards (Cox) regression is widely used in patient-based outcomes studies to determine prognostic factors and compare treatment regiment after adjustment for imbalances (covariates) between the treatment groups.[14]

Outcomes studies are prone to *data dredging* and post hoc hypotheses, because of the large number of variables often involved. When a large number of statistical tests are performed, some will be significant by chance alone because each test has a 5% chance of error. This "multiple P value problem" is compounded by extensive subgroup comparisons, but can be avoided by using multivariate analysis. Even with multivariate analysis, however, problems can still arise when hypotheses are formulated post hoc—after even the briefest glance at the data—thereby invalidating the probability basis for statistical testing. This is similar to the Texas sharpshooter who shoots an arrow at a barn wall, then runs and draws a bulls-eye around it. The friends who arrive later may applaud his incredible accuracy, but his post hoc cleverness invalidates its significance.

A statistical test is valid only when the *study sample* (Table 9–4) is random and representative. Unfortunately, these assumptions are frequently violated or overlooked. A random sample is necessary because most statistical tests are based on probability theory—playing the odds. The odds apply only if the deck is not stacked and the dice

TABLE 9–4. Glossary of Statistical Terms Related to Sampling and Validity

Term	*Definition*
Target population	Entire collection of items, subjects, patients, observations, etc., about which we want to make inferences; defined by the selection criteria (inclusion and exclusion criteria) for the study
Accessible population	Subset of the target population that is accessible for study, generally because of geographical or temporal considerations
Study sample	Subset of the accessible population that is chosen for study
Sampling method	Process of choosing a sample from a larger population; the method may be random or nonrandom, representative or nonrepresentative
Selection bias	Error caused by systematic differences between a study sample and target population; examples include studies on volunteers, and those conducted in clinics or tertiary care settings
Internal study validity	Degree to which conclusions drawn from a study are valid for the study sample; results from proper study design, unbiased measurements, and sound statistical analysis
External study validity (generalizability)	Degree to which conclusions drawn from a study are valid for a target population (beyond the subjects in the study); results from representative sampling and appropriate selection criteria

are not rigged; that is, all members of the *target population* have an equal chance of being sampled for study. Investigators, however, typically have access to only a small subset of the target population because of geographical or temporal constraints. When they choose an even smaller subset of this *accessible population* to study, the method of choosing (sampling method) affects our ability to make inferences about the original target population.

Of the sampling methods listed in Table 9–5, only a random sample is theoretically suitable for statistical analysis. Because outcomes research is observational, random samples are rarely feasible. Nonetheless, a *consecutive sample* or *systematic sample* offers a relatively good approximation, and provides data of sufficient quality for most statistical tests. The worst sampling method occurs when subjects are chosen based on convenience or subjective judgments about eligibility. Applying statistical tests to the resulting convenience (grab) sample is the equivalent of asking a professional card counter to help you win a blackjack game when the deck is stacked deck and cards are missing—all bets are off because probability theory will not apply.

Separating the Meaningful from the Meaningless

A meaningful outcomes study is *valid* not only for the subjects studied, but for similar subjects outside the study. *Internal validity* exists when the study results are credible for the specific sample of subjects studied. The preceding sections describe several features of internal validity, including 95% confidence intervals to measure precision, *P* values to control for chance (random error), and multivariate analysis to adjust for the effects of multiple predictor variables. More important, bias should be minimized by protocol-driven data collection using valid and reliable outcome measures. *External validity* exists when the study results are credible for subjects outside the study. Consecutive or systematic samples that are representative of the target population ensure that this goal is achieved.

A meaningful outcomes study uses outcome measures that are valid and reliable. For example, the following steps are necessary to construct a quality of life measure: (1) select the items, (2) choose response options, (3) determine reproducibility, (4) determine validity, and (5) determine responsiveness.[15] These issues will be discussed later in greater detail, but for now let it suffice to say that good outcomes measures rarely arise by divine providence. At a bare minimum the measure should make sense (face validity), should be approved by expert clinicians (content validity), should be reproducible (test-retest validity), and should measure what it is supposed to measure (construct validity). Finally, if the survey is used to measure clinical change, it must be capable of detecting differences when they occur (responsiveness to longitudinal change) (see Table 9–6).

A meaningless outcomes study ignores the laws of statistical and epidemiological gravity (if you missed these laws, reread the two preceding sections). These studies lack control or comparison groups, are conducted without a specific protocol, and often rely on biased data that were not collected in a systematic fashion (e. g., chart review or administrative data bases). Patients are selected using judgmental or convenience samples. Outcome measures are limited to simple surveys or questionnaires of unknown validity and reliability. Follow-up is sporadic and incomplete, with low response rates. Comparative

TABLE 9–5. Methods for Sampling a Population

Method	*How It Is Performed*	*Comments*
Brute force sample	Includes all units of study (charts, patients, laboratory animals, or journal articles) accessible to the researchers	Time consuming, and unsophisticated; bias prone because missing units are seldom randomly distributed
Convenience (grab) sample	Units are selected on the basis of accessibility, convenience, or subjective judgments about eligibility	Assume this method when none is specified; study results cannot be generalized because of selection bias
Systematic sample	Units are selected using some simple, systematic rule, such as first letter of last name, date of birth, or day of week	Less biased than a convenience sample, but problems may still occur because of unequal selection probabilities
Consecutive sample	Every unit is included over a specified time interval, or until a specified number is reached	Excellent method when intake period is long enough to adequately represent seasonal and other temporal factors
Random sample	Units are assigned numbers, then selected at random until a desired sample size is attained	Best method because all units have a known (and equal) probability of selection; rarely feasible for outcomes studies

TABLE 9–6. Essentials of Outcomes Research

1. Most outcomes studies use observational data collected during routine patient care, not specifically for research. Consequently, they are prone to biases that randomization avoids including allocation bias, detection bias, transfer bias, and sampling bias.
2. Outcomes studies without a control or comparison group provide descriptive data only; no statements can be made about effectiveness, regardless of how encouraging the results appear.
3. The same laws of statistical gravity apply to outcomes research that apply to all other medical data; random error, uncertainty, and sampling problems. Check for 95% confidence intervals, *P* values, and representative sampling schemes.
4. Patient-based outcomes studies are nothing more than cohort studies with a quality of life twist. Adjustments must be made for baseline covariates, co-morbidity, unequal periods of follow-up, and patients who drop out or are lost to follow-up.
5. Records-based outcomes studies are limited by the quality and completeness of the source material, which was originally collected for administrative (not clinical) reasons. Important clinical covariates may not be recorded, creating biased and misleading results.
6. Outcomes studies of process are always dynamic. Resulting recommendations and guidelines are subject to constant revision as new studies are published.

statements are made without statistical tests for association or correlation to control for random error. Conclusions tend to reflect the a priori biases of the investigators, and are not supported by the data.

■ Outcomes and Otolaryngology: the Good, the Bad, and the Ugly

As an example for all physicians, this section presents an overview of outcomes research efforts in otolaryngology. No attempt is made to provide a systematic review of all published studies. Rather, examples are selected to illustrate the virtues, limitations, and embryonic nature of outcomes efforts to date. For consistency with the AAO-HNS grant application guidelines, this section will be divided into patient-based studies, record-based studies, and studies of process assessment.

Patient-Based Outcomes Research

Several authors have reported improved quality of life for adult[16–17] and pediatric[18] patients after endoscopic surgery for chronic sinusitis. Hoffman and colleagues observed reduced headaches, nasal drainage, nasal congestion, sinus infection, and breathing difficulties in 31 adults 6 months after the procedure was performed. Similarly, Gliklich and Hilinski described reduced sinus pain, nasal drainage, nasal congestion, antibiotic use, and antihistamine-decongestant use in 63 adults after 3 months. Both studies also showed improvement in one or more subscales of a general health status measure, the Medical Outcomes Study (MOS) Short Form 36-item Health Survey (SF-36).[19]

Rosenfeld treated 41 children with chronic or recurrent sinusitis with a stepped protocol of additional antibiotics, adenoidectomy, and sinus surgery. After 12 months, over 80% of children reported improvement or cure of all major symptoms, and 85% of caregivers felt their expectations had been met or exceeded. The results reflect the stepped protocol as a whole, not the comparative value of the three management options. No general health status measure was included in this study.

The above studies suggest that quality of life improves *after* sinus surgery, but not necessarily *because* of sinus surgery. Since none of these studies had an untreated comparison group, we cannot exclude chance, natural history, placebo effect, halo effect, or regression to the mean as explanations for the favorable results (Table 9–3). We *can* say that patients are better after treatment, but we *cannot* say with certainty exactly what components of the protocol (e. g., surgery, physician attention, perceived efficacy of sinus surgery, passage of time) caused this outcome. The methodology and questionnaires developed in these uncontrolled studies, however, set the stage for larger investigations of comparative treatment effectiveness.

An interesting mix of outcomes research and basic science is demonstrated in a study by Lee and Rosenfeld.[20] The authors hypothesized that the adenoid may serve as a reservoir for bacterial pathogens that cause sinonasal symptoms. A quality of life questionnaire was given to 84 caregivers of children undergoing adenoidectomy, with 7-point questions to assess the frequency and severity of sinonasal infectious symptoms, ear infection symptoms, and nasal obstructive symptoms over the preceding 6 months. Good validity was demonstrated. Multivariate analysis showed that 48% of the variability in pathogenic bacteria levels within the adenoid core was explained by the sinonasal symptom impact score. Adenoid size (weight) did not correlate with pathogen levels, similar to what has been observed for otitis media.

An active area of patient-based outcomes research concerns efforts to develop quality of life measures for common disorders. Gliklich and Metson[21] developed a 6-item Chronic Sinusitis Survey based on symptom duration and medication use over the past 8 weeks. Despite its brevity, the survey proved reliable, valid, and sensitive to longitudinal change. Several validated questionnaires are also available to measure quality of life and functional status in patients with head and neck cancer.[22] Quality of life surveys are under development for otitis media, sleep apnea, and adenotonsillar disease, but have not yet been validated.

The information obtained from disease-specific surveys is complemented by data from general measures of health profiles, constructs, and behaviors. For example, data from Gliklich and Metson[23] suggest that the national health impact of chronic sinusitis is far greater than currently appreciated. Patients with chronic sinusitis scored significantly poorer on the SF-36 subscales for bodily pain and social functioning than did patients with angina, back pain, congestive heart failure, or chronic obstructive pulmonary disease. In addition to the SF-36, other validated measures are available to assess the impact of chronic disease on adults.[24] These include measures of pain, coping, function, fatigue, depression, medication taking, and global health and quality of life.

Record-Based Outcomes Research

A productive area of record-based outcomes research in otolaryngology has been meta-analysis of RCTs for acute otitis media (AOM) and otitis media with effusion (OME). Meta-analysis is a form of literature review in which studies are systematically assembled, appraised, and combined using a predefined protocol to reduce bias and subjectivity.[25] The emphasis is often on numbers over narrative, in order to increase statistical power and improve estimates of effect size—an index of how much difference exists between two groups. A traditional literature review emphasizes narrative, with strengths and weaknesses of individual studies discussed selectively and informally by one or more experts. Varying degrees of credibility result because of potential bias in selecting source articles. The differences between narrative reviews and meta-analyses are summarized in Table 9–7.

Meta-analysis has helped define what to expect from medical treatment of otitis media, based on the more than 200 clinical trials already published.[26] A consistent finding has been the relatively modest impact of therapeutic antibiotics on clinical control of AOM and OME: about 7 children must be treated to improve one child above and beyond what would occur from natural history alone. Further, natural history (spontaneous resolution) is a formidable opponent: about 80% of AOM resolves with placebo "treatment," and recurrent AOM decreases by 1.5 to 3.0 annual episodes with placebo "prophylaxis." Prophylactic antibiotics also had a marginal impact on control, requiring treatment for 9 months to prevent a single episode of AOM. Finally, no comparative benefits were seen for expensive extended-spectrum drugs (e. g., cephalosporins) over amoxicillin or trimethoprim-sulfamethoxazole.

Studies of cost effectiveness and decision analysis often begin where meta-analysis ends. The "bottom-line" efficacy estimates derived in the meta-analysis are combined under various clinical scenarios to determine which offers the highest probability of a successful outcome. For example, Berman and co-workers[27] determined the most cost-effective treatment for persistent OME to be corticosteroid plus an antibiotic 6 weeks after diagnosis of AOM. The average reader is unlikely to contest this conclusion after trying to decipher the 11 dense numeric tables in the article. Unfortunately, the 16 efficacy estimates in the decision tree are biased, imprecise, and make several unproven assumptions for intervention combinations with no published data. The 11 tables, therefore, suffer from the garbage-in garbage-out phenomenon, to which many well-intentioned cost-effectiveness studies succumb. Further, the study occurs in a clinical vacuum, with no discussion of steroid risks, such as behavioral changes, immune suppression, flare-ups of AOM, and disseminated varicella infection.

A widespread clinical practice that has its roots in records-based outcomes research is the mandatory second opinion for tonsillectomy required by many insurance carriers. After Wennberg and colleagues[28] reported in 1969 that Vermont hospital service areas had a 13-fold difference in tonsillectomy rates, the State

TABLE 9–7. Comparison of Narrative (Traditional) Reviews and Meta-analyses

	Narrative Review	Meta-analysis
Research design	Free form	A priori protocol
Literature search	Convenience sample	Systematic sample
Focus	Broad; summarizes a large body of information	Narrow; tests one or two specific hypotheses
Emphasis	Narrative	Numbers
Validity	Variable; high potential for bias in article selection	Good, provided articles are of adequate quality and combinability
Bottom line	Broad recommendations, often based on personal opinion	Estimates of effect size, based on statistical pooling of data
	Provides quick overview of a subject area	Provides summary estimates for decision analysis,

Medical Society and local physicians adopted a second opinion procedure. Four years later, the average rate for all areas had declined 46% and most of the prior small-area variations were eliminated. Small-area variations in tonsillectomy rates are not confined to the United States; similar trends occur in England and Norway.[29] Differences among physicians in either their diagnostic style or their belief in the efficacy of tonsillectomy are believed responsible for the observed variance. The largest small-area variations generally occur for elective procedures with controversial indications, providing inspiration to writers of record-based outcomes studies.

Process Assessment

A notable example of process assessment is the clinical practice guideline on OME released by the AHCPR in 1994.[30] Clinical guideline development is a major emphasis of recent health policy efforts, driven by economic pressures and a desire to achieve a baseline level of practice in clinical settings. Guideline development is an explicit process, based on highly organized and critical review of the literature, extraction of raw data from primary research sources, and data review by a multidisciplinary panel of experts. Of the 3600 OME articles identified for initial study, 1200 were selected for comprehensive review, and 250 were considered appropriate for evidence-gathering. The final guideline required several years of sustained effort to produce, cost approximately one million dollars, and was scrutinized by nearly 100 expert peer reviewers before publication.

The target population for the OME guideline is a child age 1 through 3 years who is otherwise healthy except for OME, and has no craniofacial, neurological, or sensory deficits. Pneumatic otoscopy was endorsed as the preferred method for detecting OME, and a hearing evaluation was recommended when bilateral effusions persist for 3 months. Antibiotics were considered *optional* therapy, because of the minimal impact on resolution seen in meta-analysis. Antihistamine and decongestant preparations were found ineffective, and oral steroids were not recommended based on limited scientific evidence and panel majority opinion. Tympanostomy tubes were *recommended* for bilateral OME lasting at least 4 months with an associated hearing loss (20 decibels hearing threshold level or worse in the better hearing ear), but were *optional* at 3 months. Adenoidectomy was a clinical option for children age 4 years or older, but tonsillectomy was not recommended at any age for control of OME.

Although the OME guideline is imperfect, it is the most systematic, readable, and clinically relevant overview of the OME literature available. Criticisms raised reflect more the inherent uncertainty of the primary data, not the integrity of the guidelines process. Guidelines are an imperfect way of coping with imperfect data. Readers may debate whether a cut-off of 20 decibels is appropriate for "normal" hearing, whether oral steroids may or may not benefit selected children, and whether children younger than 4 years derive any benefit from adenoidectomy for OME. What is not debatable, however, is the lack of definitive research to support one opinion over the other. The strength of guideline development lies as much in its ability to identify holes in our knowledge base, as in its ability to define rational—and irrational—treatment paradigms.

A delightful example of process assessment run amuck is the attempt by Kleinman and colleagues[31] to assess the appropriateness of tympanostomy tube insertion. After studying a utilization review database for three private insurers, the authors concluded that with "generous clinical assumptions" surgical recommendations were appropriate for 41% of children, equivocal for 32%, and inappropriate for 27%. Not surprisingly, the sensational results received widespread attention in the lay press despite numerous methodological flaws in study design. Unfortunately, these flaws readily escaped the casual reader who was bombarded with terminology such as "expert panel," "two-round modified Delphi method," and "smart-logic branching algorithms" as an assurance of validity.

Scrutiny of the proprietary criteria cited by Kleinman to judge appropriateness show them to be inconsistent and biased. For example, a child with OME for 120 days and untested hearing is an "equivocal" surgical candidate, but becomes "appropriate" after an audiogram is performed, regardless of whether the results are normal or abnormal. What is being assessed here is the presence or absence of an audiogram, not the appropriateness of surgery. Further, a child with hearing loss is an "equivocal" surgical candidate when OME lasts 91 to 120 days, but paradoxically becomes "inappropriate" when the effusion lasts longer. Surgery was also "inappropriate" when no antibiotics were prescribed beyond those for AOM, in spite of the AHCPR conclusion that antibiotics are a clinical option, not a mandate (or even a recommendation) before surgery. Finally, tube insertion was never judged appropriate for *recurrent* AOM—even after breakthrough infections while on antibiotics—despite several RCTs showing efficacy that matched or exceeded antimicrobial prophylaxis.

The most serious problems with this appropriateness study, however, is that the authors do not compare the utilization review process with a gold standard, and hence the sensitivity and specificity are unknown. Some tape-recorded conversations were reviewed for validity, but the reviewer was the lead author of the article, a prior paid consultant for the insurance firm, and someone who is obviously biased against surgery by the negative editorial tone of the article. A meaningful gold standard would incorporate information from physician- or patient-initiated appeals, second opinions by impartial physicians (who actually examined the child), and direct interviews of caregivers and their children. Not only was this information not sought, it was never even determined if the proposed surgeries were performed.

I have elaborated on this article to illustrate what happens when outcomes research is initiated by insurance companies seeking to cut costs, rather than by concerned physicians seeking to increase effectiveness. What can the critical reader conclude from the Kleinman article? That when data are collected with a utilization review process of unknown sensitivity and specificity, and judged for appropriateness against biased and inconsistent criteria, a lot of surgical recommendation appear inappropriate or equivocal. In the words of Mark Twain, "Get your facts first, then you can distort them as you please."

Simple studies of process assessment can be performed easily during routine clinical care. For example, Rosenfeld and Sandhu[32] determined the prevalence of injury counseling opportunities in children referred to a pediatric otolaryngologist by surveying caregivers as part of office registration. A random sample of 300 surveys stratified by age showed that the hottest water temperature was unknown by 72% of caregivers, smokers were present in 25% of households, bicycle helmets were not used by 22% of children, car seats or seat belts were not used by 11% of children, and 10% of homes did not have working smoke alarms. Although 98% of caregivers had a regular pediatrician, 91% of families still offered one or more counseling opportunities. This suggests substantial opportunities for surgical specialists to reinforce the prevention foundation laid by PCPs.

A final example of process assessment concerns the practice of sending patients a copy of the medical report letter sent to the referring doctor. When copies of letters are sent to parents of children after pediatric consultation, nearly all parents respond favorably and note less worry or concern.[33] Information is important to patients, and doctors are often poor communicators. Consequently, the written transfer of information can greatly improve quality of care. Since 1992, I have routinely forwarded a copy of my medical report letter to parents of all children, along with a satisfaction survey that includes a question concerning the value of such a letter. Responses are universally favorable, with many patients asking why this practice has not been adopted by all physicians.

Using Quality of Life Measures to Enhance Clinical Practice

Physicians can participate in the outcomes movement by using quality of life measures in their everyday practice. As noted previously, quality of life reflects the patient's subjective perception of health status. When quality of life improves after physician contact, all stakeholders in the health care process are more likely to view the situation favorably. In the absence of physician-generated effectiveness data, process-based studies (like the Kleinman fiasco described above) will be the only source of outcomes "data" to judge the medical profession.

Outcomes research is more interested in *health-related quality of life* (HRQL) than in overall, or general, quality of life. HRQL excludes other widely valued aspects of life that are not typically considered as "health," including income, freedom, and quality of the environment. Although these aspects are important, they are rarely affected by health interventions. In contrast, a HRQL survey focuses on the physical, social, and emotional impact of disease on the individual. Most surveys are self-administered questionnaires, composed of *items* or questions grouped into *domains* that reflect a particular focus of attention. The focus of an HRQL instrument may be generic or disease specific. Generic measures are of particular interest to policymakers; disease-specific measures are of particular interest to patients and clinicians.

This section will show clinicians how to develop, validate, and use a disease-specific HRQL survey in their routine practice. For the remainder of this section, the term "quality of life survey" will be used for simplicity instead of "disease-specific HRQL survey." Even if you never design your own survey, you will benefit from a little insight into what makes a good survey good and a bad survey bad. Although the approach is purposefully simplistic, curious readers will find more in-depth information in the numerous articles[15,34] and books[35–36] published on survey development.

What Makes a Meaningful Survey?

A quality of life survey is judged by its purpose, reliability, validity, and responsiveness (Table 9–8).When the purpose of the survey is to evaluate change over time (e. g., effectiveness), the instrument is called an *evaluative* measure. Surveys may also be designed to predict prognosis or discriminate among individuals with different levels of disease.[15] Because effectiveness research is of great interest to physicians, I will focus on evaluative measures.

Reliability refers to the stability or reproducibility of a survey result. All measurements possess some degree of unavoidable random error, and survey results are no exception. We are more likely to discount random error when a self-administered survey shows similar results at two time points for a subject with stable disease (test-retest reliability), or when an oral survey is administered twice by the same interviewer (interobserver reliability) or by different interviewers (intraobserver reliability). A survey should have a test-retest coefficient of at least 0.70 before

TABLE 9–8. Comparison of Discriminative, Predictive, and Evaluative Surveys

	Evaluative Survey	*Discriminative Survey*	*Practice Survey*
Purpose	Evaluates within-person change over time in effectiveness studies	Discriminates among individuals along a continuum of illness	Predicts outcome or prognosis
Content	Emphasizes aspects of the domain that respond to clinically significant change	Emphasizes aspects of the domain that are stable over time	Emphasizes items that correlate well with a gold standard measure
Reliability	Requires good test-retest reproducibility; internal consistency less important	Requires good internal consistency and test-retest reproducibility	Requires good internal consistency and test-retest reproducibility
Validity	Degree to which the survey measures what it is supposed to measure	Degree to which the survey measures what it is supposed to measure	Degree to which survey results correlated with a gold standard measure
Responsiveness	Ability of the survey to detect a clinical difference when one is present	Not applicable	Not applicable

it can be recommended for clinical use (a coefficient of 1.00 indicates perfect reliability). The coefficient is calculated in the same manner as for Pearson correlation, but instead of two independent samples the test versus retest results are compared. About 100 subjects must be tested to achieve a precision of ±0.05 (95% confidence interval) for the coefficient.

Another form of reliability often mentioned for surveys is *internal consistency*. When measuring a trait, behavior, or symptom, we usually want the scale to be homogeneous—all the items should be tapping different aspects of the same attribute. If we are measuring the emotional impact of chronic sinusitis on a child, then each item should relate to emotional impact (e. g., irritability, frustration, embarrassment). Therefore, the items should be moderately correlated with each other, as well as the total score for the emotional impact domain omitting that item. Items with Pearson correlation scores less than 0.20 should be discarded or rewritten.

Validity refers to how well the survey is measuring what we think (or hope) it is. Validation is actually a process of hypothesis testing, in which we seek correlations between survey items or results and external measures of similar properties (e. g., a gold standard test or a previously validated survey). For example, we are most likely to believe results of a pain question on a sinusitis survey if the response correlates with radiographic disease or with a pain subscale on a general quality of life measure like the SF-36. Similarly, a question on hearing loss should correlate with audiogram results. Correlation coefficients (R) need not be large, but should be about 0.20 to 0.50. Although statisticians have described a veritable grab bag of validity subtypes (construct validity, criterion validity, etc.), the distinctions are subsidiary to the basic principles already noted.

Responsiveness is the ability of a survey to detect change in a patient's condition. An evaluative measure is typically administered before *and* after some intervention of interest, and the difference in scores is noted. The larger this *change score,* the larger the degree of clinical change, regardless of whether the intervention was watchful waiting, an educational program, or medical or surgical treatment.

An astute reader may wonder "Why bother with change scores? Why not simply ask people how to rate how much they have changed?" Although this is a time-honored approach, people simply do not remember how they were at the beginning. They tend to systematically overestimate their initial symptoms, creating exaggerated effectiveness results. Additional bias occurs because retrospective estimates of initial state are highly correlated with the present state, not the true initial state. Consequently, change should not be assessed directly, but indirectly with change scores.

Creating a Meaningful Survey for Office Use

Disease-specific HRQL outcome surveys are essentially nonexistent for common disorders seen by physicians. Clinicians are ideally positioned to create new instruments, because of their intimate familiarity with patients and diseases. Although innovation is easy when the existing terrain is barren, enthusiasm must be tempered by the principles of survey design enumerated in the preceding section. An evaluative survey must not only look good and make sense, it must have a known amount of reliability, validity, and responsiveness. In the remainder of this section I will illustrate this process by showing how to develop a disease-specific HRQL survey for otitis media.

The first step in creating a disease-specific outcomes survey is to define the domains and items (questions) of interest. For example, the Otitis Media Impact Survey (OMIS) in Figure 9–1] consists of 6 items representing the domains of physical suffering, hearing loss, speech impairment, emotional distress, activity limitations, and caregiver concerns. Each domain has only a single item, although multiple related items could also have been used. Item content is determined by caregiver interviews, consensus among health providers (physicians, audiologists, etc.), and expert review. Ideally the items are unambiguous, ask only a single question, and are comprehensible to the target population (Table 9–4). The target population for the OMIS is children age 6 months or older with chronic OME (3 months or longer) or recurrent AOM (3 or more episodes on past 12 months).

Having defined the items, the next step is to specify the measurement scale for the response. A response s categories is an efficient way to measure change.[37] Using a 7-point scale, a change score of 0.5 indicates minimal clinical change, 1.0 suggests moderate change, and 1.5 is consistent with large change. When fewer than 5 levels are used, reliability and efficiency decrease dramatically. Examples of 7-point Likert scales are shown in the OMIS (Figure 9–1). Likert scales permit a discrete number of continuous responses that are framed on an agree-disagree continuum. At the bottom of the figure is a global ear-related quality of life question, which is scored using a 10-point visual analog scale.[38] Although this survey includes only a global disease-specific question, some investigators recommend that all instruments contain two global ratings: one for overall quality of life and one for health-related issues.[39]

The pilot version of the survey should be tested on a small group of representative patients. If it takes too long to complete, or appears too confusing, it must be rewritten. For each question the frequency of the individual responses should be tallied. Responses chosen less than 20% of the time, or more than 80% of the time, must be reassessed. Similarly, if certain questions routinely get a minimal response level, they should be replaced. A final aspect of the pilot test is to check for internal consistency as described earlier.

When the final version of the survey is ready for testing, thought must be given as to what other data will be collected concurrently for validation. For example, a quality of life survey for sinusitis should show some moderate correlation with results of intranasal examination and CT scan staging. An otitis media survey should correlate with middle ear status, otoscopy results, and prior disease burden (antibiotic use and physician visits). The specifics will vary according to the survey purpose, but the basic principle is to show that the survey behaves the way it should correlating items and domains with appropriate external measures. Another approach is to administer a previously validated general quality of life measure and compare survey findings with appropriate subscale values on the general measure. During the validation process, a subset of patients with stable disease should complete a second survey *within 2 to 14 days* to determine test-retest reliability.

As an example of survey validation, I will briefly present results on 186 patients who received the OMIS, 60 of whom were retested for reliability. Adequate test-retest reliability was obtained both for the survey score ($R = .87$) and the quality of life rating ($R = .85$). Internal consistency was shown for the related domains of speech impairment versus hearing loss ($R = .37$, $P < .001$) and activity limitations versus physical suffering ($R = .48$, $P < .001$). Validity was shown by significant correlations ($P = .002$) between middle ear status (by algorithm) with both the survey score and the caregiver estimate of hearing loss. Significant correlations ($P < .001$) were also observed between survey score and quality of life rating ($R = .64$), doctor's visits past month and physical symptoms ($R = .47$), and antibiotics past months and caregiver concerns ($R = .27$).

The final aspect of testing an evaluative survey—and perhaps the most important—is to demonstrate responsiveness to change. An easy method for assessing responsiveness is to have both the patient estimate the perceived degree of clinical change on a 7-point scale, using positive values for improvement and negative values for deterioration. The survey change score (difference between pre- and post-intervention results) is then tested for correlation with the perceived change levels. An alternate way is to calculate the *standardized response mean* by dividing the mean change score by its standard deviation.[40] Values less than 0.2 denote insensitive instruments, and values greater than 0.8 indicate large sensitivity. For the OMIS, the change score showed good correlation with the degree of reported change ($R = .66$, $P < .001$) and the standardized response mean after tympanostomy tube insertion was 1.7. These preliminary results suggest good responsiveness to longitudinal change.

There is no right or wrong way to design an evaluative survey. The principles and practices outlined above along with the pointers in Table 9–9 should help guide the motivated reader. Using outcomes measures in your practice will not only help demonstrate the effectiveness of the care you provide, but will give greater insight into the way common disorders impact your

OTITIS MEDIA IMPACT SURVEY

Instructions: Please help us understand the impact of ear infections or fluid on your child's quality of life by checking one box [x] for each question below. Thank you.

PHYSICAL SUFFERING: Ear pain, ear discomfort, ear discharge, ruptured ear drum, high fever, or poor balance. How much of a problem for your child during the past 4 weeks?

[ ] Not present/no problem
[ ] Hardly a problem at all
[ ] Somewhat of a problem
[ ] Moderate problem
[ ] Quite a bit of a problem
[ ] Very much a problem
[ ] Extreme problem

HEARING LOSS: Difficulty hearing, questions must be repeated, frequently says "what," or television is excessively loud. How much of a problem for your child during the past 4 weeks?

[ ] Not present/no problem
[ ] Hardly a problem at all
[ ] Somewhat of a problem
[ ] Moderate problem
[ ] Quite a bit of a problem
[ ] Very much a problem
[ ] Extreme problem

SPEECH IMPAIRMENT: Delayed speech, poor pronunciation, difficult to understand, or unable to repeat words clearly. How much of a problem for your child during the past 4 weeks?

[ ] Not present/no problem (or not applicable)
[ ] Hardly a problem at all
[ ] Somewhat of a problem
[ ] Moderate problem
[ ] Quite a bit of a problem
[ ] Very much a problem
[ ] Extreme problem

EMOTIONAL DISTRESS: Irritable, frustrated, sad, restless, or poor appetite. How much of a problem for your child during the past 4 weeks as a result of ear infections or fluid?

[ ] Not present/no problem
[ ] Hardly a problem at all
[ ] Somewhat of a problem
[ ] Moderate problem
[ ] Quite a bit of a problem
[ ] Very much a problem
[ ] Extreme problem

ACTIVITY LIMITATIONS: Playing, sleeping, doing things with friends/family, attending school or day care. How limited have your child's activities been during the past 4 weeks because of ear infections or fluid?

[ ] Not limited at all
[ ] Hardly limited at all
[ ] Very slightly limited
[ ] Slightly limited
[ ] Moderately limited
[ ] Very limited
[ ] Severely limited

CAREGIVER CONCERNS: How often have you, as a caregiver, been worried, concerned, or inconvenienced because of your child's ear infections or fluid over the past 4 weeks?

[ ] None of the time
[ ] Hardly any time at all
[ ] A small part of the time
[ ] Some of the time
[ ] A good part of the time
[ ] Most of the time
[ ] All of the time

OVERALL, HOW WOULD YOU RATE YOUR CHILD'S QUALITY OF LIFE AS A RESULT OF EAR INFECTIONS OR FLUID?
(Circle one number)

0 1 2 3 4 5 6 7 8 9 10

0 = Worse Possible Quality-of-Life; 5 = Half-way Between Worst and Best; 10 = Best Possible Quality-of-Life

FIGURE 9–1. Example of a disease-specific quality of life measure for evaluating longitudinal change in outcomes studies of treatment effectiveness.

patients' lives. The more that patients perceive physician interest in their quality of life, the more enthusiastic they will be about completing outcomes surveys in the office setting.

Measuring Patient Satisfaction

"X rays are a hoax," proclaimed the nineteenth-century physicist Lord Kelvin. If you feel the same way about satisfaction surveys, guess again—learning how patients feel about your practice is essential for thriving under managed care. Why? Because gatekeepers and referring physicians are happiest when the anxious, neurotic, and sick patients they send you return calm, tranquil, and salubrious. If you do not return satisfied patients in that condition, they will find someone else who will. Moreover, physicians who breed satisfaction are at least risk for being sued.[41]

Satisfaction surveys are designed to discriminate (Table 9–8) among patients with different perceptions regarding the quality of care received. Reliability and validity are important when measuring satisfaction because most patients have an inherent tendency to respond favorably. Only rarely do studies performed without standardized measures show satisfaction rates below 90%.[42] Examples of such measures occur commonly in the otolaryngology literature, such as "Are you satisfied with the surgical results?" or "Would you recommend the surgery to a friend or relative?" In contrast, published or standardized measures are developed and tested so that they discriminate among upper levels of satisfaction.

A valid and reliable survey for evaluating office encounters is the nine-item Patient Visit Rating Questionnaire used in the Medical Outcomes Study.[43] Response categories for the items are poor, fair, good, very good, and excellent. The questionnaire instructs patients "Here are some questions about the visit you just made. In terms of your satisfaction, how would you rate each of the following:"

1. The visit overall
2. The technical skills (thoroughness, carefulness, competence) of the person you saw
3. The personal manner (courtesy, respect, sensitivity, friendliness) of the person you saw
4. How long you waited to get an appointment
5. Convenience of the location of the office
6. Getting through to the office by phone
7. Length of time waiting at the office
8. Time spent with the person you saw
9. Explanation of what was done for you

Ware and Hays[44] have shown that optimal validity and reliability are obtained for satisfaction surveys with five-point response scales of "poor, fair, good, very good, and excellent." In contrast, scales ranging from "very satisfied" to "very dissatisfied" are less valid. When scoring the survey, responses may be dichotomized to "excellent" and "not excellent" because current theories of quality management and improvement recommend comparisons to best practices rather than minimal standards.[43] In the Medical Outcomes Study, for example, 64% of solo practitioner's patients rated their visit overall as excellent compared with only 49% of patients in health maintenance organizations ($P < .001$).

TABLE 9–9. Essentials of Designing an Evaluative Quality of Life Survey

1. Keep it simple. A beautifully crafted reliable, valid, and responsive survey is of little use if it is too cumbersome for seamless integration into routine clinical care.
2. Choose questions that fully reflect the diverse physical, emotional, and social impact of the disorder on the target population. Focus on items likely to change with treatment.
3. Use a 7-point response scale to measure change; scales with fewer than 5 options or more than 10 options are not recommended
4. A survey needs more than good looks and common sense; it must be tested for reliability and validity. Determining test-retest reliability is particularly important.
5. Retrospective patient estimates of change are prone to numerous biases; measure change by the difference in survey scores before and after the intervention of interest.
6. Survey findings are subject to the same uncertainty as all medical data; 95% confidence intervals are required to show the range of results consistent with the data

Although using a standardized satisfaction survey allows comparison with published norms, the most useful feedback for your practice will come from adding customized questions. When I survey new patients in my pediatric otolaryngology practice, I include questions about registration, audiology, the play area, and the medical report letter (a copy of which is sent along with the survey). After surgery I send a survey asking patients to grade the preadmission visit, anesthesia experience, nursing staff, operating physician, and initial surgical results.

Written mail surveys encourage anonymity, and the response rate is generally good when a self-addressed stamped envelope is enclosed. Limiting the survey to a single side of an 8½ by 11 inch page with ten or fewer questions will also improve the response rate. I also recommend including several lines at the bottom for comments, and a final question asking the respondent if they wish to be called to discuss their responses. Unsolicited comments provided by patients can be a veritable gold mine of information about your practice.

Surveys are useless if they end up in a circular file; results must be tabulated, prioritized, and taken seriously. The physician or staff member should follow up all negative comments by telephone to solicit additional information and show that the office is sincerely interested in the patient's opinion. Staff meetings are an ideal place to present results and address any issues or problems that need improvement. They also present a wonderful opportunity to acknowledge or reward employees who receive favorable mention in the survey's comments section.

Getting Started in Outcomes Research

In this chapter, I have provided an overview of outcomes research, its virtues and limitations, and its potential impact on practicing physicians. Several points deserve reemphasis. Outcomes research is nothing new; it simply places a quality of life twist on old-fashioned cohort studies. As an observational endeavor, however, outcomes studies are subject to all of the biases and distortions that randomized studies so beautifully prevent. Records-based studies and studies of process assessment face the added problem of garbage in, garbage out. Because these studies rely on data collected for routine patient care or for administrative purposes, important clinical information related to decision making, prognosis, or outcome is often absent.

Outcomes research and randomized trials are synergistic. There is a need for both the realism of experimental studies and the empiricism of personal experience. Outcomes studies are simply a means for systematically recording and interpreting personal experience. As noted by the U.S. physician Alvan Barach, we must "Remember to cure the patient as well as the disease." Randomized trials focus on disease, but outcomes studies emphasize patients and their subjective perceptions of health status. As Tannenbaum[6] so astutely noted, outcomes research is not "a new foundation for clinical medicine; it is raw material for the artful practitioner."

By systematically recording their own clinical experience, practicing physicians can participate proactively in the outcomes movement. Table 9–10 offers some suggestions for involvement. Given the existing void of physician-collected outcomes data, almost any effort will produce new and useful data. A project is most likely to succeed if it is simple, focused, easily understood, and seamlessly integrated into normal office flow. For example, surveys can be completed during registration or while waiting in a room for the physician to enter. As health care providers we cannot afford to delegate responsibility for monitoring effectiveness to insurers and governmental agencies whose overriding objectives are to manage cost—not improve patient care.

TABLE 9–10. Getting Started in Office-Based Outcomes Research

1. Administer satisfaction surveys to all new patients after their initial office visit; keep tract of results on a computerized spreadsheet or simple database.
2. Assess health-related quality of life before and after interventions using previously validated general or disease-specific questionnaires.
3. Develop your own disease-specific quality of life survey to help evaluate outcomes in your particular area of surgical or clinical expertise.
4. Send copies of medical report letters to patients to improve communication; solicit and record feedback on the value of such letters.
5. Form a network with one or more colleagues dedicated to collecting simple outcomes data on clinical disorders or surgical procedures of mutual interest; alternatively, join a large established group such as Project Solo.
6. Gain a better grasp of outcomes research through self education and committee involvement; beware of the numerous problems and pitfalls outlined in this chapter.

REFERENCES

1. Ellwood PM: Outcomes management: a technology of patient experience. *N Engl J Med* 1988; 318:1549–1556.
2. Guadagnoli E, McNeil BJ: Outcomes research: Hope for the future or the latest rage? *Inquiry* 1994; 31:14–24.
3. Maklan CW, Greene R, Cummings MA: Methodological challenges and innovations in patient outcomes research, *Med Care* 1994; 32(Suppl):JS13–JS21.
4. Moses LE: Measuring effects without randomized trials? Otions, problems, challenges *MedCare* 1995; 33 (Suppl): AS8–AS14.
5. Last JM, ed: *A dictionary of epidemiology.* 3rd ed. New York: Oxford University Press, 1995.
6. Tanenbaum SJ: Knowing and acting in medical practice: The epistemological politics of outcomes research. *J Health Politics* 1994; 19:27–44.
7. Moses LE: The series of consecutive cases as a device for assessing outcome of intervention. *N Engl J Med* 1984; 705–710.
8. Turner JA, Deyo RA, Loeser JD, Von Korff M, Fordyce WE: The importance of placebo effects in pain treatment and research. *JAMA* 1994; 271:1609–1614.
9. Feinstein AR: Fraud, distortion, delusion, and consensus: The problems of human and natural deception in epidemiologic science. *Am J Med* 1988; 84:475–478.
10. Feinstein AR: Epidemiologic analysis of causation: The unlearned scientific lessons of randomized trials. *J Clin Epidemiol* 1989;42: 481–489.
11. Gardner MJ, Altman DG: Confidence intervals rather than *p* values: Estimation rather than hypothesis testing. *Br Med J* 1980; 292:746–750.
12. Gustafson TL: *TRUE EPISTAT reference manual.* Richardson, TX: Epistat Services, 1994.
13. Mehta C, Patel N: *StatXact: Statistical software for exact nonparametric inference.* Cambridge, MA: Cytel Software Corporation, 1991.
14. Katz MH, Hauck WW: Proportional hazards (Cox) regression. *J Gen Int Med* 1993; 8:702–711.

15. Jaeschke R, Guyatt GH. How to develop and validate a new quality of life instrument. In: Spilker B, ed: *Quality of life assessments in clinical trials.* New York: Raven Press, 1990:47–57.
16. Hoffman SR, Mahoney MC, Chmiel JF, Stinziano GD, Hoffman KN: Symptom relief after endoscopic sinus surgery: an outcomes-based study. *ENT J* 1993; 72:413–420.
17. Gliklich RE, Hilinski JM: Longitudinal sensitivity of generic and specific health measures in chronic sinusitis. *Quality Life Res* 1995; 4:27–32.
18. Rosenfeld RM: Pilot study of outcomes in pediatric rhinosinusitis. *Arch Otolaryngol Head Neck Surg* 1995; 221:729–736.
19. Ware JE, Sherbourne CD: The MOS 36-Item Short-Form Health Survey (SF-36). *Med Care* 1992; 30:473–483.
20. Lee D, Rosenfeld: Adenoid bacteriology and sinonasal symptoms in children. *Otolaryngol Head Neck Surg;* in press.
21. Gliklich RE, Metson R: Techniques for outcomes research in chronic sinusitis. *Laryngoscope* 1995; 105:387–390.
22. D'Antonio LL, Zimmerman GJ, Cella DF, Long SA: Quality of life and functional status measures in patients with head and neck cancer. *Arch Otolaryngol Head Neck Surg* 1996; 112:482–487.
23. Gliklich RE, Metson R: The health impact of chronic sinusitis in patients seeking otolaryngologic care. *Otolaryngol Head Neck Surg* 1995; 113:104–109.
24. Lorig K, Stewart A, Ritter, et al: *Outcome Measures for Health Education and other Health Care Interventions.* Thousand Oaks, CA: SAGE Publications, 1996.
25. Rosenfeld RM: How to systematically review the medical literature. *Otolaryngol Head and Neck Surg* 1996.
26. Rosenfeld RM: What to expect from medical treatment of otitis media. *Pediatr Infect Dis J* 1995; 14:731–738.
27. Berman S, Roark R, Luckey D: Theoretical cost effectiveness of management options for children with persisting middle ear effusions. *Pediatrics* 1994; 93:353–363.
28. Wennberg, JE, Blowers L, Parker R, Gittelsohn AM: Changes in tonsillectomy rates associated with feedback and review. *Pediatrics* 1977; 59: 821–826.
29. McPherson K, Wennberg JE, Hovind OB, Clifford P: Small-area variations in the use of common surgical procedures: An international comparison of New England, England, and Norway. *N Engl J Med* 1982; 307:1310–1314.
30. Stool SE, Berg AO, Berman S, et al: *Otitis media with effusion in young children. Clinical practice guideline.* Number 12. AHCPR Publication No. 94-0622. Rockville, MD: Agency for Health Care Policy and Research, Public Health Service, US Dept. of Health and Human Services. July 1994.
31. Kleinman LC, Kosecoff J, Dubois RW, Brook RH: The medical appropriateness of tympanostomy tubes proposed for children younger than 16 years in the United States. *JAMA* 1994; 271:1250–1255.
32. Rosenfeld RM, Sandhu S: Injury prevention counseling opportunities in pediatric otolaryngology. *Arch Otolaryngol Head Neck Surg* 1996; in press.
33. Waterson T, San Lazaro C: Sending parents outpatient letters about their children: Parents' and general practitioners' views. *Qual Health Care* 1994; 3:142–146.
34. Kessler RC, Mroczek DK: Measuring the effects of medical interventions. *Med Care* 1995; 33(Suppl):AS109–AS119.
35. Streiner DL, Norman GR: *Health measurement scales: A practical guide to their development and use.* 2nd ed. Oxford: Oxford Medical Publications, 1995.
36. Fink A: *The survey handbook.* Thousand Oaks, CA: SAGE Publications, 1995.
37. Juniper EF, Guyatt GH, Willan A, Griffith LE: Determining a minimal important change in a disease-specific quality of life questionnaire. *J Clin Epidemiol* 1994; 47:81–87.
38. Hadorn DC, Uebersax J: Large-scale health outcomes evaluation: How should quality of life be measured? Part I—calibration of a brief questionnaire and a search for preference subgroups. *J Clin Epidemiol* 1995; 48:5:607–618.
39. Gill TM, Feinstein AR: A critical appraisal of the quality of quality-of-life measurements. *JAMA* 1994; 272:619–626.
40. Gliklich RE, Hilinski JM: Longitudinal sensitivity of generic and specific health measures in chronic sinusitis. *Qual Life Res* 1995; 4:27–32.
41. Levinson W: Physician-patient communication: a key to malpractice prevention. *JAMA* 1994:272:1619–1620.
42. Health Services Research Group: A guide to direct measures of patient satisfaction in clinical practice. *Can Med Assoc J* 1992; 146:1727–1731.
43. Rubin HR, Gandek B, Rogers WH, Kosinski M, McHorney CA, Ware HE Jr: Patients' ratings of outpatient visits in different practice settings. Results from the medical outcomes study. *JAMA* 1993; 270:835–840.
44. Ware JE Jr, Hays RD: Methods for measuring patient satisfaction with specific medical encounters. *Med Care* 1988; 26:393–402.

Dr. Rosenfeld is an Associate Professor of Otolaryngology at the State University of New York Health Science Center at Brooklyn, and Director of Pediatric Otolaryngology at The Long Island College Hospital and the University Hospital of Brooklyn. He is a regular contributor to the American Academy of Otolaryngology—Head & Neck Surgery (AAO-HNS) Instruction Course Program, where he teaches biostatistics, otitis media, and reading the medical literature. Dr. Rosenfeld is a member of the AAO-HNS Research Review Committee, Outcomes Task Force on Otitis Media, Task Force on New Materials, and Instructional Course Advisory Committee. He has authored over 50 articles and book chapters and given over 150 scientific presentations. Dr. Rosenfeld's clinical and research interests include all areas of pediatric otolaryngology, with emphasis on sinusitis, otitis media, meta-analysis, and outcomes research.

10

Improving Health Care: Measuring Outcomes and Implementing Change

EUGENE C. NELSON, JULIE J. MOHR, PAUL B. BATALDEN, STEPHEN K. PLUME, AND CHRISTINE C. MAHONEY

Part 1: The Clinical Value Compass

Health care providers still don't get it. What other industry asks you to pay more for its defects? DRG's are higher for complications than for uncomplicated events. If an infection occurs during a hospital stay, the cost goes up and the buyer is expected to pay it. When we sell a computer, if there is a problem we have to fix it, at no cost to the customer. We need to pay for the health achieved, not the work done.

Robert Hungate, formerly of Hewlett Packard

Health care providers are getting a wake-up call. The message is to improve value—rapidly. This chapter aims to provide practical, user-friendly *tutorials* that busy clinicians can use to improve the value of health care quickly and successfully. Real improvement will come only when we link the measurement of outcomes with the understanding and change of the processes and systems related to the production of those results. These tutorials build on prior work by the authors and others and focus on "how to." Each one will include a worksheet to guide the clinician team through a particular aspect of clinical improvement work, plus case examples to illustrate how the concepts can be applied in the real world.

Part 1 introduces the quality/value paradigm in health care and offer instruction on how to construct a clinical value compass. Part 2 provides guidance on the total process of making improvements, beginning with aim and clarification of the clinical process and proceeding with the generation of change concepts and the subsequent tests of high-leverage changes by running a PDCA (Plan-Do-Check-Act) cycle. Part 3 offers an approach for conducting clinical benchmarking to identify the "best of the best" in the provision of care and learn how new processes might be adapted and tested in one's own delivery system. Part 4 presents generalizable techniques and change concepts that can be applied to many different clinical processes to generate testable ideas for improving outcomes and lowering costs.

Health Care Value: The New Paradigm

The most pressing current problem with the nation's health care delivery system has little to do with traditional health professional views of quality; however, it does involve the costs of care (and to a lesser extent, access to care for all segments of the population). There is widespread sentiment that the costs for delivering health care—now approximating 15% of gross domestic product—have been rising too fast and consume too much of our nation's wealth. Runaway health care costs terrify consumers who are uninsured and create worry about losing coverage for those who are insured. They erode the profits of business and industry, jeopardize the nation's competitiveness in a global economy, and contribute to the upward spiral of the national debt. Health care reform is moving ahead rapidly even without new government legislation. Market forces are propelling the health care industry in the direction of integrated, managed care systems and away from fee-for-service, piecework delivery systems.

What this means is that a new paradigm for *good* health care is rapidly gaining momentum and widespread acceptance. The motto might be put simply: "best quality at lowest cost." The era of *value* in health care is now upon us. Value can be thought of as quality in relationship to the cost and the volume of services.[1,2] A value equation might look like this:

$$\text{Value} = f\left(\frac{\text{Quality}}{\text{Costs}} \times \text{Volume}\right)$$

That is, the value of a service is a function of the service's quality divided by its cost and multiplied by the number of services provided (volume). Improving the value of health care is a matter of increasing quality while decreasing or holding costs and volume constant, or decreasing costs and volume while increasing or holding quality constant. Those who pay for health care—particularly employers/purchasers—are focusing on care that is based on value: quality in relationship to price per unit of service and volume of services provided.

Making Improvements: Measuring and Improving Value

There is skepticism in some quarters about whether quality and value can be accurately measured or improved using continual improvement principles and methods.[3] Great advances have been made in the measurement of clinical status, health status, health risk, and patient satisfaction during the past decade.[1,4–7] We believe that measurement of quality and outcomes is no longer an insurmountable barrier to documenting whether value is improving or declining.

Moreover, the evidence showing that providers can use continual improvement to systematically enhance outcomes and cut costs is growing. Here are a few examples of what clinical teams can accomplish given both time and expertise:

- *Reduce postsurgical wound infection rates from 1.8% in 1985 to 0.4% in 1991, saving the hospital $500,000 per year.*[8]
- *Decrease adverse drug reactions from 5.0% to 0.2%, saving the hospital $450,000 per year.*[9]
- *Cut mortality rate for CABG surgery by 26% from 1990 to 1993, representing 82 fewer deaths in northern New England.*[10]

It is clear that wise application of continual improvement methods can generate better value health care, just as it has succeeded in other sectors of the economy.[11] We believe that the main challenge is to *accelerate* durable clinical improvement work and to *disseminate* it throughout our health care delivery system.

The Clinical Value Compass Approach

Four assumptions about the aim of health care, quality, and value follow:

1. *The* ***aim*** *of health care is to prevent or diagnose and treat disease and thereby reduce or limit the burden of illness by restoring or maintaining healthy functioning.*[12,13,14–15]
2. *Human* ***functioning*** *is made up of biological, physical, mental, and social health.*[3,13]
3. *Quality health care provides services (i.e., clinical care processes) that are most likely to achieve the health* ***outcomes desired*** *by the patient.*[6,16]
4. *The* ***value*** *of health care is a function of quality, costs, and volume.*[1,4,15,17]

How might these assumptions be put together into a useful, understandable whole? There are probably many ways to do this, but one approach that we have found to be helpful is illustrated in Figure 10–1; it's called the "clinical value compass."

First, the figure starts with people who experience a health need: an individual patient (or a population) who has a health need (such as a fractured leg in need of repair, heart attack in need of treatment, child with need to manage asthma and prevent diseases through immunization). These patients can be described—at "baseline" or before a treatment episode starts—in terms of their clinical status, functional health status, and expectations (what they hope that health care can accomplish for them in terms of pain relief, symptom reduction, freedom from physical and mental limitations, etc.). They can also be characterized by the amount of health-related costs they have experienced up to this point due to prior utilization of health care. In a sense, the cost "meter" for each individual starts running at birth and continues rising until death.

Second, it illustrates the flow of the delivery process—accessing system, assessing patient, diagnosing patient, treating patient, following up with the patient. Third, these process steps create a result, for each patient or a population, that can be measured in a set of quality-related *outcomes* and *costs*. Once again, the patient (or population) can be described posttreatment or at the end of the illness episode with respect to their clinical status, functional status, and satisfaction against fundamental need and pretreatment expectations. The patients can also be characterized, again, with respect to the incremental health-related costs they have incurred as a result of this new treatment episode. Note that the health "outcomes" are, in fact, transitions in quality-related outcomes (clinical status, functioning, satisfaction), and the "costs" are, in fact, incremental costs associated with treatment.

We call the circular display of measures—which is shown twice in Figure 10–1 at time 1 (pre-episode) and

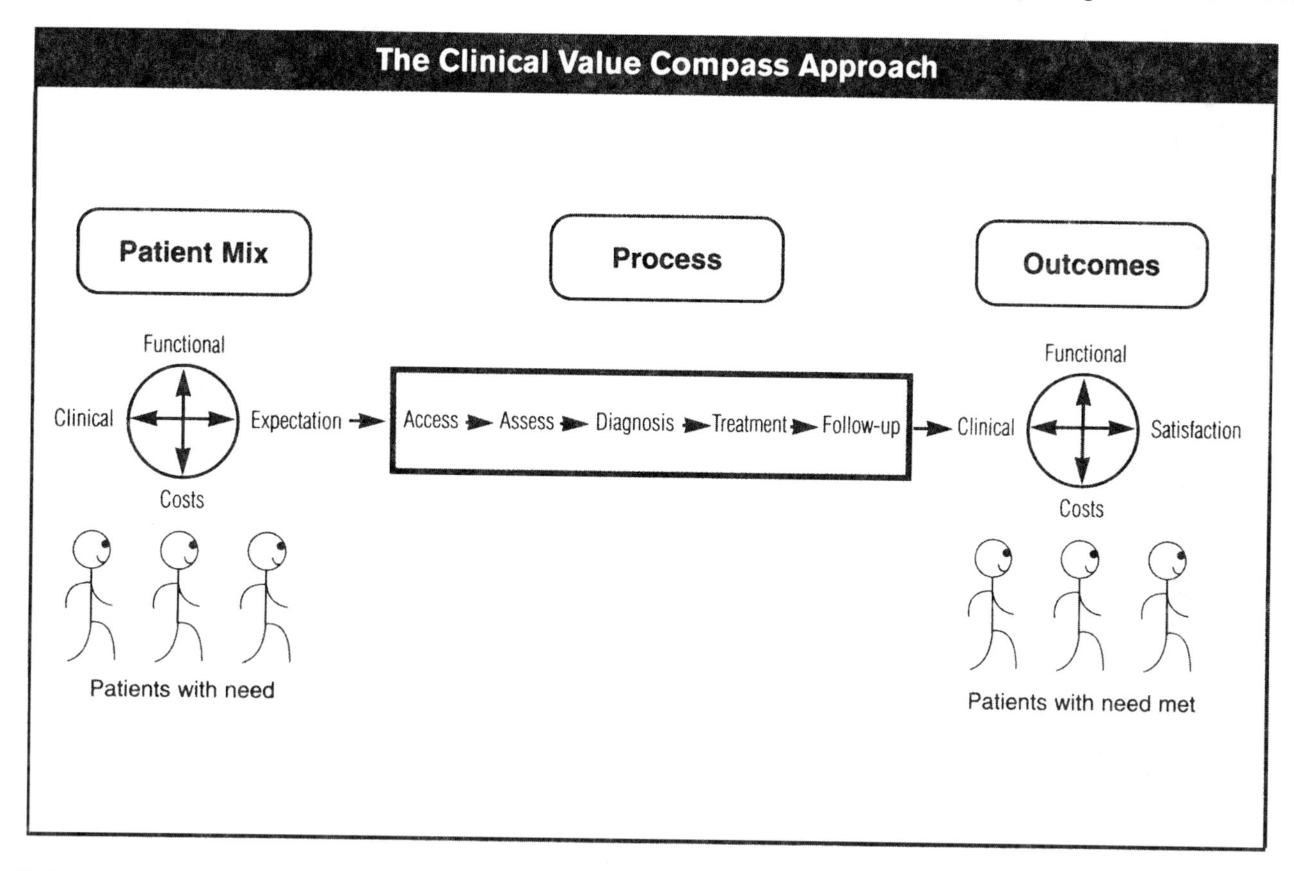

FIGURE 10–1. Patient care processes and outcomes: the clinical value compass approach.

time 2 (post-episode)—a clinical value compass, because the layout resembles an old-fashioned, directional compass used for navigation. It has four cardinal points:

- North—*Functional health status, risk status, and well-being*
- South—*Costs (direct health care costs for physicians, hospitals, drugs, etc., and indirect social costs incurred by the family, employer, and community)*
- East—*Satisfaction with health care and perceived health benefit*
- West—*Clinical outcomes (such as mortality, morbidity and complications)*

All four compass points are important. The territory in each respective direction needs to be more fully explored, documented, and mapped.

The following logic underpins the value compass approach. If providers wish to manage and improve the value of the services they provide, they will then need to: (1) measure the value of care for similar patient populations; (2) analyze the internal delivery processes that contribute significantly to the current levels of measured outcomes and costs; (3) run tests of **changed** delivery processes; and (4) deter-mine if these changes lead to better outcomes and lower costs.

It is apparent that, if one were to take all **recognized** dimensions of *structure* and *process quality* (such as facilities, equipment, supplies, appropriateness, availability, continuity, effectiveness, efficacy, respect and caring, safety, and timeliness) and *outcomes quality* (such as biological function, physical function, mental health, social/role function, health risk status, and health-related quality of life) and apply them to the care for almost any particular health problem or condition (such as low back pain, depression, chemical dependency, pregnancy, and childbirth), then it would be complicated and costly to conceptualize, define, and measure the quality of care in a truly comprehensive manner.[17]

The clinical value compass approach allows us to select some critical indicators of process and outcome that are known to be significant and are of the greatest interest to the group in evaluating or judging quality and focus attention on these vital, few dimensions of quality that hold the most interest.

Clinical Value Compass Worksheet

The Clinical Value Compass Worksheet is shown in Figure 10–2 (worksheet front) and Figure 10–3 (worksheet back). This worksheet aims to help clinicians move

Clinical Value Compass Worksheet, Side A

① **Outcomes:** Select a population. *Patients with confirmed acute MI, direct admits only, from time of admission to Emergency Department to 8 weeks post discharge.*
(specify patient population)

② **Aim:** **What is the general aim? Given our desire to limit/reduce the illness burden for "this type" of patient, what are the desired results?**

We aim to find ways to continually improve the quality and value of care for acute MI patients.

TIPS: Path Forward →

Worksheet purpose: to identify measures of outcomes/costs that contribute most to the value of care.

1. Select a clinically significant population.
2. Assemble small interdisciplinary team.
3. Use brainstorming or nominal group technique to generate "long" list of measures.
4. Start with West (Clinical) on the compass and go clockwise around the compass.
5. Use multi-vote to identify "short" list of 4-12 key measures of outcomes and costs.
6. Determine what data is needed vs. what data can get in real time at affordable cost.
7. Use Side B of worksheet to record the names and definitions of selected measures of value.

③ **Value:** Select starter set of outcomes/cost measures.

Clinical
- Mortality
- Morbidity
- Complications

Death
Angina

Functional
- Physical Function
- Mental Health
- Social/Role
- Other (eg, Pain, Health Risk)

Physical function
Overall health status

Satisfaction
- Health Care Delivery
- Perceived Health Benefit

Patient satisfaction with hospital
Change in overall health

Costs
- Direct Medical
- Indirect Social

Total hospital charges
Length of stay
Days lost from work/routine

Eugene C. Nelson, DSc, MPH; Paul B. Batalden, MD; Stephen K. Plume, MD; Julie J. Mohr, MSPH
© February 1995, Lahey Hitchcock Clinic

FIGURE 10–2. Clinical Value Compass Worksheet: Side A.

Clinical Value Compass Worksheet, Side B

TIPS: Conceptual & Operational Definitions →

A conceptual definition is a brief statement describing a variable of interest. It should tell people what you want to measure and who "owns" it.

An operational definition is a clearly specified method for reliably sorting, classifying or measuring a variable. It should be written as an instruction set, or protocol, that would enable two different people to measure the variable, using the same process, and thereby, producing the same result. It should explain to people how a variable should be measured.

④ Specific Operational Definitions for key outcome and cost measures.

Variable Name & Brief Conceptual Definition (see "TIP" to the left)	Source of Data & Operational Definition (see "TIP" to the left)
A. *Death: patient dies during hospital stay or within 8 weeks post discharge.* *Owner:* ______	*Medical record review indicates patient died, or follow-up by mail/telephone at 8 weeks indicates patient died.*
B. *Angina: angina pectoris – pain in chest associated with coronary artery disease (Rose scale).* *Owner:* ______	*Patient's answers to four questions at 8 weeks coded to form scale:* *27. Do you ever have any pain or discomfort in your chest?* • *Yes* • *No* *28. If no, do you ever have any pressure or heaviness in your chest?* • *Yes* • *No* *36. Do you have this pain, discomfort, pressure or heaviness when you walk up hill or hurry?* • *Yes* • *No* *37. Do you have these symptoms at an ordinary pace on level ground?* • *Yes* • *No*
C. *Physical function: the ability to perform physical activities associated with normal living (COOP scale).* *Owner:* ______	*Patient's answers to one question at 8 weeks:* *26. During the past 2 weeks, what was the most strenuous level of physical activity you could do for at least 2 minutes?* • *Very heavy, e.g.,* ______ • *Light, e.g.,* ______ • *Heavy, e.g.,* ______ • *Very light, e.g.,* ______ • *Moderate, e.g.,* ______
D. *Overall health: patient's general perception of his/her health status (COOP Chart).* *Owner:* ______	*Patient's answers to one question at 8 weeks:* *1. During the past 2 weeks, how would you rate your overall physical health and emotional condition?* • *Excellent* • *Very Good* • *Good* • *Fair* • *Poor*
E. *Patient satisfaction with hospital: patient's overall rating of inpatient care and services (HQT item).* *Owner:* ______	*Patient's answers to one question at 8 weeks:* *33. How likely would you be to return to this hospital if you ever needed to be hospitalized again?* • *I'm 100% sure that I'd return* • *I probably would not return* • *It's very likely that I'd return* • *It's very unlikely that I'd return* • *I probably would return* • *I'm 100% sure that I would not return* • *I'm not sure if I'd return* • *Does not apply to me, because I do not live near hospital*
F. *Change in overall health: patient's perception of the health benefit received from care.* *Owner:* ______	*Patient's answers to one question at 8 weeks:* *7. Overall, is your health better or worse than you expected it to be at this point?* • *Much better than expected* • *Somewhat worse than I expected* • *Somewhat better than expected* • *Much worse than expected* • *About what I expected*
G. *Total hospital charges: the sum of all inpatient charges to the patient for the stay, excluding physician charges.* *Owner:* ______	*Search of hospital's billing records to determine total sum of charges billed to the patient's account for the hospital stay.*
H. *Length of stay: number of days patient stayed in hospital.* *Owner:* ______	*Medical record review used to determine date of admission and date of discharge; length of stay computed based on interval.*

Eugene C. Nelson, DSc, MPH; Paul B. Batalden, MD; Stephen K. Plume, MD; Julie J. Mohr, MSPH
© February 1995, Lahey Hitchcock Clinic

FIGURE 10–3. Clinical Value Compass Worksheet: Side B.

efficiently through the process of identifying key measures of outcomes and costs (Side A) and serves as a place for recording the operational definitions of key measures that are actually selected for measurement (Side B). (Single copies of this worksheet are available from the authors on written request at no charge.) This worksheet is related to the *Clinical Improvement Worksheet.* A Users Manual for the Clinical Improvement Worksheet will be provided in Part 2 of this chapter. Both worksheets are based on the Serial Vee approach to improving clinical care.[18]

The Clinical Value Compass Worksheet begins with the selection of a clinical population and an outcomes-based aim statement that becomes the focus of improvement work. The core of the worksheet is the clinical value compass. As compared to the clinical value compass shown in Figure 10–1 the four cardinal points have prompts or cues for categories of measures that should be considered early in the outcomes/costs measurement idea generation process.

- Clinical—*mortality and morbidity (such as signs, symptoms, treatment complications, diagnostic test results, laboratory determinations of physiologic values).*
- Functional—*physical function, mental health, social/role function, and other measures of health status (such as pain, vitality, perceived well-being, and health risk status).*
- Satisfaction—*patient/family satisfaction with health care delivery process, patient's perceived health benefit from care received.*
- Costs—*direct medical costs (ambulatory care, inpatient services, medications, etc.) and indirect social costs (days lost from work/normal routine, replacement worker costs, caregiver costs).*

The Clinical Value Compass Worksheet follows Russell Ackoff's advice on problem solving. His counsel is: "Think up. Think down. Think up again."[19] Ackoff is suggesting that we should first think about the big picture and take the long view before honing in on the specifics of a problem to be solved. After working on the specifics and arriving at a sound plausible solution, one should then think again about the specific solution in light of its fit with the larger issues and longer term aims. This is akin to starting with strategy before going to tactics and then checking tactics and actions against strategic intent. Side A of the worksheet invites the user to "think up," Side B to "think down."

How to Make a Clinical Value Compass: Case Example. Acute MI

The Clinical Value Compass Worksheet, shown in Figures 10–2 and 10–3, can be used to design a method for measuring outcomes and costs in the real world. (See the Side Bar case study for information on how this approach was used in a community hospital to begin the work of measuring value for the purpose of improving care.)

An approach for making a clinical value compass is illustrated next using acute myocardial infarction (MI) as a case example and is illustrated in Figures 10–4 and 10–5.

Side A—Getting Started: Outcomes and Aim

The process begins with a statement of aim that's linked to desired outcomes for a target population. This is an invitation to "think up." The aim statement answers the question, "What are we trying to accomplish?"[20]

In this case, the team selects an acute MI population for observation over a certain time period: *Patients with confirmed acute MI who are directly admitted to the hospital (that is, nontransfer patients). The clinical process starts at the time of admission to the Emergency Department and ends at 8 weeks post discharge.*

In general, it's best to select a clinical population and time period over which the clinical team has primary responsibility for patient care. Next, the team clarifies its aim and writes down the answer to the question, "Given our desire to limit/reduce the burden of illness for acute MI patients, what are the desired results? What's the aim?" In this case, the team describes their aim in this way: *to find ways to continually improve the quality and value of care for acute MI patients.*

Although it is often helpful to start with a general aim statement (as illustrated above), over time, most teams will want to revise their aim statement to make it more specific. The increased specificity tends to result from the team's work to: (1) describe the current clinical care process; (2) identify potential changes that are expected to lead to improvement; and (3) select specific "high leverage" changes to test using a plan-do-check/study-act cycle. Part 2 in this series will introduce this process of winnowing down the aim from general to specific.

Value Measures: Select a Set of Outcome/Cost Measures

If a team is designing a value compass, it can then proceed to select important measures of outcomes and costs by circling the value compass, beginning with clinical status and followed by functional status, satisfaction, and costs, respectively. Subcategories of measures are bulleted under each value compass point as reminders of the types of variables that might be considered under each broad area. Knowledge of the appropriate literature is the place to begin. A shared knowledge base from that literature, combined with the daily experience of patient care, will usually yield a large number of potential measures. Decision-making skills—such as brainstorming and nominal group technique to generate ideas along with multivoting to reduce a long list to a manageable number of measures—can be helpful.[21]

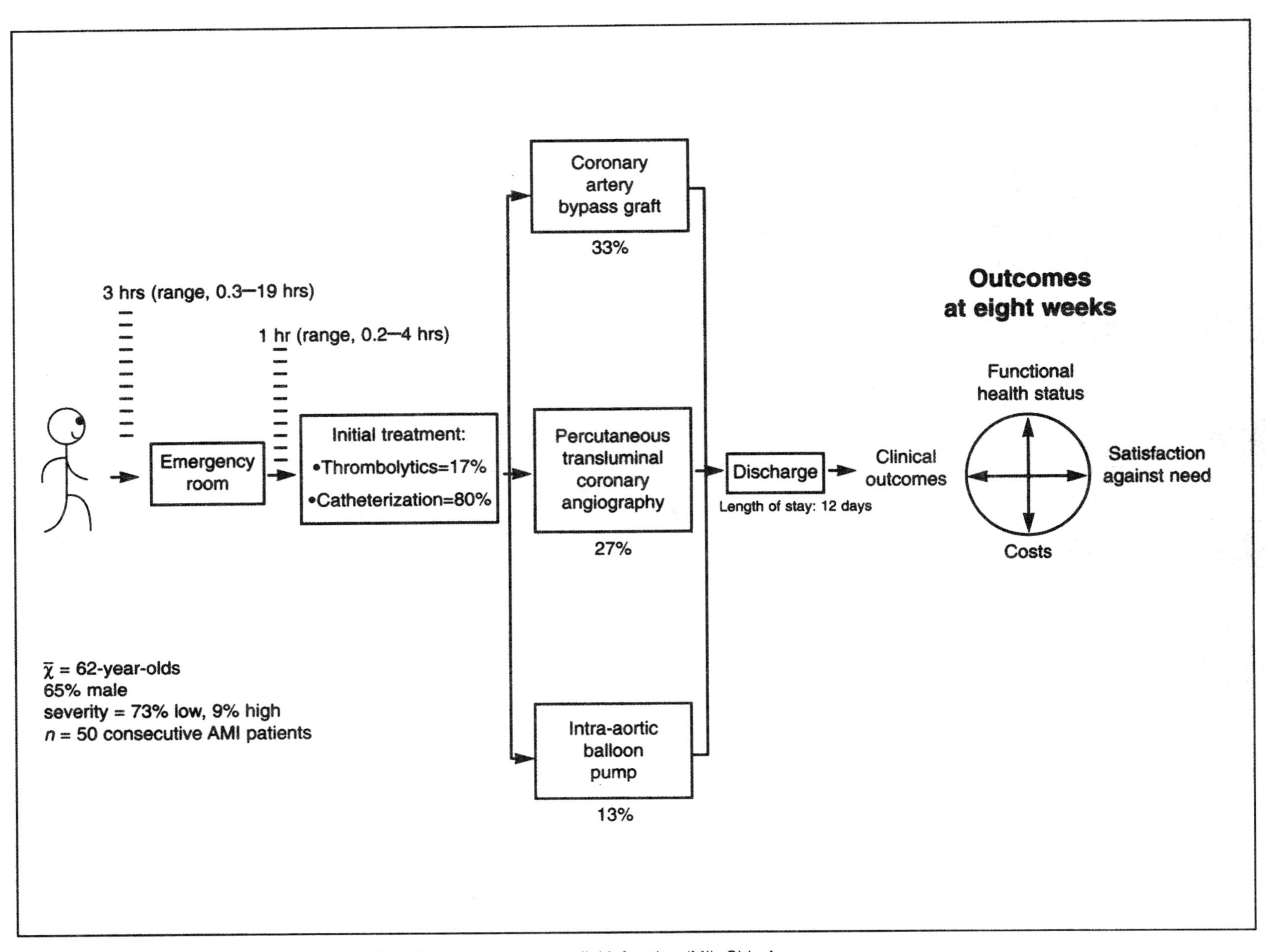

FIGURE 10–4. Clinical Value Compass Worksheet for an acute myocardial infarction (MI): Side A.

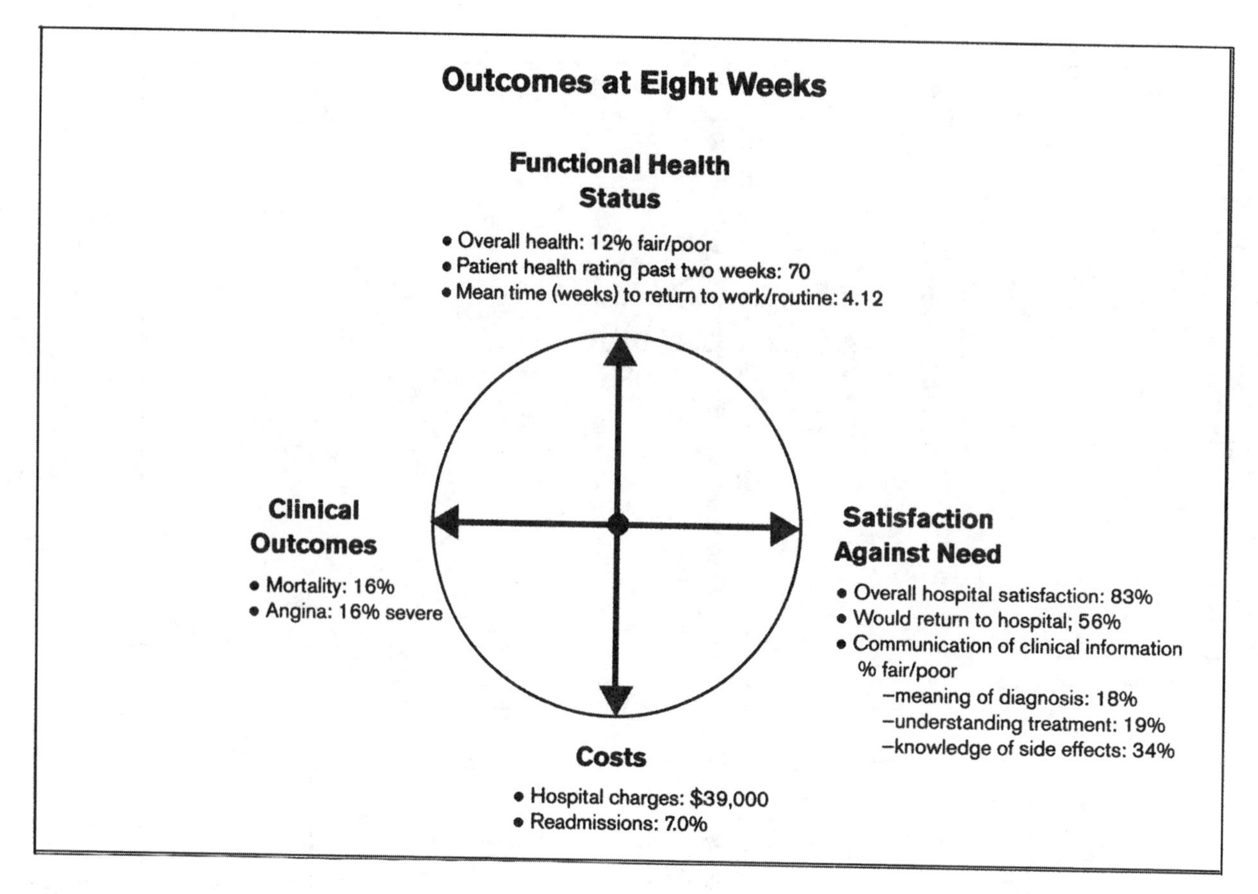

FIGURE 10–5. Clinical Value Compass Worksheet for an acute myocardial infarction (MI): Side B.

It is extremely important to note that the Clinical Value Compass Worksheet starts with a statement that intends to capture the ethical values of clinical professionals. This statement reads: "Given our desire to limit/reduce the illness burden for this type of patient, what are the desired results? What's the aim?" If we wish to enlist busy clinicians in the work of improving care, then it is essential to start the work off with an explicit tie to the ethical canons of the helping professions and the personal value set of clinicians—to find the best ways to help patients.

A word of caution. Although the list of potential outcome/cost measures can be very long, *it is usually prudent to start measurement work with a small number of key measures for which it is possible to collect reasonably accurate information at a cost that's affordable.* Recall that our intention is to improve (make better than in the immediate past) our ability to characterize the results of care from the perspective of value. As a rule of thumb, 4 to 12 carefully chosen outcome/cost measures are sufficient to get started. More measures can always be added as time passes, experience is gained, and needs for data change.

This list summarizes the *starter set* of key measures selected by the team for initial monitoring on all acute MI patients:

Clinical Status
- Death in hospital or within 8 weeks post discharge
- Angina symptoms

Functional Status
- Physical function
- Overall health

Satisfaction Against Need
- Patient satisfaction with hospital
- Change in overall health

Costs
- Total hospital charges
- Length of stay in hospital
- Days lost from work/normal routine

The clinical team used nominal group methods and brainstorming to produce a long list of potential measures of outcomes/costs, then used multivoting to reduce the list to a smaller, more manageable number for which data could be gathered from one of three sources: (1) medical record review; (2) administrative and billing data; or (3) patient-based data gathered by mailed questionnaire (with telephone follow-up of nonrespondents) at 8 weeks post discharge. Although the list of value outcomes is small, the team did (and this is a critical point) have one or more measures for each quadrant of the compass.

Side B: Operational Definitions of Measures

Side B of the Clinical Value Compass Worksheet provides space for recording "think down" ideas in the form of specific definitions of key outcome/cost measures. For each measure, the name is listed, along with a conceptual definition of the measure (a brief description of the dimension or phenomenon of interest) and a specific operational definition (a specific, reliable, understandable process for turning the concept into a specific observation on each patient). If a measure is based on a previously published or validated measure, the source can be listed along with the name of the measure. Figure 10–5 provides definitions for most of the measures selected by the acute MI team. It is very important to state operational definitions clearly and correctly.[22] Reliability and validity of measures are critically dependent on clear operational definitions that are applied consistently. As shown in Figure 10–5 the measures will be based on information from the medical record, administrative/financial records, and patient reports and ratings at 8 weeks post discharge.

Once the plans for the value compass measures have been laid out and recorded on the Clinical Value Compass Worksheet, the next steps involve designing: (1) the data collection plan (a simple graphic of who, what, where, when, and how for each measure may be helpful); (2) analysis plan for different users; (3) display of information; (4) distribution of results; and (5) use of the results for managing patients and improving care.[23] The displays should include graphical approaches for showing summary information (e.g., results for first 50 patients) and/or comparative information (such as results for this quarter versus prior quarter, or the organization's results compared with other organizations' results) and control charts for displaying variation and trends over time for individual measures (e.g., control chart showing length of stay for past 24 months).

Comments on Clinical Value Compass Worksheet and Approach

Some discussion and a few words of warning may be helpful before moving to concluding comments. We have used the Clinical Value Compass approach and Clinical Improvement Worksheet for several years and offer these provisional insights and advice.

Be Flexible

The overall aim is to accelerate clinical improvement, not to slavishly follow any one method for making improvements. There are two flaws to avoid in making improvements: going too fast ("ready, fire, aim") or going too slow ("Ready . . . ? Ready . . . ? Are you sure you are ready?"). Sometimes, it is prudent for a clinical team to work quickly through Side A of the Clinical Value Compass Worksheet and skip the step of constructing precise definitions (Side B) until a specific test of change has been selected. Often, the very occasion of coming together to discuss a common patient care problem will yield many different ideas for improvement. In this case, it is often helpful to proceed with some test of change that everyone agrees is worth doing, even if they do not agree about its relative priority. Making improvements is more important than arguing about which improvement should be attempted first.

Once a test of change has been decided on, the team can create operational definitions for key outcome/cost measures of the specific test of change, and these measures can be obtained in real time at affordable cost. If a clinical group is committed to long-term improvement and repeated tests of change, it may be wise to begin developing a clinical value compass data set that can be gathered and analyzed continuously to spot favorable trends, monitor progress, and detect adverse events quickly.

Start Small

The Clinical Value Compass approach reminds us that there are many facets to quality and value. It is easy to feel overwhelmed after discovering a multitude of facets, and to be tempted to measure everything from the start. This is generally a mistake. It is usually best to start with a small, balanced set of important outcome/cost measures that can be measured reasonably well and that "hit" each of the four value compass quadrants. New and better measures can be added at any point in future.

Build Measurement into Delivery Process

Measurement systems that quantify the quality of processes and results of care are all too often add-ons to routine care delivery. This offers the opportunity for customized design and standardization, but has a major drawback—it adds new costs and thereby reduces value, unless the new measures generate better quality. The process of measurement should be intertwined with the process of care delivery. This approach is likely to be efficient and durable (measure the right thing at the right time and use it in multiple ways) and effective, because front-line providers are involved in both managing the patient and measuring the process and related outcomes/costs. The new measures can be used, in real time, to improve care for the individual patient, and, if combined with continuous improvement models, can also be available immediately to redesign care for future patients.[24] This means that one must select measures that are actionable by those involved in providing the service, and are proximal to (upstream from) the result and drive the desired quality characteristic of the result.

Here are two examples of building measurement into the delivery process. First, primary care clinicians in the Dartmouth COOP Project have found that building standardized assessment of their elderly patients' functional status into the beginning of the visit improves the appropriateness of the regimen and patient satisfaction. In addition, the standardized measures of function can be aggregated to analyze functional status of the clinician's entire panel of patients compared to other similar panels of elderly patients.[24] Second, the cardiac services team at Dartmouth-Hitchcock Medical Center have discovered that coronary artery bypass graft (CABG) patients who must be "returned to pump" have a much higher mortality rate. Therefore, the pump clinicians and cardiac team keep running counts of the frequency of returning patients to the pump and attempt to manage each patient in a way that minimizes the need to do so.[25]

Compass Metaphor: Clear or Confusing

No metaphor is perfect or works equally well for all individuals. We have used the "compass" as a metaphor to bring to mind four key aspects of health care value—clinical status, functional status and well being, satisfaction, and costs—just as a compass brings to mind four cardinal points—north, south, east and west. As a compass is used for navigation on the open seas or for orienteering in the north woods, there is no inherent hierarchy of the points. All are important. Clinical value for a patient, or for defined patient/member populations, is the territory to be explored and understood. If one wishes to explore the southern region of the clinical value territory, one would be learning about the direct and indirect costs of care. If one seeks to explore the northern region of the territory, then one would be evaluating the functional health status, risk status, and well-being domains of the territory. The idea is to understand that there is an entire "territory" of value that should be explored, understood, mapped, and improved over time in ways that meet the customers' needs and expectations.

Having said this, some people have found the compass metaphor confusing. Thinking, for example, that if one wishes to go due north, that north is the only important point on the compass and the other directions are to be avoided to reach the desired destination. This is a legitimate viewpoint and can cause misunderstanding. We, however, use the value compass as a way of bringing rapidly to mind cardinal points of value and to encourage use of the value compass to explore, manage, and improve the territory just as one might use a directional compass to explore, map, and manage a particular piece of property that one held in stewardship.

Recognize Limitations

Although the Clinical Value Compass approach can be a useful way of analyzing the value of health care and identify areas for improvement, it doesn't do everything that's needed. It has several limitations that merit recognition. First, it does not provide prospective information about patient preferences or identify excess capacity in the system. Second, unless it is supplemented with appropriate control charts, showing variations in trends over time, it is not possible to separate important "signals" from random noise. (See article by Nugent, Schults, Plume, et al. for further information on how to construct a clinical value compass and allied control charts.)[25] Third, if one wished to pursue the most rigorous, most expert, most advanced state-of-the-art application of the clinical value compass approach, it would require mastery of several related measurement methods (the measurement of clinical outcomes, functional status and well-being, patient satisfaction with care, cost accounting, and financial burden of illness assessment), as well as the application of technical analytic techniques (such as creation of summated rating scales, clinical indices, risk adjustment/stratification, and cost-effectiveness analysis).

Indeed, the value compass idea builds on advances in all these fields of measurement and analysis, and they can be used with more or less rigor as circumstances permit. We have observed, however, that many people have found the value compass framework and way of thinking to be: (a) useful in providing a logical and balanced framework for measuring and improving care; (b) appealing to diverse stakeholders—doctors, nurses, consumers, purchasers, and planners; and (c) flexible and robust insofar as it can be used, in the real world, in a more or less sophisticated manner depending on needs, circumstances, resources available, level of experience, and technical knowledge.

Conclusion

Key stakeholders—clinicians, patients, and employers/purchasers—are interested in the information that is summarized in the Clinical Value Compass. Clinicians are curious about outcomes, but want to focus on process measures because this might help them monitor and improve delivery of care and thereby impact outcomes and costs. Patients are keenly interested in outcomes (such as clinical symptoms, functional health status, and satisfaction with health care) because their health is at stake. Employers/purchasers, who foot the health care bill, demand financial data; they are curious about process and interested in outcomes, but they must learn about the difference in what it costs them to have their employees/members treated in one system versus another.

Conflict or Cooperation

There is potential for conflict and also opportunity for new cooperation to align the interests of these stakeholders. Conflict can arise if there is disagreement about the tradeoffs made between the quality indicators (clinical outcomes, functional outcomes, and patient satisfaction) and costs. Providers and patients might accuse employers/purchasers of fixating on just one compass point—costs—without regard to quality. Employers/purchasers might castigate patients and providers for demanding free choice of provider and care options, regardless of whether it is needed or cost effective. On the other hand, cooperation flourishes if both parties gain a deeper appreciation for their common interests in high-value care and the interdependencies of the points on the Clinical Value Compass. Most stakeholders want to minimize the burden of illness and have patients maintain their ability to work and enjoy an active, independent life (functional health status), receive the right care (appropriateness) at the right time (access) in a satisfying and efficient manner. In addition, controlling unnecessary costs—including health care costs that don't add value—meets the needs of providers, patients, and employers/purchasers.

Final Comment

Real improvements in the quality and value of care require time to change systems and processes, constant vigilance by leaders, and full involvement of front-line clinicians.[26] However, as change-making skills increase and as pressures for change intensify, we expect to shorten the time needed to make changes and accelerate improvement of health care value. Real, durable improvements and innovations also require know-how—what Deming called "profound knowledge."[27] This know-how is increasing rapidly within health care just as the pressures to change and innovate are mounting.[28,29] It is our hope that this four-part chapter will help clinicians, as well as other stakeholders in the health care delivery system, to gain new insight and tools that they can readily apply to benefit the patients and the populations they serve.

ACKNOWLEDGMENTS

The authors wish to thank Diane Hall for her design work on the figures and for her efforts in preparing the manuscript.

REFERENCES: PART 1

1. Joint Commission on Accreditation of Healthcare Organizations: *The measurement mandate: On the road to performance improvement in health care.* Oakbrook Terrace, IL: JCAHO, 1993.
2. Grumbach K, Bodenheimer T: Painful vs. painless costs control. *JAMA* 1994; 272:1458–1464.
3. Meier B: Hurdles await efforts to rate doctors and medical centers. *New York Times*, Mar 31, 1994, p. B1.
4. Greenfield S, Nelson EC: Recent developments and future issues in the use of health status assessment measures in clinical settings. *Med Care* May 1992; 30(suppl):MS23–MS41.
5. U.S. Congress, Office of Technology Assessment, ed: *The quality of medical care: Information for consumers*, OTA-H-386. Washington, DC: US Government Printing Office, June 1988.
6. Lohr KN, ed: *Medicare: A strategy for quality assurance.* Washington, DC: National Academy Press, 1990.
7. Ellwood PM: Outcomes management: A technology of patient experience. *N Engl J Med* 1988; 318:1549.
8. Classen DC, Evans RS, Pestotnik SL, Horn SD, Menlove RL, Burke JP: The timing of prophylactic administration of antibiotics and the risk of surgical-wound infection. *N Engl J Med* 1992; 326(5):281–286.
9. Brent James, MD, Intermountain Health Care, personal communication, 1995.
10. O'Connor GT, Plume SK, Olmstead EM, Morton JR, et al: Results of a regional study to improve the in-hospital mortality associated with coronary artery bypass grafting. Northern New England Cardiovascular Disease Study Group, in press, *JAMA*.
11. Womack JP, Jones DT, Roos D: *The machine that changed the world.* New York: Harper Collins, 1991.
12. Dubos R: *Mirage of health.* New York: Doubleday Anchor, 1959.
13. World Health Organization: *Constitution of the World Health Organization.* Geneva, Switzerland: WHO Basic Documents, 1948.
14. Susser M: Health as a human right: An epidemiologist's perspective on the public health. *Amer J of Pub Health* 1993; 83:418–426.
15. Rice D, Feldman J, White K: The current burden of illness in the United States. Presented at the annual meeting of the Institute of Medicine, October 27, 1976, Washington, DC.
16. Wennberg JE, Barry MJ, Fowler FJ, Mulley A: Outcomes research, ports, and health care reform in doing more harm than good: The evaluation of health care interventions. *Annals of NY Acad of Sciences* vol 703, December 1993.
17. Donabedian A: *The definition of quality and approaches to its assessment.* Vol 1: Explorations in quality assessing and monitoring. Ann Arbor, MI: Health Administration Press, 1980.
18. Batalden PB, Nelson EC, Roberts JS: Linking outcomes measurement to continual improvement: The Serial "V" way of thinking about improving clinical care. *Jt Comm J Qual Improv* April 1994; 20(4):167–180.
19. Ackoff RL: *The art of problem solving.* New York: John Wiley & Sons, 1978.
20. Langley GJ, Nolan KM, Nolan TW: The foundation of improvement. *Quality Progress* June 1994; 27(6):81–86.
21. Scholtes PR: *The team handbook: How to improve quality with teams.* Madison, WI: Joiner Associates, 1988.
22. Deming WE: *Out of the crisis.* Cambridge, MA: MIT Press, 1986.
23. Nelson EC, Batalden PB: Patient-based quality measurement systems. *Quality Management in Health Care* Fall 1993; 2(1):18–30.
24. Nelson EC, Wasson JH: Using patient-based information to rapidly redesign care. *Healthcare Forum Journal* July/August 1994; 37(4):25–29.
25. Nugent WE, Schults WC, Plume SK, Batalden PB, Nelson EC: Designing an instrument panel to monitor and improve coronary artery bypass grafting. *JCOM* December 1994; 1(2):57–64.
26. Batalden PB, Stoltz PK: A framework for the continual improvement of health care: Building and applying professional and improvement knowledge to test changes in daily work. *Jt Comm J Qual Improv* October 1993; 19(10):424–447.
27. Deming WE: *The new economics for industry, government, education.* Cambridge, MA: MIT Press, 1993.

28. Berwick DM, Godfrey AB, Roessner J: *Curing health care: New strategies for quality improvement.* San Francisco, CA: Jossey-Bass Publishers, 1990.
29. Brennan TA, Berwick DM: *New rules: Regulation, markets, and the quality of American health care.* San Francisco, CA: Jossey-Bass Publishers, 1996.

■ Part 2. A Clinical Improvement Worksheet and Users Manual

Every system is perfectly designed to get the results it gets.

The aim of this portion of the chapter is to provide a useful and flexible guide for improving the value of clinical care by *redesigning* the delivery process and testing the impact on quality and costs. Clinical improvement work begins with setting the aim and clarifying the clinical delivery process and then proceeds with generating change concepts and subsequent tests of change. Though not commonly done, small tests of change can be conducted in everyday clinical practice, thereby turning the health care delivery team into reflective practitioners who can learn from, and improve on, their work.

The Core Clinical Process: An Overview

One can think best about the clinical improvement process by beginning with the basic or "core" clinical delivery process, and then overlaying a clinical *improvement* approach on top of this process. Fundamental to this way of thinking is the idea of an episode of care that runs over time; it may involve multiple patient/clinician encounters in both ambulatory and inpatient settings, and must be actively and seamlessly managed as providers move to capitation.

Figure 10–6 illustrates the core clinical process. The figure shows a care seeking episode that has three phases: before, during, and after. The episode begins and ends with the individual patient's "clinical value compass" (see Part 1), which captures both quality and cost. The process typically begins with a person living in the community who experiences a health need such as prevention, treatment, or rehabilitation. Before the care seeking episode, the individual already has a clinical status and functional status (which can be assessed at any point in time). Though not always analyzed, documented, or managed, the patient also has expectations to be satisfied and a prior health care cost history. For example, most people have expectations regarding the way care should be delivered and a set of desired or "hoped for" health outcomes (based on prior personal experiences or on the health care experiences of others). In addition, people build a lifetime health care *cost profile* based on their utilization of medical care; each episode adds costs on the margin. Sometimes, the

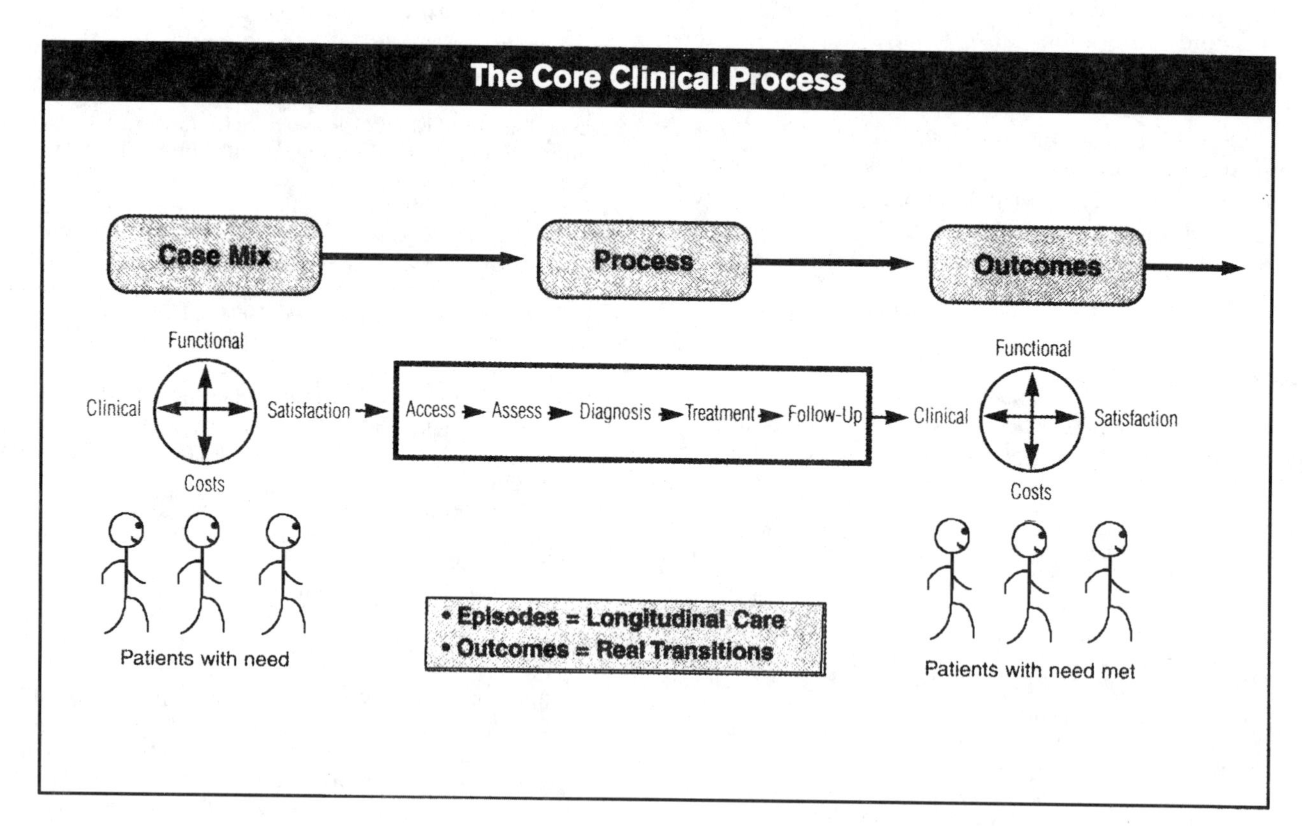

FIGURE 10–6. The core clinical process for an episode of care.

health need prompts the individual to take action and access the health care delivery system. This triggers a sequence of actions, the clinical process, which can be characterized as patient assessment (based on data collection obtained from history taking, physical examination and diagnostic tests), diagnosis (the classification of the patient based on the information gleaned from the history, physical, and diagnostic tests), treatment (the regimen that is designed for the patient based on the diagnosis), and follow-up (the process of monitoring the patient over time by repeating the preceding steps to ensure that the regimen matches the patient's clinical status). At some later point, the quality and costs of care for the individual who started the episode with an initial health care need can be analyzed, formally or informally, in terms of the impact of the care on the person's clinical status, functional status and well-being, satisfaction, and costs. As noted on the bottom of Figure 10–6, results that are often called health *outcomes*—measures of clinical, functional, and satisfaction results—are, in truth, health *transitions*. The practitioner's challenge is to take action to enable the patient to obtain the most favorable transitions in health, in the most satisfying manner, and at the least cost.

The Core Clinical Process: A Case Study

Tim S., a 43-year-old computer systems analyst and avid tennis player, called his friend and primary care physician, Dr. Clark, on a Sunday night complaining of severe hand and wrist pain. He tells Dr. Clark that his hand pain, a progressive problem over the preceding 6 months, has "gotten worse . . . it's killing me" and he thinks something more might have to be done in addition to the medication, splints, and physical therapy he has already tried. Dr. Clark tells Tim to come to his office at 9:00 A.M. on Monday and that he will work him into the schedule. The next morning, Dr. Clark sees Tim at 9:45, takes a brief history, performs a directed physical examination, and concludes that the exacerbation of Tim's pain represents further progression of carpal tunnel syndrome. He refers Tim to his colleague, Dr. Valiant, for consultation regarding surgery, since prior conservative treatment has failed. Dr. Valiant sees Tim a few days later, confirms the diagnosis, recommends surgery to Tim, and schedules the surgical procedure for two weeks later—the next available open slot. Tim is unhappy that he has to wait so long since he would like to "get it over with sooner, rather than later" now that he has decided on surgery.

On the appointed day, Tim and his wife go to the hospital at 7:00 A.M. to prepare for surgery, which was scheduled for 9:00 but was pushed back to 11:00 due to emergency cases that took priority. At 11:30, he undergoes a carpal tunnel release procedure under general anesthesia and is discharged at 3:30 P.M. with instructions from Dr. Valiant to: (a) visit his office for a brief wound healing check with his clinical assistant, (b) schedule an appointment with him for a progress check in four weeks, and (c) call if he experiences any trouble during the next week. Tim's wife drives him home (she has taken the day off from teaching to be with her husband). Tim, feeling a little weak from the anesthesia effects, stays home from work for the next few days. He returns to work the next Monday, but has some limitations on his job for a few weeks because he can't comfortably use his computer keyboard for extended periods of time.

At the four-week follow-up visit, Dr. Valiant asks Tim how he is doing. He learns that Tim still suffers some hand symptoms (pain and tingling, no numbness), but has begun using his computer again. When Tim asks when he can start playing tennis again, he is told he cannot yet resume tennis, but, with some hand therapy and the tincture of time, he most likely will be able to return to his game in several months. On his way out, Tim says that he is fairly happy with the surgery results and really appreciates Dr. Valiant's "great care," but wishes that his recovery would go quicker; taking time off from work and being limited on the job is tough and has put him "way behind" on a big project. He tells Dr. Valiant that he appreciates his friendly "down-to-earth" manner and his genuine concern, and believes that, from a technical point of view, the surgeon and the staff did a "great job." However, he says that he is glad he doesn't have to "foot the bill" because the whole thing was much more costly than he thought it would be.

Tim explained that, being a systems analyst, he had calculated a rough and ready estimate of the total costs of his care and had estimated the costs to be almost $4,000! The size of this figure surprised Dr. Valiant, so he asked Tim to break the costs down. Tim had estimated that medical care charges totaled about $2660: $150 for physician office visits, $1140 for surgical fees, $800 for the hospital facility charge, $320 for anesthesia, and $250 for laboratory test charges. The costs for time lost from work were roughly $1250: Tim's three days out of work @ $900, his wife's one day loss from work @ $200, and the substitute teacher cost of $150. Later that day, Dr. Valiant started thinking about trying out a better way to do carpal tunnel releases that might be faster, better, and cheaper.

Clinical Improvement Worksheet and Users Manual

How might we fit clinical improvement work into busy doctors' offices and hospitals in a way that does not interfere with the smooth delivery of care and builds on clinicians' professional values of science and healing, their intrinsic curiosity about cause and effect, and their personal desire to find the best way to care for their patients?

The Clinical Improvement Worksheet

The Clinical Improvement Worksheet has been designed to be a simple tool that front-line practitioners can use to blend clinical improvement work with their core clinical delivery process. Figures 10–7 and 10–8 show the front and back sides, respectively, of the Clinical Improvement worksheet for improving clinical care. (Copies of the worksheet are available from the authors.) The worksheet is based on a sequential approach to improving clinical care, which is described in a previously published article.[2] It outlines a logical way of thinking about clinical improvement and blending measured health outcomes and costs with underlying knowledge of the process and with small pilot tests of changes designed to reduce costs and increase quality.

Side A of Worksheet: READY . . . AIM

The front of the Worksheet (Side A, shown in Figure 10–7) poses a set of four questions about the core clinical process. These four questions address:

1. Outcomes—*Select a population and set aim*
2. Process—*Analyze the clinical process that produces the outcomes*
3. Changes—*Generate a list of change ideas to improve outcomes*
4. Pilot—*Select a change for pilot testing*

The purpose of Side A is to provide a high level view of these four, very basic questions. Working through Side A helps the clinical team get READY to make a change and begins the process of taking AIM by honing in on a high leverage area for testing a change—after having had the opportunity to discuss desired outcomes, care processes, and potential changes.

Side B of Worksheet: AIM . . . FIRE . . . HIT/MISS

The back of the Worksheet (Side B, shown in Figure 10–8) focuses down on a specific test of change. It continues the process of sharpening the AIM with a set of questions (placed on the left-hand half of Side B) about the team, the specific aim, measures, and the selected change.

- Team Members—Who should work on this improvement?
- Specific Aim—What are we trying to accomplish with "this" test of change?
- Measures—How will we know that "this" change is an improvement?
- Selected Change—How would you describe the change you have selected for testing?

The right-hand half of Side B of the Worksheet includes the basic Improvement Cycle (Plan/Do/Check/Act). Working through the following four questions helps the team to FIRE in a more accurate way and to determine if it was a HIT or a MISS.

1. Plan—How shall we plan the pilot?
2. Do—What are we learning as we do the pilot?
3. Check—As we check and study what happened, what have we learned?
4. Act—As we act to hold the gains or abandon our pilot efforts, what needs to be done?

The worksheet meets several needs. Side A provides a picture that blends "improvement thinking" with the core clinical process in a way that is easy for practitioners to understand and tailor to their patient care delivery routines. Side B reinforces the basic model for improvement (Aim—Measures—Selected Change—Plan/Do/Check/ Act) that we use throughout our healthcare delivery system for making improvements and innovations.[3] Taken as a whole, the Worksheet provides a graphic, flexible tool for helping clinicians make improvements and offers a simple format for teams to use to visualize their path forward, to record their progress, and to share their work in a standard format. **Appendix** (p.) presents the Clinical Improvement Worksheet User's Manual. This was written to provide brief "just-in-time instruction" to people that want further guidance on how to make use of the Clinical Improvement Worksheet. In the next section, a case study is presented to illustrate use of the Worksheet and Users Manual.

Using the Clinical Improvement Worksheet: Carpal Tunnel Surgery Case Example

No real-life team will ever follow all or only the ideas listed in the Users Manual completely, nor should they. The Users Manual works like a clinical guideline—it provides guidance about what to do under many circumstances, but cannot fit every situation perfectly.

The Carpal Tunnel Team

The person responsible for starting the team was the orthopedic surgical section chief in the southern region of the Lahey Hitchcock Clinic delivery system. He had a strong interest in outcomes measurement and clinical improvement and wanted to get some hands-on experience. The team had progressed to step E ("Do") at the time of this writing. Figure 10–9 shows a completed Clinical Improvement Worksheet to highlight their progress. A more detailed account of this case follows below and is built around the Worksheet and Users Manual.

> ***TEAM MEMBERS:* Who should work on this improvement?**
>
> *The Carpal Tunnel Team consisted of five surgeons, one hand therapist (added later), one nurse, two managers, one statistician, one mentor, and one team facilitator. To begin with, they agreed to schedule two-hour meetings every other week and follow structured*

Side A of the Clinical Improvement Worksheet

Clinical Improvement Worksheet

Aim: Accelerate clinical improvement by linking outcomes measurements and process knowledge with the design and conduct of pilot tests of change.

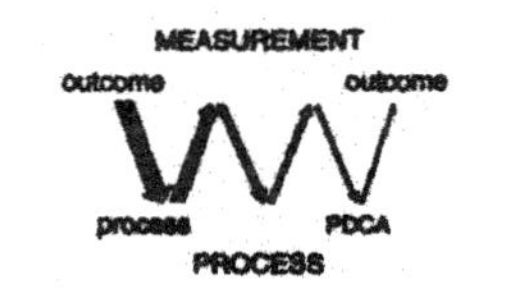

② ***PROCESS*** ➡ **Analyze the process**

What's the process for giving care to this type of patient?

① ***OUTCOMES*** ➡ **Select a population**

What's the general aim? Given our wish to limit/reduce the illness burden for "this type" of patient, what are the desired results?

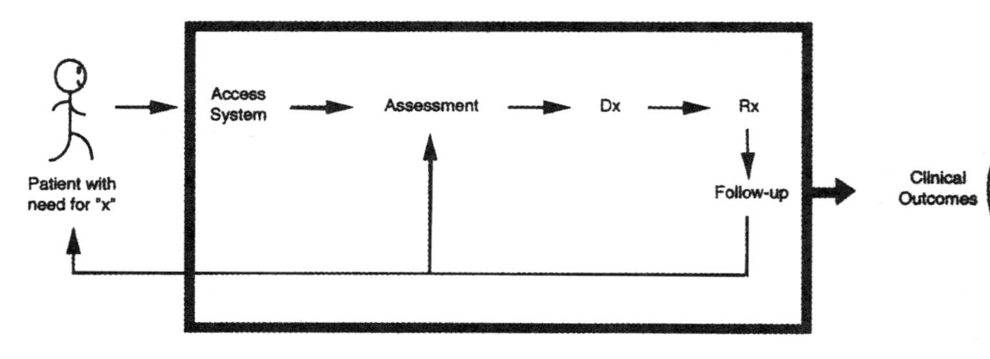

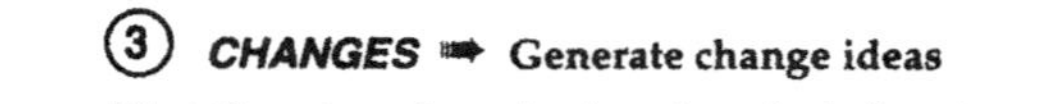

③ ***CHANGES*** ➡ **Generate change ideas**

What ideas do we have for changing what's done (process) to get better results?

-
-
-

④ ***PILOT*** ➡ **Select first/next change for pilot testing**

How can we pilot test an improvement idea using the Plan-Do-Check-Act method?

Eugene C. Nelson, DSc, MPH, and Paul B. Batalden, MD
© July 1995, Lahey Hitchcock Clinic

SIDE A

FIGURE 10–7. Side A of the Clinical Improvement Worksheet.

Side B of the Clinical Improvement Worksheet

Making Improvements: Clinical Improvement Worksheet

TEAM MEMBERS ➡ Who should work on this improvement?

1. Leader ______ 5. ______
2. Facilitator ______ 6. ______
3. ______ 7. ______
4. ______ 8. ______

Coach ______ Admin Support ______

A. ***SPECIFIC AIM*** ➡ What are we trying to accomplish? (more specific AIM)

B. ***MEASURES*** ➡ How will we know that a change is an improvement?

C. ***SELECTED CHANGE*** ➡ How would you describe the change that you have selected for testing?

D. ***PLAN*** ➡ How shall we PLAN the pilot?

- Who? Does what? When? With what tools and training?

- Baseline data to be collected?

E. ***DO*** ➡ What are we learning as we DO the pilot?

F. ***CHECK*** ➡ As we CHECK and STUDY what happened, what have we learned?

- Did original outcomes improve?

G. ***ACT*** ➡ As we ACT to hold the gains or abandon our pilot efforts, what needs to be done?

SIDE B

FIGURE 10–8. Side B of the Clinical Improvement Worksheet.

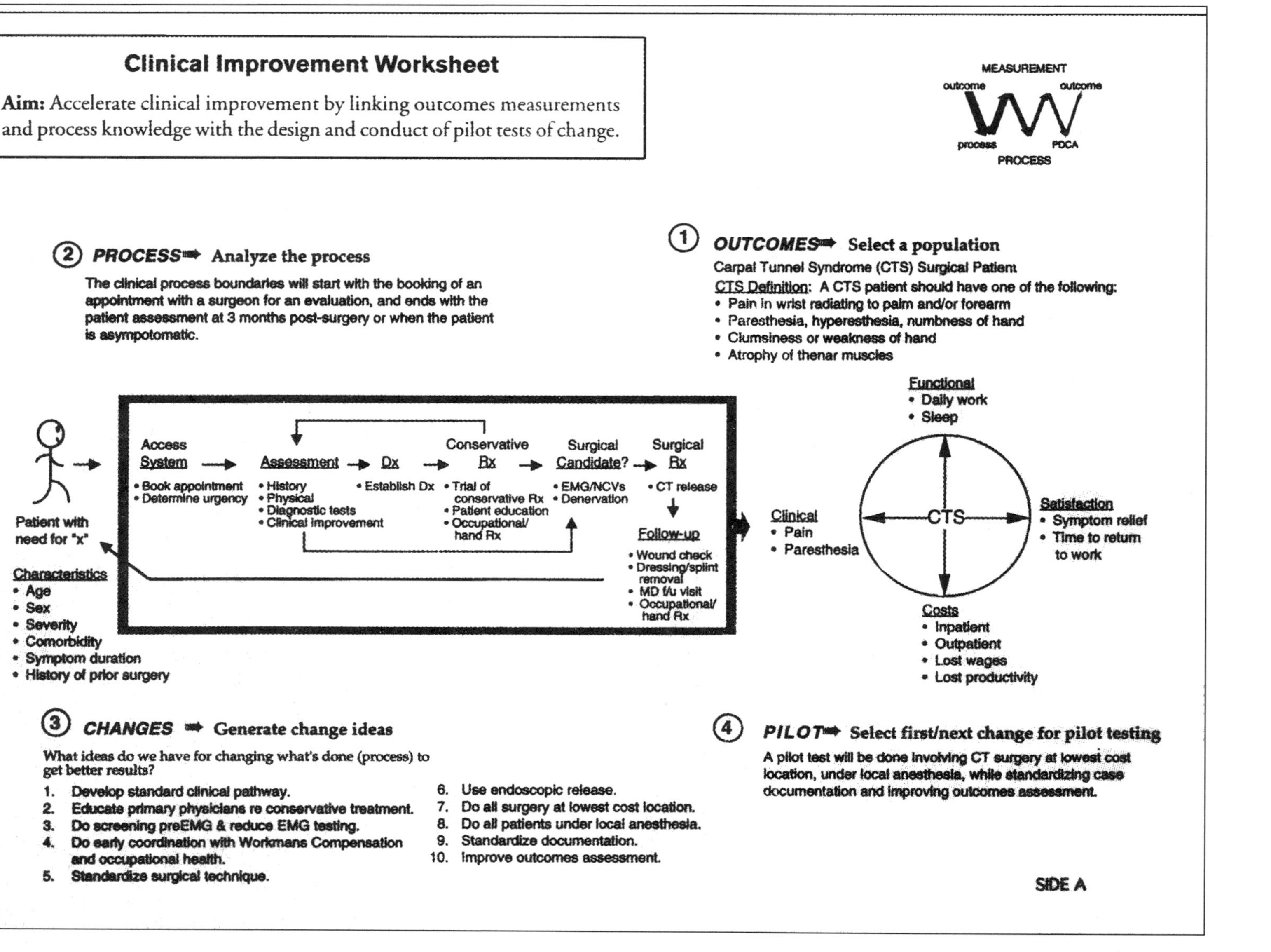

FIGURE 10–9. Carpal tunnel surgery improvement team.

meeting agendas, designating the roles of leader, timekeeper, recorder, and facilitator.

1. *OUTCOMES:* Select a population (meeting 1)

Carpal tunnel syndrome (CTS) was selected because it is a high-volume, significant problem for patients and employers, because current care is expensive, because many aspects of the process and its outcomes can be measured easily, and because optional management strategy is "not too controversial" among our surgeons. This population appeared to offer a good "starter" learning experience with high likelihood of worthwhile improvement.

"What's the general aim?" *The team was formed for the dual purpose of (1) improving outcomes and reducing costs for CTS patients, and (2) increasing capacity to make improvements in quality and value using the clinical improvement process.*

"Given our wish to limit/reduce the illness burden for 'this type' of patient, what are the desired results?" *The team brainstormed "hoped for" results for each of the four value compass points and then reduced the list by multivoting to identify the two most important measures for each value compass point. The final results were:*

- Clinical outcomes: *pain, paresthesia*
- Functional status: *daily work ability, sleep*
- Satisfaction: *perceived symptom relief and satisfaction with time to return to work*
- Costs: *direct costs—inpatient charges, outpatient charges; indirect costs—lost wages and lost productivity.*

A CTS clinical value compass annotated with selected measures was created on a flip chart. The CTS value compass flip chart page was displayed at each subsequent meeting to help maintain focus (see Figure 10–9).

2. *PROCESS:* Analyze the process (meeting 2)

"What's the process for giving care for this type of patient?" *The team flowcharted the CTS care delivery process. This was done by establishing an arbitrary start and end point and by asking each team member to write down on "stickies" (self-sticking note paper) phrases that describe their work for each point in the core delivery process. All the stickies were put on a flip chart on the wall, and the team organized them into a logical flow, analyzed the resulting flowchart, and refined it by adding missed steps and eliminating redundancies.*

Then, the team broke into two groups: one to define patient characteristics that impact process and outcomes (such as age, sex, severity, comorbidity, symptom duration, history of surgery), and the other to construct an agreed upon operational definition for the CTS patient that presents with a health need (see Figure 10–9).

3. *CHANGES:* Generate change ideas (meeting 3)

"What ideas do we have for changing what's done (process) to get better results?" *The team reviewed the general aim, the CTS value compass measures of quality and costs, the operational definition of a CTS patient, and the clinical process flow that produces the current set of results for the target population. Next, team members took about five minutes to think on their own (silent idea generation) about changes that could be made—either small changes or large innovations—that might produce better results. The team ideas for change were generated, the list was clarified, and the team multi-voted to select a change for pilot testing (see Figure 10–9).*

4. *PILOT:* Select a change for pilot testing (meeting 4)

"How can we pilot test an improvement idea using the Plan-Do-Check-Act method?" *The team selected two main ideas to combine into a pilot test: (1) perform the CTR (release) surgical procedure under local anesthesia, and (2) perform CTR procedure at the lowest cost location. It was recognized that while testing this change, it would be essential to adopt two more change ideas: (1) standardize documentation, and (2) improve assessment of patient outcomes. It was expected that this change was "doable" in all three locations by all surgeons in the southern region; and it was hypothesized that it would result in greater patient satisfaction, lower direct and indirect costs to patients, employers, and the delivery system.*

AIM: What are we trying to accomplish? (meeting 4)

The team sharpened their aim statement to be:

> *"Our aim is to improve our care of patients with Carpal Tunnel Syndrome (CTS) and to improve our ability to study clinical processes. This clinical process begins with the presentation of the patient to the surgical specialist and ends when a patient is (a) 12 weeks post-op, or (b) asymptomatic, whichever is later. Our plan is to see if surgical patients treated with local anesthesia in a low-cost location for their carpal tunnel release have superior satisfaction with care, comparable clinical and functional outcomes, and lower medical (and social) costs."*

MEASURES: How will we know that a change is an improvement?

The team decided to develop operational definitions for selected measures that related to (a) clinical outcomes (such as pain, paresthesia), (b) functioning (such as daily work, sleep), (c) satisfaction (with speed of recovery, convenience, treatment timeliness), and (d) costs (such as medical charges to patient, days lost from work).

SELECTED CHANGE: How would you describe the change that you have selected for testing? (meeting 4)

In session #3 the team had generated a working list of possible changes (Side A, Step 3 of the Worksheet). The change trial will include the asterisked items from the list of potential changes:

1. *Design standard clinical pathway*
2. *Communicate with PCPs about optional conservative therapy*
3. *Do clinical screening before EMG and eliminate unnecessary EMGs*
4. *Coordination with Workman's Compensation and occupational health early in the course of care*
5. *Standardize surgical technique*
6. *Use endoscopic CTR*
7. *Do all surgery at lowest cost location***

8. *Do all surgery under local anesthesia***
9. *Standardize documentation of care* **
10. *Improve outcomes assessment***

The team worked with providers in each of the three communities in which CTR was performed. The basic change to be tested was to do the procedure at the lowest cost location in each of the three communities using local anesthesia. Furthermore, for the first time, standardized assessments of patient case-mix, treatment processes, and health outcomes were designed into the delivery process by gathering data from the patient and from the surgeon (pre surgery, post surgery 4 weeks, and post surgery 12 weeks) using self-coding data collection forms.

PLAN: How shall we PLAN the pilot? (meetings 4-10)

"Who? Does what? When? With what tools and training?" *The change was to be piloted in all three locations in the region in which CTR was performed. The team brainstormed a task list and then developed a critical path of steps that must be taken to prepare for the pilot test. Some of the steps were:*

- *Set up and define measures.*
- *Obtain cost estimates from potential outpatient surgical centers.*
- *Estimate cost for current system versus new system.*
- *Make detailed protocol using flowchart method.*
- *Determine budgetary implications of plan.*
- *Gain agreement from surgeons in all locations.*
- *Develop data analysis plan and review relevant literature.*
- *Design self-coding data forms for use by patients and surgeons.*
- *Establish microcomputer-based analysis system.*
- *Identify and purchase needed equipment.*
- *Determine plan for using surgical procedure room.*
- *Select and train staff to assist in new CTR method.*
- *Collect cost and utilization data on old method.*
- *Begin new method by conducting CTR in lowest cost location, using local anesthesia and gathering standardized measures.*

"Baseline data to be collected?" *The team planned to collect data prospectively from both patients and surgeons. The patient-based data included measures of clinical status, functional status, satisfaction, and indirect costs associated with time lost from work. The data to be collected from the surgeons included information on prior history, clinical status, the CTR procedure, surgical findings, and postoperative care. Information from patients was to be gathered at three points in time: presurgery, 4 weeks postsurgery, and 12 weeks postsurgery using patient self-completed questionnaires. Information from surgeons was to be completed at the same time points plus time of surgery. Considerable effort was put into constructing operational definitions for variables and designing pre-coded questionnaires for the patients and data collection forms for the surgeons that could be used with minimal interruption to care delivery. In the course of several drafts, the questionnaires and forms were color coded for ease of use. One person was identified to oversee the entire data collection process—from identification of a patient as meeting CTR protocol criteria through obtaining complete follow-up data.*

DO: What are we learning as we DO the pilot?

The team is currently in the "Do" phase of its work. The pilot will be performed on 50 to 100 consecutive CTR patients and will take several months to complete. The first thing that was learned in "doing" was that the data collection process did not automatically get inserted cleanly into the delivery process without some fine tuning, reminders, and adjustments. The key to success, here, was for the data coordinator to identify incomplete or missing information early in the implementation process and to return the forms to the clinicians/patients to get complete information before much time had passed. The team held periodic "reunions" to review the results for the first series of patients and plan more, new improvement work while this first change cycle continues.

CHECK: As we CHECK and STUDY what happened, what have we learned? Did original outcomes improve?

At time of writing, the team analyzed their results for the first series of 49 patients cared for in the "new way" to determine the impact of their first test of change (i.e., PDCA Cycle #1: CTR done at lowest cost location under local anesthesia and using standardized measurements over time). The team gathered "before" and "after" data on costs (old method vs. new method) and "after-only" patient-specific longitudinal data on patient outcomes (clinical, functional, and satisfaction outcomes pre surgery and post surgery). Selected results are illustrated on the clinical value compass that appears in Figure 10–10. Outcomes improved and costs decreased:

- *Clinical—The percentage of patients who rated their hand pain as "moderate" or "severe" decreased from 77% pre surgery to 37% at 4 weeks post surgery and to 20% at 12 weeks post surgery.*
- *Functioning—35% were able to return to work immediately; 15% returned in less than 1 week; 20% in 2 to 4 weeks; and 30% took 5 or more weeks.*
- *Satisfaction—85% of patients were dissatisfied with hand ability before surgery, and 14% were dissatisfied 12 weeks postoperatively. Patient satisfaction with local anesthesia was high (88%).*
- *Costs—Total direct costs for providing care were reduced by more than 50%, from $937 to $405. These savings resulted from: (a) replacement of same day inpatient surgery with ambulatory surgery under local anesthesia, (b) elimination of the preoperative appointment and some ancillary tests, and (c) elimination of "handoffs" from the clinic to the hospital for scheduling the procedure, transferring patient information, and transporting the patient. Because over 70% of CTR patients are prepaid, these reductions in costs were associated with better financial margins for this clinical activity.*

The team is now finishing the follow-up of their initial cohort of patients who went through OPDCA Cycle 1.0 OPDCA Cycle 20 is likely to target: (a) upstream processes of testing patients who are candidates for surgery in an effort to design the most cost-effective method for identifying patients who would benefit from treatment, or (b) the approximately 30% of patients who were out of work five or more weeks to attempt to decrease time lost from work or normal activities.

Comments

This section discusses some of the specific lessons learned by the Carpal Tunnel Team and some general observations on using the Clinical Improvement Worksheet.

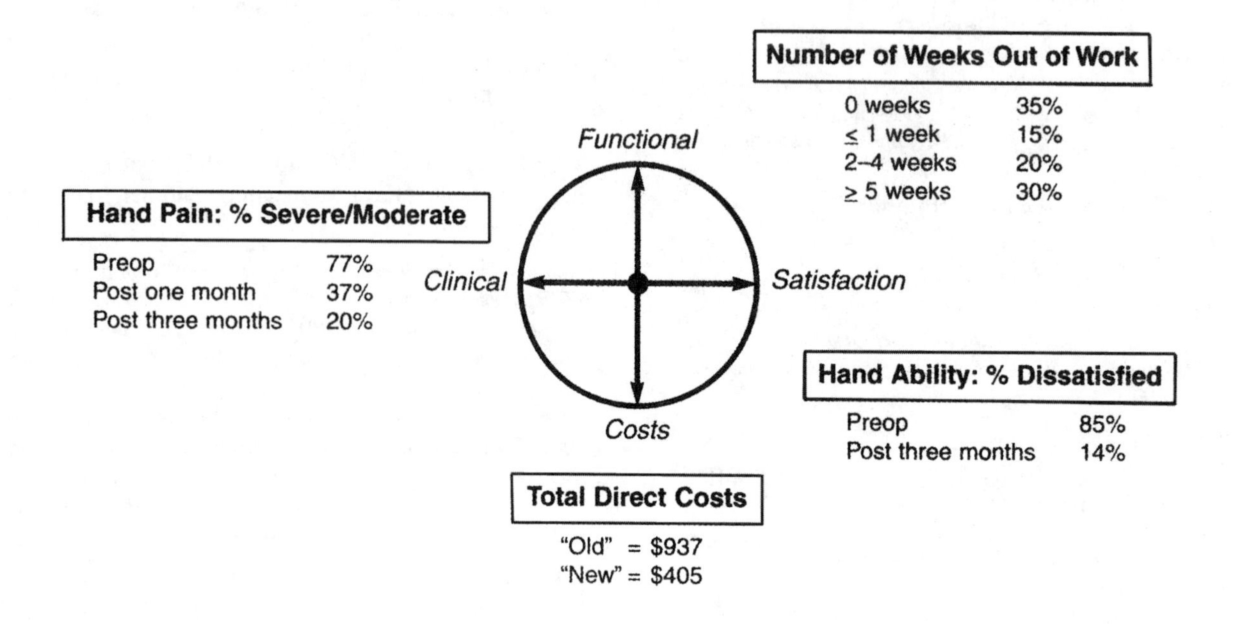

FIGURE 10–10. Carpal tunnel value compass results.

Carpal Tunnel Team: Lessons Learned

The team has already learned some important lessons. First, the clinical improvement process is fun and challenging. The team is energized and ready to move on to more challenging, controversial, and costly areas of work such as total joint replacement.

Second, progress was rapid at first—the team moved through Side A of the Worksheet in only three meetings, but slowed down when they hit the implementation phase. It took more than three months to plan and implement the change. Change can be fast, but not instant; it is important to *not* become discouraged when slowdowns are encountered.

Third, even though CTS was selected to be a quick, noncontroversial opportunity, they discovered that considerable effort had to be expended to ensure that all clinicians and other affected staff would understand and support the new method. The team began to handle two key processes: (1) process redesign (designing and testing a new way), and (2) change management (managing the human, political, cultural, and logistical factors that will determine the success or failure of the *new way* in the *old setting*).

Fourth, there is the potential to become overwhelmed by data collection. The team was warned about the problems associated with "just doing it" and forgetting about any quantitative assessment of impact and the opposite problem of overdoing it and drowning in a sea of excessive measurement. Using a few carefully targeted new measurements that can be inserted into the routine patient/clinician care process is the ideal, along with wise use of currently gathered information.

Finally, it is expected that this clinical change will result in better value for consumers—lower costs, less surgical risk, and better patient satisfaction, with clinical/functional results as good or better than before. Preliminary estimates suggest that the charges to patients will be reduced substantially—approximately $650 per case—and that time lost from work/normal routine should plummet. While this is occurring, surgeon time will be used more efficiently and operating margins for the delivery system will go from a loss of approximately $90 per patient to a profit of over $500 per patient because payments to hospitals and anesthesiologists for prepaid members will be eliminated. This case, when completed, is expected to demonstrate how higher quality reduces costs while improving patient safety and provider margins.

Carpal Tunnel Team: Limitations Observed

This team made real progress, yet critics could easily point out some real limitations. First, it could be argued that the changes selected for the first improvement cycle were "no brainers" that primarily targeted cost reductions. These changes could have been identified without all the fuss and bother of forming a team. For example, a managed care plan or capitated group practice could simply mandate local anesthesia at the lowest cost location and have saved physician time in attending meetings.

This may be true. It is our belief, however, that improvement work should not be a spectator sport for clinicians. They should be actively involved in finding ways to both reduce costs and maintain or improve quality. Changes in clinical practice are more likely to be accepted if they are instigated by physicians who are looking to find ways to improve outcomes and reduce costs for the patients they serve. Also, if cost cutting measures are taken without building in some measurement of their impact on quality (i.e., clinical, functional, and satisfaction outcomes), then it will not be possible to determine the real costs and benefits of the newer/cheaper method.

Second, it could be argued that the team made a mistake by testing out a change in clinical process—local anesthesia at lowest cost location—without gathering baseline data on clinical, functional, and satisfaction outcomes. In fact, the real innovation was to modify the care process to include routine gathering of data on patient mix, treatment process, and outcomes based on patient and physician-reported information.

The team did in fact seriously consider gathering baseline "outcomes" data on a series of patients before proceeding with the clinical process change. This option was rejected, however, because: (a) it would have delayed the testing of the change by several months, (b) there was anecdotal evidence from a local surgeon that this practice change would be preferred by many patients (local anesthesia favored over general anesthesia), (c) there was the belief that this change would not have a positive or negative effect on clinical outcomes but, if anything, would probably have a positive impact on role function (i.e., time lost from work or normal activity), and (d) that the idea was to begin making repeated tests of change (in an already changing world) so that the outcomes data gathered in change cycle 1 could serve as baseline data for change cycle 2.

General Recommendations

By providing the Clinical Improvement Worksheet, Users Manual, and Carpal Tunnel Team case example, this second part in a four-part series has demonstrated a flexible method for stimulating clinical improvement. Before concluding, we offer a few general recommendations.

1. Think of ramping up improvements. A group that's working on improvement may benefit from having a longer-term picture in mind that features running repeated tests of changes over time—all for the purpose of reducing costs and improving quality. Figure 10–11 shows a continual improvement ramp with small tests of change strung together to illustrate this concept.[3] The idea is to run test after test of change. As time passes, more and more change trials are conducted and the complexity of the attempted changes increases (e.g., going from simple, small improvements with a real but modest impact on value, to total process redesign and radical reengineering with a very large impact on value). People often arrive at the first meeting with many ideas for changes—these are usually the obvious changes. Beyond the obvious changes, are the changes that result from process knowledge and an understanding of systems theory.[4]

2. Accelerate tests of change. The aim should be rapid redesign—to make tests of change on things that need improvement quickly and effectively. Redesign work takes practice. With experience, both the number of change attempts and the speed of the change cycles can increase. In the case example we just discussed, it is possible that the team could run a more powerful test of change more quickly in their second attempt than they were able to do in their first effort. Cutting the cycle time from conceptualization of a change concept to the conclusion of a small-scale pilot test should be an objective. Setting out an ambitious timetable early on in the work can help to pick up the pace of change.

3. Think of multiple ways to make improvements. The Clinical Improvement Worksheet is quite versatile. Question #3—"What ideas do we have for changing what's done to get better results?"—invites people to think broadly about change concepts that may produce better outcomes. A change concept is a general notion or approach to change that is useful in developing specific ideas for changes that lead to improvement.[5] For example, if the change concept is "standardization," ideas for change may include developing clinical guidelines, or designing a critical pathway.

In our system, the Clinical Improvement Worksheet is being applied to ambulatory and inpatient care on topics ranging from primary prevention to inpatient care and rehabilitation. The Worksheet has been found to apply as long as there is a specific clinical population that undergoes a more or less predictable clinical process.

4. Implementation. The work of implementing changes in the real world under everyday circumstances can be challenging. Most of us suffer from "change process illiteracy." Here are some hints that may smooth the path forward:

- *Diagram core process "components" and attach measures.* Have the clinical team divide the activities that form the core process (access, assess, diagnose, treat, follow-up) into components using these headings (Side C of Worksheet). Attach performance measures to each component of the core process map. Consider gathering data on

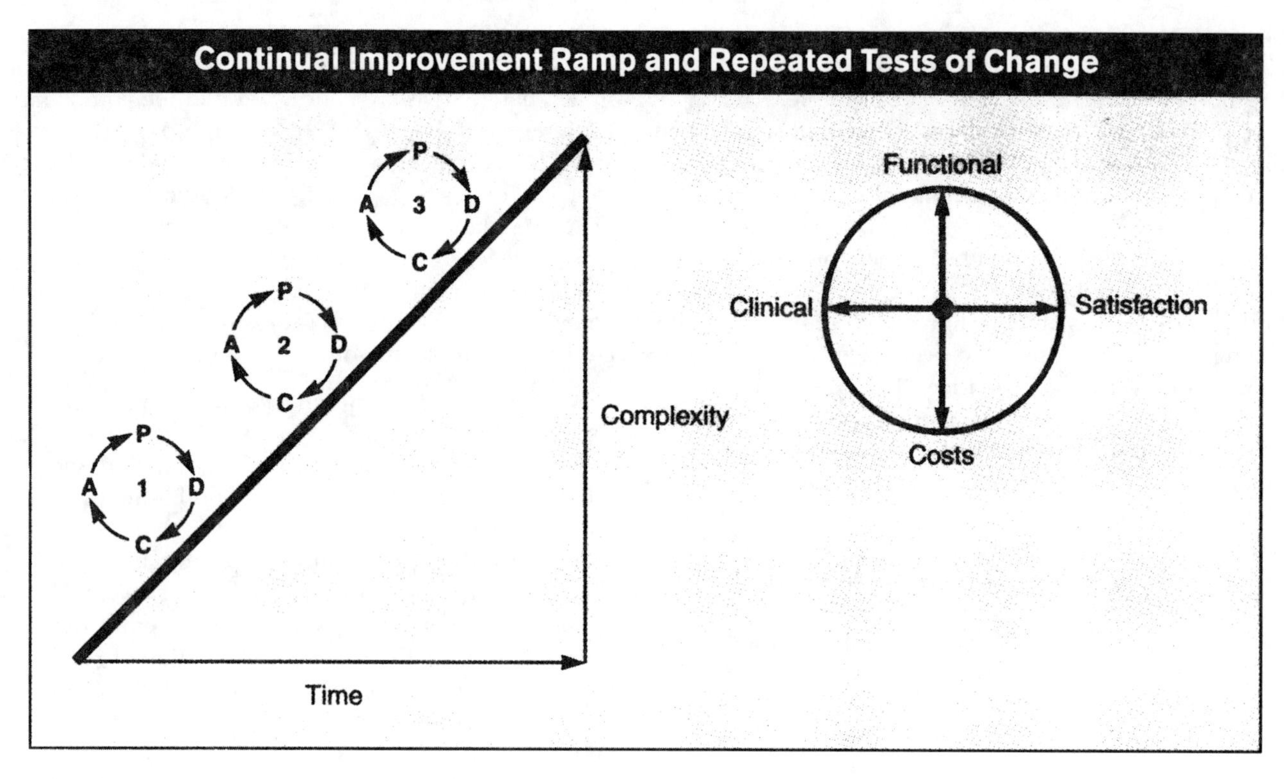

FIGURE 10–11. Continual improvement ramp and repeated tests of change.

some of these key "upstream" performance measures to enable you to determine if they relate to "downstream" measures of outcomes. The point here is that if no changes occur with the pilot test, then one can analyze the core process to learn what failed to work.

■ *Use deployment flowcharts to plan and monitor implementation process.* It often takes considerable time to plan the details that will lead to a successful launching of the test of change (Side B, Step D of Worksheet). Constructing a specific "deployment-style" flowchart that shows who will do what to implement the "change"—embedded within the process of care—can be very helpful. This deployment flowchart can be annotated to include specific, simple measures (or indicators) of implementation steps to show, for example, how many people were contacted in advance of the change and how much time was spent educating clinicians and support staff about the test of change.

■ *Use change management thinking to help sharpen plan and anticipate problems.* The preceding two suggestions can help ground the change in the process and connect the change with key people within the process. Yet another aspect of implementation merits special attention; this is the work of managing change. Much has been written about this and the subject will be specifically addressed in the fourth part of this chapter. Based on the work of consultants to the American Group Practice Association, Jim Reinertsen has suggested, and we (as members of the AGPK) have used and modified, some change management guidelines. These guidelines, along with selected examples from the Carpal Tunnel team, follow:

1. Understand and communicate the cost of the status quo: team compared current costs with expected new costs.
2. Develop and communicate the specific vision of a "better way": team discussed and diagramed the "new way."
3. Obtain the commitment of those with the power to make the new way legitimate: team members "jawboned" all effected surgeons to gain cooperation,
4. Make sure the change agents have the skills to achieve both human and technical objectives and have support and recognition for their work: team provided support and recognition for one another and ensured that each surgeon felt comfortable with new location and anesthesia.
5. Anticipate, understand, and manage the resistance to achieve commitment: negotiated with surgical facilities concerning "new way" and discussed the rationale behind the change with all affected surgeons.
6. Align the change with the organization's culture: organization is working to emphasize high-value clinical care and this activity fit with the value theme.
7. Leave enough organizational "change reserve" to handle unexpected events: team did not wish to bite off more than it could chew for Cycle 1 change.

8. Prepare a thorough change management plan: team developed flowchart, time line, and critical path listing of what was involved with testing the new way.

It is hoped that the Worksheet, Users Manual, and case study presented in this part of the chapter will help clinical teams to sharpen their improvement know-how and accelerate their own improvement work. The next part will provide further guidance on performing clinical benchmarking analyses to locate and study the "best practices" that achieve highest quality and lowest costs.

ACKNOWLEDGMENTS

The authors wish to thank Diane Hall for her design work on the figures and for her assistance in preparing the manuscript. The authors are deeply indebted to the Clinical Carpal Tunnel Improvement Team, which includes the following members: Kim Doherty, Cara Eckstein, Kelly Goudreau, J. Gerald Kennedy, M.D., Linda Lascelles, Kim Lenihan, Mary Lee Sole, M.D., Dennis Stepro, M.D., William Swartz, Winona Thompson, James Vailas, M.D., Loren Vorlicky, M.D., Wesley Wallace, M.D., John Wolf, M.D., Suzanne Zimmerman, M.D.,and Lisa Johnson, M.B.A., C.P.A., who performed the cost analysis.

REFERENCES: PART 2

1. Nelson EC, Mohr JJ, Batalden PB, Plume SK: Improving health care: Part 1. The clinical value compass. Submitted for publication, 1995.
2. Batalden PB, Nelson EC, Roberts JS: Linking outcomes measurement to continual improvement: the Serial "V" way of thinking about improving clinical care. *Jt Comm J Qual Improv* April 1994; 20(4):167–180.
3. Langley GJ, Nolan KM, Nolan TW: The foundation of improvement, *Quality Progress* June 1994; 27(6):81–86.
4. Nolan TW: The design of change. Presentation given at the 1995 Summer Symposium: *Building the Knowledge for the Leadership of Improvement of Health Care,* Sponsored by the Institute for Healthcare Improvement, the Health Care Improvement Leadership Development section of the Dartmouth Medical School, and the Bureau of Health Professions; Woodstock, VT, July 11, 1995.
5. Langley GJ, Nolan TW, Nolan KM, Norman C, Provost L: *Change Directions—the science and art of improvement.* In press, San Francisco, CA: Jossey-Bass.
6. Reinertsen J: American Group Practice Association annual meeting, New Orleans, LA, January 20, 1995.

Copying permission: The authors grant readers permission to copy and use the Clinical Improvement Worksheet© and the Clinical Improvement Users Manual©. Single copies are available on written request to the authors.

Reprints: Address reprint requests to Dr. Nelson, Office of the President, Lahey Hitchcock Clinic, One Medical Center Drive, Lebanon, NH 03756-0001.

Appendix: Clinical Improvement Worksheet: Users Manual

Introduction

This manual is intended to be used by clinical work groups (such as neonatal intensive care unit [NICU] staff, a family practice patient care team, or an obstetrics [OB] team) or special "ad hoc" clinical teams that are working to find ways to improve quality and reduce costs for certain types of patients.

Instructions

The following paragraphs offer brief instructions and comments for each part of the Clinical Improvement Worksheet. *The steps of Side A (Figure 2, p 535) are numbered 1 through 4, and Side B (figure 3, p 536) are lettered A through G.* Although the instructions and comments are provided in a typical linear sequence, it is not necessary to strictly follow this order of steps.

Getting Started

The top section of Side B has space for recording team members and designating a leader, facilitator, coach, and administrative support.

TEAM MEMBERS: Who should work on this improvement?

Consider these guidelines when assembling a team:
a. Limit the number of members to eight or fewer people.
b. Select people who are familiar with different elements of the core process.
c. Reflect diverse areas of expertise and knowledge by including interdisciplinary members.
d. Designate a leader who is credible and responsible for the clinical process.
e. Early on, choose an experienced team facilitator.

Tips

Select a set time and day of the week to meet on a regular basis to plan and oversee the first improvement cycle. Structured meeting agendas are recommended.[1] The *team* can be a naturally occurring work group (people who normally work together such as NICU staff, a family practice patient care team, or an OB team) or a special "ad hoc" clinical team specifically assembled or chartered to work on a specific clinical improvement topic (such as urinary tract infection, adolescent asthma, total joint replacement). The team cannot be selected until there is a good sense of the patient population that will be targeted for improvement. In practice, it is usually necessary to make a preliminary determination of the "selected population" and the broad "aim" (see step 1) before assembling a team.

Side A: Ready . . . Aim

1. Outcomes: Select a population

To select a patient population, identify several criteria to help narrow the focus. Potential criteria include procedures or diagnoses that have high volume, high cost (including long lengths of stay), high improvement potential per case, market competition, high probability of achieving change, importance to stakeholders, and clinician interest.

Tips

To start the process, it is helpful to select an area where there is both a *business need* and strong *clinician interest.* Investment of improvement work in one topic may mean forgoing work on another topic. Reviewing strategy, mission, and data on current performance versus best-known performance can help target populations for improvement work.

"What's the general aim?" Start with a broad statement concerning the general, long-term aim for the selected patient population. The aim statement might touch on multiple aspects of quality and costs. This aim statement can be made more specific when preparing for the pilot test of change.

Tips

The aim statement can indicate the name of the process, where the process starts and finishes, and what some of the expected benefits of improvement will be.

"Given our wish to limit/reduce the illness burden for 'this type' of patient, what are the desired results?" Based on the general aim statement, brainstorm to identify potentially important clinical, functional, satisfaction, and cost outcomes for the selected patient population. Start with clinical outcomes on the value compass (west) and proceed to functional (north) and satisfaction (east), and finish with costs (south). After clarifying the meaning of each brainstormed suggestion, use multivoting to identify the one to three most important results in each area.

Tips

See "Improving health care, part 1: The Clinical Value Compass"[2] for more detailed instructions on this step. Make a wall-sized illustration of the Clinical Value Compass (use flipchart paper) and place the brainstormed ideas and highest-priority results on the wall. This will build a clear, graphic model for all the team to review and refine.

2. Process: Analyze the process

"What's the process for giving care to this type of patient?" Construct a flowchart of the care delivery process. Begin by specifying the process boundaries, or where the process should start and finish for the selected patient population (the process starts when patients . . . and the process ends when patients . . .). Have the team construct a first-draft flowchart of the delivery process. It is often wise to begin with a simple high-level flowchart (5 to 20 steps) and then refine the flowchart over time. Use basic conventions of flowcharting—ovals at the beginning and end of the process, rectangles for main action steps, diamonds for important decision points, and so on.

Specify the patient characteristics that are most likely to have a direct impact either on what's done for the patient in terms of the clinical process that matches care with patient characteristics, or what happens to the patient in terms of outcomes. Common patient descriptors that tend to influence processes or outcomes are demographics (age, gender, education), health factors (diagnosis, severity of primary diagnosis, comorbidity), and other factors such as lifestyle, patient expectations for treatment, and results valued by the patient.

Tips

Make the flowchart big enough for team viewing and include space for comments. Consider posting it in a place for team and nonteam members to review between meetings. Ask each team member to discuss the improvement work in general, and the flowchart specifically, with one or two colleagues (who are not on the team) to refine the flowchart and gain better understanding of improvement work rationale and methods. Also make a wall-sized illustration (using flipchart pages) of the graphic elements of Side A of the worksheet showing:

- patient with need,
- care delivery process, and
- outcomes.

3. Changes: Generate change ideas

"What ideas do we have for changing what's done (process) to get better results?" Use brainstorming or nominal-group-type methods to generate a long list of change ideas. Use multivoting or another method to reduce the list to the top priority for actually testing in a pilot study.

Tips

Set up a task by asking team members to step back for a moment and to think about the aim, the desired results (clinical, functional, satisfaction, costs), and the delivery process (which has been represented as a flowchart). Then, based on their own ideas and analysis (or based on some other person's/expert's ideas or analysis), ask team-members to write down (silently and on their own) as many changes as they can think of that they believe may result in better care and/or lower costs. Ask each team member to read one idea, rotating around the team to develop an exhaustive list of change ideas. Clarify these concepts and combine those which are redundant. Use multivoting or another method to help determine the most promising change idea for pilot testing.

4. Pilot: Select first/next change for pilot testing

How can we pilot test an improvement idea using the Plan-Do-Check-Act method?" It's essential to know if a change results in an improvement; thus, it is wise to pilot test most proposed changes. The most common design for pilot testing is a simple before/after study comparing the old way with the new way. If possible, it's best to test the change quickly on a small scale. Any logistic, political, or timing issues that support or hinder a pilot test should be identified now.

Tips
Not all changes will necessarily be pilot tested. Some may be "quick and easy" to accomplish, produce obvious and immediate improvements, and obviate the need for a pilot test (for example, giving patients an accurate, legible written regimen can improve understanding of the treatment plan). It is sometimes possible to use a more powerful design than a simple before-and-after trial (for example, controlled trials, randomized designs, or factorial designs).

Side B: Aim . . . Fire . . . Hit/Miss

A. Aim: What are we trying to accomplish? (more specific aim)

Make a more specific aim statement that is consistent with the original, general aim statements and serves as a clear aim for the proposed pilot.

Tips
A *structured* aim statement is often helpful. For example: "An opportunity exists to improve [*name the process*]. The process starts [*insert start point*] and ends when [*insert end point*]. It is expected that improvement in this process will [*insert likely improvements in outcomes/costs*]. It is important to work on this process now because [*state clinical/business/learning need for selecting this process now*]."

B. Measures: How will we know that a change is an improvement?

Select three or four counterbalanced measures that can be used to evaluate the pilot's success (outcomes and costs).

Tips
Measures should flow from the specific aim statement cited in step A and from the more general, higher-level list of outcomes/costs that came from step 1. It is often wise to

- include fewer rather than more measures to avoid data overload, and
- select a few patient descriptors to characterize case mix, a few process measures to indicate how the process is changing/staying the same, and a small, counterbalanced set of measures of quality and costs.

C. Selected Change: How would you describe the change that you have selected for testing?

List here the most promising change ideas that came from completion of step 3 (or that have been identified since then) and provide a general description of the change that has been selected for testing.

Tips
This is a "holding pool" of potential changes to be tried out in future. (The essence of continual improvement is to run repeated, increasingly effective, and increasingly rapid tests of changes.) It also is a place to record a brief description of the selected change before proceeding to a detailed plan.

D. Plan: How shall we plan the pilot?

"Who? Does what? When? With what tools and training." Write a brief change protocol that answers these questions. Illustrate the protocol with a simple flowchart.

Tips
A good plan must be executed well to succeed. This means that everyone involved should know what they are doing and why they are doing it. Write down the specifics—illustrating them with a flowchart is a good start. Discuss the plan with all those who will be executing it, and be prepared to make refinements and changes as needed.

"Baseline data to be collected?" Write a brief data collection protocol indicating who will gather and analyze what data from what sources based on operational definitions.

Tips
Specify the key questions that will be answered by the pilot and show a "dummy" version of how the data will be

displayed to answer the key questions. Include the operational definitions to be used for each variable included in the data-collection plan. Whenever possible, build the data collection into the flow of the work and design self-coding data-collection forms that can be used by people as care is delivered. Often a pocket-sized, preprinted card can be used to gather values on variables that are not routinely recorded or accurately recorded in normal clinical or administrative databases. (Note: "Improving health care, part 1"[2] contains more information and a worksheet on operational definitions.)

E. Do: What are we learning as we do the pilot?

Keep a diary of the pilot. Jot down notes on how the pilot is going and include information on whether the pilot is going as planned.

Tips

Work is full of unanticipated events that positively or negatively influence the results of the pilot. Also, the results of the pilot will be no better than the care with which the planned change was executed. Observations on the process of making the change happen can help prepare the way for making bigger, more powerful changes in future.

F. Check: As we check and study what happened, what have we learned?

"Did original outcomes improve?" Analyze the results of the pilot test of change in a way that answers the main question—did the change lead to the predicted improvement?

Tips

Consider summarizing the key results graphically and leading off each graph with a question that is answered by the data display. One method of summarizing the results (that links case mix with process changes with outcomes/cost results) is to put before–after measures on key points in the process–outcome flowchart. This creates a process-based instrument panel.[3–5]

G. Act: As we act to hold the gains or abandon our pilot efforts, what needs to be done?

If successful, and if the pilot was done on a small scale or a temporary basis, determine what will be required to build the successful change into daily work routines in an efficient and effective manner. Make a plan for "mainstreaming" the change into daily work and begin to implement it. If unsuccessful, analyze the source(s) of the failure. Was this due to a change concept that did not work or a change concept that was not properly implemented? If the former is most likely to be true, consider going back to the "holding pool" of promising changes and select another for a pilot test.

Tips

Many tests of change fail to produce the desired results. Do not be discouraged; much can be learned from failures. Use this new knowledge to feed into more effective, next-phase change attempts.

REFERENCES

1. Scholtes PR: *The Team Handbook: How to Improve Quality with Teams.* Madison, WI: Joiner Associates, 1988.
2. Nelson EC, et al: Improving health care, Part 1: The Clinical Value Compass. *Jt Comm J Qual Improv* 22:243–258, 1996.
3. Nelson EC, Batalden PB: Patient-based quality measurement systems. *Quality Management in Health Care* 2(1):18–30, 1993.
4. Nelson EC, et al: Report cards or instrument panels: Who needs what? *Jt Comm J Qual Improv* 21:155–166, 1995.
5. Nugent WE, et al: Designing an instrument panel to monitor and improve coronary artery bypass grafting. *Journal of Clinical Outcomes Management* 1(2):57–64, 1994.

■ Part 3. Clinical Benchmarking for Best Patient Care

There is always one best result and one best process for achieving that result . . . and they can always be improved.

Brian Joiner

The Concept of Benchmarking and its Use in Health Care

Why has benchmarking created such interest in health care? Increased competition, the certain knowledge that similar patients are treated very differently, and better communication about measurable differences in outcomes and costs are just a few catalysts that have pressured practitioners to learn about "what works best." By learning that a much better way of doing something may be possible, one can stimulate local changes that previously were not thought necessary.

It is useful to review the generally accepted definitions of benchmarking in business and industry before discussing how the approach has been adapted to health care. Xerox Corporation, a recognized leader of business process benchmarking, formally defines *benchmarking* as "the continuous process of measuring products, services and practices against the company's toughest competitors or those companies known as leaders."[1] Robert Camp simplifies this definition as "finding and implementing best practices."[2] Thus, benchmarking is a search to find what works best and put this knowledge to work in one's own organization. The concept of benchmarking, which has spread rapidly throughout the United States, draws from the Japanese industrial practice termed "dantotsu." In Japan, the phrase "dantotsu" refers to a method for finding the "best of the best"—the best practice that consistently produces best in world results.[2]

Often the terms "benchmarking" and "benchmarks" are used interchangeably. Clarifying the differences between the two terms is important, because it is through combining them that an effective improvement strategy can be designed.

> ***Benchmarking*** is a systematic process of searching to identify best practices, and ***benchmarks*** are statistical measures.[3]

Benchmarking, without considering statistical *benchmarks,* does not allow the merits of different practices to be evaluated. On the other hand, only looking at the benchmarks, or the statistical measures of the results of a process, does not provide insight into the process identified as a best practice. It is rather obvious that benchmarking would be pointless without a comparison of the benchmarks. However, teams often forge ahead after finding benchmarks without an understanding of the underlying process responsible for producing the results—essentially, they are limited to a simple comparison of data (their results versus benchmark results).[4] It is through combining the two (*benchmarking* plus *benchmarks*) that an improvement strategy can be developed.

Growth in the use of benchmarking, first in industry and now in health care, has given benchmarking its place among other common "buzzwords." However, if a benchmarking process is defined and followed systematically, benchmarking can be used as a powerful tool to

- *Create tension for change.*
- *Build awareness of current capability versus best known capability.*
- *Encourage people to move from a position of inertia to positive action.*

The aim is both to get good ideas for change that can result in improvement[5] and to produce meaningful tension for change for those who are already interested in doing their best and are willing to try a new method.

For some organizations, an early step in benchmarking is to identify benchmarking partners or someone to benchmark against. One advantage of building a relationship with benchmarking partners is that it provides an opportunity to compare outcomes while gaining an understanding of the underlying process. However, if these benchmarking partners are not the "best of the best" in the area targeted for improvement, then the potential increase in performance will not approach best achievable levels. Furthermore, if the partnership only offers a comparison of the results, the partners might do just as well by selecting arbitrary performance targets.

Nonclinical aspects of providing health care—such as billing, payroll, and training—can undoubtedly benefit from benchmarking. Benchmarking partners for nonclinical areas should not be limited to other health care facilities; excellent benchmarking partners exist in other industries. More than two-thirds of revenue streams, however, flow through clinical, not administrative, processes.[6] Given this fact, plus our aim to reduce the illness burden and improve the value of patient care, this chapter focuses on using benchmarking to improve important clinical processes.

Benchmarking and the Clinical Value Compass

The Clinical Value Compass (shown in Figure 10–12) is a good starting point for thinking about best results, because it essentially provides a guide for determining what to look for in the benchmarking process. The cardinal points on the top portion of the Clinical Value Compass—west, north, and east—show clinical outcomes, functional health status, and patient satisfaction. The lower half of the Clinical Value Compass represents total costs (direct medical care costs plus indirect social costs). As a starting point, total charges paid by purchasers makes sense, but, as improvement work progresses, it is wise to include other costs—such as indirect social costs, time lost from work, workmans compensation—so as to find ways to minimize the real total costs of illness. (See earlier publications for further details on the Clinical Value Compass concept[7,8] and how to develop a Clinical Value Compass.[9])

Our process for clinical benchmarking, described in the following section, uses the Clinical Value Compass as the "jumping off point." This has the advantage of starting with a clearly defined target population and a related set of outcome and cost measures. Parallel processes occur between learning about what others outside one's own organization are doing through benchmarking and systematically examining internal processes with the help of the Clinical Improvement Worksheet. The results of the initial benchmarking work then feed back into the Clinical Improvement Worksheet to provide additional ideas for making changes.

Benchmarking for Best Practices—A Planning Worksheet

Numerous models have been defined for benchmarking.[10] For example, Motorola uses a 5-step process, Florida Power & Light has a 7-step process, AT&T has a 9-step process, and Xerox uses a 10-step process. While it seems that everyone involved in benchmarking has developed their own process, there are some elements that successful processes share. To begin with, each process

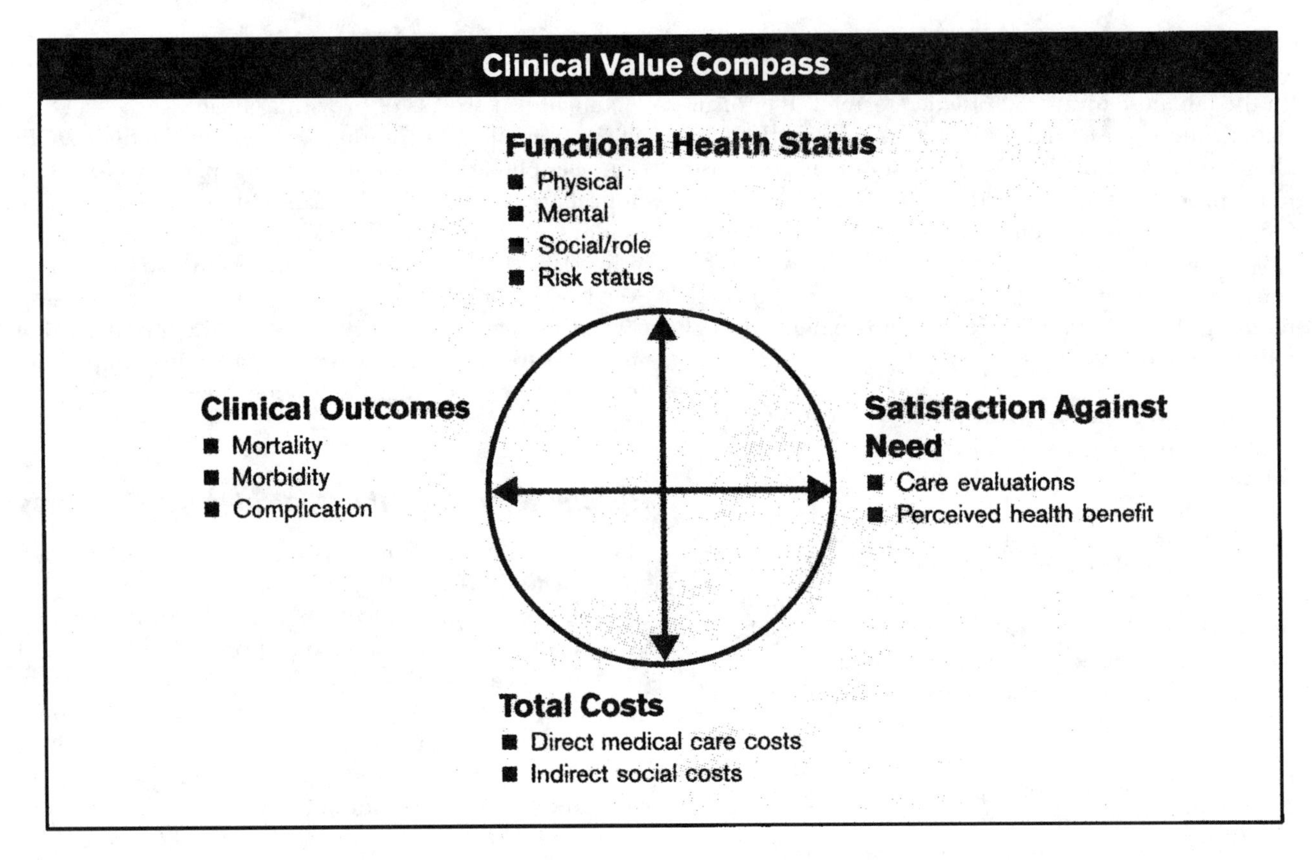

FIGURE 10–12. Clinical Value Compass.

reflects a systematic, measured approach to benchmarking that follows a basic—plan, collect, analyze, and improve—format.[11] Our model, which is described in the following paragraphs, shares this format.

The Benchmarking Worksheet developed for use with the Clinical Value Compass approach is shown in Figures 10–13 and 10–14. This worksheet, along with the other worksheets in this series, was designed to be used as a tool to guide the process, keep track of the results, and document the work accomplished by the team. The aim of the benchmarking process is to develop testable ideas about best practices. The Worksheet has five basic steps:

1. *Identify measures.*
2. *Determine resources needed to find the best of the best.*
3. *Design data collection method and gather data.*
4. *Measure best against own performance to determine gap.*
5. *Identify the best practices that produce best in class results.*

Step 1: Identify Measures

This step identifies the statistical measures, or benchmarks, that will focus the external scan (the search outside one's own organization for best practices). Using the Clinical Value Compass as a guide, the team reaches consensus on two to three measures for clinical outcomes, functional health status, satisfaction against need, and total costs. Generally, many measures are identified early in the improvement process. It may be valuable to start the improvement work by examining numerous outcomes; however, when beginning the benchmarking process, it is wise to reduce the number of measures and focus the search on a few key measures that are likely to (a) reflect variability of performance across facilities, and (b) be available as valid comparison data. An appropriate benchmark enables measurement and comparison across locations.

Step 2: Determine Resources Needed to Find the Best of the Best

This step determines the resources that will help find the best of the best. These resources include the best data, the best people, and the best literature currently available. The best data include sources of internal *and* external data because, to make a valid and reliable comparison, there must be confidence in the accuracy of both internal and external data. Furthermore, internal data may need to be reformatted to allow comparison to external data. Valuable people resources include in-house experts most familiar with the clinical process, the data, and the benchmarking and improvement processes. Usually, the in-house experts can identify external experts through their professional contacts. The measures identified in the first step should be used as "key words" to focus the literature

Appendix: Benchmarking Worksheet (Side 1)

Benchmarking for Best Practices

Aim: Develop ideas about best practices.

1. Identify measures

Using the Clinical Value Compass as a guide, reach consensus on 2 - 3 statistical measures, or benchmarks which will be the focus of the external scan. Consider availability of valid comparative data and the variability of performance across facilities. (An appropriate benchmark enables measurement and comparison across systems.)

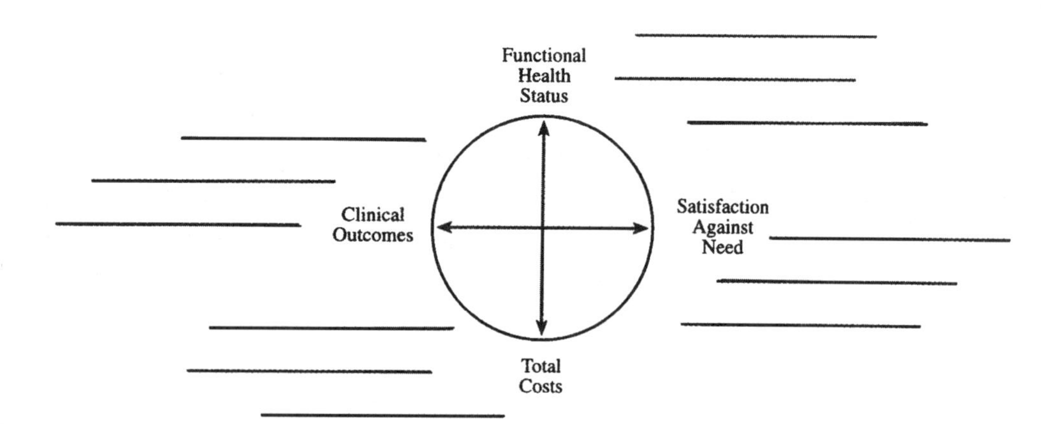

2. Determine resources needed to find the best of the best

Given our desire to limit/reduce the illness burden (cost, resource use, excess morbidity, mortality) for our patients, think about the information needed for finding the best of the best.

The Best Data to use?	The Best People to ask?
internal?	*in-house?*
external?	*out-of-house?*

The Best Literature?

© December 1995, Lahey Hitchcock Clinic

Identified measures and needed resources are recorded on Side 1, above; the data collection method and data, the performance gap, and best practices producing best-in-class results are recorded on Side 2, p 616.

FIGURE 10–13. Benchmarking Worksheet (Side 1).

Appendix: Benchmarking Worksheet (Side 2)

3. Design data collection method and gather data

Who will collect the data? How will the data be analyzed? Who will review the literature?

Tasks:	Person completing:	Date to be completed:

4. Measure best against own performance to determine gap

Based on the measures identified in Step 1, and the results of an internal and external scan of the data, how does our performance compare to the best of the best?

Summary Data	
Number of cases	______
Total revenue	______
Revenue rank	______

Benchmark: ____________
Our results ______
Nat'l avg ______
"Best" ______

Benchmark: ____________
Our results ______
Nat'l avg ______
"Best" ______

Functional Health Status

Clinical Outcomes

Satisfaction Against Need

Total Costs

Compared to what we found, how good is our quality and value?

Benchmark: ____________
Our results ______
Nat'l avg ______
"Best" ______

Benchmark: ____________
Our results ______
Nat'l avg ______
"Best" ______

Benchmark: ____________
Our results ______
Nat'l avg ______
"Best" ______

Benchmark: ____________
Our results ______
Nat'l avg ______
"Best" ______

5. Identify the best practices that produce best in class results

© December 1995, Lahey Hitchcock Clinic

FIGURE 10–14. Benchmarking Worksheet (Side 2).

search. Most teams find it helpful to create a bibliography of those articles constituting the best literature.

Essentially, this step involves "secondary research."—searching for information about a subject from indirect sources.[12] In general, the secondary research methods described here—the best data, people, and literature—won't reveal the processes that the best of the best use to accomplish their results. However, secondary research can help guide the way to the best.

Step 3: Design Data Collection Method and Gather Data

This step keeps the project on track by establishing a method and a timeline for collecting and analyzing data and reviewing the literature. There is space on the Benchmarking Worksheet for recording the tasks to be completed, who will be completing them, and the date for completion.

Step 4: Measure Best against Own Performance to Determine Gap

In this step, the team compares the best of each of the identified measures—through data, literature, and people resources—to their own performance to determine the gap. The goal is to create tension for change by showing that the gap in one's performance, when compared to the best of the best, is substantial. For the benchmarks where comparative data are available, the Benchmarking Worksheet includes space for internal results, national average results, and the best of the best. To provide some interpretive context, there is also a place to record summary data for the number of cases, total revenue, and revenue rank.

Step 5: Identify the Best Practices That Produce Best in Class Results

At this point in the benchmarking process, it is time to start identifying the processes that produce the best results. This adds to people's understanding of measurement and the relationship between process and outcomes, and creates tension for change. This step is generally accomplished through identifying potential benchmarking partners and working to establish a symbiotic learning relationship. It is important to understand your own processes and have gained as much information as possible through secondary research prior to contacting potential benchmarking partners.

Case Example: Bowel Surgery

This case example is from the Accelerating Clinical Improvement Bowel Surgery Team at Dartmouth-Hitchcock Medical Center (DHMC). This team was formed in November 1994, after a kickoff event was held to accelerate clinical improvement for this patient population (DRGs 148 and 149: major small and large bowel procedures with and without complications) in the Dartmouth-Lahey Hitchcock delivery system. The steps defined in the Benchmarking Worksheet—(1) identify measures, (2) determine resources needed to find the best of the best, (3) design data collection method and gather data, (4) measure best against own performance to determine gap, and (5) identify the practices that produce best in class results—are part of a larger process for developing a strategy for improvement encompassed in the Serial Vee approach.[13] The Clinical Improvement Worksheet (see Figures 10–15 and 10–16) provided the framework within which the work of the team was organized and guides the case discussion below.

TEAM MEMBERS: Who should work on this improvement?

The Bowel Surgery Improvement Team consists of two general surgeons, one senior general surgery resident, one gastroenterologist, one clinical nurse specialist, one enterostomal nurse, one clinical nurse leader, two general surgery clinical administrators, a process consultant, a data specialist, and a team facilitator. They agreed to schedule 60 minute meetings every week and followed structured meeting agendas, designating roles of leader, timekeeper, recorder, facilitator, and group process.

1. _OUTCOMES:_ Select a population

The team formed because DRGs 148 and 149 represent a large patient population at DHMC. In addition, initial review of external comparative data suggested that DHMC is higher than some other academic medical centers on length of stay, mortality, and costs.

"What's the general aim?" *The aim is to decrease the overall average length of stay (ALOS), decrease the mortality rate, increase patient satisfaction, and create the opportunity to better characterize the clinical practices involved in the care of these patients.*

"Given our wish to limit/reduce the illness burden for 'this type' of patient, what are the desired results?" *The team brainstormed many important measures on the Clinical Value Compass:*

- Clinical outcomes: *mortality, readmissions, success/cure, resumption of diet, and morbidity measures—intra-abdominal, cardiac and pulmonary complications, wound infection, reoperation*
- Functional health status: *physical and mental health based on SF-36 or SF-12*[14]
- Satisfaction: *patient/family education, RN caring and concern, diet/nutrition, timeliness/access from clinic visit to OR date, ease of transition (from office to hospital, one hour after surgery, hospital to home), congruence of outcomes with expectations*
- Costs: *direct costs—preoperative, operative, hospital charges, professional (surgical fees), visiting nurses; indirect costs—loss of work, family, child care, and out-of-pocket expenses*

Clinical Improvement Worksheet, Side A

Clinical Improvement Worksheet

Aim: Accelerate clinical improvement by linking outcomes measurements and process knowledge with the design and conduct of pilot tests of change.

① OUTCOMES ➡ Select a population DRG 148/149 pts

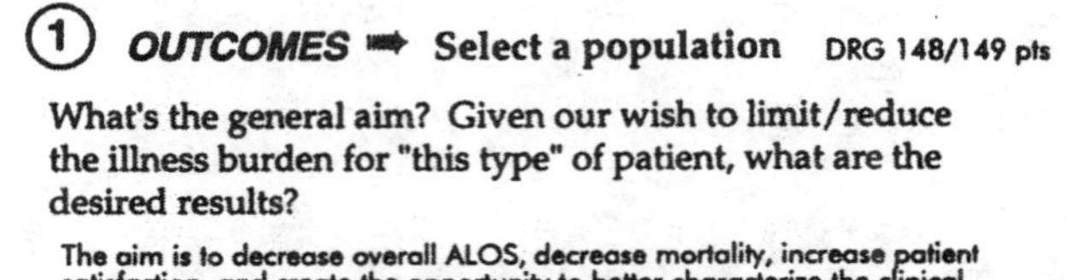

What's the general aim? Given our wish to limit/reduce the illness burden for "this type" of patient, what are the desired results?

The aim is to decrease overall ALOS, decrease mortality, increase patient satisfaction, and create the opportunity to better characterize the clinical practices involved in the care of these patients.

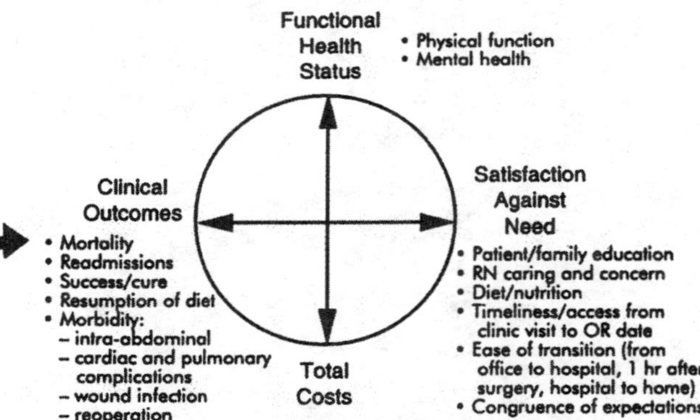

② PROCESS ➡ Analyze the process

What's the process for giving care to this type of patient?

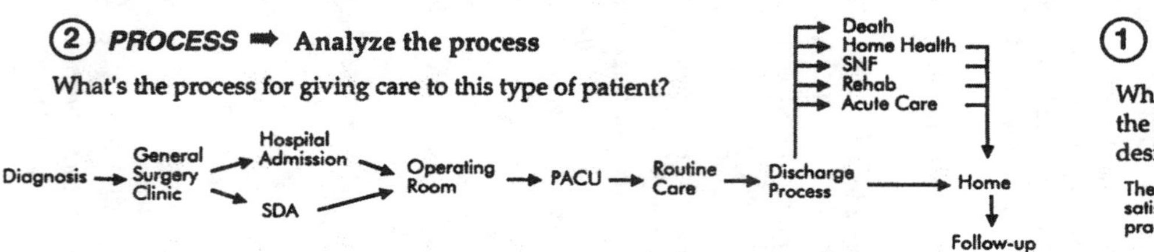

③ CHANGES ➡ Generate change ideas

What ideas do we have for changing what's done (process) to get better results?

- Focus on high-leverage processes within overall process: general surgery clinic, same day service, routine care
  1. Reduce lab/rad use
  2. Begin discharge planning in out-patient clinic
  3. Admit all elective cases through same day services
  4. Standardize bowel prep
  5. Standardize post-op routine care

④ PILOT ➡ Select first/next change for pilot testing

How can we pilot test an improvement idea using the Plan-Do-Check-Act method?

1. Use same day service for all
2. Establish standardized pre-op bowel prep
3. Use standardized pre/post-op routine care orders

Eugene C. Nelson, DSc, MPH, and Paul B. Batalden, MD
© July 1995, Lahey Hitchcock Clinic

SIDE A

FIGURE 10–15. Clinical Improvement Worksheet (Side A) for Bowel Surgery Improvement Team.

Clinical Improvement Worksheet, Side B

Making Improvements: Clinical Improvement Worksheet

TEAM MEMBERS ➡ Who should work on this improvement?

1. Leader
2. Facilitator
3. 2 surgeons
4. 1 general surgery resident
   1 process consultant
   1 gastroenterologist
5. 1 clinical nurse specialist
6. 1 enterstomal nurse
7. 1 clinical nurse leader
8. 2 gen surg clin administrators
   1 data specialists

Coach ____________ Admin Support ____________

A. ***AIM*** ➡ What are we trying to accomplish? (more specific AIM)

An opportunity exists to improve the surgical care of patients undergoing surgery of the small and large bowel beginning with diagnosis and ending
30 - 60 days after discharge

B. ***MEASURES*** ➡ How will we know that a change is an improvement?

- Decreased LOS
- Decreased mortality rate compared with DHMC 1992 data and AMCC data
- Increased patient satisfaction

C. ***SELECTED CHANGE*** ➡ How would you describe the change that you have selected for testing?

First Cycle:
1. Admit all elective cases through same day services
2. Standardize the outpatient bowel preparation process
3. Develop and implement a standard order set for the first post-operative day

Second Cycle:
1. Develop a clinical pathway for bowel surgery patients
2. Implement clinical pathway for the elective surgery population

D. ***PLAN*** ➡ How shall we **PLAN** the pilot?

- Who? Does what? When? With what tools and training?

For the clinical pathway trial, inservice training was provided by the nursing members of the bowel surgery team to the outpatient General Surgery staff, the Same Day Services program, and the two in-patient surgical units. The participating surgeons provided orientation to the General Surgery Section attendings and housestaff. A Resource Binder was developed to provide housestaff and nursing staff an overview of the pathway and articles which support the clinical content of the pathway's order set.

- Baseline data to be collected?

Length of stay, total charges, charges categorized by medications, laboratory tests, PACU and OR charges, proxies for functional health status and patient satisfaction.

E. ***DO*** ➡ What are we learning as we **DO** the pilot?

- Shading the physician's order set made it difficult for the pharmacists to read the medication orders.
- The tracking sheet used to identify elective patients scheduled for surgery needed to be optimized so that their progress could be better monitored by a team member.
- Compliance with use of the pathway was higher on the unit where the team member followed the patients each day to answer nursing and housestaff questions and to follow up on incomplete documents.
- The goal of mobilizing the patient immediately after surgery was general delayed until the first post-operative day.

F. ***CHECK*** ➡ As we **CHECK** and **STUDY** what happened, what have we learned?

- Did original outcomes improve?

Yes, summarized and illustrated in the text

G. ***ACT*** ➡ As we **ACT** to hold the gains or abandon our pilot efforts, what needs to be done?

The team continues to meet on a monthly basis to discuss progress of pathway patients.

FIGURE 10–16. Clinical Improvement Worksheet (Side B) for Bowel Surgery Improvement Team.

After identifying the points on the Clinical Value Compass, the team began the benchmarking process described next.

Benchmarking for Best Practices: Using the Benchmarking Worksheet

The team's use of benchmarking is described in this section. The completed Benchmarking Worksheet is shown in Figures 10–17 and 10–18. To get started, a clinician member of the team involved in providing care to bowel surgery patients was selected as the person to lead the benchmarking process.

Step 1: Identify Measures

The team reached consensus on 2 to 3 benchmarks for each of the Clinical Value Compass points:

- Clinical outcomes: *mortality, morbidity, infection rate, surgical technique*
- Functional health status: *pain management, physical function, psychosocial health*
- Satisfaction against need: *patient/family satisfaction, patient/family perspective*
- Total costs: *length of stay, total charges, indirect social costs*

Step 2: Determine Resources Needed to Find the Best of the Best

For the best internal data, the team focused on the statistical measurement and graphical display of key data points related to the surgical patient care process. The best sources of external data available to the group were the large, administrative databases of the New Hampshire Hospital Association and the Academic Medical Center Consortium. The results of scanning the internal data suggested areas of process variability for further investigation.

Dartmouth-Hitchcock Medical Center physicians and other "experts" most familiar with the clinical process were recruited for the team. The team discovered that clinical experts (nationally recognized surgical leaders) existed within their system and were now active members of the improvement team. Furthermore, these internal experts had been networking with their national colleagues for years prior to this improvement effort. It is interesting to note that the team decided to delay formally contacting the external regional and national experts regarding best practices until later in the improvement process. Doing so enabled them to become completely familiar with current sources of variation within the existing medical care delivery before moving on to identifying the gaps between their own delivery process and the delivery process used by the best known surgical teams.

Working with a clinical reference librarian, the benchmarker focused on the measures identified in Step 1 to search the literature using available on-line databases: MEDLINE and CINAHL. As the benchmarker scanned the results of the literature searches to identify those articles that constituted the best literature about bowel surgery, she created a bibliography that could be shared with the improvement group and could be updated easily over time. A commercially available bibliographic database was used to create and maintain the bibliography.

Step 3: Design Data Collection Method and Gather Data

Assigned tasks included running internal data reports, constructing graphic displays of the data, periodically updating the literature review, and creating a condition-specific bibliography. The team also set a date for a "state of the union" address (the kickoff event) for presenting the results of the benchmarking process to the improvement team. A reunion was scheduled for 6 months following the kickoff as a time to come together to report on progress made to date and share lessons learned with others involved in similar improvement efforts within the Dartmouth-Lahey Hitchcock system.

At this point, the team hit a roadblock that many improvement teams experience—they became paralyzed by the amount of data that was available. The volume of data and discussions of different methods of analysis slowed the team's progress at this step. They also found that there were long turnaround times from requesting data to receiving something in a format that could be discussed during a team meeting. The team resolved this issue, in part, by setting realistic expectations about the time involved in data analysis. It takes time to sort through questions about validity of the data and the best way to format the analyses. In addition, during the course of the project, the medical center made available GQL, graphical query language, which allows individual users to access databases and display results on spreadsheets as well as graphically. This has reduced the turnaround time involved in analyzing data. Finally, the team found it helpful to focus on the Clinical Value Compass measures identified earlier to limit their data requests and analyses.

Step 4: Measure Best against Own Performance to Determine Gap

Finally, the benchmarker identified how internal quality and value measured up to the best of the best. It was difficult to find comparable data for both the functional health status and satisfaction measures, but data were available for mortality, length of stay, and total charges. The literature also revealed that gains could be made in pain management.

Step 5: Identify the Best Practices That Produce Best in Class Results

The work accomplished prior to step 5, the secondary research, revealed a clear path to the "best of the best." An important point to remember as potential benchmarking

Benchmarking Worksheet, Side 1

Benchmarking for Best Practices

Aim: Develop ideas about best practices.

1. Identify measures

Using the Clinical Value Compass as a guide, reach consensus on 2 - 3 statistical measures, or benchmarks which will be the focus of the external scan. Consider availability of valid comparative data and the variability of performance across facilities. (An appropriate benchmark enables measurement and comparison across systems.)

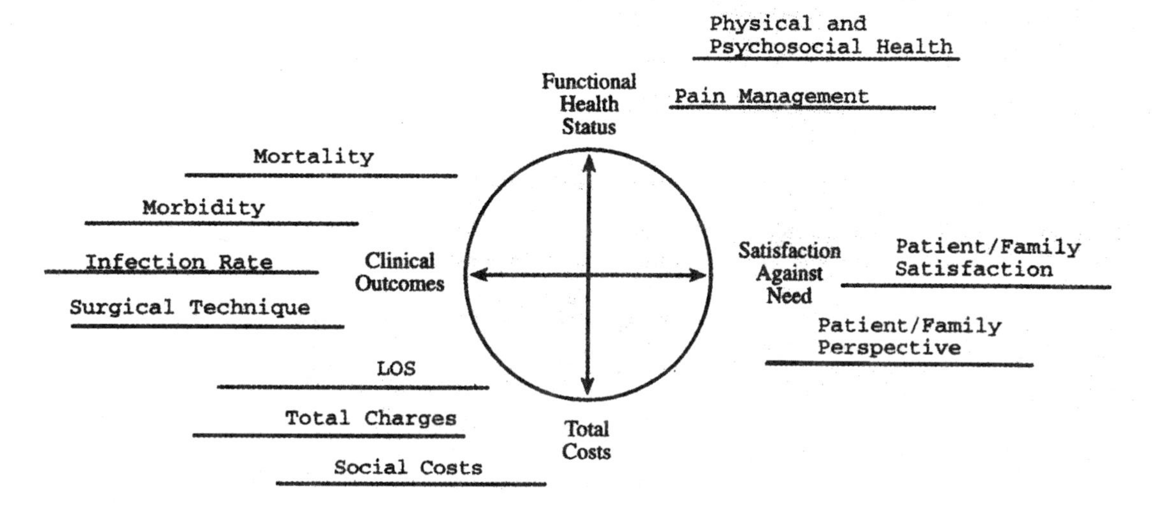

2. Determine resources needed to find the best of the best

Given our desire to limit/reduce the illness burden (cost, resource use, excess morbidity, mortality) for our patients, think about the information needed for finding the best of the best.

The Best Data to use?

internal?

Focus on statistical measurement and graphic display of key data points related to patient care process

external?

NHHA Database
AMCC Database

The Best People to ask?

in-house?

Focus on developing multi-disciplinary team

out-of-house?

Identify key clinical experts in the field for future consultation

The Best Literature?

Search the literature using MEDLINE, CINAHL.
Create electronic bibliographic database.

© December 1995, Lahey Hitchcock Clinic

FIGURE 10–17. Benchmarking Worksheet (Side 1) for Bowel Surgery Improvement Team.

Benchmarking Worksheet, Side 2

3. Design data collection method and gather data

Who will collect the data? How will the data be analyzed? Who will review the literature?

Tasks:	Person completing:	Date to be completed:
Produce data reports	A. Hinkle	
Create data displays	A. Hinkle, B. Swartz	
Search literature	C. Mahoney	
Create bibliography	C. Mahoney	

4. Measure best against own performance to determine gap

Based on the measures identified in Step 1, and the results of an internal and external scan of the data, how does our performance compare to the best of the best?

Benchmark:	Surgical Technique
Our results	Not available
Nat'l avg	Not available
"Best"	Not available

Benchmark:	Pain Management
Our results	Not available
Nat'l avg	Not available
"Best"	Not available

Summary Data	
Number of cases	170
Total revenue	> $5 Million
Revenue rank	#8

Benchmark:	1993 Total Hospital Charges
Our results	$34,000
Nat'l avg	$33,000
"Best"	$14,000

Compared to what we found, how good is our quality and value?

Benchmark:	Pt/Fam Satisfaction
Our results	Not available
Nat'l avg	Not available
"Best"	Not available

Benchmark:	1993 Mortality**
Our results	> 3%
Nat'l avg	3%
"Best"	< 1%

**NOTE: This illustrates results of initial benchmarking effort done in November 1994, comparing DHMC to other major medical centers. Data have been adjusted for case-mix, but include both urgent and elective cases as well as complicated and uncomplicated cases.

Benchmark:	1993 LOS
Our results	16
Nat'l avg	14
"Best"	10

5. Identify the best practices that produce best in class results

© December 1995, Lahey Hitchcock Clinic

FIGURE 10–18. Benchmarking Worksheet (Side 2) for Bowel Surgery Improvement Team.

partners are identified is that the team should wait to contact benchmarking partners until they have answered as many of their questions as feasible through the secondary research achieved in Steps 2 and 3. Furthermore, as the team becomes more knowledgeable about their own processes, they can make better use of time spent with benchmarking partners.

The benchmarking results (see Figure 10–18) show that a substantial gap existed between results that are currently produced by our own bowel surgery delivery process and the best known results among comparable organizations. When the team studied the results, they rapidly came to the following conclusions:

- *All the data were far from perfectly accurate, and fair, careful comparisons were difficult to make; nevertheless, they were still useful for identifying potential improvement areas. The team decided to break out elective cases from urgent cases to clarify the results for each perspective strata.*
- *Reduction in average length of stay (ALOS) was a high-priority improvement opportunity.*
- *The exact survival rate was not known, but it was possible that a gap existed between the current team's rate and the best survival rate. However, even the best survival rate could probably be improved.*
- *While hospital charges to payors are not necessarily related to actual costs of care, there was a very large difference in charges between DHMC and the lowest charge provider. The team suspected that there were many unnecessary costs built into their own system for providing bowel surgery.*
- *Accurate comparative data on functional health status and patient satisfaction were scarce. Unpublished data suggest that some medical centers were doing substantially better, yet none appeared to have reached maximum achievable levels of performance.*
- *The team recognized that benchmarking should be an ongoing process; as they continued to identify improvement strategies, they continued to assess best practices.*

As the benchmarking work was proceeding (described above), the Bowel Surgery Team continued pushing ahead using the Clinical Improvement Worksheet as a path forward. The team's progress on this is summarized below.

2. *PROCESS:* Analyze the process

"What's the process for giving care for this type of patient?" *The team flowcharted the bowel surgery process (see Figure 10–15), beginning with the diagnosis and ending 30 to 60 days after discharge (at the first follow-up clinic appointment).*

3. *CHANGES:* Generate change ideas

"What ideas do we have for changing what's done (process) to get better results?" *Using the flowchart developed for analyzing surgical care, the team identified the high-leverage steps within the overall process: General Surgery Clinic, Same Day Service, and routine care. Ideas for changing the General Surgery Clinic process included reducing utilization of laboratory and radiology resources preoperatively and beginning the discharge planning process in the outpatient clinic. In the Same Day Services area, some ideas for change included admitting all elective cases through Same Day Services and standardizing the bowel preparation procedure. Finally, the team decided that standardizing orders for postoperative routine care could influence more appropriate utilization of medications and laboratory, NG tube management, resumption of feeding, ambulation, and utilization of ancillary consultations (for example, PT and OT). These changes are being incorporated into the development of a clinical pathway for this patient population. To address the issues of patient satisfaction and functional health status, the team collaborated with an existing internal consulting group that is responsible for performing patient surveys by telephone. Under the negotiated agreement, all patients undergoing large and small bowel surgery will be surveyed 4 weeks post discharge to gather feedback on functional status and satisfaction. In addition, the team has continued to review current tools used to measure the health status and satisfaction points on the Clinical Value Compass, and is exploring the development of a condition-specific survey for this surgical population.*

4. *PILOT:* Select a change for pilot testing

"How can we pilot test an improvement idea using the Plan-Do-Check-Act method?" *The team planned three successive PDCA cycles, beginning with the least complex change and progressing toward the changes the team perceived as more difficult (see Figure 10–19). The first three initiatives have now been implemented and data related to these steps has been collected. The first three initiatives are:*

- *Utilization of Same Day Services for all elective surgery patients.*
- *Establishment of a standardized preoperative bowl preparation.*
- *Utilization of standardized pre and postoperative routine care orders.*

Results for 1995 elective patients ($N = 97$)—in contrast to 1994 elective patients ($N = 83$)—are encouraging. The findings show that the average LOS has been reduced by one day, that readmission within 30 days have been reduced by more than 50%, and median hospital charges have been cut by over $1000. Figure 10–20 shows a control chart that is an example of how the team has monitored data. The chart shows that in 1994 average LOS was 9.66 days and in 1995 it was 9.98 until the improvement cycles were implemented in June of that year. The improvement cycles resulted in a reduction in LOS to 8.29 days. As the team continues to analyze data and make improvements, they will want to look at data over time through the use of control charts, as shown in Figure 10–21 While the summary measures shown on the benchmarking worksheet in Figure 10–17 are helpful to create the tension for change, other

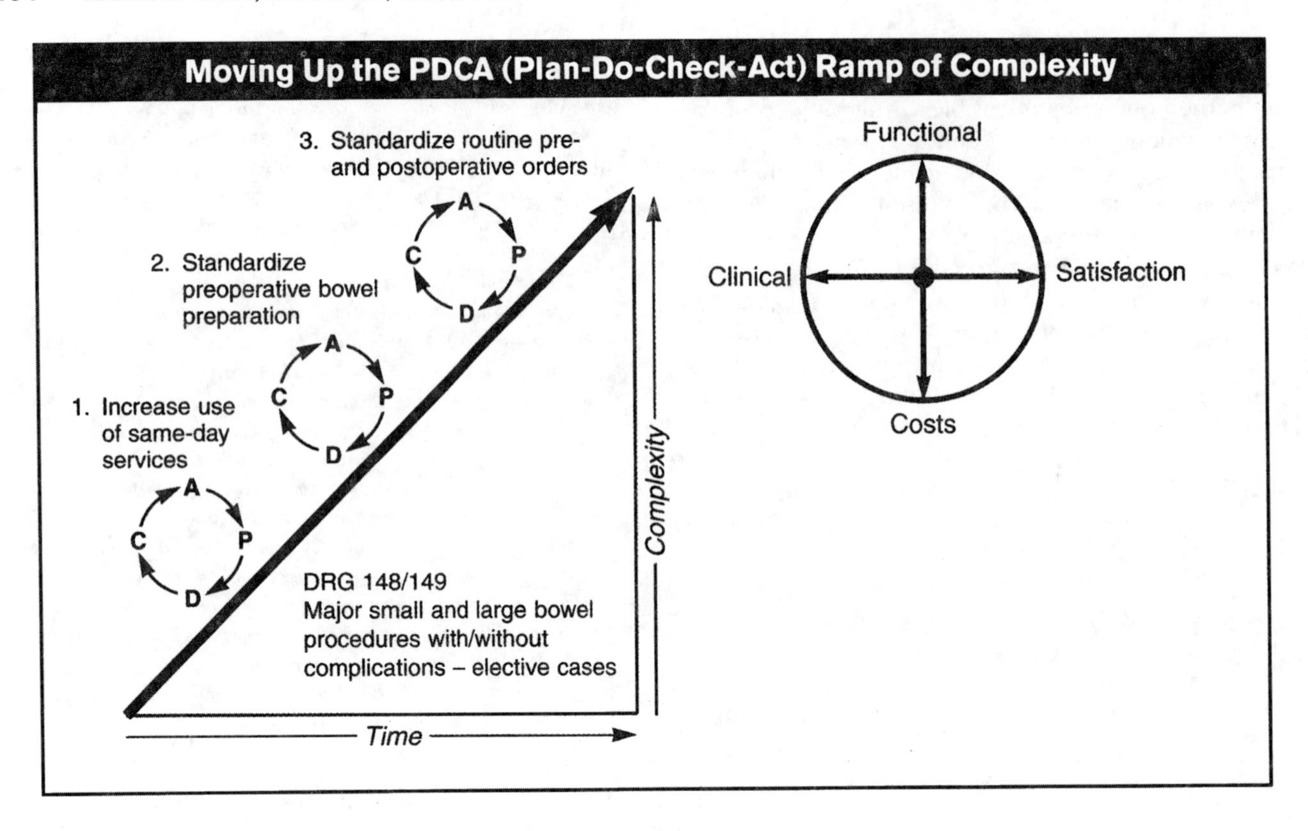

FIGURE 10–19. Testing three changes in Bowel Surgery care: moving up the PDCA Ramp of Complexity.

techniques, such as control charts, are more appropriate for monitoring change.

After the time spent working through this process, the team discovered that many barriers to implementation had been eliminated. Key to successful implementation was the initial selection of team members. Including the most senior attending surgeons eliminated any resistance that those surgeons might have had. Furthermore, their support decreased resistance among other attendings and house staff. Other team members who were directly involved in patient care were able to anticipate resistance and work to resolve any problems with implementation before they arose. Finally, the team obtained section input into the major changes and had achieved consensus prior to formalizing the planned changes.

The team is now identifying the next areas for improvement. Overall and surgeon-specific instrument panels have been created to show trends in patient mix, key process variables (e.g., OR hours, PACU hours, OR charges, and counts of medications and laboratory tests), and outcomes and cost-related variables (mortality, readmissions, functional health status, LOS, and hospital charges). Data are compiled every six months comparing surgeons to each other and to the section average. Each surgeon is able to identify him or herself, but not other surgeons. Currently the reports have just been used to create awareness and have been received without animosity. It isn't clear how helpful they will continue to be, given the team's focus on using process measures to monitor outcomes.

Substantial effort has gone into developing and implementing a critical pathway. Several "generic" references were used to guide the team's understanding of pathway development and use.[15–24] Despite the success with implementation of earlier changes, resistance to implementing a pathway has been experienced regardless of the team's efforts to reach consensus and provide education and support. Many of the barriers seem to be cultural, for example the appearance of "cook book medicine." Furthermore, there have been issues about how to handle patients who "fall off" the pathway. The team decided early on not to have on person accountable for the pathway, which may have added to the implementation difficulties. Even with these difficulties, results for elective patients since implementing the pathway have been a 3-day reduction in LOS (as shown in Figure 10–19) and an additional $3000 reduction in total charges. The next step will be to add nonelective patients to the pathway. The team's effort at pathway development has now become part of a broader effort to determine development, documentation, and use of critical paths at DHMC.

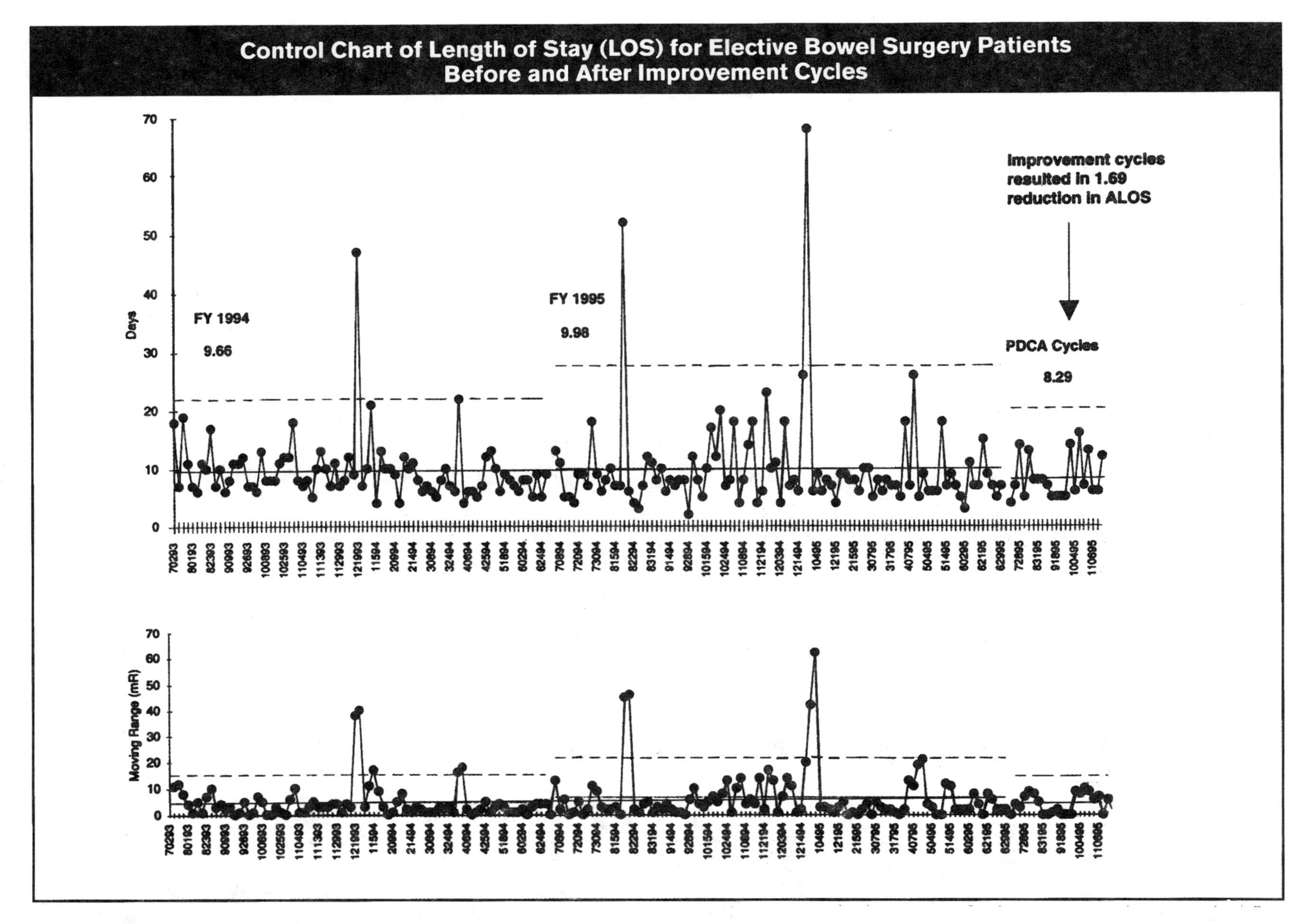

FIGURE 10–20. Control Chart of LOS for Elective Bowel Surgery Patients.

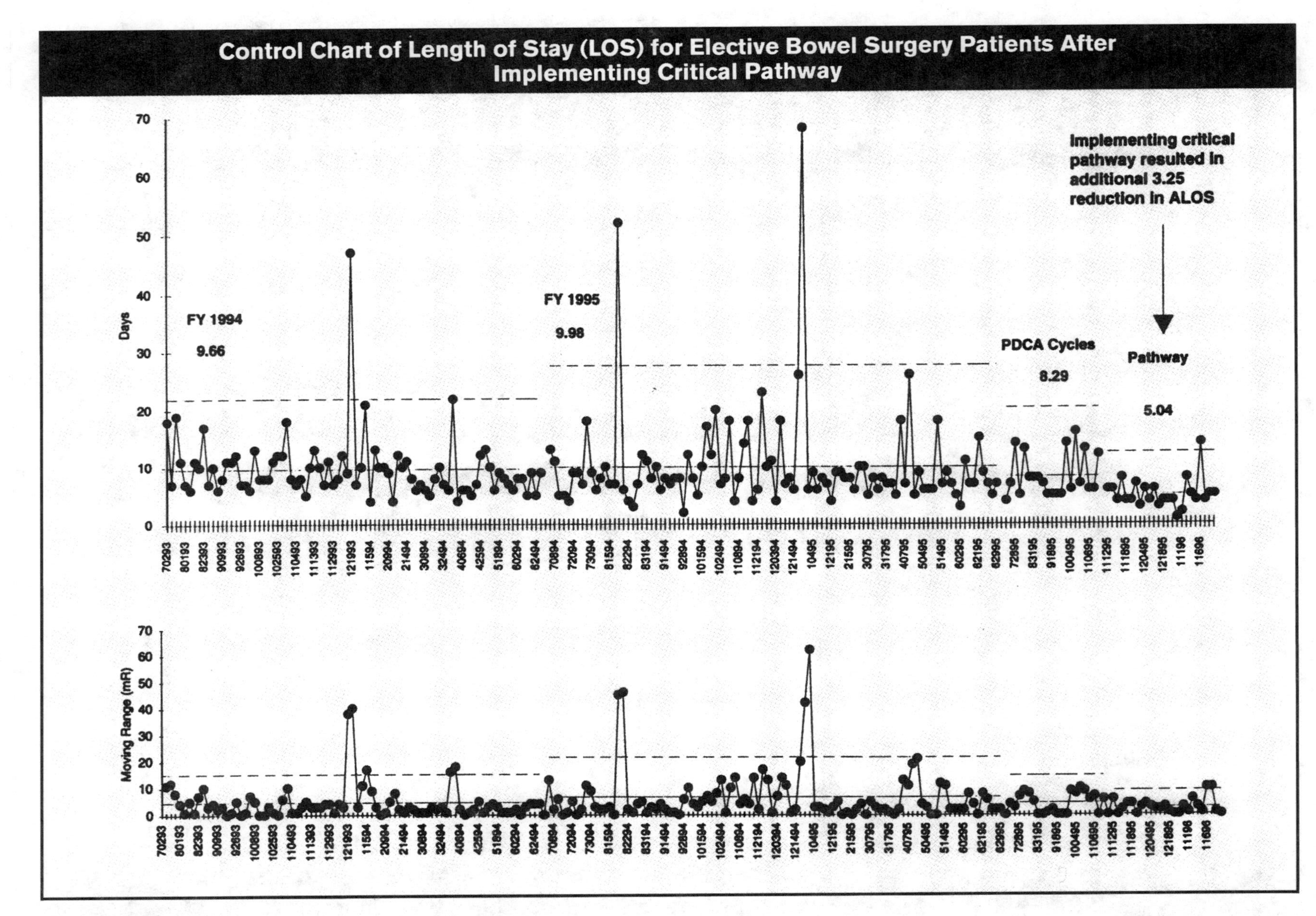

FIGURE 10–21. Control Chart of LOS for Elective Bowel Surgery Patients after Implementing Critical Pathway.

■ Comments and Conclusion

The bowel surgery case illustrates some important points that should be kept in mind as a clinical team prepares to use benchmarking to help them improve care.

- *While it may not be an individual provider, someone somewhere does practice in a way that produces the best results in clinical outcomes, functional status, satisfaction, and costs. Learning about those best practices is the aim of the benchmarking process.*
- *The desired health system—knowledge about relevant treatment options freely and accurately communicated to patients, shared decision making (patients and clinicians) regarding therapeutic actions, continual improvement of the process of care, continual assessment and reassessment of conventional treatment modalities, and identification and reallocation of excess capacity[25]—is usually somewhere beyond one's own current performance as well as beyond existing best known practices.*
- *While benchmarking is a useful tool for understanding and learning about current best practices, it is important to realize that it's a just one step in the journey. Benchmarking goes beyond replicating what others are doing to achieve similar outcomes. Benchmarking can be used to create the tension for change that will lead to innovative performance and breakthrough results.*
- *Benchmarking is an ongoing process. As the best results, and the practices that produce them, continue to evolve, using a benchmarking process will help assess the external environment.*

This approach assigns the benchmarking leadership role to a clinical member of the condition-specific improvement team, then supports the benchmarking leader with data analysts and other familiar with the benchmarking process. The improvement team includes those familiar with the process of patient care that is the focus of the improvement work along with a benchmarker—someone familiar with both the processes of patient care involved and the processes of comparative analysis and improvement. Understanding the process of care, including the results of patient outcomes, gives the benchmarker the insight needed to look for best practices. Camp and Tweet emphasize the importance of team members actively involved in the process conducting their own benchmarking. "When the process owners conduct their own benchmarking, they develop a commitment to the process and the resulting best practices."[2] Finally, both carefully designed communication to the organization and concerted management support are essential to the benchmarking process.[26] In conclusion, benchmarking can stimulate wise clinical changes and promote measured improvements in quality and value.

Reprints: Address reprint requests to Ms. Mohr, Center for the Evaluative Clinical Sciences, Dartmouth Medical School, Hanover, NH 03755.

ACKNOWLEDGMENTS

The authors wish to thank Diane Hall for help in preparing the manuscript and its figures, and would like to express our appreciation for the work done by the Accelerating Clinical Improvement Bowel Surgery Team at the Dartmouth-Hitchcock Medical Center—John Birkmeyer, M.D., Thomas A. Colacchio, M.D., F.A.C.S., Judith Dixon, R.N., B.S.N., Stuart R. Gordon, M.D., Wendy Manganiello, R.N., C., B.S.N., C.E.T.N., William Mroz, B.S.N., M.B.A., Cathy Pallatroni, Frederick C. Pond, B.A., M.L.S., John E. Sutton, Jr., M.D., F.A.C.S., Gayle Thomson, and Charles L. Townsend, M.A.

REFERENCES: PART 3

1. Camp RC: *Business process benchmarking: Finding and implementing best practices.* Milwaukee, WI: ASQC Press, 1994.
2. Camp RC, Tweet AG: Benchmarking applied to health care. *Jt Comm J on Qual Improv* May 1994; 20(5):229–238.
3. Bogan CE, English MJ: *Benchmarking for best practices: Winning through innovative adaptation.* New York: McGraw-Hill, Inc, 1994.
4. Mosel D, Gift B: Collaborative benchmarking in health care. *Jt Comm J on Qual Improv* May 1994; 20(5): 239–249.
5. Nolan T: *Cost reduction while maintaining quality.* Seminary at Dartmouth-Hitchcock Medical Center, May 4, 1995.
6. Campbell B: Benchmarking: a performance intervention tool. *Jt Comm J on Qual Improv* May 1994; 20(5):225–228.
7. Nelson EC, Greenfield S, Hays RD, Larson C, Leopold B, Batalden PB: Comparing outcomes and charges for patients with acute myocardial infarction in three community hospitals: An approach for assessing "value." *Int J Qual Health Care* 7(2):95–108.
8. Nugent WE, Schults WC, Plume SK, Batalden PB, Nelson EC: Designing an instrument panel to monitor and improve coronary artery bypass grafting. *JCOM* December 1994; 1(2):57–64.
9. Nelson EC, Mohr JJ, Batalden PB, Plume SK. Improving health care, Part 1: The clinical value compass. *Jt Comm J on Qual Improv* April 1996; 22(4):243–258.
10. American Productivity & Quality Center. *The benchmarking management guide.* Portland, OR: Productivity Press. 1993.
11. Ibid.
12. Ibid.
13. Batalden PB, Nelson EC, Roberts JS: Linking outcomes measurement to continual improvement: The Serial "V" way of thinking about improving clinical care. *Jt Comm J on Qual Improv* April 1994; 20(4)167–180.
14. Ware JE, Jr, Snow KK, Kosinski M, Gandek B: *The MOS SF-36 Health Survey and the MOS SF-12 Health Survey.* Boston, MA: The Health Institute, New England Medical Center, April 1995.
15. Coffey RJ, Richards JS, Remmert CS, LeRoy SS, Schoville RR, Baldwin PJ: An introduction to critical paths. *Quality Management in Health Care.* 1992; *1,* 45–54.
16. Zander K: Toward a fully-integrated CareMap (R) and case management system. *The New Definition,* 1993; 8(2):25–27.
17. Zander K: Focusing on patient outcome: case management in the 90's. *Dimension of Critical Care Nursing,* 1992; *11*(3), 127–129.

18. Zander K: Qualityfing, managing, and improving quality. Part I: How CareMaps™ link CQI to the patient. *The New Definition,* 1992; 7(2), 12–14.
19. Zander Z: CareMaps™: The core of cost/quality care. *The New Definition,* 1991; *6*(3), 5–7.
20. Zander K: Nursing case management: resolving the DRG paradox. *Nursing Clinics of North America,* 1988; *23*(3), 503–520.
21. Zander K: Nursing case management: Strategic management of cost and quality outcomes. *Journal of Nursing Administration,* 1988; *18*(5), 23–30.
22. Zander K: Second generation primary nursing: a new agenda. *Journal of Nursing Administration,* 1985; *15*(3), 18–24.
23. Zander K, Blaney C, Hayes J, et al: Nursing group practice: "The Cadillac" in continuity, 1988; *Definition, 3*(2), 29–31.
24. Zander K, McGill R: Critical and anticipated recovery paths: only the beginning. *Nursing Management* 1994; *25*(8), 34–37, 40.
25. Wennberg JE, Barry MJ, Fowlder FJ, Mulley A: Outcomes research, PORTs, and health care reform in doing more harm than good: the evaluation of health care interventions. *Ann N Y Acad Sci* December 1993; 703(31):52–62.
26. Camp RC: *Benchmarking: The search for best practices that lead to superior performance.* Milwaukee, WI: American Society for Quality Control, Quality Press, 1989.

Part 4. Concepts for Improving Any Clinical Process

"Until you can see a different reality, you are hard-pressed to do anything differently."

John Kelsch

The Context of Clinical Improvement

The outcomes of health care work are caused by processes and methods that interact in a specific place with the underlying biological, psychological, genetic, and social status needs of patients and their families. Understanding patient need → health care process → results as a linked graphical model can help us "see" relations between and among the elements of the model. When explicitly connected to this linked model, measurement can help describe, learn, and accelerate the job of designing and inventing better methods for delivering care. The approach to improvement presented in this four-part chapter invites participation in the application of these ideas and understandings.

Today's challenge is to make changes that will improve the value of clinical care—removing cost while adding quality. This must be done well, rapidly, and with some measurable confirmation of improvement. Clinicians, however, are acutely aware that they work in complex environments that often resist (and only rarely promote) efforts to change and improve. Consider the following case.

Dr. Emily Bohn, an orthopedic surgeon, has been invited to join a small group of people, from various disciplines, who are working to improve care for patients undergoing total hip replacement surgery. Mr. Ken Johnson, an orthopedic nurse, is the leader of the group. Following the method suggested by Argyris and Schön,[1] the conversation is mapped into two columns in Table 10–1. What was actually said is on the right side of Table 10–1. What Dr. Bohn was *thinking, but didn't say,* is on the left side and is written in italics.

This type of dialogue about designing and testing clinical changes probably never occurs in your setting, but you may have heard of this happening elsewhere. How might this conversation be different? How might health professionals working in clinical teams proactively consider making changes when they aren't busy "fixing a problem"? How can we **decrease the time** getting to good ideas for improving care? One promising method for streamlining the generation of "good ideas" is to formulate what are sometimes called *change concepts.* We discuss the notion of change concepts in the next section.

Change Concepts

The ability to design and rapidly test change is at the heart of a learning environment for work. But, a *new* design idea—with sufficient merit to be tested—is the output of a process for producing new, good, feasible ways of doing something. DeBono offers insight into the importance of identifying an underlying **concept** as a generator of ideas.[2] He suggests that if we understand the underlying concept on which a specific idea is based, then we can use that underlying concept as a cue to develop numerous ideas or options. Consider the following simple analogy:

Having a fun Saturday afternoon

Mandy and Zach have three or four hours of free time on a Saturday afternoon. They start to think about doing something for fun. The "main route" that they begin with is to think of something fun to do (route "X"). It's a fall weekend, and they quickly come up with several specific ideas for having fun:

A. Go to a college football game.

B. Ride mountain bikes to the copper mine and look at the fall foliage.

C. Go canoeing down the Connecticut River.

Zach quickly selects option "B"—mountain biking—since he has waited all week for a chance to try out his new bike. However, as they start to prepare for the mountain bike outing, Mandy discovers that her daughter, Phoebe, has borrowed her bike (without asking), and recalls that her last bike trip left her lame for several days. At this point, it might be prudent for Mandy and Zach to "pull back" to the underlying concept "X"—find something fun to do—and select an alternate path forward: "A"—the football game, "C"—canoeing, or even a new idea, "D"—apple picking at the nearby orchard.

TABLE 10–1. Dr. Bohn's Conversation Map

What Dr. Bohn thought, but did not say	*What was said*
This is my first meeting with this weird team that wants to fix up our hip replacement surgery. I wonder what they think the problem is.	Dr. Bohn: "What's the problem?"
Hmm. Johnson's answer wasn't what I expected. I think I'll just listen for a bit.	Mr. Johnson: "No problem."
Fuzz talk. I'm wondering if I'm about to be attacked. Could this be "code talk" about my surgical work? I wonder where in the heck they are coming from?	Mr. Johnson: "We're trying to improve our results by working on those processes that produce them."
Maybe they're talking about efficiency. I'm not against that.	Mr. Johnson: "The first thing our team tried was to consolidate the pre-op workup steps to make it easier for the patient, the doctor, and the hospital. It worked. Patients get less confused now. We just work with the office nurses to set it up."
It won't hurt to explore the issue a bit.	Mr. Johnson: "We'd like to turn our attention to the actual clinical care we give the patient and wanted your help." Dr. Bohn: "I'm not sure I understand what you are after, what do you expect of me?"
Where have these people been? I've let everyone around here know about my pet peeves and I've "carried on" about the 100's of ideas I have had.	Mr. Johnson: "What ideas do you have for improving the care of hip replacement patients?"
	Dr. Bohn: "Where have you been when I've made all my suggestions?"

DeBono illustrates the value of a generic concept ("X") and its relation to specific ideas ("A," "B," and "C") as indicated in Figure 10–22. This might be thought of as a path forward or a main route, "X," with three specific branches labeled "A," "B," and "C." A core concept labeled "X" in Figure 10–22 may lead to many ideas labeled "A," "B," and "C."

Both Figure 10–22 and the Zach and Mandy story illustrate a basic point about concepts. When traveling down a road or pursuing a chain of thought, a junction point comes and offers choices for different routes, or ideas. Once in pursuit of a specific idea, we tend to think in that "channel." It is often more helpful, however, to engage in what DeBono calls "lateral thinking" which is made easier if we "pull back" to the underlying concept, clarify what that underlying concept is by giving it a descriptive name, and find an alternate path forward.

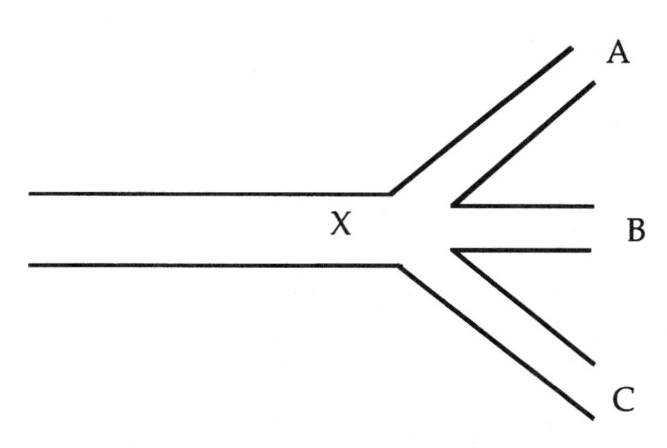

FIGURE 10–22. The change concept—idea relationship.

Langley, Nolan, et al. have incorporated DeBono's "concepts" into an approach for developing changes that lead to improvement.[3] They defined a "change concept" as a general notion or approach to change that has been found to be useful in developing specific ideas for changes that lead to improvement.

We believe that change concept thinking applies to health care. An application of change concept thinking might be seen in current efforts to reduce health care costs by discounting provider charges. In this situation, the underlying generic concept is "reducing health care costs," and the specific idea is "discounting provider charges." Short-term gains in health care cost reduction can occur by the vigorous pursuit of discounts. After some time, however, limits to discount-induced reduction in costs are experienced. Persevering and continuing to travel down the "discounting provider charges" path is less likely to produce further substantial improvement than returning to the basic concept of "reducing health care costs." Similar thinking opportunities present themselves when designing changes in clinical processes for the improvement of health care value.

Langley, Nolan, et al. have built extensively on DeBono's concept strategy and have identified 70 generic change concepts that can be applied to designing improvement across a wide spectrum of work settings, including health care.[3]

■ Using Change Concepts to Improve Clinical Care: The Hip Replacement Case

Imagine that you are working with an interdisciplinary team that aims to reduce costs while improving the quality of care for patients in need of hip joint replacement. Your team has used the Clinical Improvement Worksheet approach (described in previous parts)[4,5,6] and agreed on the following:

1. ***OUTCOMES:* Select a population.** The team's aims were specified with respect to achieving clinical, functional health status, satisfaction, and cost outcomes that are superior to current outcomes.
2. ***PROCESS:*Analyze the process.** The team analyzed the current delivery process that is producing current results by constructing a flowchart. This gave them a picture of the steps involved in providing joint replacement care. Figure 10–23 illustrates their high-level flowchart.

The team is now ready to tackle the third issue—ideas for making changes that will improve care:

3. ***CHANGES:* Generate change ideas.** "What ideas do we have for changing what's done (process) to get better results?"

While the team was constructing their flowchart, they developed several hunches about changes that they might make to improve care. For example, some of the team started aggressive physical therapy very early in the presurgical process to prepare the patient for surgery, while others waited until after the procedure had been done before initiating physical therapy. The team jotted down their ideas on a "potential changes" list, but, after they had finished their flowcharting, they wanted to think bigger and more creatively before selecting their first PDCA change cycle.

To make rapid headway on this critical third step on the Clinical Improvement Worksheet—"What ideas do we have for changing what's done (process) to get better results?"—the team worked through the following activities:

■ *First, each person silently wrote down their improvement ideas and pinpointed each idea on the flowchart that had been constructed in step 2. The ideas for improvement came from many sources: personal experience, professional knowledge, direct observation, literature review, and clinical benchmarking.*

■ *Second, the team created a simple matrix listing specific ideas in the right column, then moved back to the underlying change concept listed in the left column. Table 10–2 is an example of what one team member's list looked like.*

■ *Third, these specific ideas and the underlying change concepts were discussed by pairs of team members to clarify thinking and prompt even more ideas for improvement. This was done by using the generic change concepts as the generator of additional ideas that might be used in other parts of the delivery process—either upstream or downstream from the original, specific location on the flowchart.*

■ *Fourth, the team generated both a master list and a long list of ideas by putting all of them into an "idea pool." The idea pool was discussed and generated much excitement; people came to believe that what was currently going on was no longer an option and they now had some concrete ideas to test in the days ahead. (Notice that the team started with a specific idea, then "moved back" to identify the underlying change concept, and finally used their insight to generate many more ideas, now that they were aware of the generic concept of change. Another approach that could have been used after becoming comfortable with the use of generic change concepts, was to* ***start*** *with some generic change concepts that have widespread applicability, and use them to generate ideas for testing change.)*

■ *Fifth, as a homework assignment, two people volunteered to take the top 10 ranked ideas for change—those voted most powerful/feasible by the team—and display them on a high-level flowchart of their joint replacement care process. This was done to help all the team visualize where they might exert greatest leverage, and where they might run specific pilot tests to evaluate the impact of their change on outcomes and costs.*

Figure 10–24—the ten concepts for changing any process—illustrates the results from this last activity and offers another way of thinking about the practical things that can be done to design change in a clinical process. This figure represents a generic clinical process consisting of several steps; imagine it to be a somewhat stylized, high-level flowchart of hip replacement care. Generic change concepts and specific improvement ideas for changing the inputs, action steps in the process, outcomes, or the entire process are superimposed on the core clinical process. These generic change concepts have been used repeatedly as people have redesigned work and clinical care. Using them can help save time in generating many powerful ideas for improving care. As an example, each change concept listed below, and referred to in Figure 10–24, is related to a specific idea for improving the value of hip joint replacement.

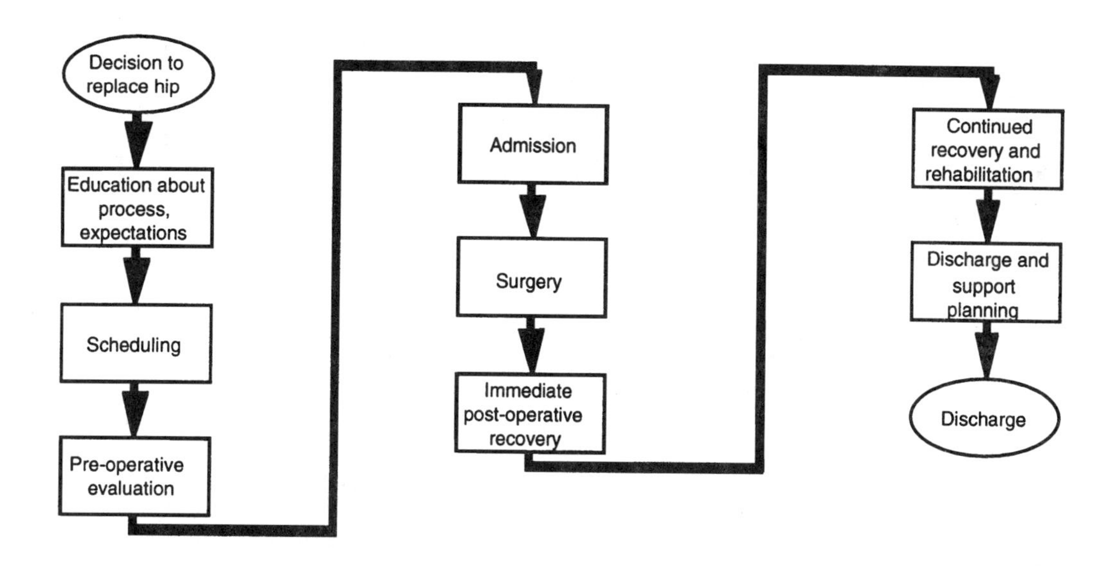

FIGURE 10–23. High-level flowchart of a hip replacement process.

TABLE 10–2. A Matrix of Specific Change Ideas and the Underlying Change Concepts for a Member of the Hip Replacement Care Team

The underlying, generic change concepts are . . .	*My specific ideas are . . .*
1. Modify input	Let's start a physical conditioning program in advance of surgery to make our patients "fit" for surgical procedure and thereby reduce risk and speed up recovery.
2. Combine steps	Let's bring together the pre-op workup and the basic label work and make one step out of two, as we currently do it.
3. Replace a step with a better value alternative	We could save money by standardizing our decision making about which prosthesis to use and always selecting the lowest cost, clinically appropriate one.

Concept #1. Modify input. Increase the ability of the patient to successfully withstand the intervention and recover more quickly by operating on "fit" patients.

Concept #2. Combine steps. Decrease the work and waste associated with doing things as multiple steps by combining the steps into a single step, such as combining the preoperative laboratory work and preoperative evaluation.

Concept #3. Eliminate failures at hand-offs between steps. By making the egress from one step become the explicit ingress to the next, the "coupling" of steps can occur with less errors, such as redesigning the format of the discharge planning forms and the orders for admission to home health and follow-up physical therapy care.

Concept #4. Eliminate a step. Stop doing things that do not add significant value to the desired result, such as eliminating epidural pain control and covering the need by extending the use of the other analgesics.

Concept #5. Reorder the sequence of steps. By placing a later step in an earlier position in the process, achieve a smoother overall flow of the care, such as having the physical therapist teach patients to manage their own post-op rehabilitation care before admission—when they are alert and ready to learn.

Concept #6. Change an element in the process by creating an arrangement with another party (customer, supplier, other) to change the concept of the process. By combining a step with something extrinsic to the current process, it is possible to create a new possibility

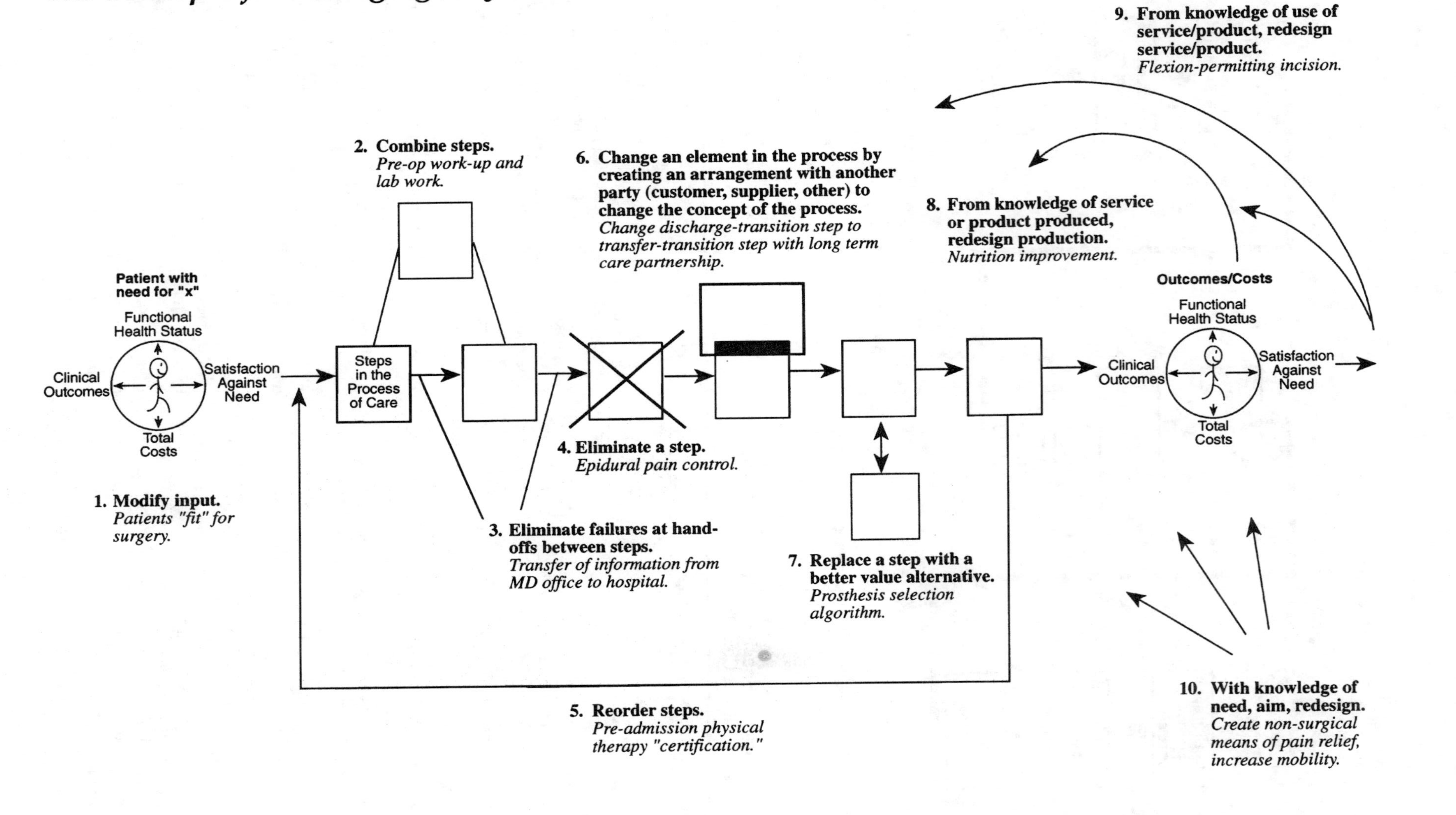

FIGURE 10–24. Ten concepts for changing any process applied to a hip replacement case.

altogether, such as combining discharge with admission to a transition care setting, thus making the discharge step into a transfer step and the entire process into one of hip replacement and rehabilitation.

Concept #7. Replace a step with a better value alternative. Identify a better method or technology to perform a given step, such as the use of a decision algorithm for prosthesis selection that results in a recommendation for the lowest cost, clinically appropriate device.

Concept #8. From knowledge of service or product that is produced, redesign production. Redesign the process once the full nature of the result and its possible contributors are known, such as creating optimal nutritional status prior to surgery after recognizing the value of good nutritional status for prompt healing,

Concept #9. From knowledge of use of service/product, redesign service/product. Knowing the next uses of the end result of the process allows consideration of further process changes such as the creation of a flexion-permitting incision for the joint replacement after recognizing the need for early ambulation,

Concept #10. With knowledge of need and aim, redesign. If the need is clearly known, entirely different services can be considered and designed, such as when the need for pain relief is clarified as the purpose of the intervention, alternative approaches to achieve that aim, with or without the intervening surgery could be developed.

When the joint replacement team reviewed their work (see Figure 10–24), they realized that they had achieved several important benefits. They had:

- *Built up a "savings account" of great ideas that could be used to run a series of small tests of change—PDCA Cycle 1, PDCA Cycle 2, etc.*
- *Linked their understanding of current process with very specific ideas for improving discrete elements within the process—incremental first order change—and for redesigning the entire process—innovation, second order change.*
- *Discovered 10 different generic clinical change concepts that could be applied more thoroughly to joint replacement care and could also be transferred to other clinical conditions—the team speculated that using these generic change concepts early in the improvement process might generate ideas even more quickly if they started directly with these concepts and worked to connect them to the clinical process at hand.*

They believed that, by deepening their understanding of "change concepts," they could accelerate wise improvement attempts and supercharge the impact. The team quickly proceeded to step four on the Clinical Improvement Worksheet to select their first test of change.

4. *PILOT:* Select a change for pilot testing

To select their first pilot test, the team first reviewed the 10 change ideas listed in Figure 10–24 and then asked themselves, "Where is the leverage for change?" What changes will have the largest effect on patient safety? Resource use? Undependability? Other subprocesses (influence or ripple effects on the whole collection of interlinked subprocesses)? Next, the team reminded themselves to think about the ramp of complexity[7] and to answer this query: "What's the largest, feasible change that we can test, that we predict will lead to improvement, **and** that we can test by a near certain date?"

In light of all the above, the team elected to combine 3 ideas into a pilot test: (1) patient fit for surgery, (2) prosthesis selection algorithm, and (3) nutrition improvement. The team chose to defer the remaining 7 improvement ideas until they were ready to run their next change cycle.

Comments and Conclusions

To survive, health care systems must be able to improve. Learning about making change, encouraging change, managing the change within and across organizations, and learning from the changes tested will characterize the sustainable, thriving health systems of the future. Setting goals were once enough, but it's clear that goals must be coupled with the *concepts and specific methods* to produce sustainable change. This chapter of papers suggests an approach to the design and testing of change in the clinical care of patients. This approach is based on the following "fundamentals":

- ***Aim for Better Value:*** *Common aim for the improvement of health and the reduction of the burden of illness in people's lives—including excess mortality, morbidity, dissatisfaction, cost, and suboptimal functioning in daily life.*[8]
- ***Systems Thinking:*** *An understanding of the overall system of care within which the desire for change may arise.*[9]
- ***Cultural Mindedness:*** *An awareness of the habits, traditions, policies, and values that promote or impede taking the risk of introducing change;*
- ***Change Management:*** *A grasp of the tension and pressure needed to promote change, the creation of a customized and locally sensible, actionable alternative to the status quo, the skills and knowledge necessary to execute the change and the social support required for sustaining the change efforts.*[10]
- ***Clinical Improvement Model:*** *An understanding of a flexible, basic format (the Clinical Improvement Worksheet*

and the PDCA cycle) for thinking about outcomes/costs, the underlying process, designing new processes, and testing changes.[11,12]

The approach suggested in this four-part chapter is intended to be illustrative of a path forward. It is emphatically *not* a definitive or exhaustive exposition of all the possible ways to improve the quality and value of patient care. We would appreciate hearing from you as you experiment with these methods and discover new ways to accelerate the improvement and innovation of high-value health care in your setting.

Reprints: Address reprint requests to Dr. Batalden, Lahey Hitchcock Clinic, One Medical Center Drive, Lebanon, NH 03756-0001.

ACKNOWLEDGMENTS

The authors wish to acknowledge their intellectual debt and encouragement of their friend and colleague, Tom Nolan, Ph.D., who has championed the use of powerful, elegant, simple, and linked methods for testing change—such as the use of change concepts linked to the design and testing of rapid pilots of change.

REFERENCES: PART 4

1. Argyris C, Schön D: *Theory in practice.* San Francisco, CA: Jossey-Bass, 1974.
2. DeBono E: *Serious creativity.* New York: HarperCollins Publishers, 1992.
3. Langley GJ, Nolan KM, Nolan TW, Norman CL, Provost LP: *The improvement guide—A practical approach to enhancing organizational performance.* San Francisco: Jossey-Bass, 1996.
4. Nelson EC, Mohr JJ, Batalden PB, Plume SK: Improving health care: Part 1: The clinical value compass. *Jt Comm J on Qual Improv* April 1996; 22(4):243–258.
5. Nelson EC, Batalden PB, Plume SK, Mohr JJ: Improving health care: Part 2. A clinical improvement worksheet and users manual. *Jt Comm J on Qual Improv,* August 1996.
6. Mohr JJ, Mahoney CC, Nelson EC, Batalden PB, Plume SK: Improving health care: Part 3. Clinical benchmarking for best patient care. *Jt Comm J on Qual Improv,* September 1996.
7. Langley GJ, Nolan KM, Nolan TW: The foundation of improvement, *Quality Press* June 1994; 27(6):81–86.
8. Gustafson DH, Peterson Helstad C, Hung CF, Nelson G, Batalden PB: the total cost of illness: A metric for health care reform. *Hospital & Health Services Administration* Spring 1995; 154–171.
9. Batalden PB, Stoltz PK: A framework for the continual improvement of health care: Building and applying professional and improvement knowledge to test changes in daily work. *Jt Comm J on Qual Improv* October 1993; 19(10):424–447.
10. Gustafson DH, Cats-Baril W, Alemi F: *Systems to support health policy analysis.* Ann Arbor, MI: Health Admin Press, Chapter 2, pp 43–50, 1993.
11. Moen RD, Nolan TW: Process improvement. *Quality Progress* pp 63–68, September 1987.
12. Batalden PB, Nelson EC, Roberts JS: Linking outcomes measurement to continual improvement: The Serial "V" way of thinking about improving clinical care. *Jt Comm J on Qual Improv* April 1994; 20(4):167–180.

Paul B. Batalden, M.D., is board certified by the American Board of Pediatrics. He is Director, Healthcare Improvement Leadership Development, Center for Evaluative Clinical Sciences, Dartmouth Medical School. He is a charter member and Chairman of the Board of the Institute for Healthcare Improvement. Dr. Batalden is the Ernest Breech Chairman, Department of Health Care Quality Improvement Education and Research, Henry Ford Health Services Center, Detroit, Michigan. He serves on the Board of Directors for Allina Health System, Minneapolis, Minnesota. He is the author of numerous book chapters and scientific articles on quality, and co-authored *Quality Assurance in Ambulatory Care,* (1980), and a videotape with W. Edwards Deming, *A New Way of Thinking for Health Care* (1994). Dr. Batalden's research interests include: systems for managing the improvement of health and value of health care for a panel of patients' systems for assessing the burden of illness in a defined population; and systems for assessing the degree to which health care workers can learn their work setting.

Christina C. Mahoney, R.N., M.S.N., is Clinical Nurse Specialist, Surgical Specialties Unit, Dartmouth-Hitchcock Medical Center, Lebanon, NH. Christina has her Bachelor of Arts degree from Vassar (1982) and her Master's of Science in nursing from MGH Institute of Health Professions (1992).

Julie J. Mohr, M.S.P.H., is Research Associate, Health Care Improvement Leadership Development, The Center for Evaluative Clinical Sciences, Dartmouth Medical School. Julie has a bachelor of arts in economics and industrial relations (1987) and a Master's of Science in Public Health from the University of North Carolina at Chapel Hill, (1993).

Eugene C. Nelson joined the Dartmouth-Hitchcock Medical Center, Lebanon, New Hampshire, in August 1992 as the Director of Quality Education, Measurement and Research for the Office of the President, Lahey Hitchcock Clinic. In September 1992, he was appointed Professor of Community and Family Medicine at the Dartmouth Medical School in Hanover, New Hampshire.

From 1987 to 1992, Nelson was the Director of Quality Care Research at the Hospital Corporation of America in Nashville, Tennessee. He led the design of HCA's systems for obtaining consistent feedback from its customers (patients), physicians, employees, and the community. He designed new quality measurement systems for specific types of patients (e.g., myocardial infarction), major payers, and automated the "anytime, anyplace" analysis of quality surveys.

From 1986 to 1987, Nelson served as Associate Professor and Vice Chairman of Community Medicine at Dartmouth Medical School's Department of Community and Family Medicine in Hanover, New Hampshire. He was also executive director of the Dartmouth Institute for Better Health and director of the Dartmouth Cooperative Information project, a regional medical practice research network.

Nelson serves on the Steering Committee of the Medical Outcomes Study, and on the Board of Directors for the Institute for Healthcare Improvement. He is a member of the Editorial Review Board for *Quality Management in Healthcare* (*QMHC*), and is a consultant to organizations such as the American College of Physicians, the Midwest Business Group on Health, RAND Corporation, and the World Organization of National Colleges of General and Family Practitioners. He has authored over 50 publications. Nelson received his bachelor of arts degree in sociology from Dartmouth College, his masters in public health related to medical care planning and administration from Yale Medical School, and a doctorate in health services administration from the Harvard School of Public Health.

Stephen K. Plume is President of Lahey Hitchcock Clinic, an 830-physician group practice system serving residents of New Hampshire, Vermont, and Massachusetts. Plume, a cardiothoracic surgeon, Professor of Surgery, Dartmouth Medical School, joined The Hitchcock Clinic in 1977. He served as Chief of Cardiothoracic Surgery for twelve years before assuming his responsibilities as President of the Hitchcock Clinic in 1990. His long-standing interest in systems of care and an increasing awareness of outcomes research led to the founding, with Gerald O'Connor, of the Northern New England Cardiovascular Disease Study Group. This group has embarked on a multicenter, multidisciplinary effort to understand and reduce variation in health care practices and outcomes.

Plume has served as consultant to institutions interested in bringing a continuous quality improvement approach to their cardiac surgery services and to others wishing to understand alternatives in the organization of academic group practices.

A 1964 graduate of Harvard College, Plume received an M.D. from the University of Rochester in 1969, where he completed a residency in Surgery in 1975. He was then a Fellow in Cardiovascular and Thoracic Surgery at the University of Toronto for two years before joining the Hitchcock Clinic.

11

Project Solo/Physicians' Information Exchange: Organizing Physicians Around Quality

STEVEN F. ISENBERG

Project Solo (PS) was founded in 1994 as a grassroots organization of independent physicians united for quality, autonomy, patient advocacy, and cost containment. It utilizes a benchmarked, confidential patient satisfaction measurement process to assess the perception of quality from the patients' viewpoint. Physicians, assured of confidentiality and confident in PS's peer supervision, share information with each other and compare their overall percentage of excellent responses within the group and with national data. This focus on perceived quality allows patients to anonymously inform physicians about their perceptions. Project Solo's Confidential Self Assessment of Quality allows physicians to assess these perceptions, benchmark these perceptions against their peers, and initiate quality improvement in a nonpunitive, continuous quality improvement technique.

Organizing physicians from different specialties with diverse socioeconomic and demographic backgrounds is a challenge. Project Solo approached the problem by focusing on the following strategic points:

- Explaining why it is important, proving it, and implementing it.
- Organizing around a central vision and mission.
- Keeping it simple.
- Keeping it confidential.
- Using peer development and direction.
- Producing results.

Explaining Why It Is Important, Proving It, and Implementing It

Explaining the importance of perceived quality to physicians requires an organized presentation from a peer. This is accomplished utilizing a three-step process:

Step 1. Physicians are initially presented with their position as perceived by consumers in the health care marketplace. An example is the sequential presentation of graphics demonstrating that physicians receive $0.19 of the healthcare dollar[1] (Fig 11–1) This is followed by a graphic demonstrating the large increase in administrative personnel compared to physicians and nurses (Figs.11–2, 11–3).[2,3] Of the one trillion dollar annual health bill, 1500 private insurers kept about $50 billion of the $300 billion in insurance premiums.[4] Another $200 billion can be attributed to substance abuse and addiction; $20 billion to violence; $50 billion to smoking and $68 billion to teen pregnancy.[5] The physician audience is then asked: Who's Responsible? (Fig. 11–4) At this point, physicians are shown a 1993 *Los Angeles Times* survey demonstrating that the majority of people feel that physicians are responsible for rising health care costs. (Fig. 11–5)[6] Data is then presented that demonstrates how highly patients value physicians choice (Fig. 11–6),[7], how vulnerable they feel on the quality issue as it

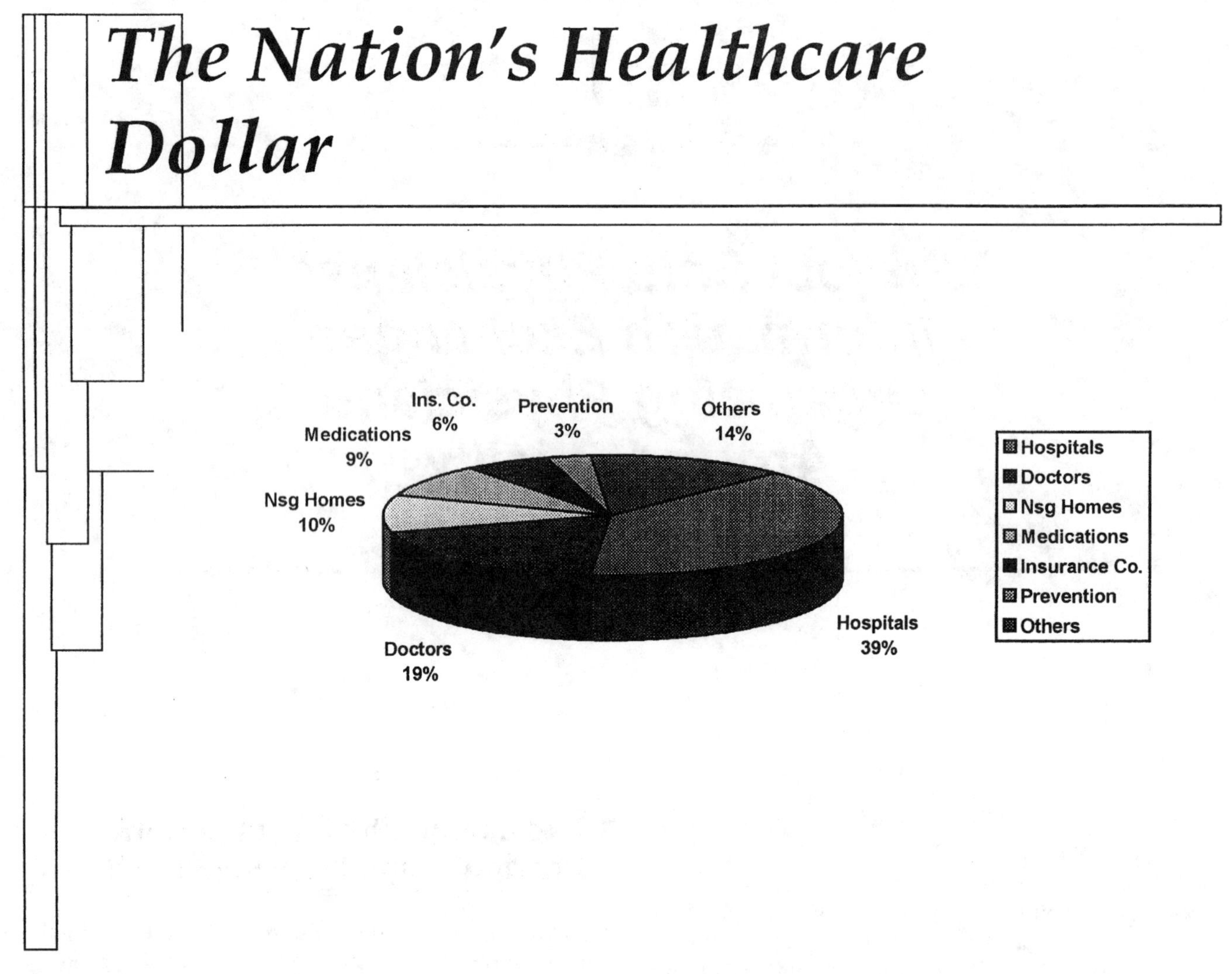

The Nation's Healthcare Dollar
Ins. Co.
6%
Prevention
3%
Others
14%
Medications
9%
Nsg Homes
10%
Doctors
19%
Hospitals
39%
Hospitals
Doctors
Nsg Homes
Medications
Insurance Co.
Prevention
Others

FIGURE 11–1.

BETWEEN 1968 - 1993

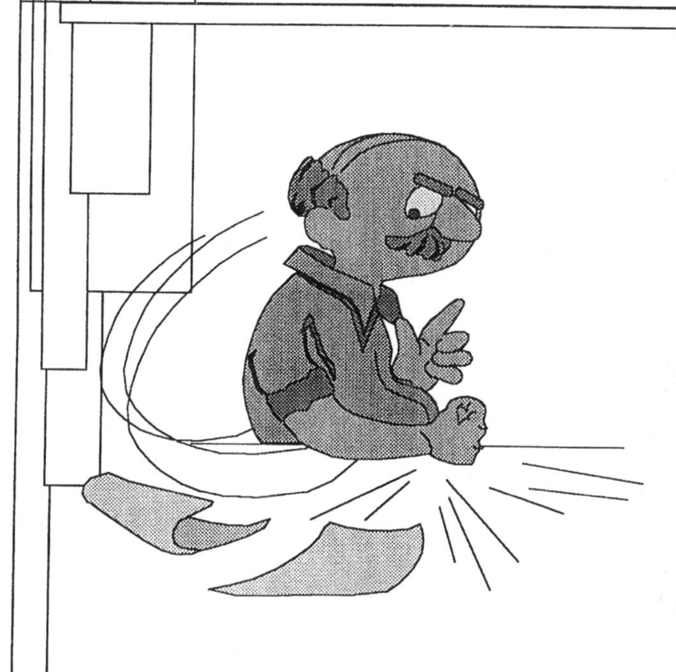

- The numbers of administrators 693%

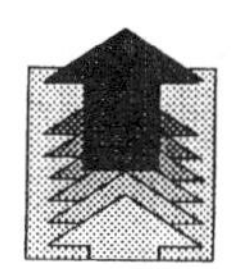

- The number of doctors 77%

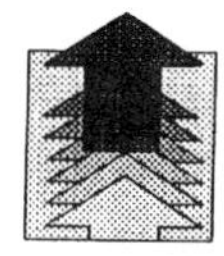

- The number of nurses 164%

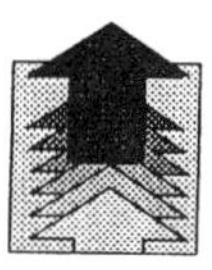

FIGURE 11–2.

HOSPITALS

1968

- *435,100 MANAGERS OVERSAW 1,378,000 PATIENTS*

1990

- *1,221,600 (3x) OVERSAW 853,000 PATIENTS (38%)*

FIGURE 11–3.

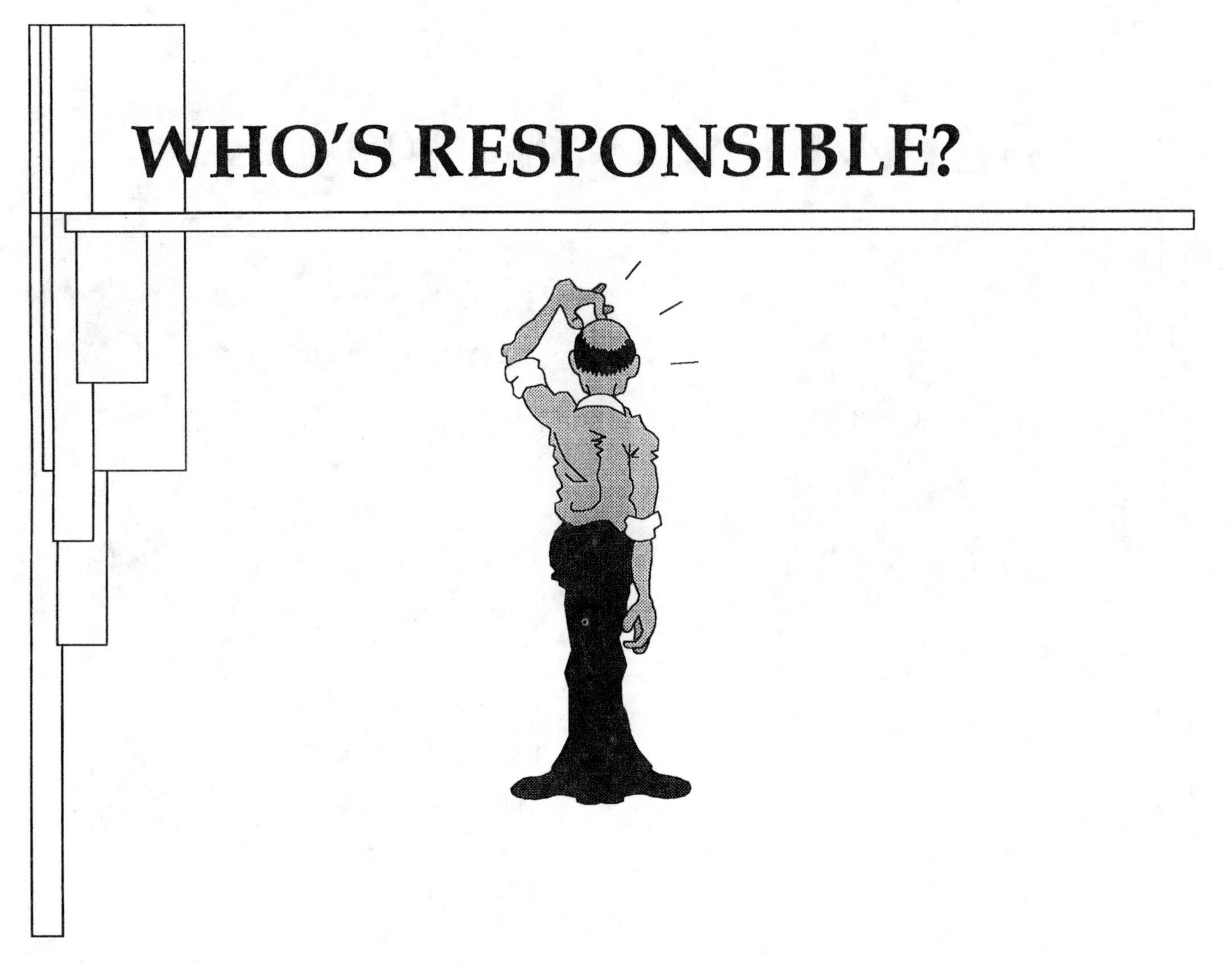

FIGURE 11–4.

OUTMARKETED!

1,500 ADULTS SURVEYED : Who is responsible for rising healthcare costs?

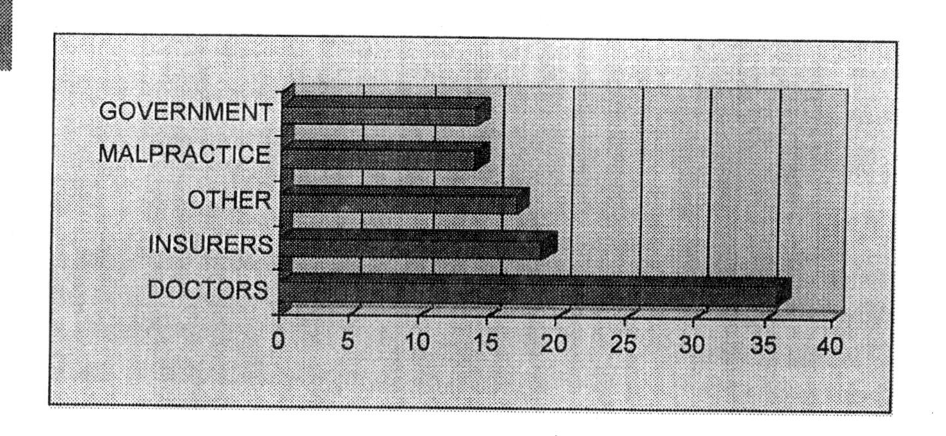

FIGURE 11–5.

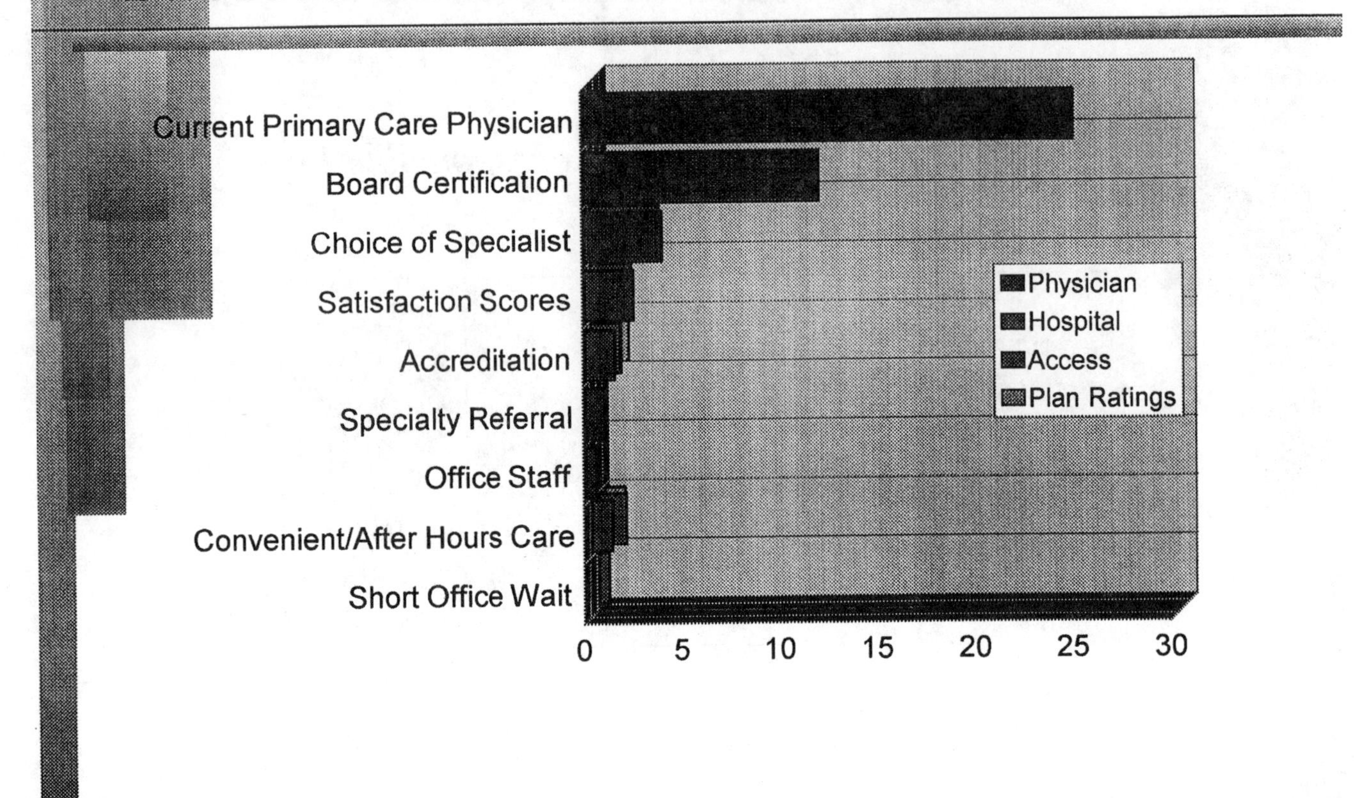

FIGURE 11–6.

PATIENT SATISFACTION

With Quality

	very satisfied	very dissatisfied
FFS	97%	4%
PPO	93%	6%
HMO	87%	14%

With Cost

FFS	67%	32%
PPO	73%	27%
HMO	81%	18%

FIGURE 11–7.

WHY DO PATIENTS FIRE THEIR DOCTORS?

- No Bedside Manners
- Vague and Evasive
- Never on Schedule
- No diagnosis given
- Does not respect confidentiality
- Does not "listen" to what I say
- Unpleasant office staff

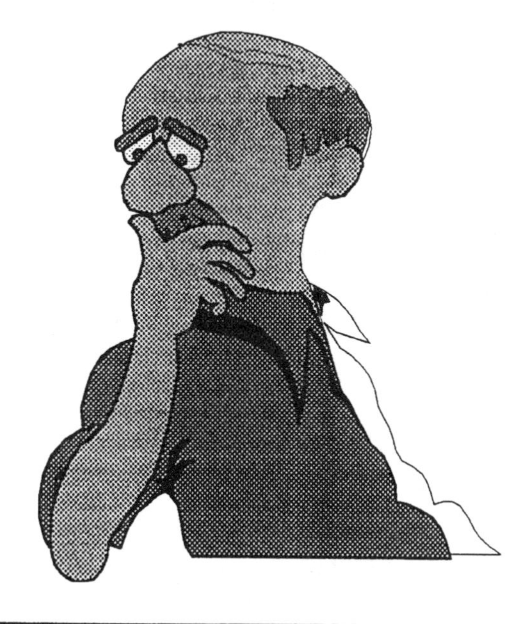

Source: American Academy of Family Physicians, 1987.

FIGURE 11–8.

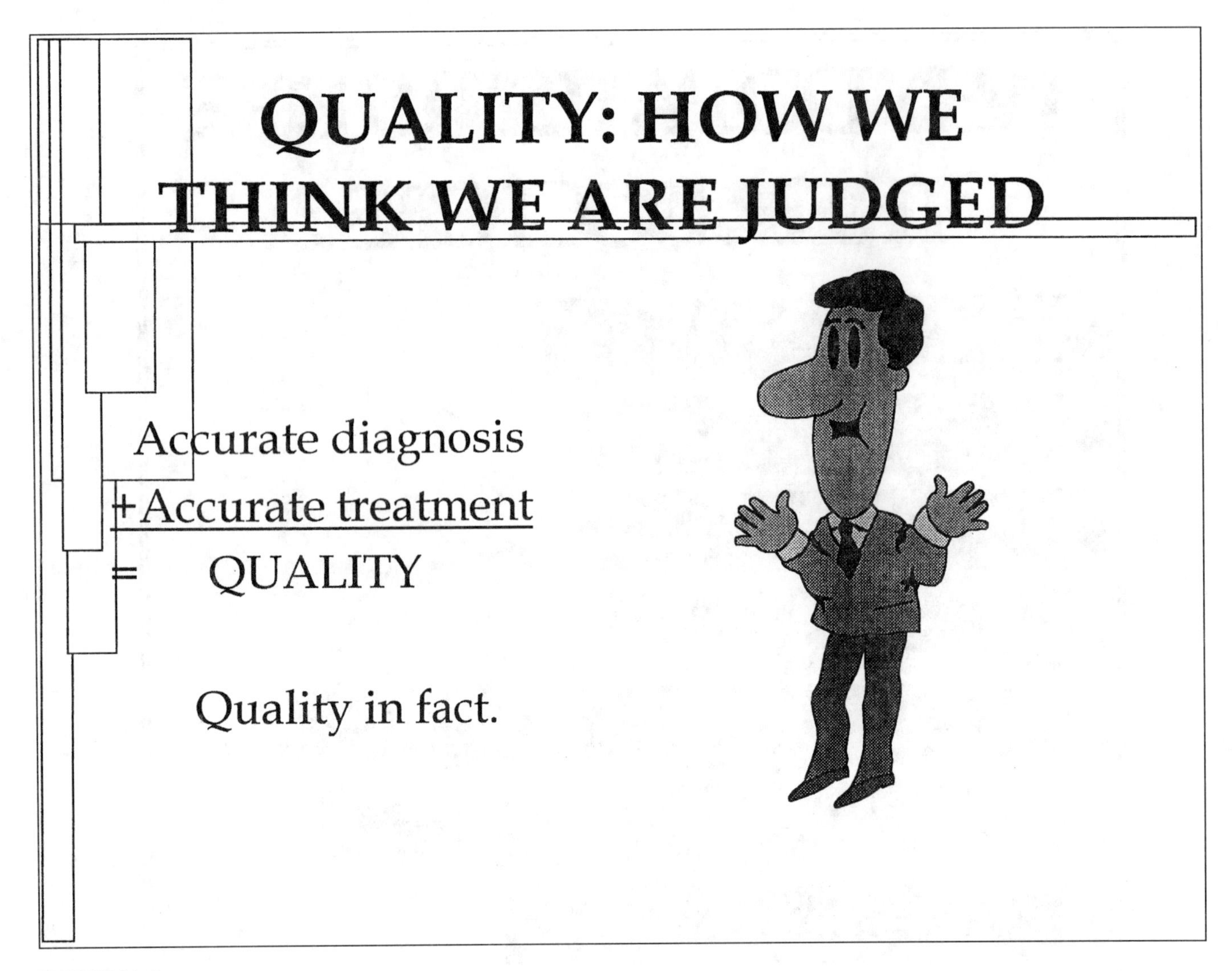

FIGURE 11–9.

relates to managed care (Fig. 11–7),[8] and exactly how important perceived quality is to patients when they consider firing their doctor (Fig. 11–8).[9] It is demonstrated that patients fire their doctors primarily because of problems with quality as perceived by the patients (quality in perception), *not* because of quality in fact (Figs. 11–9, 11–10). Physicians are encouraged to regain control of healthcare through joint data collection emphasizing quality (Figs. 11–11, 11–12).

Step 2. Physicians, now open to the discussion that problems with patient perceived quality might result in loss of patients, and become receptive to the theory that improved patient perceived quality has personal, professional, and marketing potential. As physicians, however, they still must be convinced of the scientific basis for the interpretation of perceived quality as a measure of overall quality of care. This is reinforced with scientific documentation that in the last 20 years research has demonstrated that patient judgments of their medical care can be measured reliably and accurately.[10–14] In addition, standard reports of quality or quality report cards are prepared on a regular basis by many health care plans.[15,16] It is further emphasized that since measuring patient satisfaction is generally easier than performing other outcomes measurements, patient satisfaction has assured a dominant role in quality measurement. Additional importance is emphasized with the prominent role that patient (customer) satisfaction plays in continuous quality improvement and total quality management.

Step 3. Physicians, now convinced of the importance of continuously measuring customer satis-faction, must be directed into an effective implementation of the process. The credibility of peer presentation is amplified again in this instance. Some of the mechanics of implementing the process in a busy practice are outlined and scientific methods of surveying, as presented by the Health Services Resource Group, are provided:

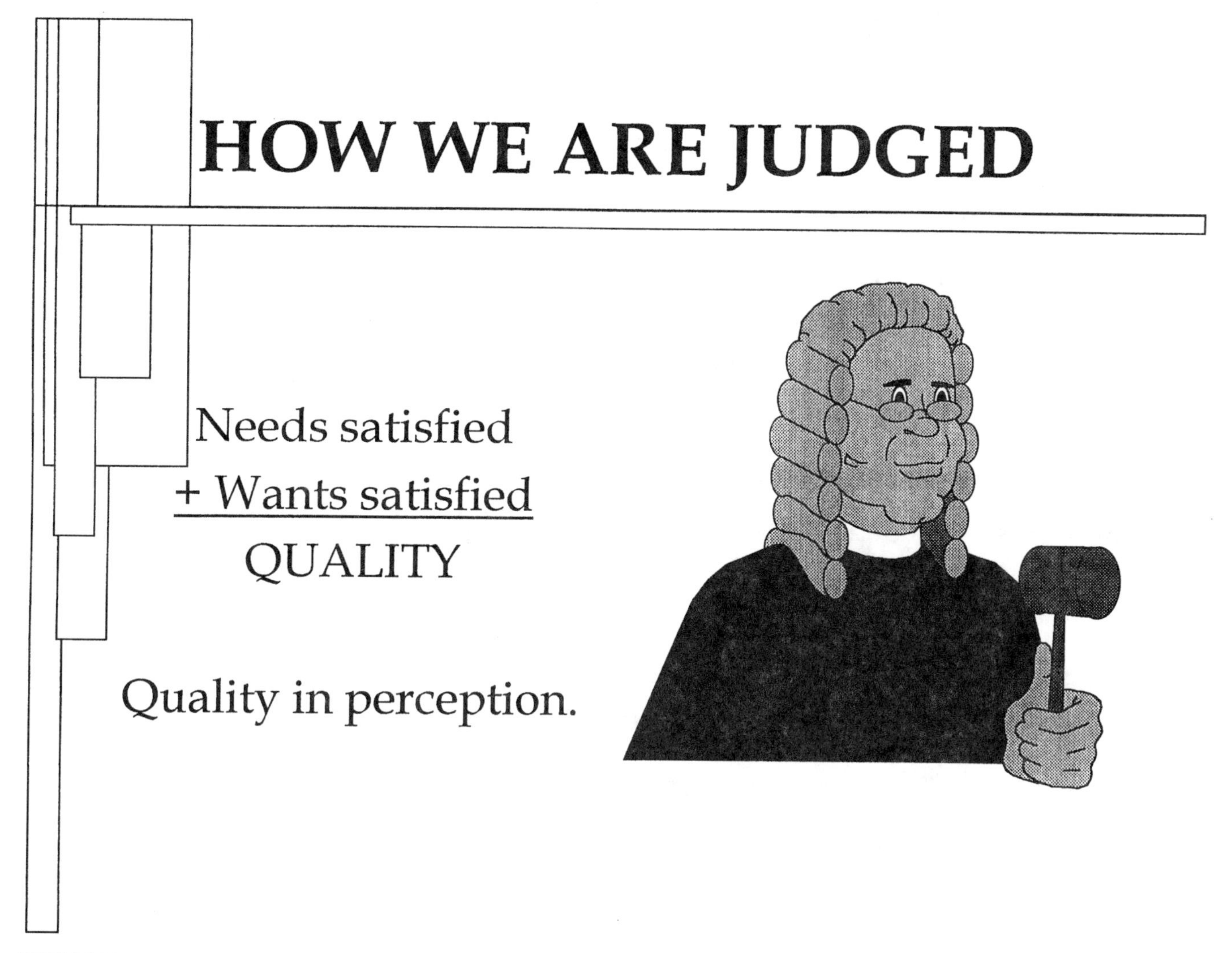

FIGURE 11–10.

- Surveyed patients should be informed why their opinion is of interest, how they were chosen, how the information will be used, the procedure that will be followed, and an assurance of anonymity.
- The surveyed patients should be assured that there are no wrong answers, their doctor will not know their individual ratings, and that the purpose of the study is not to evaluate the providers but improve services.
- Patients should be given the surveys and complete them on site. Project Solo's protocol is introduced: the surveys are deposited in a sealed, confidential box, mailed to the database, opened, and compiled at the database. This is justified based on the research that mailed surveys have low rates of response (30%) and are biased positively.[17]
- PS's method of surveying focuses on new patients or those completing a course of therapy. This is justified based on the theory that demonstrates that patients who stay in a practice generally already have a higher level of satisfaction. In addition, surveying new patients focuses on continuous quality improvement.
- Physicians are informed of the importance of implementing a benchmarked surveying process so that they can accurately compare their data. For this reason, the 9-item Visit Rating Questionnaire is utilized. (Fig.11–13).[18]

Organize Around a Central Vision and Mission

Quality Is the Focus

The ageless value of the patient–physician relationship is the foundation upon which patient-perceived quality displays its importance. Physicians are provided adequate proof that patients still value the patient-physician

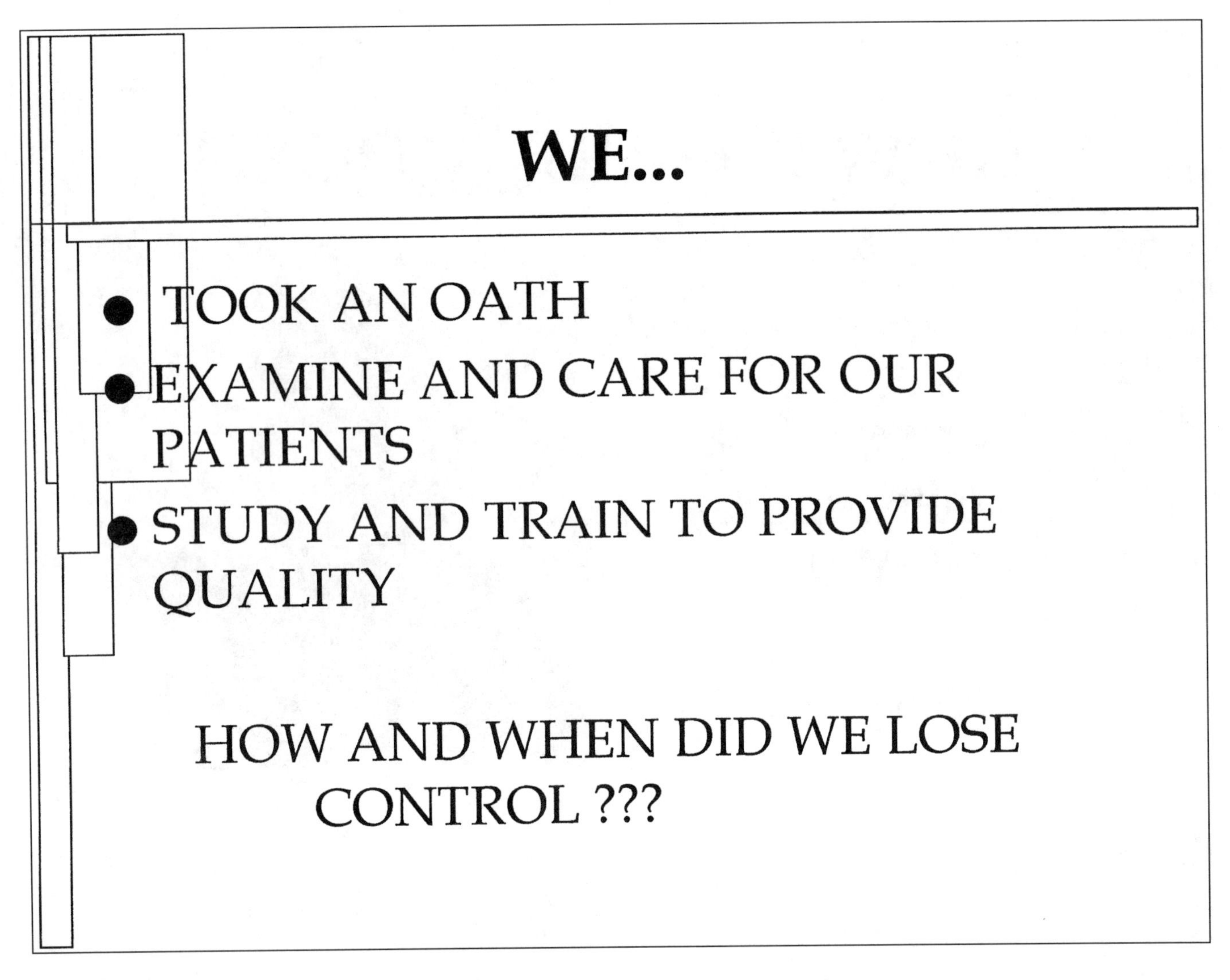

FIGURE 11–11.

relationship (Fig. 11–6) and remain unsure about quality guarantees from third parties (Fig. 11–7). As a result, physicians efforts at *quality insurance* provide the opportunity for physicians to ensure a dominant role in health care management.

■ Keeping It Simple

The implementation process described above is focused on simplicity. Processes are field tested in busy community-based practices and finalized after extensive review by practicing physicians and office personnel. Continuous quality improvement in the medical office requires physician leadership. This is why the physician must be convinced of the importance of patient perceived quality. The three basic parts of Total Quality Management (TQM) are illustrated with the emphasis on listening to the voice of the consumer. The second part of management by data is emphasized to encourage physicians to measure and compare their patient perceived quality of care (Fig. 11–14).

■ Keeping It Confidential

In 1996, PS received an Honorable Mention PINNACLE Award sponsored by the American College of Physician Executives. Confidential Self Assessment of Quality (CSAQ), described as a Model for Medical Management, provides a method for the individual physician to confidentially identify his or her individual performance relative to the group. It therefore encourages confidential self-directed quality assurance. As a part of PS's program, when patient results have been compiled for return to the physician, information is also provided about suggested methods of improvement. These methods are those already used effectively by managers, as well as those meth-

- They have it and we don't.
- The Science of Medicine will be controlled by those who capture and analyze data, such as outcomes.

SUMMARY:

Our Best Ally: Our Patients
Our Best Method: Quality

FIGURE 11–12.

ods obtained from suggestions confidentially provided by exemplary performers within PS. Confidential Self Assessment of Quality, therefore, links the two integrally related modalities of quality assurance and continuous quality improvement. It permits quality assurance without defensive posturing, and continuous quality improvement with standard methods of quality improvement and new input from the group itself. As an additional benefit, confidential self-assessment of quality facilitates the collection of "unbiased" data. Because each physician is assured anonymity, there is less temptation to send biased data, which could be a temptation to participants not assured of confidentiality.[19]

Peer Development and Direction

A key to physician participation is peer development and direction. Project Solo was developed by me in 1994. I have been in solo practice since 1979 as an otolaryngologist (ear, nose, and throat physician). I am very careful to identify my similarities, as well as my differences, to the audience of physicians who are usually composed of diverse demographics. While I am a specialist in solo practice, the central focus of information sharing for the purpose of measuring and improving patient perceived quality serves the needs of all practicing physicians. As a result, PS continues to grow with representation from all 50 states, several foreign countries, nearly every specialty, and a wide variety of practice styles. In 1996, PS initiated Physicians' Information Exchange (PIE); PIE continues the PS methodology of measuring patient perceived quality utilizing the 9-item Visit Rating Questionnaire. In addition, PIE offers physicians the opportunity to benchmark practice management data with each other through a process termed DOCSHARE. Figure 11–15 illustrates a portion of the response obtained within 48 hours when members of PIE were surveyed and asked 5 questions:

- Percentage of managed care in the practice.
- Number of employees in the practice.
- Number of patients seen per week.
- Type of software utilized by the practice
- Percentage overhead in the practice.

Benchmarking practice management parameters is an important part of total quality management. As membership in PIE grows, physicians' chances of achieving a demographic match increase. PIE, funded currently by research and corporate grants, currently requires only that physicians complete a membership application (Fig. 11–16). Physicians from all practice styles and specialties continue to join.

Producing Results

Physicians are historically and justifiably suspicious of new ideas. While it is difficult to prove, this probably reflects the beneficial reluctance of physicians to accept new ideas that are not substantially scientifically based. With this in mind, I set out to scientifically and methodically create a method that would produce meaningful results. In November 1996, the *American Journal of Medical Quality* published *Project Solo: An Independent Practitioner's Initiative for Confidential Self Assessment of Quality*. The case editor noted: "The case featured in this issue is presented for its notable educational value. It demonstrates a laudable effort by a group of independent practitioners to fulfill their role as patient advocates—by gathering, analyzing, and confidentially sharing data on patent satisfaction, with the goal of improving quality of care. The case also has merit in that it provides data from the *perspective of the patient*. . . . The reader is encouraged to note the potential of the model for future research and development in the field of quality assurance."

Project Solo's research efforts have provided helpful data about the idiosyncrasies of community-based

Satisfaction Survey

For Office Use Only

Date: | || | | || |

Month Day

Location: | || |

Please fill this out, fold it, and return it to the special mailbox in your physician's office. Thank you.

Please consider your visit to the doctor and answer the following questions by circling the number in each line.

	Poor	Fair	Good	Very Good	Excellent
1) How long you waited to get an appointment	1	2	3	4	5
2) Convenience of the location of the office	1	2	3	4	5
3) Getting through to our office by phone	1	2	3	4	5
4) Length of time waiting at the office	1	2	3	4	5
5) Time spent with the person you saw	1	2	3	4	5
6) Explanation of what was done for you	1	2	3	4	5
7) The technical skills (thoroughness, carefulness, competence) of the person you saw	1	2	3	4	5
8) The personal manner (courtesy, respect, sensitivity, friendliness) of the person you saw	1	2	3	4	5
9) The visit overall	1	2	3	4	5
10) In general, would you say your health is	1	2	3	4	5

11) Are you (patient) male or female? Male Female

12) How old were you (patient) on your last birthday? (write in) | || | years

Comments:

Adapted with the permission of the American Association of Health Plans

FIGURE 11–13.

TOTAL QUALITY MANAGEMENT (TQM)

- Listening to the voice of the consumer
- Management by data
- Analysis of the process of care

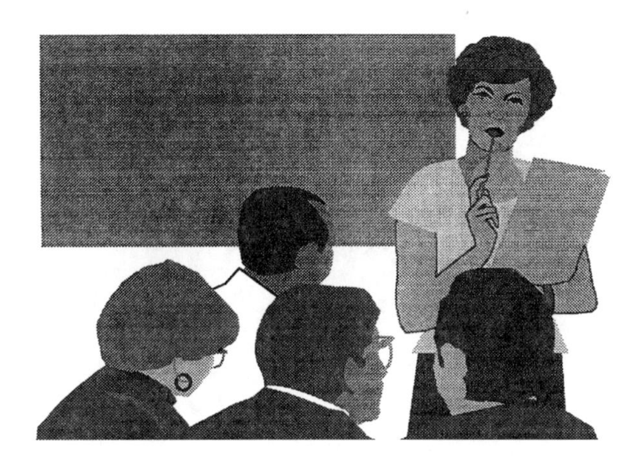

FIGURE 11–14.

Project Solo 5 ?'s
June 1996

Managed Care %	Employees Full/part time	# Patients per week	Software	Barcode #
95%	9/1	120	Med One	10957208
40%	2/2	150	Med Mgr	09225595
20%	3/1	75	Lytec	10076195
59%	13	255	C.D.S.	08275295
80%	9/4	120	Med One	10045895
20%	4/1	71	M.O.M.S.	09015395
70%	1/4	115	Med Mgr	42183478
25%	3/1	75	Windows	03027396
5%	4/1	70	Med Mac	92772173
0%	6/1	140	Versys	10206795
15%	6	200	Versys	18267861
20%	10/1	80	P.C.N.	03197496
20%	10/1	65	P.C.N.	49103452
70%	2/1	75	Medic	18434111
35%	8/22	130	Medic	02067296
45%	2/1	—	Medisoft	69508745
15%	8/1	250	ABS Med	10055995
15%	10	35	I.D.X.	82124232
40%	2/2	75	Medisoft	10316895
70%	4/2	112	Med Mgr	29798226
20%	7	180	Micro D.	10025695
95%	7	110	Windows	63215028
25%	2/2	60	Med Mgr	17834335
60%	10/1	200	Elcomp	31876358
30%	14/2	250	Medic	10066095
2%	5/4	—	Med Mac	37289589
60%	6/2	250	M.S.M.	10785431

FIGURE 11–15

Membership Application for PHYSICIANS' INFORMATION EXCHANGE

Physician's Name ____________________

Address ____________________

City ____________________ State ____________

Zip Code ____________ Email ____________________

Phone Number ____________________ Fax ____________________

Manager's Name ____________________

1) Type of Practice (Please circle only one)

01 Solo
02 Specialty group with shared expenses only
03 Specialty group with shared income and expenses
04 Multi-specialty group with shared expenses only
05 Multi-specialty group with shared income and expenses
06 Other

2) Number of Physicians in group

3) Location of practice where majority of patient visits occur (please circle only one)

01 Rural (certified as medically underserved area)
02 Small town/city fewer than 25,000 residents
03 Small city between 25,000 and 100,000 residents
04 City 100,000 to 500,000 residents
05 City 500,000 to 1,000,000 residents
06 City 1,000,000 or more residents
07 Suburban, metro area 500,000 to 1,000,000 residents
08 Suburban, metro area 2,500,000 to 5,000,000 residents
09 Suburban, metro area 2,500,000 to 5,000,000 residents
10 Suburban, metro area greater than 5,000,000 residents

4) State (Postal Abbreviation)

5) Gender M / F Year of Birth

6) Board Certified? Y / N Board Eligible? Y /N Year Certified/Eligible?

7) How many patients do you see in an average week?

8) Primary specialty:

Sub-specialty

9)Self Employed Y / N

10) Employee? Y / N

11) Independent Contractor? Y / N

Physicians' Information Exchange is the opportunity to build our own database. Your input is needed and guaranteed to be confidential. It is time we joined together to benefit our businesses and our patients. THERE IS NO FEE TO JOIN P.I.E. SIMPLY COMPLETE THIS FORM THEN MAIL OR FAX AND WE WILL SEND YOU YOUR CONFIDENTIAL BAR CODE.

PHYSICIANS' INFORMATION EXCHANGE
1400 N. RITTER AVENUE, SUITE 221
INDIANAPOLIS, IN 46219–3046
FAX: (317) 335-1992 E-MAIL: projsolo@iquest.net

FIGURE 11–16

outcomes research.[20] Patient satisfaction is an expanded area of outcomes research. Project Solo/PIE has recently begun studying clinical outcomes research utilizing disease specific and general health status outcomes measurement instruments. The organization and mobilization of physicians around the quality issue offer the opportunity for studing patient perceived quality of life, functional status, and satisfaction in community-based physician offices throughout the world.

REFERENCES

1. Califano J: The medicine men and women: 19 cents of every dollar. In: *Radical Surgery*. New York: Times Books, 1994, p. 27.
2. More people pushing paper. *Am Med News* 1996; Vol. 39 (10):2.
3. Califano J: Temples of the medicine men and women: 39 cents of every dollar. In: *Radical Surgery*. New York: Times Books, 1994, pp. 21–25.
4. Ibid. The money changers and cherry pickers: 6 cents of every dollar, p. 42.
5. Ibid. pp. 53–73.
6. Ibid. Patient, heal thyself, p. 73.
7. Jensen J: Consumers put a premium on keeping physician choice. *Healthcare* November 21, 1994:74.
8. Clinical Research Services Survey ABC/Washington Post. Presented November 20, 1995, on American Agenda.
9. American Academy of Family Physicians, 1987.
10. Davies AR, Ware JE Jr. Involving consumers in quality of care assessment. *Health Aff* 1988; 7:33–48.
11. Maloney TW, Paul B: The consumer movement takes hold in health care. *Health Aff* 1991; 10:268–279.
12. Cleary, PD. McNeil BJ: Patient satisfaction as an indicator of quality care. *Inquiry* 1988; 25:25–36.
13. Ware JE Jr., Hays RD: Methods for measuring patient satisfaction with specific medical encounters. *Med Care* 1988; 26: 393.
14. Rubin HR: Can patients evaluate the quality of hospital care? *Med Care Rev* 1990; 47:267–326.
15. Department of Quality and Utilization: Quality Report Card. Oakland, CA: Kaiser Permanente; 1994: 1–9.
16. Harvard Community Health Plan: Planwide Report: HEDIS 2.0. Wellesley, MA: Howard Community Health Plan: 1993; 1–18.
17. Nguyen TD, Attkinsson CC, Stegner BL: Assessment of patient satisfaction: development and refinement of a service evaluation questionnaire. *Evaluation and Program Plann* 1983; 6(3–4):299–313.
18. Rubin HR, Goundek B, Rogers WH, Kosinji M, McHorney C, Ware, JE, Jr: Patients' ratings of outpatient visits in different practice settings: results from the Medical Outcomes Study. *JAMA* 1993; 270:835–840.
19. Isenberg SF, Davis C, Keaton S: Project Solo: An independent practitioners initiative for confidential self assessment of quality. *Am J Med Qual* 1996; 11(4):1–8.
20. Isenberg SF, Rosenfeld R: Problems and pitfalls in community based outcomes research. *Otolaryngol-Head and Neck Surg;* 1997:662–665.

Steven F. Isenberg, M.D., has been a self-employed, independent Otolaryngologist practicing at the same location in Indianapolis, Indiana, since completing his residency in Otolaryngology-Head and Neck Surgery in 1979. He is a Fellow of the American College of Surgeons, the American Academy of Otolaryngology-Head and Neck Surgery (AAO-HNS), the American Academy of Otolaryngic Allergy (AAOA), the American Rhinologic Society, the American Society for Head and Neck Surgery, and the American College of Physician Executives. He is a Diplomat of the American Board of Otolaryngology. He has passed the written and the oral examinations of the American Board of Facial Plastic and Reconstructive Surgery, and submitted his cases for acceptance as a fellow. Dr. Isenberg has been selected to serve as an oral examiner for the American Academy of Otolaryngic Allergy. He serves on the Editorial Review Board of the *Journal of the American Medical Writers Association*.

Dr. Isenberg's interest in community-based outcomes research and quality led to his founding of Project Solo (PS) in 1994. Project Solo is a grassroots organization of independent physicians organized for quality, autonomy, patient advocacy, and cost-containment. Recently, PS completed its first phase. The data was published in the *American Journal of Medical Quality*, Vol. 1, No. 4, Winter 1996. The editorial preface to the article notes that Project Solo "demonstrates a laudable effort by a group of independent practitioners to fulfill their role as patient advocates-by gathering, analyzing, and confidentially sharing data on patient satisfaction, with the goal of improving quality of care." The editor goes on to point out the potential of Project Solo as a "model for further research and development in the field of quality assurance." Dr. Isenberg co-authored "Problems and Pitfalls in Community Based Outcomes Research," Otolaryngology-Head & Neck Surgery, in press. Project Solo has been endorsed by the Indianapolis Medical Society, the Indiana State Medical Society, and several national organizations. In 1996, Dr. Isenberg's unique methodology entitled "Confidential Self Assessment of Quality" was listed in INNOVATIONS '96 as a model for medical management by the American College of Physician Executives. Since 1979, Dr. Isenberg has served as the President of Steven F. Isenberg, MD, Inc. He is the author of the instructional workbook "Surviving as an Independent Practitioner" and the Course Director of "Outcomes, the Best Tool in your Bag." In 1996, St. Vincent's Foundation, Indianapolis, Indiana, provided a grant to Dr. Isenberg to study "Quality Improvement Utilizing Project Solo." This was the first grant St. Vincent's awarded for outcomes research, and further funding by St. Vincent's and others is currently supporting Phase II of Project Solo's research: Quality Improvement and Benchmarking. Dr. Isenberg has presented Project Solo's Physicians' Information Exchange to physicians in Washington, D.C. (AAO-HNS), (AAOA), Chicago (American Medical Writer's 56th Annual Convention), San Francisco (American College of Surgeons), Paris (2nd Forum on Quality Improvement) and Orlando (American Society of Dermatology).

Dr. Isenberg is a member of the Outcomes Subcommittee, Professional Liability and Practice Management Committees of the AAO-HNS. Since 1994, he has published scientific articles on Fibrous Dysplasia (*ENT Journal*), Endoscopic Sinus Surgery, Thyroid Needle Aspiration, Thyroid Cancer, Bullous Pemphigus, Relapsing Polychondritis (*Otolaryngol Head and Neck Surgery),* Chondromyxoid Fibroma, Osteogenic Sarcoma, and Cystic Hygroma (*American Journal of Otolaryngology*). He has also been featured on a practice management audiotape series entitled "Utilizing Outcomes to Market Your Practice."

Dr. Isenberg serves on the faculty of the Community-St. Vincent's Family Practice Residency Program. In 1989, he was selected as Teacher of the Year. He is an associate professor of Otolaryngology at Indiana University and serves on the Indianapolis Medical Society's Committee for Professional Standards. He is a member of the national medical honorary Alpha Omega Alpha. Dr. Isenberg's interests lie in the community based involvement in outcomes research, benchmarking, continuous quality improvement, practice management, and physician directed organizations.

■ SECTION THREE ■

Quality in the Front and the Back Office

12

Improving Office Efficiency in a Managed Care Environment

CHERYL TOTH

Theoretically, managed care is forcing physicians to run their business more efficiently; but is this theory a reality? With increased paperwork, lengthy phone hold time with plans, and a flurry of cumbersome rules—which seem to be different for each contract—physicians and staff need to focus on improving the efficiency in the office so that they can effectively manage managed care.

Is there a way for physicians to improve the efficiency in their operation *and* deal with managed care? Simply put, the answer is yes. But doing so requires a monumental shift in the way staff and physicians have historically run their business operation. This shift—both in mindset and process—isn't always easy. Physicians may find that long-time staff have difficulty accepting the change that comes with increased efficiency because it means a significant change to that individual's job description. Training, increased use of computer software, and maybe even full scale reengineering will need to take place before the practice can function at optimal efficiency.

> *We cannot attempt to fix the problems of today with the same level of thinking that created the problem.*
>
> William Kenneth Galbraith

■ "Flowchart" Your Operation

Before you can become more efficient, you've got to diagnose where your inefficiencies are. A good way to start is by "flowcharting" the main operational processes in the office. That way you can visualize the steps it takes to complete a process. What are you looking for? When you begin to map out each process, you'll discover certain steps that are redundant or require manual or paper-intensive systems. For example, to register a new patient, staff might have to construct a chart, ask the patient to complete their paperwork, and type out the patient's name, address, phone, and account number on a small Rolodex card (in addition to entering the information in the computer). The Rolodex card is a good example of a system, left over from pre-computer days, that really is no longer necessary.

You don't have to ascribe to perfect flowcharting methodologies—circles or squares are sufficient. Start by flowcharting the following processes:

- **Patient Services:** From the time a patient schedules an appointment, to the time he or she checks out or schedules surgery.
- **Reimbursement Services:** From the time the charge is posted, to the time an account balance is settled.
- **Administrative Services:** The process of pulling, filing, and using a chart; and the process of getting physician dictation to and from transcription.

■ Identify the Problem Areas

Look at your flowcharts. Do you see anything that could use improvement? You might find any one of the following inefficiencies:

- Lots of forms and papers
- Little, or ineffective, use of the computer system; a reliance on handwritten processes
- Steps for which no one can answer the question "Why do we do this?"
- Tasks that are completed by more than one person (redundant)
- Lack of proper equipment to do the job right (i.e., poor telephone system, not enough printers)

Now that you recognize the problem areas (in graphic form, no less), it's time to think about updating your operations to meet the needs of a managed care environment.

Update Your Operations

The key to efficiency is continuously improving the way you do business. For example, systems that used to work quite well can become redundant or ineffective with the advent of new technology. (Remember the old pegboard and ledger card system?) Use the following efficiency goals to develop operations that minimize staff time and ensure effective operations.

Efficiency Goal: Get Organized!

More than anything, the issue that impedes staff's ability to be efficient in a managed care environment is the lack of organization when it comes to contracts, plan rules and reimbursement guidelines. The physician's philosophy of "Sign them all!" typically results in uninformed staff, reimbursement errors, and lost revenue. The first step to becoming an efficient practice is to know the *exact* contracts the practice has signed, along with the details of each one. If your manager and staff can't answer these questions, provide them the Get Organized! project shown in Figure 12–1, and set a deadline for its completion.

Efficiency Goal: Better Use of the Telephone

If you haven't yet considered voice mail, you should. While most patients indicate they don't like an automated menu system, they do prefer to leave a confidential, detailed message. Offering the voice mail option allows your telephone answerer the opportunity to answer and route calls quickly.

Efficiency Goal: Improved Appointment Scheduling

If staff still use a paper appointment book, they've been equipped with an outdated management tool. Not only is a paper appointment book messy and inefficient (what if two people need to schedule at the same time?)—it also limits the practice's ability to set automated physician schedule templates, run a centralized scheduling system, generate encounter forms with essential information, and maintain audit control for cash handling. If you are computerized, use at least the following features of the appointment scheduling module:

- **Physician time templates.** This allows each physician in the group to hold hours as he or she wishes. Patient "appointment types" can vary by physician. If Dr. Smith likes 25 minutes with a new patient, and Dr. Jones prefers 35 minutes, these differences can be accommodated. The next step is to design your own "perfect schedule." For example, you only like to see three new patients on Tuesday and you'll only take one dizzy patient. These preferences can be input into the computer so that when a patient calls, staff type in the code for "dizzy" and the computer searches for the next appropriate slot that fits that criteria.
- **Encounter form generator.** At the touch of a button, staff can generate a day's encounter forms; information comes directly from appointments already scheduled.
- **Computer-generated audit control numbers.** The system will generate a number for each encounter form printed. At day's end after all payments are posted, a "missing encounter form" report is printed. If encounter forms have not been "closed" with a payment, staff must look for the strays. This is a great feature for controlling embezzlement.

The "Domino Effect" and Cost of Bad Scheduling

Problems such as long patient waiting times, "front desk frenzy," and overbooking are nearly always a result of poorly designed—or outdated—physician office schedules. A great deal of staff time is then spent "catching up," calming patients, and dealing with irate physicians and nurses; this ultimately costs the practice in dollars and cents from overtime or lost patients.

When was the last time you took a look at the physician office schedule? Below are some common problem areas; and why they need to be revised.

What if you're following these recommendations and you schedule is *still* inefficient? Maybe it's time to expand your patient hours to evenings and weekends. Or quite possibly the practice could use the services of a physician extender to see some of the established patients; leaving the new patient appointments and consultations for the physicians.

Efficiency Goal: Preregistration of All New Patients

Efficient patient flow always includes a preregistration regime. Gone are the days where staff only ask "name,

Get Organized!

Stop the Confusion!

#1: Inventory your plans: Develop a definitive list of all the plans you contract with and *how you are contracted with them.*

St. Mary's IPA	Direct	OtoNet
National HMO Aetna HMO PruCare PPO HealthNet Preferred Health Partner PPO County Employees	National HMO WeCare HMO PruCare PPO HealthNet Preferred GoodPlan PPO PHCS	National HMO Aetna HMO PHCS

Get Business and Clinical Staff Organized

#2: Develop a **Quick Reference Grid** that shows, at a glance, whether the plan requires a referral, what the co-pay is, etc. Provide this to the front desk.

#3: **Flag the charts,** so clinical staff and physicians are informed.

#4: Design a **Plan Summary Sheet** for each plan that includes the following information:

- **Address, phone, and fax of the plan**
- **Provider Relations contact, and other appropriate contacts, with their respective titles and direct lines, if applicable**
- **Date the contract was signed, and date of renewal**
- **Listing of which physicians within the group are contracted with the plan**
- **Provider number for the plan, and for each physician**
- **Payment schedule methodology, if available**

#5: Develop an **Insurance Reference Guide:** a three-ringed binder that's updated regularly and kept at the front desk, in the billing office, and in the clinical area. It should include the Plan Summary Sheet and Quick Reference Grid, as well as any other pertinent plan information such as copies of benefit cards, co-pay amounts, covered/noncovered service, or preauthorization/preverification phone numbers.

#6: Develop an individual hanging file for each contract. Include in it the payment schedule, Summary Sheet, and all correspondence from the plan.

#7: Establish a tickler system to track the date each contract is up for renewal.

Plan Name	Expiration Date	Schedule Re-Negotiation
St. Mary's IPA	July 29, 1996	June 29, 1996
National HMO-Direct	December 2, 1996	November 2, 1996
WeCare HMO	March 1, 1997	February 1, 1997
GoodPlan PPO	February 1, 1997	January 3, 1997

FIGURE 12–1.

Quick Reference Grid: Associated Otolaryngologists

Plan	Through	OV Copay	Referral?	Pre-Cert: Specify Procedures	Eligibility Phone Number	Approved Lab	Approved Hospital(s)
National HMO	St. Mary's IPA	$10	Yes	800.321.4567 All surgeries, all tests, all lab	800.123.4567	Metro	St. Mary's
National HMO	Direct	$10	Yes	800.333.3333 All surgeries, CT, MRI	800.123.4565	Metro	General
National HMO	SurgNet	$10	Yes	800.222.2222 All surgeries, CT, MRI	800.555.1212	Metro	General
WeCare HMO	Direct	$5	Yes	800.999.9999 All surgeries, all tests	800.123.5555	Pathology Associates	St. Mary's
Good Plan PPO	Direct	$20	No	800.999.8888 Surgeries only	800.222.5555	Pathology Associates	St. Mary's
PHCS	Direct	$10	No	800.666.6666 Surgeries, CT	800.123.4444	Pathology Associates	St. Mary's
PHCS	St. Mary's IPA	$10	No	800.555.5555 All surgeries	800.123.4567	Pathology Associates	St. Mary's

FIGURE 12–1. ***(Continued)***

TABLE 12–1 Solutions to Common Scheduling Problems

Problem	*Result/Solution*
Patients scheduled every 10 or 15 minutes—regardless of presenting complaint	You know you can't see a new Medicare or dizzy patient in 10 minutes—why schedule that way? Instead, design the automated template for *appointment type,* and prompt staff to ask the right questions during scheduling.
"I've always had Wednesday afternoons off."	Times have changed, and physician schedules must change too. If four out of five physicians take Wednesday afternoon off, yet all four want to see patients from 9–12 on Tuesday, staff become inefficient. Space office schedules so no day is "underdoctored" or "overdoctored."
Bottleneck at the front desk—many new patients arrive simultaneously.	All new patients should be *preregistered.* This 1990s style of patient registration is key to getting rid of the "patient crunch."
Overbooking because of work-ins.	It's common knowledge that work-ins happen daily. Failure to recognize this—and leave open appointment slots to accommodate it—means the schedule will always run behind and you'll be inefficient. You have to feel confident that leaving slots open does not mean you'll be sitting in the back reading *Time* magazine. *They will fill.*
Physicians who consistently arrive late for office hours.	While emergencies do arise for surgeons, it's disrespectful to patients to start patient hours behind right from the start. You expect patients to arrive on time to see you. Extend the same courtesy to them.

phone, and social security number" when scheduling patient appointments. A way to control congestion at the front desk, as well as improve the shape of your accounts receivable, is to implement a system of *preregistration for all new patients.* Then when the patient arrives, there are no forms for them to complete—only signatures to gather. Preregistration not only makes patient flow more efficient, it also considerably decreases no-show rates. Here's how it's done:

1. When the appointment is scheduled, the patient is asked for name and home and work telephone number.
2. *Several days or one week prior to the appointment,* a staff person calls the patient directly and asks each question in the computer system's patient registration and insurance screens—completing each field as the information is provided. (A telephone headset for staff is a wise investment.)
3. The patient is told about the practice's financial policy, range of possible charges, and whether the patient needs to bring a referral or test results to the visit.
4. Staff call the patient's insurance company to verify eligibility and coverage. Referral authorization is obtained if needed—or the appointment is rescheduled.
5. A clinical history form and patient brochure are mailed to the patient.
6. A chart is constructed.

Efficiency Goal: Smooth and Effective Check-in

Checking patients in involves more than a smile. Ensuring that the proper referral has been brought to the visit and gathering accurate insurance information are crucial to ultimately being reimbursed. If your check-in staff miss any of the items on the following protocol (Fig. 12–2), their efficiency needs improvement.

Efficiency Goal: Reimbursement Systems That Get You Paid

Efficient reimbursement systems are a direct result of the efficiency goals of complete preregistration and smooth check-in. This accurate information gathering on the front end will eliminate nearly all the work on the back end. To play their part, physicians need to select CPT and ICD-9-CM codes, for both office visits and surgeries, so staff can post the patient transactions correctly. What takes the physicians literally seconds to do (code a surgical case) can take staff up to 20 minutes after they read the operative report, consider the codes, and add modifiers. Then there's the risk that the staff didn't accurately code for what the physician did—after all, he or she wasn't in the OR.

What about claims follow-up? Are staff still generating accounts receivable reports alphabetically, by patient name? To be efficient under managed care, they must review A/R by payor *and* patient. Running A/R reports in descending balance order is a much better use of time. For optimum efficiency of claims follow-up, staff should organize their time like this:

1. Generate the aged accounts receivable by payor, detailed by patient, in descending balance order.
2. Start with commercial claims, since they are still the best paying. Follow these claims with PPOs, HMOs, then Medicare.
3. Look at the high dollar balances in the 60-day aging column. Follow up on the largest balances first, and group the follow up by payor type to organize the time spent on the phone with the insurance company.
4. Call the insurance company to determine why the claim has not been paid. Do not send tracers or ambiguous letters requesting the insurance company to "reconsider" the claim—you must call.
5. Correct the problem, copy medical records, or complete whatever task is necessary to properly refile the claim.
6. Type in "notes" in the computer system about what you did. Include the date and your initials.
7. Send refiled surgical claims by certified mail if the insurance company said they "did not receive claim."

Efficiency Goal: Medical Records Management

Known affectionately as "The Great Chart Hunt" in many surgical practices, management of the medical record is essential to operational efficiency. If staff can't find a patient chart, the patient waits unnecessarily and the physician is unable to effectively treat the patient. Are staff spending hours looking for charts each day? Do patients sometimes arrive and there's no chart to be found? Although it's a common problem, The Great Chart Hunt can be brought under control. Here's how:

1. **Only one individual is in charge of the chart room.** Treat the chart room as a library. The "librarian" is the only one who can pull and file charts. That way, one person is accountable for chart whereabouts. Everyone else: hands off. (That goes for physicians too.) Chart requests for prescription refills and patient callbacks are facilitated by the "librarian."
2. **Use "out guides."** Out guides are plastic inserts that get placed where charts have been pulled. The out guide designates who has checked out the chart.
3. **Dictate so a chart is not necessary for transcription.** If you speak clearly, and provide the correct spelling of the patient's name, as well as the referring physician,

Sample Check-in Protocol

Protocol: **Checking in a Patient**

Last Updated: **May 1997**

Summary: **Greet the patient in a customer-focused manner and verify that all information is correct in the patient account.**

NOTE: The following protocol assumes charts and encounter forms were pulled one day ahead of time, and encounter forms have been attached to each patient's chart.

1. Greet each patient pleasantly, and with a smile.

Note: A patient at the window *always* takes precedence over anything else you are doing at the time. If you are on the telephone when the patient arrives, at least acknowledge his or her presence, and let the patient know you will be with him or her momentarily. Think about how you feel in a restaurant when you've been seated for 10 minutes and the waitress or waiter has not greeted you. We treat our patients with extra special care—they are our customers. Do not ignore them, turn your back to them, or make them wait unnecessarily.

2. Register the patient.

New Patients—Already preregistered (encounter form is attached to chart):

- Make a copy of the patient's benefit card, front and back.
- Pull up the patient's account in the computer and ask the patient to tell you his or her full name, address, telephone number, and insurance plan. Verify that this information is correct in the computer. Look at the benefit card, and verify that the plan and group number match.
- Provide the patient a copy of the financial policy, assignment of benefits, and release of medical records statements. Once the patient has signed these, print a copy of the demographic face sheet from the computer, and place it, the benefit card copy, and financial policy statement in the chart.
- Obtain appropriate signature for Medicare.
- Put the chart up for the clinical staff.

New patient—Not Preregistered, and Work-in Patient:

- Make a copy of the patient's benefit card, front and back.
- Provide the patient with registration forms.
- Provide the patient a copy of the financial policy, assignment of benefits, and release of medical records statements. Once the patient has signed these, print a copy of the demographic face sheet from the computer, and place it, the benefit card copy, and financial policy statement in the chart.
- Enter the new patient data into the computer system.
- Print a revised encounter form for the patient and attach it to the chart.
- Obtain appropriate signature for Medicare.
- Put the chart up for the clinical staff.

Established patient, seen within the last year (encounter form is attached to chart):

- Make sure a copy of the patient's current benefit card, front and back, is in the chart.
- Pull up the patient's account in the computer and ask the patient to tell you his or her full name, address, telephone number, and insurance plan. Verify that this information is correct in the computer. Look at the benefit card, and verify that all information is correct in the computer system.
- Put the chart up for the clinical staff.

FIGURE 12-2.

Sample Check-inProtocol

Established patient, over one year (encounter form is attached to chart):

- Make a copy of the patient's benefit card, front and back.
- Print out a copy of the patient's demographic information, and ask patient to review and edit for changes in information.
- Enter all corrected data into the computer system.
- Print an updated copy of the demographic face sheet from the computer, and a benefit card copy, in the patient's chart.
- Obtain appropriate signature for Medicare.
- Put the chart up for the clinical staff.

3. **Direct any patients with large outstanding balances to the Patient Account Specialist.**

4. **Monitor the length of time patients wait for the physician(s).** If the physicians are running behind schedule, let the patients know this and ask if they wish to reschedule. Keep all patients in the waiting room abreast of any changes in the amount of time the physicians are running behind.

FIGURE 12–2. ***(Continued)***

if there is one, the transcriptionist will not need a chart. This being the case, charts can get filed within 24 hours of patient visit.

Efficiency Goal: Clinical Systems That Incorporate "Highest and Best Use"

If your practice still employs an RN to clean instruments and put patients in rooms, you're not making the best use of that individual's time. Use each clinical staff to their "highest, best, and most cost effective use." A Certified Medical Assistant can room patients, take vital signs, and review clinical histories in addition to keeping the exam rooms stocked. Degreed staff such as RNs are useful in managing clinical triage and assisting with patient care.

Consider also the efficiency brought by a physician extender such as a Physician Assistant. These trained individuals are *revenue generating,* and can make physicians more efficient by seeing established patients and post-ops—freeing the surgeons to see potential surgical cases in consultation.

■ Automate, Automate, Automate!

Selection of new chart numbers from a chronological log book begun in 1965, manual accounts payable, paper insurance claim submission, handwritten encounter forms—all are real-life examples of inefficient or wasted staff time in a physician practice. The "old way" of doing things is probably not the best way anymore. Every one of the manual systems from 1970s medicine can now be done more quickly in the computer.

Are Your Staff "Held Hostage?"

Staff's ability to be efficient can be impeded by even the best intentions. Review your practice to be sure you're clear of "hostage crises":

Unreasonable or impossible job descriptions
Do you have a receptionist who is also responsible for checking patients in, running messages back to the clinic, and performing some transcription? You can't reasonably assume that the combination of these tasks could ever be efficient! How is this staffer supposed to prioritize her time when she's jumping in and out of her seat and pulling headsets in and out of her ears?
Don't place roadblocks in front of your staff. Develop sets of tasks that make sense and have similar functionality. If you demand great customer satisfaction, which you should, your "greeter" should never have to leave her chair during patient hours. She should display the pleasant smile and personality you hired to welcome patients and gather necessary managed care information.

Get organized before you give orders
Think carefully about how you give instruction to staff. Do you come out of an exam room and announce what's on your mind to the closest individual within hearing range? If this declaration requires the staff person to drop everything he or she is doing to facilitate the request, you've just made the staff inefficient.
Instead, be clear about which requests are STAT, and which can wait. STAT requests are given immediately. All others are held and then provided to staff in an organized fashion at the end of office hours, or the end of the day.

Inadequate information system and office equipment
If you haven't invested in a computer terminal for each staff person, they will literally have to schedule time on the computer to get their work done! And just how old is your fax machine? If it requires thermal paper—the kind that rolls up as it prints from the machine—staff will be forced to cut it apart and make a plain paper copy. This is a waste of time, not to mention that thermal paper costs four times as much as the plain copy paper used in today's fax machines.

If you've invested in a contemporary computer system, and your goal is efficiency, be sure staff are aware of all the computer's capabilities and are well trained. If you're not using the computer system to do at least the following things, call your vendor to find out how quickly you can.

1. Automated appointment scheduling using customized templates and connected to the "countdown" of authorized referrals for each patient.
2. Automatic encounter form generation, with audit control numbers.
3. Automatic calculation of Medicare secondary insurance and automatic crossover for secondary billing.
4. Electronic claims submission through a clearinghouse for all claims (not just Medicare).
5. Patient statements generated through a mailinghouse.
6. Managed care management features: the computer screen contains copays, referral and preauthorization numbers, eligibility date ranges, contracted labs and hospitals, and so on.
7. Transcription using an industry standard word processing system, integrated into the patient's account.
8. Collections module that maintains "notes" and "tickler" files about the follow-up on patient accounts.
9. Automated surgery scheduling (if available).
10. Electronic data interchange (EDI) to connect with the hospital and lab for information.
11. Electronic claims remittance for Medicare (if available).
12. Internal electronic mail.

■ Use Process Reengineering and Process Improvement Techniques to Increase Efficiency

Process Reengineering is a fundamental rethinking and redesigning of existing process tasks and operating structure to achieve dramatic improvement in process performance. It involves a complete disassembly of current processes and procedures and then reassembly to meet the needs of a new environment.

You may have discovered while reading this chapter that your practice must undergo a great deal of operational change before it can be truly efficient. If that's the case, reengineering is for you. To facilitate this process, select a "cross-functional work team." A cross-functional work team is composed of each staffer or physician who "touches" part of the process in need of improvement. So, if you are reengineering the patient services process, you would need the Appointment Scheduler, Registrar, Cashier, a clinical staffer, and a physician on the team. This team is then charged with solving the efficiency issue in the process.

To complete the steps for process improvement, equip the team with a full-sized flip chart, and colored markers.

1. Select a "scribe" to stand at the flip chart with a marker.
2. Select a "project leader" who will lead the team discussion (this could also be the scribe).
3. The project leader leads the team through the process, from beginning to end, and asks the team for input about *exactly* what happens, which pieces of paper are used, at *each step*.
4. The scribe writes down each step throughout the discussion.
5. When everything is recorded on the flip chart, the team assesses which steps are unnecessary, redundant, or could be made easier.
6. The use of automation must enter the discussion regularly; if it is not known whether the computer system could automate a particular process, the project leader is responsible for finding out the answer.
7. Ultimately, the team agrees on a streamlined, efficient process.
8. The process is submitted in writing to the physicians.
9. After final edits, the new and improved written process is explained to the entire group and staff are trained, if necessary.

As the team goes through the 9 steps, team members should focus on the following:

- **Could the process be made simpler?** For example, are there multiple forms that could be consolidated into one?
- **Are we asking for items or data that no one pays attention to?** An example is a report you asked your manager for five years ago; now she runs it every month, but you never look at it.
- **How can we better use the computer system to do this?** Most physician groups have a computer system that's only used to a fraction of its capacity. The team should interface with your computer vendor to determine whether manual systems can be automated.
- **Can we reduce the time it takes to complete a process?** There may be unnecessary steps to a process that can be eliminated—such as a daily meeting of three staff to discuss the balances of the patients coming in that day. If one person were trained to look up that information, the meeting wouldn't be necessary.

A good source for operational reengineering techniques is *Process Re-Engineering in Action,* by Richard Y. Chang, Richard Chang Associates Publishing. It can be purchased for $12.95 at local bookstores and provides excellent "road mapping" for improving efficiency in your practice.

13

Staffing Requirements in Managed Care

CHERYL TOTH

Remember the days when all physicians needed was one staffer who could do most of the work—and actually get it done by the end of the day? Scheduling appointments and surgeries, following up on overdue accounts, and transcribing dictation were key elements of this person's job description—and in a pinch, the staffer could even room patients.

The advent of managed care has changed those times. Staff in today's practice must be highly skilled and trained about the managed care issues faced by physicians. But does that always mean you need to hire more people? Not necessarily. It's what staff *do,* and how their job fits into your overall staffing plan, that counts. The *jack-of-all-trades* or *generalist* who was the backbone of an physician's practice years ago must be replaced with staff who have specialized knowledge.

■ Complete an Operations Checklist—Who Is Responsible For What?

Managed care has brought with it a variety of tasks staff must complete, that didn't exist under fee-for-service medicine. For example, surgical preauthorization requires additional staff time, but is critical if the physician wants to get reimbursed. When was the last time you took inventory of which staffer is responsible for completing managed care-related tasks? It's common in medical practices for staff to continue doing things "the way they've always done it." But this attitude will not work in a managed care environment.

Use the Responsibility Checklist shown in Table 13–1 to determine the individual responsible and held accountable for each of the following essential managed care tasks.

TABLE 13–1. Responsibility Checklist

Responsibility	*Who's Responsible?*
Maintains centralized filing system for all contracts and plan payment schedules.	
Holds an in-service, updates all software maintenance files, and trains staff on new "rules" each time a new contract is signed.	
Verifies eligibility and coverage for all new managed care patients.	
Updates established patient demographic and insurance information at every visit.	
Determines patients' financial responsibility prior to surgery; collects deductibles and coinsurance pre-operatively.	
Makes certain HMO patients present with an appropriate referral—reschedules those who don't have one.	
Obtains precertification and preauthorization for surgeries.	
Verifies that all insurance payments are accurate according to contractual agreement.	
Analyzes practice payer mix and contractual receivables, by plan.	
Monitors rejection trends by plan, and resolves them.	
Analyzes each new contract and discusses the results with the physicians.	
Analyzes each plan reimbursement schedule, and provides data for the negotiation or renegotiation meeting	
Monitors physician utilization and prescription writing habits, to conform with managed care requirements.	

194

■ Update Job Descriptions for the Times

If you haven't updated your staff's written job descriptions in the past year—or worse, if staff don't have job descriptions—the time is now. Written job descriptions help clarify the role of each employee in your practice. They are used in the hiring, training, and performance appraisal process to ensure that employees know what they are responsible for.

Well-crafted job descriptions contain the following items:

- An appropriate title for the position. "Clerk" is a meaningless position title. "Transcriptionist," or "Medical Records Assistant" more accurately describes what the staffer does.
- A summary of the job's tasks.
- The person to whom the employee reports.
- The education and experience qualifications for the position.
- A detailed listing of the key functions for the position.

The staff needed in today's practice are different from those staff needed years ago. Overall, the role of each employee has become more focused and specialized. And while cross training is certainly a good idea, on a daily basis, your staff should be assigned and held accountable for very defined duties.

In addition to the clinical staff who support you, as well as a transcriptionist, and medical records assistant, the following staff positions are essential in a managed care environment:

- **Receptionist/Registrar.** The Receptionist/Registrar is much more than a smiling face at check-in, and a pleasant voice on the phone—that person is a key information gatherer. Signatures are obtained, benefit cards copied, and established patient information verified by this individual. One hint: when you find a Receptionist/Registrar who's a gem, *don't* "promote" him or her into "billing." This person is already the first step in your billing process!
- **Preregistration Coordinator** If you are going to be successful in a managed care world, the registration process must be moved as far "up front" as possible. This includes *preregistration* of all **new** patients. The Preregistration Coordinator is responsible for completely registering new patients into the computer system *prior to their arrival at the practice.* This process typically includes verifying the patient's eligibility and coverage, explaining your financial policies, reminding the patient of the necessity of a referral, and constructing a chart. See Figure 13–1 for a sample job description.
- **Cashier.** It's more important than ever to focus on collection at the time of service. Someone has to collect all those copays—sending statements for $5 or $10 is costly. The cashier collects copays, deductibles (yes, some PPO and HMO patients still have them), and posts the day's charges and payments.
- **Reimbursement Specialist.** No longer a biller, the reimbursement specialist's role is to know the specific rules and guidelines of each plan he or she is responsible for overseeing. Unpaid claims are followed up at 45 days, and the reimbursement specialist typically posts payments too. The reimbursement specialist must continually be sent to educational courses to be sure of maintaining specialized knowledge about insurance reimbursement—rules change often. See Figure 13–2 for a sample job description.
- **Patient Account Specialist.** Collecting from insurance companies and collecting from patients are two very different tasks. The patient account specialist is responsible for following up on patient balances, and can be available to counsel patients about their bill or set up budget plans when the patient is in the office. Some practices even offer flexible hours for the patient account specialist, so that he or she can reach patients on the telephone in the evening.
- **Surgery Coordinator.** Managed care has made the amounts patients owe for surgery vary significantly from plan to plan. The surgery coordinator is responsible for explaining a patient's financial obligation, collecting a presurgical deposit, and scheduling the surgery. This staffer is a patient advocate who makes sure all tasks that go into scheduling surgery are complete prior to the physician's going to the O.R. See Figure 13–3 for a sample job description.
- **Referral Coordinator.** Remember: no referral, no payment! Depending on the size of your practice, you may need an individual exclusively dedicated to managing the referral process. The referral coordinator is responsible for checking the charts one day prior to appointment and ensuring that a valid referral is available—if not, the referral coordinator is responsible for making sure the PCP is called.
- **Clinical Coordinator.** If your practice is large enough, you may want to consider a clinical coordinator; a degreed individual who oversees chart documentation audits, ensures physicians code correctly, interprets utilization and outcomes data, hires and trains clinical staff, and runs the operations in the clinic.

JOB DESCRIPTION: Preregistration Coordinator

RESPONSIBLE TO: Manager

JOB SUMMARY: With a customer service orientation—preregister all new patients, verify insurance eligibility, and construct new patient charts.

EDUCATIONAL REQUIREMENTS:

- High school diploma
- College education/trade school preferred but not required

QUALIFICATIONS AND EXPERIENCE:

- Minimum 12 months experience in a medical office
- Minimum 50 words per minute typing skills
- Working knowledge of managed care, Medicare, and Medicaid
- Computer experience required
- Strong written and verbal communication skills
- Ability to perform multiple tasks simultaneously
- Ability to perform in a highly stressful situation
- Pleasant speaking voice and demeanor

Responsibilities include, but are not limited to, the following:

- Generates the appointment schedule 5 working days ahead of time, and preregisters new patients over the telephone before they arrive for their appointment
- Completes all fields in the patient demographic and insurance screens in the computer
- Calls patient's insurance company to verify eligibility and obtain benefit coverage for office visits, audiology tests, and surgery
- If the patient's insurance carrier requires a formal referral authorization, obtains the referral number and notes it in the computer system
- Reschedules patients who do not have a referral authorization at the time of preregistration
- Explains to patients which pieces of information they are to bring
- Provides a range of potential charges for the visit; details the patient's financial obligation, depending on insurance type
- Creates a new chart for the patient encounter
- Maintains patient confidentiality
- Attends all regular staff meetings
- Performs all other tasks and projects assigned by the Manager

---

FIGURE 13–1. Sample job description: Preregistration Coordinator

POSITION: Reimbursement Specialist

RESPONSIBLE TO: Manager

JOB SUMMARY: Posts insurance payments for specific payer types, follows up on unpaid insurance claims and rejections using EOBs and reports, and maintains relationships with specified payers.

EDUCATIONAL REQUIREMENTS:

- High school diploma
- College education or trade school preferred

QUALIFICATIONS AND EXPERIENCE:

- Minimum 18 months experience working in a physician group practice billing department
- Knowledge of third party payer reimbursement guidelines
- Experience establishing relationships with insurance companies
- Understanding of CPT and ICD-9-CM coding for otolaryngology
- Working knowledge of medical office billing software
- Pleasant speaking voice and demeanor
- Neat, professional appearance
- Strong written and verbal communication skills

Responsibilities include, but are not limited to, the following:

- Ensures all paper claims are submitted with 0% error—verifies completeness of paper insurance claim information before mailing
- Transmits all appropriate electronic claims; corrects claims that hit the "front end edit," then retransmits
- Posts all mailed-in insurance payments by line item, following up on rejections as they occur
- Notifies Manager immediately when insurance payments do not match contractual agreement
- Processes requests for refunds, and submits to Manager for approval
- Utilizes monthly aged accounts receivable report, beginning at 45 days, to contact payers regarding unpaid insurance claims
- Makes necessary arrangements for medical records requests, completion of additional paperwork, etc., if payers request this information prior to payment of claims
- Utilizes Insurance Reference Manual to support completion of assigned tasks
- Responds to written and telephone inquiries from insurance companies
- Manages relationships with personnel from assigned carrier
- Responds to patient questions about insurance-related reimbursement, as needed
- Meets with Manager regularly to discuss and solve reimbursement and insurance follow-up problems
- Attends regular staff meetings as requested
- Attends continuing education sessions as requested
- Performs any additional duties as requested by the Manager

FIGURE 13–2. Sample job description: Reimbursement Specialist

POSITION: Surgery Coordinator

RESPONSIBLE TO: Manager

JOB SUMMARY: Act as liaison between patient and physician, schedule all surgeries and preoperative tests, and counsel patients prior to surgery regarding financial responsibility.

EDUCATIONAL REQUIREMENTS:

- High school diploma
- College education or trade school preferred
- Medical Assistant certification a plus

QUALIFICATIONS AND EXPERIENCE:

- Minimum 18 months experience working in a physician group practice
- Experience in a project-oriented position preferred
- Experience establishing relationships with insurance companies
- Knowledge of medical terminology
- Ability to work with patients and make them feel comfortable
- Neat, professional appearance
- Strong written and verbal communication skills

Responsibilities include, but are not limited to, the following:

- Receives instructions from physicians about which surgery or test is recommended
- Obtains precertification/preauthorization from insurance companies prior to surgery for each procedure and test
- Verifies patient eligibility and coverage for the procedure; if patient is not eligible on date of service, or procedure is not a covered benefit, explains options to patients
- Counsels patients preoperatively regarding their potential financial obligations, and provides information about patient insurance coverage
- Discusses preoperative instructions with the patient, as directed by physicians
- Assists patients with setting up payment plans, and collects presurgical deposits
- Schedules operating room time, according to physician scheduling protocols
- Schedules all appropriate preoperative tests
- Coordinates all paperwork prior to surgery, using physician-approved forms and checklists
- Responds to written and telephone inquiries from patient and carriers regarding planned surgeries
- Maintains communication among the physician, patient, insurance company, and hospital at all times
- Posts all surgical charges within 48 hours of procedure
- Maintains patient confidentiality
- Attends continuing education courses as requested
- Attends all regular staff meetings
- Completes all other duties as assigned by the Manager

FIGURE 13–3. Sample job description: Surgery Coordinator

How Many Staff Are Needed

Many physicians wonder if they have the right number of staff, too many staff, or not enough staff. National surveys that provide the average number of "full time equivalent" employees per physician can be used as a benchmark, but be careful. These statistics do not take into consideration the following issues—which are key to determining the appropriate staffing for your practice.

1. How many patients are seen each day? How many are new? (New patients take more time to process.)
2. How many managed care contracts have you signed? If you have multiple HMOs that have a cumbersome referral authorization and precertification process, more "hands" may be necessary.
3. How many physicians see patients at the same time? If you have "three doctors" or "four doctor" days, you'll need more people during those hours.
4. How quickly do surgeons need response time? "ASAP" doctors who insist tasks be done quickly, and ask staff to drop what they're doing to complete them, will require a greater number of staff.
5. Do you have an information system that automates operational systems? The more paper intensive your business systems, the more staff you'll need.

Determine the Type of Management You Need

The amount of detail and expertise necessary to run a practice continues to increase. Only in solo practice or rare circumstances can physicians go it alone when it comes to management. In fact, many physicians relish the thought of delegating staffing, operational, and financial minutia to a capable individual. Oversight of these issues along with policy setting are where physicians should set their sights.

Many physicians wonder what type of manager is really needed for the practice. Do you have to hire an MBA, or is someone with "up through the ranks" expertise sufficient? To answer that question, physicians need to understand how manager types differ.

Three Genres of Managers

There are basically three types of managers—all of whom have different backgrounds, different skill sets, and different roles within the practice. They are referred to by any number of job titles, depending on the preference of the organization. Common titles for these manager types are:

- Office Manager
- Practice Manager
- Practice Administrator

An office manager is an often misused title, handed out in place of a raise or to reward loyalty. This person does not usually have a business background or education—often their entire career has been spent in a physician practice. A practice manager has experience in physician practice, sometimes has achieved at least a college degree, and has business experience from another industry. A practice administrator nearly always comes from a varied business background. This individual has worked in large organizations, and quite often has experience as a hospital executive.

Which manager type does your practice need? That's the million dollar question. Physicians must decide how much time they want to spend on management issues, and which tasks they want to delegate. They must also consider how much authority they are willing to extend to the manager. If you and your colleagues wish to maintain a considerable amount of managerial control, a practice administrator may not be the best fit. A cost effective choice is a manager whose skill set complements that of the physician group.

Regardless of the management expertise you select, the individual must be knowledgeable about managed care administration and operations. Higher level managers will have greater expertise in contract negotiation, but all levels must understand the impact managed care has on the practice. Use the chart in Table 13–2 to assist you in choosing the right manager for your group.

Give Your Manager the Power to Get the Job Done

Once a manager is hired, the physician team must form a united front and position the manager as the individual in charge. *Front line staff often need to hear this firsthand from the physicians.* And stand behind your manager's authority. Don't allow staff to circumvent the manager and go to a physician for a "better" answer. Without physician support, your manager will not be able to implement positive change in the organization because he or she will never be perceived by staff as a leader.

TABLE 13–2. What Kind Of Manager Do You Need?

	Office Manager	*Practice Manager*	*Practice Administrator*
Level of Authority	An Office Manager rarely initiates; he/she *responds* to heavy physician direction.	A Practice Manager is an *initiator* of projects and ideas, generated by him/her and the physician team. Physicians participate in the process.	An Administrator is a *business leader*, who directs a team of capable managers or team leaders. Physicians set policy but do little directing.
Number of Full Time Physicians	1–approximately 3	Approximately 3–approximately 10	Approximately 10 or more
Number of Physician Extenders	0	Often 1 or more	Often 2 or more
Types of Business Units	Office Practice, maybe lab	Office practice, lab, audiology, maybe hearing aid sales and/or surgery suite	Office practice, lab, audiology, hearing aid sales, probably a surgery suite
Number of Full Time Staff	Appproximately 5–10	Approximately 10+	Approximately 20+
Annual Practice Revenue	Up to $1 million	$1 million to $6 million	Over $6 million
Number of Practice Sites	1 primary site	1 primary site, maybe 1–2 satellites	1 primary site, typically multiple satellites
Maturity of Managed Care Market	**Typically, less than 20%:** Fee-for-service reimbursement still dominates, not many contracts signed yet, physicians and staff still Golden Age of Medicine mindset	**Typically, more than 20%:** Business coalitions forming, at least PCPs are capitated, physicians looking for ways to increase market share and gain exclusivity with plans	**Typically, more than 20%:** Some specialists are capitated, business coalitions hold power, employer-direct contracts and case rates used, large primary care and multispecialty groups may steer patient flow
Degree of Market Integration	Solos and small groups prevail, probably an IPA in place	Physician groups are growing in size, hospitals and physicians working together, PCPs may be owned by hospitals or national management companies, several IPAs and possibly an MSO have been developed	Physicians in groups, single specialty networks present, health "system" quite evolved, PCPs owned, IPAs and MSOs
Number of Capitated	0–1	1+	2+

Use Your Manager's Time Cost Effectively

An office manager's strength is typically in the oversight of daily operations and staffing, and accounts receivable management. They can fill in for staff as needed and implement contract details once the agreement has been signed. A practice manager or practice administrator can prepare contracts for negotiation, review reimbursement analyses, initiate expense reduction strategies in anticipation of capitation, direct the management of accounts receivables, and review staff performance. That's what you pay them for. It doesn't mean you abdicate the entire business to the manager—simply that some of the responsibility for your business is shouldered by another professional. Of course, you and your partners should be part of these projects, but the manager initiates and does the lion's share of the work.

■ Hire People with the Right Skill Set

Gone are the days when a staff member's friend or neighbor is an appropriate addition to your team. Physicians need capable, trained, employees who understand managed care and the operational changes brought about by HMOs and PPOs. Be leery, for example, of a candidate who worked for a surgeon *five years ago.* That experience doesn't necessarily "translate" into the skill set needed today. You need staff with up-to-date knowledge of managed care requirements in your market.

The job descriptions you developed will guide you in the selection process and should be part of the interview with candidates. Use them to discuss the specific responsibilities of the job, so there are no surprises when the candidate accepts your offer. And just where do you find those candidates? Putting a specific ad in the newspaper is a good start. Stay away from the generic copy: *"Busy surgeon's office in need of friendly person to answer telephone."* Instead, place an ad that will attract candidates with the skills you want:

> If you are an expert with HMO and PPO guidelines, and have experience with Medical Manager, we need you! Our busy surgical practice seeks a

customer-focused Referral Coordinator to oversee the details of our managed care plans. Knowledge of the referral process, CPT and ICD-9-CM coding a must. Fax us a commercial about yourself: 555-1234

Another option is to put the word out to colleagues and referring physicians that you are looking. Depending on the position you're hiring for, you might find that someone from another industry is a potential employee. Regardless of where you find candidates, review their credentials and experience while keeping in mind the considerations shown in Table 13–3.

In addition to the actual interview, it's smart to provide candidates with a "hiring assessment" (see Fig. 13–4) to determine the level of experience and skill set they have. Sometimes asking specific questions can weed out those who talk a good game, but aren't as knowledgeable as they would lead you to believe. The "assessment" is also useful to determine the candidate's training needs, should you choose to hire that person.

■ Pay People What They Are Worth

To hire and retain excellent staff, you're going to have to pay them well. The old adage, "You get what you pay for" accurately describes what can happen to your practice if there is no emphasis on hiring the right people and paying them for their expertise.

Set a salary range for each position in the practice. This range should indicate both the low and high end of the earning spectrum for an employee in that position. Hire employees at the low end of this spectrum. At year three of employment, the employee should be near the middle of the range, and at year five, at the high end of the range. Be clear at the time of hire that the position has a range—in other words, there are no lifetime raises. When the employee has "topped out" in the position, there may be opportunity for greater responsibilities or a promotion, but this is not a guarantee.

Where to Go for Specific Salary Information

The Medical Group Management Association (303-799-1111) provides information about hourly wage ranges for staff and salary ranges for managers. Your state may have a chapter that has done local research as well; which means you can obtain local averages.

Try also contacting a hospital's physician services section. Often these people survey local office managers about the wages in your community.

■ Check References

It's a mistake not to request and verify references for the final candidates. Hiring is always a risk, but you can minimize it by being sure you ask about a candidate's track record, and whether the physician he/she worked for would hire him/her again. For a full reference check—including commercial credit, licensure, education and driving record—outsource this task to a company such as The Omnia Group (800-525-7117). For about $100, you can buy yourself added peace of mind.

TABLE 13–3 Review of Candidate Credentials and Experience

Possible Candidate Experience	*Considerations*
Worked in a doctor's office for 10 years.	Could be good or bad. Staff who have spent this long in Doctorland may be jaded toward managed care; or worse, be "stuck" in the way things used to be done in fee for service. Be sure the "10 years" include a progressive mindset.
Has experience in the hospital billing department.	Beware: this person may not even know what a CPT code is. The language of physician billing is much different from that of a hospital. This individual may very well be trainable, but he/she will not hit the ground running.
Adjudicated claims for Blue Cross Blue Shield.	Good insight into plan operations. You'll have to train him/her, but the understanding of how an insurance company works can be an asset to your practice.
Worked in a primary care or pediatric office.	This individual is used to high volumes of patients and transactions, and can handle significant stress. Very little would "shake" a well-trained person with this experience.
Has experience in the hospital admission department.	Could be a good registrar candidate. The hospital often offers customer service training classes.
Was a waitress or bartender.	You'll have to train on the computer and medical terminology, but waitresses and bartenders typically make excellent registrars or cashiers. They are used to working with irate customers, juggling multiple tasks at the same time, and balancing their own cash transactions.
Worked in an upscale hair salon.	You'll have to train on the computer and medical terminology, but his individual could make a terrific registrar or appointment scheduler. Most likely, he/she has terrific customer service skills, and is experienced at making appointments and verifying information.

Please answer all of the following questions to the best of your ability. Your answers will assist us in determining where your skills could best be utilized.

1. Explain the difference between a CPT code and an ICD-9-CM code.
2. A CPT code has _______ digits, and an ICD-9-CM code has _______ digits.
3. What are evaluation and management codes?
4. Name all the outpatient consultation codes.
5. What is the difference between a consultation and a referral?
6. What is the difference between commercial insurance and a PPO?
7. What is a withhold? How would you post it in the computer system?
8. Why is it important to get a referral authorization in a specialist's office?
9. What is precertification? What is preauthorization?
10. Can you collect full charges from an HMO patient? Why or why not?
11. Do you need to send an operative note with all surgical claims?
12. What are *three* key things to do when scheduling a new managed care patient?
13. Explain how you would post the charges for a capitated patient.
14. Explain how the front desk staff should register an *established patient.* Define these in "steps"—i.e., Step 1: patient approaches the front desk, etc.
15. What does it mean to post by *line item?* Why is it so important?
16. When working on rejections, you encounter the following rejection types. How would you:
    1. Handle the rejection? Describe the process you'd use.
    2. *Prevent* the rejection from happening again.

    "Procedure not a covered benefit"
    1.
    2.

    "Patient not eligible on date of service"
    1.
    2.

    "Contract number does not match information on file"
    1.
    2.

    "Applied to deductible"
    1.
    2.

    "Patient has Senior HMO"
    1.
    2.
17. What could $100,000 in Happy HMO receivables in the "90 day" aging column indicate?
18. At what age should an overdue patient account be sent to an **outside** collection agency?
19. If you were discussing the status of a patient's overdue balance with him or her on the telephone, and the patient said, "I can pay you, but not until I get my paycheck next week." What would you say?
20. What is the minimum balance you think appropriate for a patient to pay under a monthly budget plan?

FIGURE 13–4. Staff Knowledge Assessment

14

Surviving and Thriving as an Independent Practitioner: The Search for Continuous Quality Improvement

STEVEN F. ISENBERG

Today's independent medical practitioners face multiple challenges. Our futures depend on our abilities to:

- Negotiate contracts with MCOs, employers, and our peers.
- Balance the financial incentives embodied within those contracts with the medical and surgical needs of our patients.
- Financially survive the risks of such contracts.
- Prove the clinical effectiveness of our treatments (outcomes).
- Implement change and continuously provide quality cost-effective care in the front and back office.

The socioeconomic, moral, and ethical debates surrounding health care will undoubtedly continue. Most practitioners, however, want to know what can be done today. How do bureaucratically burdened busy physicians, peddling frantically just to keep up, mount a proactive pragmatic response to the legions of forces surrounding them? My response is: *know your business.* It isn't likely that a single practitioner, or a group of practitioners, will dramatically change the driving force that consumes one trillion dollars a year. Therefore, the best that any of us can do is to work toward continuous quality improvement in our own practices. What follows is my solo response to today's challenges. I make no claims that it is the best response. It is, however, possible to implement it effectively in a busy practice. I can only claim to know something about running a solo ENT practice in Indianapolis, Indiana, the last 18 years. On the other hand, we all share many of the same problems. Regardless of specialty, practice style, or other demographics, I hope that you might find something useful in this chapter.

Quality

From 1970 to 1980, the Japanese captured large segments of worldwide markets with high quality, low cost products. W. Edwards Deming, Ph.D., physics, Yale University, had received Japan's Second Order Medal of the Sacred Treasure with the citation: "The Japanese people attribute the rebirth of Japanese industry and its world wide success to Ed Deming." Deming, a statistician, had been recruited by the Supreme Command for the Allied Powers to prepare for the 1951 Japanese Census. He was fascinated with process and quality control. In 1950, he lectured on quality control to the Union of the Japanese Scientists and Engineers comprising Japanese workers, scientists, and plant managers. The rest, as they say, is history.

Many analysts of the American health care revolution note that we are merely being forced to respond as other American businesses have been forced to respond. Deming became a consultant to Ford in 1981 in its quest to focus on quality. Other companies refocused themselves on product quality and customer service. The successful ones have reestablished themselves in today's worldwide markets. Deming's fundamental contribution was his insight that "customers" are created by the existence of a perceived societal need. The challenge for each independent medical practitioner is to identify and exceed that perceived need. Just as it was to American industry, Total Quality Management (TQM), with its emphasis on *management by data, analysis of the process of care,* and *continuous customer satisfaction,* is pivotal to the survival of today's independent practitioner.

■ Outcomes: The Best Tool in Your Bag

Patient Satisfaction Surveys

As Michael Stewart and Richard Rosenfeld outlined in their chapters in this book, outcomes measure morbidity and mortality (standard measures) as well as expanded measures such as quality of life, performance status, and patient satisfaction. Today's busy practitioner should begin studying outcomes by implementing patient satisfaction surveys. The lengthy list below outlines just some of the reasons why:

- Patient satisfaction surveys are easy to implement, require minimal physician staff time, and address one of the central targets of TQM (listening to the voice of the consumer).
- The definition of patient quality has shifted from patient needs, such as the correct diagnoses and treatments (quality in fact), to customer wants such as reasonable waiting times, telephone access, and office location (quality in perception). In an expert's words, the quality of care rests with both its effectiveness in improving patients' health and survival and how well it meets patients' and public standards for how care should be provided.[1]
- Businesses, picking up the tab for health care, focus on customer satisfaction and place the same quality parameters on physicians.
- The medical literature supports patient satisfaction measurement as a quality indicator. In the last 20 years, research psychologists and sociologists have demonstrated that patient judgments of their medical care can be measured reliably and accurately.[2–7]
- Patient satisfaction measurement is the current quality yardstick. Because "consumerism has become so important in health care" a 10-million-dollar federal financial study has been implemented to accelerate health plans' use of patient satisfaction data.[8]

There are multiple additional references attesting to the current acceptability of measuring patient satisfaction as an indicator of quality. Once convinced, the practitioner should use a benchmarked patient satisfaction survey process to perform meaningful surveys. Data collected is infinitely more valuable if it can be compared against data compiled from several different studies. Such a patient satisfaction survey is the 9-item Patient Visit Rating Questionnaire (VRQ) utilized by the Medical Outcomes Study and other investigators.[9, 10, 11]

The questions:

1. How long you waited to get an appointment
2. Convenience of the location of the office
3. Getting through to the office by phone
4. Length of the time waiting at the office
5. Time spent with the person you saw
6. Explanation of what was done for you
7. The technical skills (thoroughness, carefulness, competence) of the person you saw
8. The personal manner (courtesy, respect, sensitivity, friendliness) of the person you saw
9. The visit overall

Also asked:

10. In general, you would say your health is . . .
11. Are you male or female?
12. How old were you (patient) on your last birthday?
13. Comments:

Patients select an answer from 1 to 5 (1 = poor/ 5 = excellent). The percentage excellence response is used because :

- Quality management and improvement recommend comparisons to the best practices rather than to minimal standards.[12]
- In continuous quality improvement, 100% excellence is the goal.
- Research has shown that the higher the percent excellence, the more likely the physician will retain the patient.[9]

In 1994, I formed Project Solo to initially establish a national physician information gathering network. I decided to implement this benchmarked patient satisfaction survey to help myself and my peers establish a benchmarking process against which we could measure ourselves. The implementation of patient satisfaction surveying is critical to quality analysis today; it is easily done within a busy office practice, and such information sharing is critical to today's practitioner for providing quality patient care and business practice management.

The overall results of Project Solo's data accumulation are seen in Figures 14–1a, b, and c. Figure 14–2 is benchmark data provided by Project Solo. Note that Project Solo's data is benchmarked against HMO, multispecialty fee-for-service, and solo fee-for-service patient satisfaction percent excellence responses reported by Rubin.[9]

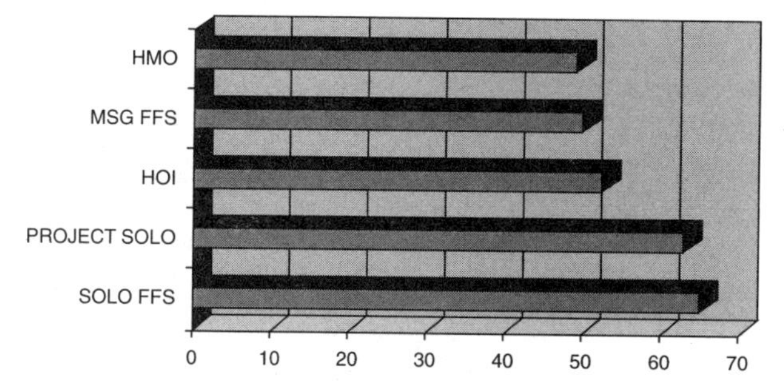

FIGURE 14–1a. Survey Results: Overall Satisfaction

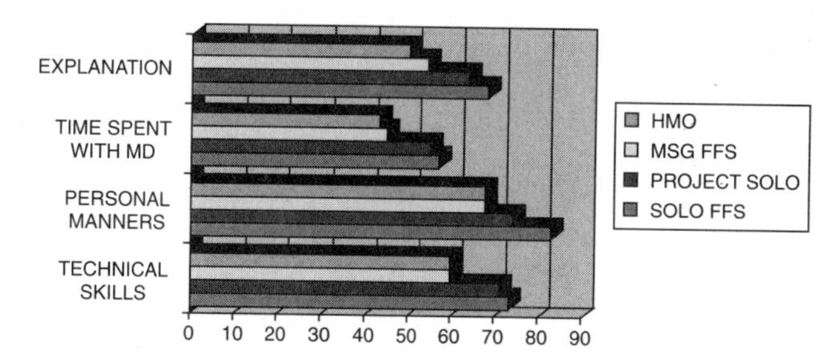

FIGURE 14–1c. Survey Results: Physician Attributes

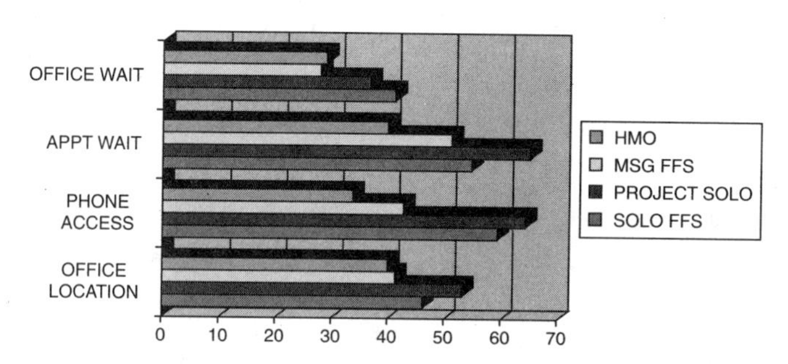

FIGURE 14–1b. Survey Results: Access

Responses are also compared to data obtained from the Health Outcomes Institute patient satisfaction survey percent excellent responses.[13] All groups utilized the 9-item VRQ. The data provided by Project Solo grows in statistical significance as the amount of data increases from greater numbers of participating physicians. The data results are probably not as significant as the data itself. Project Solo appears to be the first grassroots, peer developed and implemented effort to obtain outcomes data from a diverse socioeconomic and geographic group of physicians representing a variety of practice styles.

The physicians participating in Project Solo's data exchange were guaranteed confidentiality with the assignment of confidential bar codes on joining the organization. This methodology, termed Confidential Self Assessment of Quality, received an honorable mention in 1996 from the American Academy of Physician Executives as a Model for Medical Management. It became the foundation for DOCSHARE, the confidential physician practice management benchmarking process

Percentage of Excellent Ratings by System of Care*
% EXCELLENT (95% CONFIDENCE INTERVAL)

SURVEY QUESTION	SOLO FFS§	MSG FFS§	HMO§	HOI	PROJECT SOLO
OVERALL VISIT	65 $n = 6752$	50† $n = 1677$	49† $n = 6248$	53¥	63 $n = 2496$
TECHNICAL SKILL OF MD	75	60†	60†		71
PERSONAL MANNER OF MD	82	68†	68†		74
WAIT FOR AN APPOINTMENT	65	51†	40†		54
OFFICE LOCATION	52	41†	40†		46
TELEPHONE ACCESS	64	42†	33†		59
OFFICE WAIT	36	28†	29†		42
TIME SPENT W/PERSON	56	44†	42†		55
EXPLANATION	67	53†	5†		63

*SOLO indicates solo or single specialty; FFS, fee for service; MSG, multispecialty group; and HMO, health maintenance organization. Sample sizes for other items vary due to differing amounts of missing data: SOLO FFS, 2947–3055; MSG FFS, 882–846; and HMO, 3310–3424.
†Contrasts different from SOLO FFS at level of $P > .001$.
¥Data obtained from David Radosevich, PhD, Health Outcomes Institute. Primary Care Physicians only.
§Data obtained from Rubin, et al.

FIGURE 14–2. Benchmarked data provided by project solo to participants

utilized by Physicians' Information Exchange (PIE). I will explain more about DOCSHARE later.

I studied the survey collection process within my practice and Project Solo. Currently Project Solo is studying quality improvement utilizing patient satisfaction surveys as the measurement tool. When performing surveys in the office it is important to:

- Provide a confidential collection mechanism (Project Solo provides a sealed box that is mailed to the database when all the surveys are collected).
- Inform the patient of the reason for the survey.
- Assure the patient about the confidentiality of their response.
- Collect the surveys in the office following completion of the visit (mailing surveys results in incomplete, biased results).[14]

Piccirillo studied quality improvement efforts in an academic otolaryngology office.[10] He utilized statistical process control, including process control charts, to document that quality improvement efforts had made an import on patient satisfaction. Some of the efforts initiated by Piccirillo included:

- Physician availability for urgent office visits to see patients within 24 hours.
- A new phone triage and answering system.
- Improvement of the registration process.
- Simplified maps.

Project Solo, dealing with a geographically diverse group, is studying the ability to improve quality utilizing a posted Quality Improvement Poster in participating physician offices (Fig. 14–3). Project Solo hypothesizes that significant improvement will be obtained by:

- Involving the entire staff in the continuous quality improvement process.

Q.I.P.
Quality Improvement Process

- OUR PATIENTS ARE OUR CUSTOMERS.
- OUR CUSTOMERS ARE OUR PRACTICE. . . THEY ARE NOT OUTSIDERS.
- WE WELCOME PHONE CALLS AND QUESTIONS FROM OUR CUSTOMERS
- WE ARE DEDICATED TO TREATING AND MONITORING OUR CUSTOMERS' PROBLEMS WITH KINDNESS, EFFICIENCY, AND COST EFFECTIVENESS.
- WE LISTEN TO OUR CUSTOMERS.
- WE APPRECIATE OUR CUSTOMERS' BUSINESS AND THANK THEM FOR USING US FOR THEIR HEALTH CARE NEEDS.
- OUR CUSTOMERS PROVIDE OUR PAYCHECKS.
- PROBLEMS IN OUR PRACTICE GIVE US OPPORTUNITY FOR IMPROVEMENT IN OUR SERVICE
- WE ARE PROUD OF THE JOB WE DO EVERYDAY.
- WE STRIVE TO CONTINUOUSLY IMPROVE OUR CUSTOMERS' SATISFACTION.

FIGURE 14–3. Project solo: physicians assuring quality

- Providing the participating physician with a "report card" of patient perceived quality (Fig. 14–4). The "Hawthorne Effect" is defined in *Webster's Ninth Collegiate Dictionary:* fr. the *Hawthorne* works of the Western Electric Co., Cicero, IL. where its existence was established by experiment (1962). It is the stimulation to output or accomplishment (as in an industrial education methods study) that results from the

Total number of surveys as of 12-1-95: 152

Age range of patients completing surveys: 1–82

Percentage of males/females completing surveys: 46.7% males/52.6% females

SURVEY QUESTION	POOR—1	FAIR—2	GOOD—3	VERY GOOD—4	EXCELLENT—5
OVERALL VISIT	0	2.1	15.1	30.8	52.1
TECHNICAL SKILLS	0	0.7	7.2	30.3	61.8
PERSONAL MANNERS	0	0.7	7.9	23.2	68.2
APP'T WAIT	3.3	19.9	26.5	23.2	27.2
OFFICE LOCATION	0.7	0.7	20.8	38.3	39.6
TELEPHONE ACCESS	0	0.7	14.2	35.5	49.6
OFFICE WAIT	8.1	18.1	27.5	28.9	17.4
TIME SPENT W/PERSON	0	4	19.5	34.2	42.3
EXPLANATION	0	1.4	11.5	30.4	56.8

FIGURE 14–4. PATIENT SATISFACTION SURVEY RESULTS BAR CODE #89583271

mere fact of being under concerned observation. In other words, the Hawthorne effect is the foundation for Confidential Self Assessment of Quality. Physicians, given the opportunity to benchmark themselves, along with the knowledge of the parameters of measurement, will likely improve once they are aware of their relative positions.

The practicing physician can easily implement a sophisticated benchmarked patient satisfaction survey process as a foundation for an outcomes measurement program, and as a means of measuring continuous customer satisfaction. The 9-item Patient Visit Rating Questionnaire (VRQ) can be customized for the individual practice. The 9 questions, however, should remain the same to permit benchmarking. Physician cooperation in such a venture as Project Solo serves to benefit patients and physicians. It is also a valuable piece of data to utilize in marketing your practice, protecting yourself from inaccurate profiling of third parties, and developing a practice prospectus.

■ Utilizing Outcomes to Market Your Practice

Outcomes can be utilized to market your practice and monitor your business. A scientific outcomes study would employ a general condition survey such as the SF 36™ or HSQ 12, as well as a condition specific survey. Already clearly outlined in this book by Michael Stewart and Richard Rosenfeld, such surveys can be performed by community-based practitioners. Richard Rosenfeld and I addressed the problems and pitfalls of community-based outcomes research in our study about external otitis. Figures 14–5 and 14–6 outline our conclusions.

Within my own office I initially experimented with a less scientific approach to outcomes. I performed a Hearing Aid Business Evaluation, a Post Operative Surgery Evaluation, an Allergy Outcomes Study, and a profiling of my surgical costs compared to other surgeons performing the same procedures at the same facility.

Hearing Aid Business Evaluation

I utilized our benchmarked patient satisfaction survey questions and added some about my hearing aid business. Two hundred and ninety-eight customers who had purchased hearing aids from 1988 to 1995 were surveyed and 22% responded. Ninety-two percent responded that it was important that their hearing aids were dispensed by a board certified ENT and a master's degree audiologist. I discovered that our battery prices were slightly overpriced. I asked patients to identify what type of hearing aid they had purchased to discover if a particular brand was a problem. Sixty-two percent gave an excellent grade to the visit overall, but only 26% rated the product as excellent. I reviewed the hearing aid that had the greatest number of excellent responses. This was useful information and a strong negotiation item with suppliers. By the way, I reported a 62% excellent overall visit response. According to continuous quality improvement, we still have 38% room for improvement! See Figure 14–7 for the actual survey performed.

Postoperative Surgical Facility Evaluation

Another simple outcomes study is a postoperative outcomes sheet. We performed 163 of these over a 13 month-period. There was an overall percentage excellence response of 33%. Our ongoing office patient satisfaction surveys demonstrate a percent excellence of 63%. Therefore, it appeared that my patients' satisfaction declined substantially as they interacted with external variables such as hospital personnel. I am utilizing these results to implement change in these institutions and select the best provider for my patients. I have attempted to do this before. This time, however, I have data. See Figure 14–8 for the actual survey performed.

Allergy Outcomes Study

I listed all the allergy complaints experienced by my patients, assigned them a severity index of 0–5, and asked the patient to fill out a sheet before they started immunotherapy. Six months later they fill out the sheet again. We compiled the results of immunotherapy on 15 different patients over a 6-month period. Their pretreatment severity index was 907 and their post treatment was 408. All but two patients improved. This is certainly not a scientifically valid study. It did not employ the use of a general status survey for comorbidities nor did I measure overall improvement in quality of life or functional status. I did not calculate the effects of antihistamines, nasal sprays, other medications, or surgery. Nonetheless, it is certainly more information than I had before. I am currently implementing a more scientific study utilizing a comorbidity survey. Such a survey will employ a 7-point Likert scale, a 10-point visual analog scale, and certain modifications that make outcomes research practical and meaningful in a busy medical practice. Please see Richard Rosenfeld's excellent chapter in this book for a complete discussion of meaningful outcomes research utilizing these techniques.

Profiling of Surgical Costs

I asked for and received a list of the costs billed to my patients for surgical procedures that I had performed from 7/92 to 12/95. Fortunately, in most cases, my patients were billed less from the hospitals than other patients undergoing the same procedure. See Figures 14–9 and 14–10. In

PROBLEM or PITFALL	*SOLUTION*
1. Benefits of the proposed research are unclear to participants.	PI explains personal and societal benefits of OR with emphasis on current project.
2. Office staff are unmotivated at participating physician offices.	Encourage motivation through enthusiasm, positive feedback, and incentives for patient recruitment.
3. Communication between the PI and the data collection site is inadequate.	Physicians select a member of their staff to serve as site coordinator, who develops a feasible and ongoing contact schedule with PI.
4. Time is unavailable during office hours for completing forms and questionnaires.	PI and site coordinators define data collection methods that interfere least with pt. flow at each office.
5. Data collection at multiple time points is too cumbersome.	Limit initial projects to cross-sectional studies; defer longitudinal studies until experience has been gained.
6. Questionnaires are overly long and complex.	Eliminate all questions tangential to specific hypothesis under study; limit forms to a single page or postcard.
7. Eligible patients are not seen by a physician during the recruitment period.	Define a realistic, seasonally appropriate, recruitment period; add a 10–20% safety margin to sample size estimates.

OR = Outcomes Research
PI = Principal Investigator

FIGURE 14–5. Problems and Pitfalls in Multi-site Community-based Outcomes Research[15] (Reprinted with permission of Mosby-Year Book, Inc.)

Characteristic	*Research by Academic Physician(s)*	*Research by Independent Practitioner(s)*
Publication by volume	Large	Small
Motivation	Career advancement	Self-initiative
Predominant design(s)	Analytical & experimental	Descriptive
Target population	Hospital based	Community based
Outcomes research	Suitability varies	Excellent opportunities
Funding	Difficult, but accessible	Multiple barriers: no IRB
Support staff origin	Department & university	Private practice office
Research time	Dedicated time often available	Intermixed with pt. care
Statistical consultation	Via university	Limited access
Multi-site studies	Difficult	Extremely difficult

IRB = institutional review board
*Differences are intended to reflect broad trends; individual variations occur

FIGURE 14–6. Differences in Research by Academic Physicians and Independent Practitioners.*[15] (Reprinted with permission of Mosby-Year Book, Inc.)

Please answer as indicated:

1. If possible, please indicate the brand & model of the hearing aid you purchased.

BRAND:	MODEL:
46% Telex	12% Behind the ear
23% Starkey	34% Full in the ear
15% Microtech	29% Half size in the canal
0% Rexton	15% In the canal
2% Oticon	2% Completely in canal
5% Unitron	8% Did not know
3% Argosy	
1% ReSound	
3% other (name) ______	
2% Did not know	

2. When did you get your hearing aid and what did it cost?

1988—1
1991—3
1992—7
1993—13
1994—15
1995—11
Did not know—15

Range of prices: $500.00–$1800.00

Average Price: $750.00

3. Do you feel, comparing our price, service, and product quality to other hearing aid dispensers that you received a good value?

(Circle one)

82% Yes   0% No   18% Did not compare

4. Do you use your hearing aid?

98% Yes   2% No

5. If you need new hearing aid(s) or need service on your current aid, would you use us again?

97% Yes   2% No   1% No Response

6. How did you hear about us? (Check one)

45% Dr. Isenberg
9% Friend, relative, "word of mouth"
6% Hospital
25% Family Doctor
5% Walking by
3% Referred by union/employer
7% Other

7. Can you buy Pro-line hearing aid batteries cheaper elsewhere? (Our price is $5.00 for a 4-pack) Circle one:

38% Yes   36% No   26% Did not compare
If yes, what did you pay? $3.50–4.75

8. Our business has Master Degree Audiologists—did this matter to you when you decided to purchase your hearing aid?

92% Yes   6% No   2% No response

Please answer each question by placing a check under the most appropriate response:

	poor	fair	good	excellent	no response
a. Rate the quality & performance of the hearing aid you bought.	4%	8%	62%	26%	0%
b. How long you waited for an appointment.	0%	5%	49%	40%	6%
c. Convenience of ofc location	0%	4%	54%	42%	0%
d. Getting through to the office by phone.	0%	0%	56%	42%	2%
e. Length of time waiting at the office.	0%	3%	54%	43%	0%
f. Time spent with the person you saw.	0%	0%	40%	58%	2%
g. Explanation of what was done for you.	0%	2%	38%	55%	5%
h. The technical skills (thoroughness, carefulness, competence) of the person you saw.	0%	0%	34%	66%	0%
i. The personal manner (courtesy, respect, sensitivity, friendliness) of the person you saw.	0%	0%	27%	71%	2%
j. The visit overall.	0%	0%	36%	62%	2%

(65 of 298 Surveys were returned. A 22% return rate.)

FIGURE 14–7. PHYSICIAN'S HEARING SERVICE Patient Satisfaction Survey

Satisfaction Survey

For Office Use Only

Date: | || | | || |

Month Day

Location: | || |

Please fill this out, fold it, and return to Dr. Steven F. Isenberg's office. Thank you.

Please consider your recent surgery and answer the following questions by circling the number in each line.

	Poor	Fair	Good	Very Good	Excellent
1) How long you waited to get an appointment	1	2	3	4	5
2) Convenience of the location of the office	1	2	3	4	5
3) Getting through to our office by phone	1	2	3	4	5
4) Length of time waiting at the office	1	2	3	4	5
5) Time spent with the person you saw	1	2	3	4	5
6) Explanation of what was done for you	1	2	3	4	5
7) The technical skills (thoroughness, carefulness, competence) of the person you saw	1	2	3	4	5
8) The personal manner (courtesy, respect, sensitivity, friendliness) of the person you saw	1	2	3	4	5
9) The visit overall	1	2	3	4	5
10) In general, would you say your health is	1	2	3	4	5

11) Are you (patient) male or female? Male Female

12) How old were you (patient) on your last birthday? (write in) | || | years

Comments:

Adapted with the permission of American Association of Health Plans

FIGURE 14–8.

STEVEN F. ISENBERG, M.D.

Outpatient Procedure Efficiency

COMMUNITY HOSPITALS

7/92 - 12/95

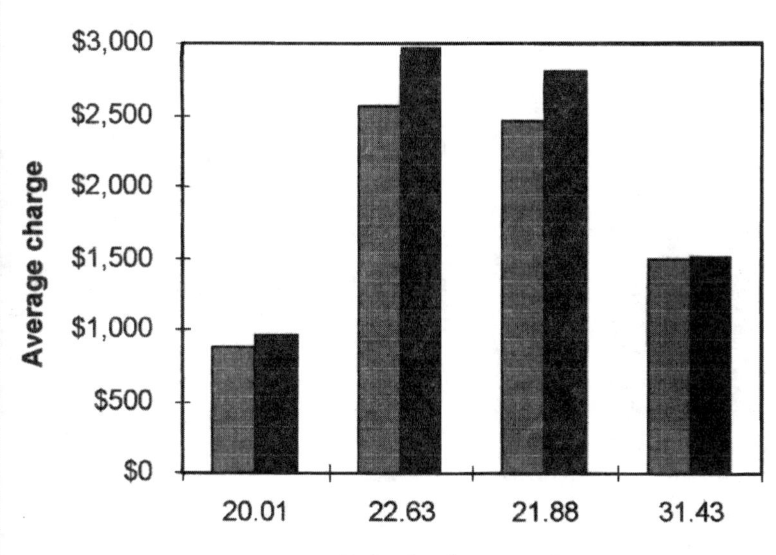

Procedure	Description	# Cases: Dr. Isenberg
20.01	Myringotomy w/insertion of tube	510
22.63	Ethmoidectomy	198
21.88	Other septoplasty	137
31.43	Closed biopsy of larynx	117

Q3, Inc.

FIGURE 14–9. STEVEN F. ISENBERG, M.D. Outpatient Procedure Efficiency

STEVEN F. ISENBERG, M.D.

Outpatient Procedure Efficiency

HOSPITAL CHARGES

7/92 - 12/95

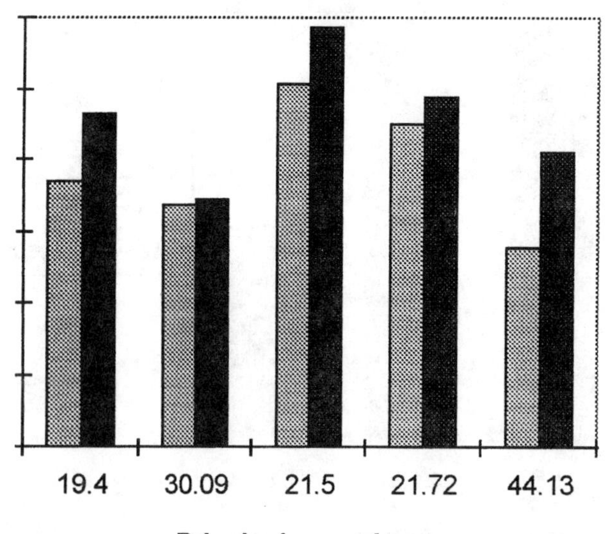

Procedure	Description	# Cases: Dr. Isenberg
19.4	Myringoplasty	75
30.09	Other excision of larynx	50
21.5	Submucous resection of nasal septum	47
21.72	Open reduction of nasal fracture	46
44.13	Other gastroscopy	31

Q3, Inc.

FIGURE 14–10. STEVEN F. ISENBERG, M.D. Outpatient Procedure Efficiency

all cases, particularly those where my patients' costs were the same or higher, I have implemented a process of reviewing my procedures. This includes:

- Checking on my surgical preference card to remove costly items that are not necessary.
- Restructuring my pre and postoperative orders and discharge criteria to reduce expenses whenever possible.
- Monitoring the use of expensive drugs and supplies.

The Practice Prospectus

My practice prospectus includes:

- Menu of services provided; my board certifications.
- Patient satisfaction benchmarked to peer group and national statistics.
- Outcomes studies, both business and clinical, e.g., hearing aid survey, allergy surveys, outpatient facility evaluation, and patient's satisfaction surveys are mentioned and available if requested.
- Continuous quality improvement practices.
- Profiling of my costs and efforts made to reduce costs.
- Free parking (very important to patients and employers).
- Preventive health programs e.g., anti-smoking.

A practice prospectus is made available to third party payers, employers in your area, and the media. I limited what I put on my practice prospectus. For example, I did not have the space, and I felt it "too much" and "too cluttered" to list my practice mission and vision statements. I also did not include office maps, office hours, e-mail address, or insurance plans accepted. These can be included in the patient pamphlet that you give to patients. The practice prospectus is different from a patient pamphlet. It is sent to *businesspeople* who are interested in continuous quality improvement, costs, and results. If you feel that you provide cost-effective quality care, then you should pose this question in your prospectus: "If your health plan or referral network does not include (your name), MD, shouldn't you ask why? (Fig. 14–11a, b) If you need help profiling your practice, please see Susan Bellile's chapter in this book.

■ Total Quality Management in a Community-Based Practice

Earlier in this chapter, I outlined how Deming's emphasis on product quality and customer focus revitalized American industry. In addition to Deming, at least two other quality gurus have influenced American business. Philip Crosby advocated a system of quality improvement that focuses on prevention rather that appraisal. The cornerstone of Crosby's quality improvement process is the commitment of top management. In our practices, of course, we *are* the top management. Dr. Joseph M. Juran emphasizes quality improvement by systematically selecting projects and working on them. Juran identified the required elements of a system to measure, design, and select processes that consistently deliver superior outcomes. He named this system *total quality management,* or *TQM.* I have found that such an approach is possible to accomplish in a busy practice. Finally, no discussion of quality in a medical practice is complete without the input of Dr. Donald Berwick.[16] The Japanese, Berwick writes, call the continuous search for opportunities for all processes to get better, *Kaizen.*[17] The epigram "Every defect is a treasure" captures this spirit. It is in such a spirit that community-based physicians must manage their practices. My search for continuous quality improvement in the office is outlined below.

- Quality commitment must come from the physicians. This cannot be considered another "program of the year."
- The office must have a mission and vision statement incorporating a continuous commitment to quality.
- The customer must be the focus. Outcomes studies such as patient satisfaction surveys and documentation of clinical outcomes must be a priority.
- Focus on the process, not the people. Problems are usually built directly into complex processes such as those that are performed in the medical office. With the philosophy that "every defect is a treasure" assume that people are already trying hard and focus everyone as a team effort to improve process failures. Please read chapter 10 by Nelson et. al., on improving health care. Implementing and measuring change on behalf of quality improvement and cost containment is possible in a busy practice. A summary of this technique is listed below:

  Find a process to improve
  Organize a team that knows the process
  Clarify current knowledge of the process
  Understand sources of process variation
  Select the process improvement
  *P*lan a change or test
  *D*o carry out the change
  *C*heck and observe the effects of the change
  *A*ct, adopt or modify the plan

Remember that change is important in continuous quality improvement. Outcomes, as I mentioned earlier, are very useful. However, they only provide knowledge about what is currently happening; they do not intrinsically inform us how to make things better.

- Involve your employees. Three different "types" of quality have been described.[18] *One-Dimensional Quality*

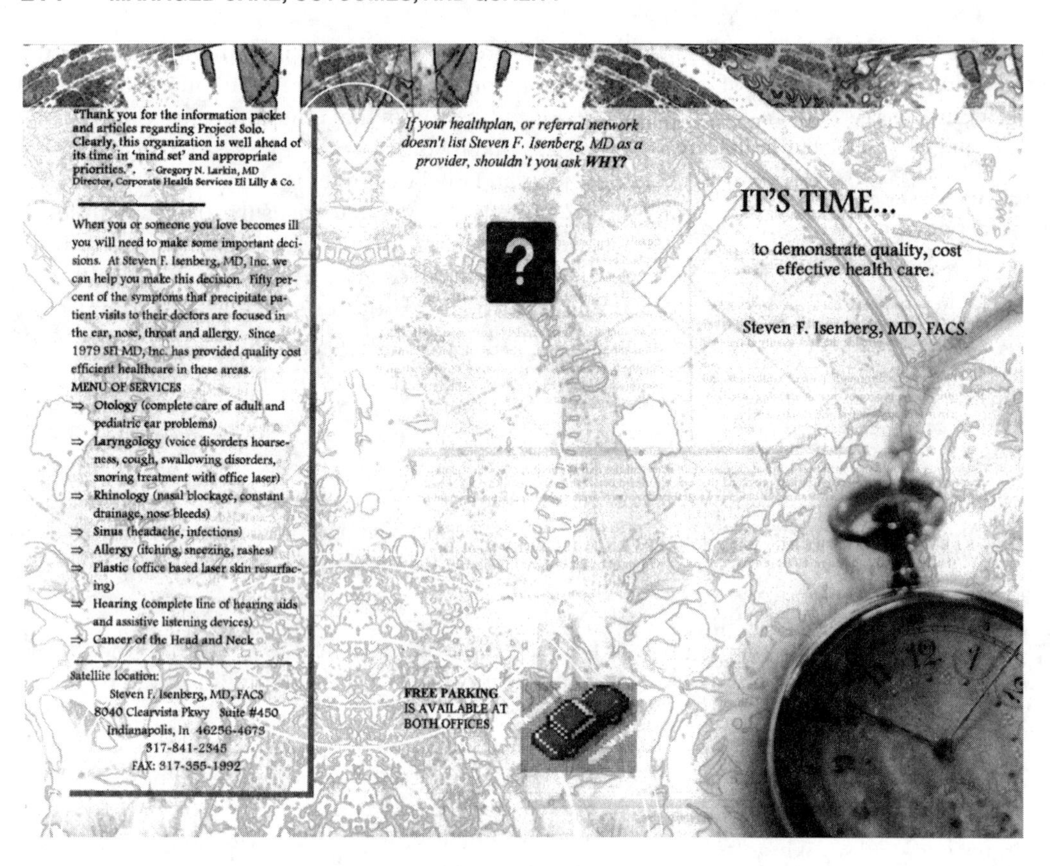

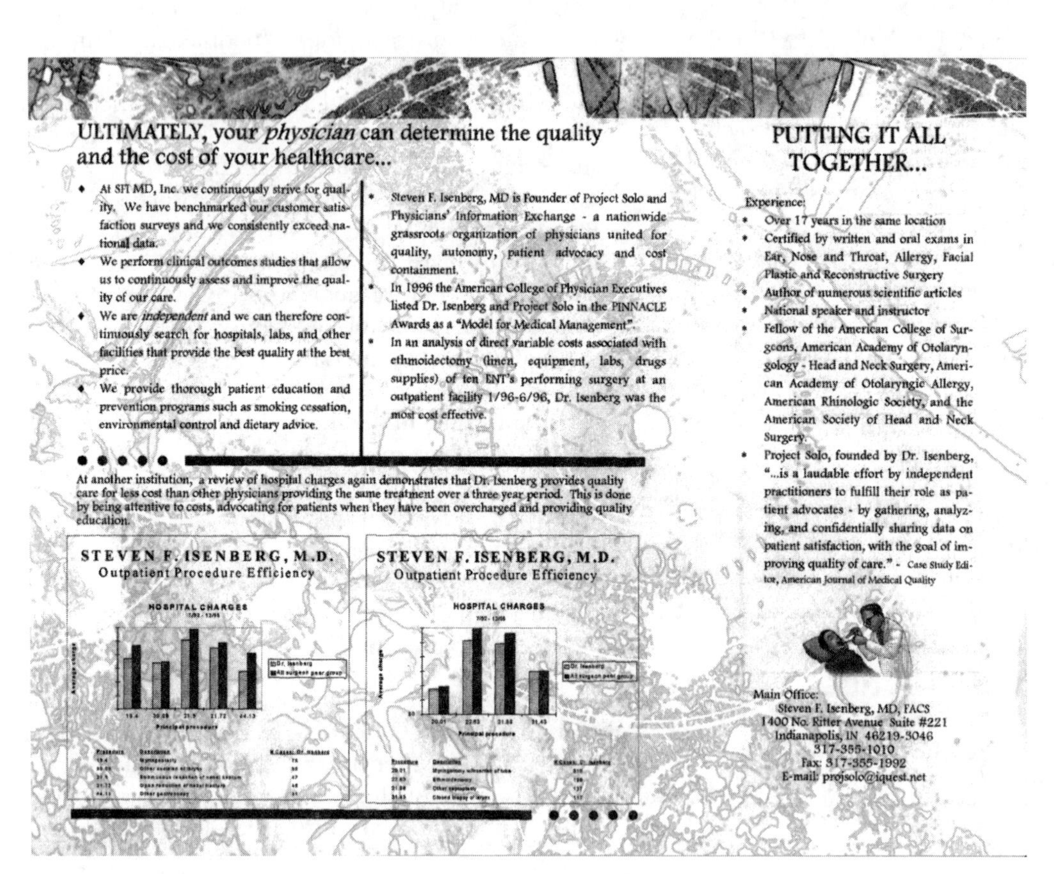

FIGURE 14–11a, b. IT'S TIME . . . to demonstrate quality, cost effective health care.

is what patients will ask for when they are questioned. *Must be or expected quality* is not voiced by patients (e.g., they do not expect to get a hospital-acquired infection). The most interesting quality is *unexpected quality*. In this situation, patients do not vocalize their desire for it, but, if it is provided, they are particularly pleased. Examples include soft drinks in the reception area when the doctor is delayed, or intervening on behalf of patients to reduce or eliminate incorrect hospital charges. I strongly encourage my employees at staff meetings to offer unexpected quality programs. The benefits are pervasive throughout the practice.

- Employee training includes an emphasis on continuous quality improvement. Employees teach TQM to subordinates or peers via a "training cascade."
- Benchmarking:

  This is a key element in TQM. Xerox, 1979, called it "a continuous process of measuring production services, practice against . . . the leaders."

To answer my need for benchmarking, I expanded Project Solo into Physician's Information Exchange (PIE). Utilizing DOCSHARE, our confidential practice management data exchange, physicians in PIE are periodically surveyed about such questions as:

Percentage overhead
Number of employees
Percentage managed care
Software utilized
Number of patients seen per week
Experience with managed care contracting, IPAS, provider service networks

These are just a few of the benchmarking questions that are compiled by PIE. The recent rulings on per se antitrust violations and physician information gathering promise to possibly expand PIE's ability to help with benchmarking. See Figure 14–12 for a portion of a

Percentage overhead	*Managed Care %*	*Employees Full/part time*	*# pat's per week*	*Software*	*Barcode #*
44%	95%	9/1	120	Med One	10957208
50%	40%	2/2	150	Med Mgr	09225595
52%	20%	3/1	75	Lytec	10076195
44%	59%	13	255	C.D.S.	08275295
62%	80%	9/4	120	Med One	10045895
40%	20%	4/1	71	M.O.M.S.	09015395
37%	70%	1/4	115	Med Mgr	42183478
NA	25%	3/1	75	Windows	03027396
32%	5%	4/1	70	Med Mac	92772173
36%	0%	6/1	140	Versys	10206795
50%	15%	6	200	Versys	18267861
50%	20%	10/1	80	P.C.N.	03197496
50%	20%	10/1	65	P.C.N.	49103452
36%	70%	2/1	75	Medic	18434111
54%	35%	8/22	130	Medic	02067296
NA	45%	2/1	—	Medisoft	69508745
61%	15%	8/1	250	ABS Med	10055995
55%	15%	10	35	I.D.X.	82124232
52%	40%	2/2	75	Medisoft	10316895
70%	70%	4/2	112	Med Mgr	29798226
51%	20%	7	180	Micro D.	10025695
65%	95%	7	110	Windows	63215028
45%	25%	2/2	60	Med Mgr	17834335
57%	60%	10/1	200	Elcomp	31876358
58%	30%	14/2	250	Medic	10066095
41%	2%	5/4	—	Med Mac	37289589
40%	60%	6/2	250	M.S.M.	10875431

FIGURE 14–12.

sample business survey performed by PIE. The results were obtained by fax within 48 hours with over 70% of the physicians responding. Since PIE has complete demographic information on each member, expanding membership will potentially permit physicians to compare practices with very similar demographics, practice style, specialty, and personal profile. The future is bright with the information exchange capabilities of the internet.

- *Profiling.* Gathering information from physician vendors such as hospitals, surgery centers, laboratories, and radiology facilities permits us to know how our patients are being charged for the services we order. Total Quality Management includes management of both intrinsic and extrinsic processes.
- *Recognition/reward.* TQM should result in rewards to the practice and those who continuously implement it within the practice. Linking employee bonuses to overall patient satisfaction and business performance as measured with the benchmarked data is a very profitable and innovative way of rewarding employees. Employees who design, implement, and measure unexpected quality improvements in the practice should be featured in practice newsletters, bulletin boards, and trade publications.

The precise details of the multifaceted management of today's community-based medical practice are presented later in this chapter. A number of excellent advisors are available, some of whom I will reference and others who have written chapters in this book. Total Quality Management with continuous quality improvement is a realistic goal for every community based practitioner. Early progress with TQM might be slow, and it is often easy to forget the continuous part of continuous quality improvement. Nonetheless, with patients as allies and quality as the focus, the community-based independent practitioner is totally equipped to survive in any health care marketplace.

Practice Management for the Independent Practitioner

"Every system is perfectly designed to get the results it gets."

As Stephen Plume has stated, this dictum attests to the wisdom that people do exactly and only what makes sense in their context. Therefore, as I outline my office procedures in this managed care environment, I am aware that many differences exist regionally, professionally, and among a wide variety of practice styles. I know that my "perfectly designed system" often yields imperfect results. It might serve, however, to allow you to "tweak" some part of your system toward improvement. You are always welcome to share some of your expertise with me.

Patient Management Services

Patient management is *the* most important part of medical practice management. According to research done by the Technical Assistance Research Project (TARP) Washington, DC, 1985, the average consumer tells 5 other people about a positive experience and 20 other people about a negative experience. Delphi Forecasts reported that 45% of urban and rural customers depend on word-of-mouth recommendations from family and friends.[19] Certainly the management of referring physicians, office accounts, managed care contracts, employees, and facility and operations management is important. Patient management services, however, are the key factor in continuous quality improvement. They serve as the heart that pumps a community-based practice.

Managing Patients

- *Practice pamphlets* should provide a menu of your services, your office hours, maps, parking instructions, and your qualifications. Don't leave out your honors, publications, and involvement in medical research (remember, performing patient satisfaction surveys is researching an expanded measure of outcomes).
- *Newsletters* are difficult to do quarterly. Establish a template using your word processing program and attempt a newsletter twice a year. Include topics of medical information pertinent to your practice. Focus on prevention—it is good quality care and very popular with patients and payers.
- *Telephone*
  - Answer over the lunch hour—many parents and patients can only call then.
  - Answer by the third ring; if you have a temporary staffing problem, take a line off the hook before you make people wait on hold.
  - Answer "Thank you for calling Dr. ________'s office. This is ______. How may I help you?"
  - Ask your phone company to perform a busy signal study and adjust your number of lines accordingly.
  - Voicemail is a nice option for referring doctors and business calls, not for patients.
  - Message while waiting on hold is a reasonable marketing technique. Emphasize services that your patients might not otherwise know: hearing aids, laser skin resurfacing, patient satisfaction analyses, free parking, credit cards, and the major payers that you accept.
- *Patient Call Back Sheet.* I instituted these several years ago. A forgotten lab report is a frequent cause for malpractice suits. The failure to call a report to a patient or miss carcinoma is a process failure. Study this carefully within your practice. Implementing change in this area is challenging because it involves outside

vendors. I have my staff attach a patient call back sheet to *every* lab report. It is then put on my desk. The sheet includes an area for *my* interpretation of the results, a written summary of what the patient should be told, and a space to report the patient's questions. These are always attached to the chart. (See Fig. 14–13) I will phone the same patients personally, but all patients are told that I will discuss the results with them if they wish. I rarely see patients abuse this. They are usually very pleased just to hear the results. Some offices have been able to design a process whereby lost lab results can be discovered. This requires a log of anticipated reports.

- *Patient Visit/Referral Letters.* Send thank you notes or letters to patients following the initial visit and to previous patients who referred someone to your practice.
- *Patient Incident Reports.* Creating an incident report file is very valuable in an office striving for TQM. These reports, embraced by the NCQA and MCOs, can be used to analyze the process of care and provide continuous efforts at improving customer satisfaction. They should be logged in, efforts at improvement noted, and kept in a file. Remember, TQM emphasizes addressing the processes, not the particular employees in your practice.
- *Employee–Patient Interaction*
  - The patient (customer) pays the staff. Link staff bonuses to overall excellent response percentage of your nationally benchmarked patient satisfaction survey process.
  - Implement employee nametags and uniform codes.

PATIENT NAME: ____________________

TEST PERFORMED: ____________________

DATE TEST PERFORMED: ____________________

NAME OF TESTING CENTER: ____________________

1) Dr. Isenberg's Interpretation: ____________________

2) What does Dr. Isenberg think should be done next? ____________________

3) Questions from the patient: ____________________

4) Results sent to PCP from test facility? YES NO
Results sent/faxed to PCP by ____________ (initials) Date: ____________

Signature of person calling the patient: ____________________

Date: ____________ Time called: ____________

FIGURE 14–13. PATIENT TEST RECALL SHEET

Always preserve patient confidentiality. Employees should know that this is an absolute requirement. They should sign a very clear statement that outlines the office's strict adherence to patient confidentiality.

Initially address patients as Mr., Mrs., Ms. Later, employees may ask permission to use the patient's first name.

Employees dealing with angry customers should listen and DO NOT INTERRUPT; thank the patient for bringing this to someone's attention; repeat the complaint as voiced by the patient; resolve that the problem will be promptly investigated while establishing a realistic time to respond; do not become defensive; accept anger, remain calm, and attempt to reach some kind of agreement.

You must attend your staff meetings. Total Quality Management and Continuous Quality Improvement *require the physician leader* to lead everyone in the practice. There should never be any doubt about the quest for 100% excellence. If the physician leader does not attend the staff meetings to emphasize the importance of quality, your practice will not achieve its potential.

- Scheduling

  Block off time when you're out. Rescheduling patients is costly and disruptive.

  Allow adequate time to process new patients. Liability can result from failure to inquire about allergies, family histories, etc.

  Set time aside for emergencies.

  Make sure the staff thanks the patient for scheduling an appointment.

  If a patient calls to cancel, reschedule while the person is on the phone.

  If you're running late, have your receptionist tell patients what is happening, and give an estimate of the waiting time.

- Maintaining Records

  Document missed or canceled appointments. If a follow-up is critical, document efforts to contact the patient. This problem can be solved by requiring your staff to give you all the charts from the day, both those seen and the no-shows.

  Document a no-show in the chart next to the date. Keep medical records indefinitely.

  Are your medical records organized? Are they identified by name/number, separate section for visits, diagnostic tests, referrals?

  Establish a filing/tracking system within the office (note that Cheryl Toth suggests assigning this to one person).

  Do you have an individual chart for each patient; are all entries legible; author identified, dated, each page with patient name?

- Physician–Patient Relationship

  Stay on time. Consider developing an average time that you spend with patients for individual presenting main symptoms. Give this to your receptionist or anyone else who schedules office appointments. See Figure 14–14.

  Note personal items of interest on the patient's chart such as previous family members or friends whom you have seen, employment information, unique hobbies pursued by your patient, or other items of personal interest. Sometimes these notes can actually help make a diagnosis.

  Physician-supervised cost containment. Whenever possible, intervene on behalf of your patient to reduce or eliminate unnecessary charges that your patient incurred as a result of a process failure at the hospital, lab, radiology facility, pharmacy, or your own practice.

  Follow the four "E's".[20]

  Engage—open-ended questions; patients rarely exceed 60-second answers; list the complaints; identify and tell which be treated now.

Procedure	Time in Minutes
Allergy Testing, skin endpoint	90
ABR	30
ENG	45
Flexible nasopharyngoscopy	15
Packing or suture removal	15
Minor surgery (lesion bx/tubes)	30–60
Office visits	
Brief	5–10
Intermediate (for acute illness)	15–20
Extended	30+
Patient teaching conference	30–60
Epistaxis	15–30
Second opinion	15–30
Hospital admission from office	30
Post op tube check	5

*The times given are approximate and may be adjusted to accommodate patient needs.

FIGURE 14–14. GUIDE TO ESTIMATE TIMES FOR COMMON MEDICAL OFFICE PROCEDURES*

Empathize—use the patient's name and maintain eye contact. I also would suggest sitting down whenever possible.
Educate—patients forget 40 to 60% and follow treatment only 50% of the time.
Enlist—patient repeats the plan; negotiate with patient to achieve goals.

■ Managing Referral Services

- Identify your best referral sources and let your staff know. They are the "gold card" referral sources and they therefore deserve "gold card" treatment such as: direct access to your voicemail; the opportunity to have patients seen sooner ; the opportunity to interrupt your meetings, other phone calls, and even patient exams if they have been informed.
- On-site visits. Attend open houses; send your key authorization person to your key referring doctor offices with breakfast to meet their staff.
- Send your referring doctors your newsletter, patient pamphlets, maps, appointment pads, and results of your outcomes studies, including patient satisfaction surveys.
- Send your referring doctors your practice prospectus, information about your honors and awards, and updates from meetings that you have attended.

■ Employee Management

- Consult a reference on this topic. There are many potential pitfalls that can be avoided by consulting a reference. (Also see Chapters 12 and 13 concerning this topic.)
- Job descriptions should define job duties, interactions with other positions, compensation, and benefits. They help recruiting and appraising performance.
- When hiring, check all references after obtaining a signed statement from the applicant authorizing former employers to supply information. Promise all employers providing information that everything is kept confidential. Fax the signed statement to the employer.
- When hiring, ask the applicant to *hand write* a spontaneous paragraph on "Why I want to work for this medical practice."
- Employee handbook—defines fringe benefits such as vacation and sick leave. It also outlines unacceptable actions and consequences. Handbooks can be viewed as enforceable employee contracts.
- Along with everything else, *the physician is responsible.* The physician employer can he held liable for exposing other patients/employees to a negligent employee. The physician employer can also be held liable for failing to deal with a negligent employee in a practice who might cause harm.
- Again, *consult a reference.* Labor law is quite complicated and a potential problem for a medical practice. The appropriate reference, however, can keep you out of trouble.
- Employee motivation. Arte Maren, a motivational speaker based in Los Angeles, emphasizes the importance of regularly scheduled staff meetings instead of crisis meetings. Staff meetings are very important:
  The physician must attend. As the practice leader, the physician must emphasize the importance and the continuous nature of continuous quality improvement.
  Ask employees to bring suggestion for "unexpected quality" additions to the practice. Staff members from all levels can be energized by this challenge.
  As mentioned earlier, link employee bonuses to overall percentage excellence patient responses as compared to benchmarked national surveys.

Cost Based Pricing→Price Based Costing

Medical practices can no longer raise prices to cover costs. We must now secure a profit from the fees we are paid. This requires improved business management.

Create a Yearly Budget (Fig. 14–15).

- Record collections and spending.
- Project how much can be spent per category in the next year.
- Plan an acceptable level of income.
- Account for seasonal variations.
- Differentiate costs: *variable* (vary with the number of patients seen) and *fixed* (remain the same despite the number of patients seen).
- Benchmark with some group to obtain national statistics. (The Medical Group Management Association, the AMA, and Physicians' Information Exchange 1-317-355-1010.)

Purchasing

- Obtain suggestions from your employees about methods to reduce purchasing costs.
- Ask vendors for "hospital prices."
- Order generics.
- Order (in bulk) nonsterile, loose, multipacked dry goods.
- Buy at year end.
- Get at least 2% discount for paying in 10 days.

Outsourcing

- Payroll service—usually cheaper when outsourced.
- Work with collections agencies that have a set fee.

	1996	*1997*	*% Change*	*1998*	*Initial Budget*	*Final Budget*	*% of Revenue*
Net collections							
Acct/legal							
Contribution							
Dues/subscr							
Equip rental							
General							
Insurance							
Health Ins.							
Malprac Ins.							
Lab fees							
Janitorial							
Medical supplies							
Office supplies							
Rent/lease							
Salaries							
Taxes—payroll							
Taxes—other							
Telephone							
Postage							
Maintenance repair							
Interest							
Depreciation							
Prof svcs.							
Profit sharing							
Other							
Total expenses							
Net Income							

FIGURE 14–15. BUDGET PLANNING WORKSHEET

- If you outsource billing, be sure that managed care billings and payments are tracked by individual plans.
- Get a bid on employee leasing as an option.

Postage

- Buy the machine; you must rent the meter.
- Investigate bulk mailing options in your area.

Insurance

- Put malpractice insurance out to bid.
- Separate health insurance policies for physicians from employees. Nonphysician employees may fit lower profiles with lower costs.
- Challenge unemployment insurance claims.
- Raise the deductible for employee health insurance and provide deductible assistance as a benefit.
- Raise the deductible on office insurance.

Inventory Control

- Formula (variables):
  1. Widgets used in a 30-day period [100].
  2. Time between order and receipt [15 days].
  3. Quantity needed during the time period in #2 [50].
  4. You should order when you have 150 widgets in stock.
  5. "Tag" your last box of 100 "*order now*"
- Ordering Log

  Date ordered

  Quantity

  Cost/item

  Always cross check packing slips with order log entries; check monthly statements with packing slips

Bartering

- If you are inclined, write to the International Reciprocal Trade Association, 9513 Beach Mill Road, Falls Church, VA 22066, 703-916-9020.

Utilities

- Ask your local utility companies to help you reduce costs. *This service is usually free.*

Legal and Accounting

- Ask for quarterly statements instead of monthly ones.
- Do in-house accounting as much as possible; utilize accountant for audit and theft control.
- Review your managed care contracts before you send them to an attorney. Ask for specific answers to specific questions. Get an estimate.
- Sign all checks; limit credit card usage to key people; examine canceled checks with the envelope unopened.

Service Contracts

- Eliminate service contracts on fax machines, telephones, personal computers, calculators, and high quality laser printers.
- No long-term service contracts.
- No automatic renewals.

Petty Cash

- Not to be used for cashing checks.
- Every disbursement must have a signed receipt.
- Use a disbursement form to track.
- One person is in charge.
- No borrowing.

General

- Yellow pages advertising is very expensive. Study how effective it is in your practice.
- If you are a corporation, insist on corporate rates for rental cars, hotel rooms, etc.

Control Employee Expenses

- Use time clocks.
- Stagger hours to increase office coverage and decrease overtime.
- Hire "prn" help for peak daytime or seasonal needs and for data entry.
- Assign jobs for off peak hours; e.g., audiology receptionist—appointment reminder calls; medical assistant—filing.
- Link bonuses to overall patient satisfaction percent excellence as compared to benchmarked national data.

You Are the Revenue

- Focus on patient care.
- Stay off the phone.
- Stay on time—post a guide to estimate times for common medical office procedures (Fig. 14–14) near your scheduling phones. Meet with your scheduling people to review this guide along with a printout of the coming week schedule. If anyone can predict an overscheduled or an underscheduled office, it is probably the physician who sees the patients.
- Assign the correct ICD-9 codes in the correct order of importance as well as the appropriate CPT codes for the services you perform.
- Write down or provide the patient with written instructions.
- Attend your staff meetings. Total Quality Management relies on the physician leader to be the leading cheerleader for quality at all times.

Tracking Revenues

- It is essential to track and analyze how much each managed care company individually contributes to your revenue. This should be cross referenced with your managed care contract and the appropriate agreed on fee schedule to verify that you are being compensated as contracted. See Chapter 15 about selecting the appropriate data management system for your practice.

Monitor Your Business

- Determine a patient cost analysis (Fig. 14–16.) Note that this uses only variable expenses. *Variable* expenses are those expenses that vary with patient volume, such as office supplies, X-ray supplies, patient treatment supplies. *Fixed* expenses do not vary with patient volume (rent, equipment leases, taxes, utilities, etc.)
- Monitor practice growth and profitability. Use Table 14–1 as a guide.
- Just as you track practice growth and profitability, it is also helpful to keep a quarterly statistics form (Fig. 14–17).

Revenues per RVU are shown in (Figure 14–18). First, create a grid of your most common CPT codes multiplied by the RBRVS units and the frequency billed in a one-year period. Then calculate your total charges for those CPTs, adjust with your collection percentage, and divide by the total RVUs calculated in your grid.

Accounts Receivable

- Inform patients of the practices' financial policy when they make the appointment and when they receive their appointment reminder call. Put the policy in written form.
- The policy should be in the Practice Brochure, New Patient Information forms and the reception area.

I. Patient Cost Analysis

1. Total number of patients seen in prior 12 months
2. Total of all expenses in prior 12 months
3. Subtract from line 2 all fixed expenses
4. Total patients expenses for prior 12 months
5. Total receipts for prior 12 months
6. Divide line 5 by line 1 to get gross revenue per patient
7. Divide line 4 by line 1 to get cost per patient
8. Subtract line 7 from line 6 to get revenue per patient

Example:

Patient Cost Analysis

1. Total number of patients seen in prior 12 months 6,000.00
2. Total of all expenses in prior 12 months 279,000.00
3. Subtract from line 2 all fixed expenses 179,000.00
4. Total patients expenses for prior 12 months 100,000.00
5. Total receipts for prior 12 months 479,000.00
6. Divide line 5 by line 1 to get gross revenue per patient 80.00
7. Divide line 4 by line 1 to get cost per patient 16.00
8. Subtract line 7 from line 6 to get revenue per patient 64.00

FIGURE 14–16. Patient cost analysis

TABLE 14–1. Growth Monitor

	Goal	*Current Month*	*Prev. Month*	*Year-to-Date*
Total Billings:				
Collections				
Collections %				
Total A/R				
A/R Monthly				
Expense ratio (total nonphys expenses ÷ total gross chgs)				
Profit <loss>				
Net income % (total net income ÷ collections)				
New patients				
Total new patient visits				

QUARTERLY STATISTICS FORM: MONTHS ________ YEAR ________

TOTAL CHARGES	
ADJUSTMENTS	
NET CHARGES	
TOTAL RECEIPTS	
ADJUSTMENTS	
NET RECEIPTS	
TOTAL PATIENTS SEEN	
DAILY AVERAGE	
COLLECTION RATIO	
ACCOUNTS RECEIVABLE	
AVERAGE PER PATIENT CHARGE	
AVERAGE PER PATIENT COST	
TOTAL MONTHLY EXPENSE	
NET INCOME	

FIGURE 14–17. Quarterly Statistics Form

Total Charges	\$1,000,000.00
Total collection	\$ 750,000.00
Total expenses (nonphysician)	\$ 300,000.00

Total RVU's =RBRV's × frequency=20,000

$$\text{Collection \%} = \frac{\text{Total collections}}{\text{Total charges} - \text{Adjustments}} = \frac{750{,}000}{1{,}000{,}000} = 75\%$$

$$\text{Expense per RVU} = \frac{\text{Non physician expense}}{\text{Total RVUs}} = \frac{300{,}000}{20{,}000} = \$15/\text{unit}$$

$$\text{Revenue per RVU} = \frac{\text{Collections}}{\text{Total RVUs}} = \frac{750{,}000}{20{,}000} = \%50 = \$37.50/\text{per RVU}$$

$$\text{Charges per RVU} = \frac{\text{Total charges}}{\text{Total RVUs}} = \frac{1{,}000{,}000}{20{,}000} = \$50/\text{RVU}$$

Negotiate managed care contract pricing between \$37.50 and \$50.00 per RVU. If < \$37.50 you will lose; if > \$37.50 you are a winner.

Negotiate higher amount for your most frequent CPTs!

FIGURE 14–18. Revenues per RVU

- Collect at the time of service. Collect co-pays at the time of service. Most managed care contracts obligate the physicians' office to collect co-pays.
- At least 90% of A/R should be 30 days or less. (May Schwartz specializes in this area; see Sources at the end of this chapter.)
- Establish a written collection policy. All accounts over 120 days go to a collection agency.
- Calculate a monthly collection ratio:

$$\frac{\text{Total collections}}{\text{Total charges} - \text{Adjustments}} = \text{Collection ratio}$$

Example:

Total charges:	$60,000.00
Total collections:	$40,000.00
Total adjustments:	$10,000.00
A/R:	$10,000.00

$$\frac{40}{60 - 10} = \frac{40}{50} = 80\%$$

Accounts Payable

- Never pay bills from a vendor's statement; always pay from an invoice attached to the check. Coordinate packing slips with invoices.
- Create a vendor by company name.
- Compare vendor prices frequently.
- Avoid rush orders.
- Create an inventory list of everything in the office.

Payroll

- Each employee should complete a new IRS W-2 each calendar year.
- All payroll records are confidential.
- Link bonuses to overall patient satisfaction; give small raises, higher bonuses.

Facility and Operations Management

Facility Management

Cleveland Clinic Foundation (Frank Weaver, Division of Public Affairs, 1986) lists five environmental factors that particularly affect patient satisfaction:

1. Cleanliness of the facility
2. Condition of the building
3. Ease of finding your way
4. Size of the facility
5. Surrounding neighborhood

Wait for 5 minutes in your own "reception area." Is it

Clean?
Comfortable? No shared armrests?
Tastefully decorated?
Like a living room?
Is the upholstery in good condition?
Are there table lamps instead of fluorescent lighting?
Are there educational videos?
TV, artwork?
Are facing seats 8 feet apart?
Are magazines current?

Business office

Uncluttered?
Clear glass window to ensure confidentiality?

Exam rooms

Soundproof?
Clean?
Hazardous items safely stored?
Prescription pads and syringes kept out of sight?

Operations Management

Office Policies

Medical records—what we charge for records; how we deal with records on unpaid accounts; how we charge for disability claims; legal requests, insurance company requests not related to a claim we have filed.
Release of information—must have a signed release from the patient.
Documentation—*all* conversations with dates and times.
Telephone advice—who is authorized, how does the physician know what was said.
Telephone technique.
Scheduling.
Lab results (check 50 charts randomly)—any not called?
Referrals/consults (top referring docs?).
Patient instructions.
Patient confidentiality.
Medication storage and dispensing.

Emergency

Each staff member's responsibility.
CPR certification of office staff.
Fire extinguisher visible, accessible, and fire disaster evacuation plan written out.
Oxygen supply if medically indicated.

General

Bloodborne Pathogens Exposure Control Plan
OSHA Record Keeping and Posting
OSHA Personal Protective Equipment
Hazard Communication and Training

Reception

Greet patients by name (Mr., Ms.).
Have all patients sign in.

Complete a patient information sheet.
Superbill attached.
See driver's license; insurance card; copy each.
Renew membership card at each visit to see changes.
Reconfirm telephone numbers and addresses.

EXAMPLE:

- Tina will make all new appointments. If Tina is not available, Heather will make new appointments. All new appointments are reviewed by Tina.
- Tina will keep a cancellation list.
- New patients are allotted 25 minutes.
- Routine follow-up appointments are allotted 5 minutes (e.g., tube check) to 20 minutes (f/u cancer, dizzy, sinus). See Guide to Estimate Time for Procedures.
- Allergy office visits are allotted 10 minutes.
- All patients are reminded of office payment policy; need to collect co-pays the day of the visit; need to bring authorization for visit; insurance card. Request 48-hour cancellation.
- Each day a copy of the day's appointments are posted in the back office.
- For each appointment, list: name of patient, phone number, age (if a child), chief complaint, new or old pt, work number (OK to call @ work?), car phone; pager. Special requests such as confidentiality.

Software

- Refer to Chapter 12 in this book, "Improving Office Efficiency in a Managed Care Environment."
- Software must provide quick access to managed care plan data.
- Software is needed to analyze managed care discounted fee-for-service offers and capitation offers.
- Software helps to track managed care results.
- You need a system to analyze outcomes and develop cost-of-service profile.
- Information needs of front and back office (Table 14–2):
  Do we participate?
  Authorizations?
  Co-pays?
  Deductibles?
  Number of visits authorized?

The Contract

I am not an attorney. However, good business requires all of us to do our homework before we seek legal advice. Before you send a contract to an attorney, ask yourself these questions:

General Clause:

- The law of endless servitude: will it automatically become part of a new plan? How will I know? Will I be dropped from the entire plan if I refuse? Will the fee

TABLE 14–2.

MANAGED CARE INFORMATION SHEET

Name of the Plan____________________
Special Plan ID #________________ Authorization required? Yes No

Referring physician name:________________
Address:________________
Phone:________________

Deductible? Yes____ No____ Deductible met? Yes No
Co-pay? Yes No ____ Amount? $____

Allergy Rx authorized? Yes ____No ____RAST? S.E.T.

Second opinion required? Yes No
Phone number for authorization:________________
Fax number for authorization:________________
Phone number for benefits: ________________

Address of the plan:________________

Special:

Audiology Services

1. ABR/ENG
2. Tymps
3. audiogram

Laboratory Services

Radiology Services

schedule be the same? Can the contract be assigned without the prior written consent of both parties?

- How long must I perform after I terminate the contract?
- How are the disputes resolved? Legal/Arbitration? Who pays?
- Are written amendments required to alter the contract?
- Terminate with/without cause by either party? Which "causes" lead to breach and termination?
- Who notifies the patients in the event of termination?
- Are patients held "harmless" even if MCO becomes insolvent—i.e., can I collect what is owed?
- Does the contract incorporate amendments "by reference"? Do I get to see them? Am I bound by them?
- Must I indemnify the MCO against liability? If so, CHECK WITH YOUR MALPRACTICE CARRIER.
- What happens when treatment I prescribe is wrongfully denied or delayed by the MCO?
- Can peer review decisions be appealed? Is the specialist local?
- If I am required to do peer review, am I protected from liability?
- Can I refer patients to the physician best able to treat them?
- Can I continue to see an unlimited number of non-plan patients?
- Can I refuse to treat plan patients if they are threatening, abusive; fail to comply with directions; refuse to make co-pays?

Financial Terms (Before you send it out and incur legal fees)

- Withholds, risk pools? When they are paid; can and may that be audited ; am I liable for increased payback if the budget is not met?
- When will the MCO pay; what happens if they're late; will they question "valid" submitted claims? (Give them 10 days.)
- Obtain a complete and specialty specific fee schedule. If not, provide the MCO with your 20 most frequently used CPT codes with fees. Are they covered? What will they pay for discount off "physicians charges" or "usual and customary"? How will they pay for uncovered procedures?
- Withhold/incentives—should bear interest: paid yearly.
- Define the protocol for claim demands.

Terms and Conditions

- Services covered
- Limits/exclusions of benefits
- Enrollment verification and eligibility status—what is the process?
- Malpractice coverage requirement of physician? Does the MCO have malpractice? What are the limits?
- What is the authorization process? Preauthorization requirements? Referral requirements?
- Physician's financial liability? MCO's financial liability? Insolvency insurance? What are my obligations in the case of insolvency?
- Must I accept every patient referred? Is there a maximum/minimum?
- What is the range of the obligations of the PCP?

BEWARE !

- Is there a program notification? Do you accept a contract if you do not "affirmatively reject" within 10 days with a written notice?
- Termination period the same: 30 days for each party.
- Do not allow the MCO to advertise in your office.
- Beware of automatic contract renewals. Seek a one-year term, with annual negotiation of payment rate.

You probably should not join if:

The contract requires you to assume the obligation of the MCO.
The contract contains a "hold harmless" clause for the physician only.
The contract can be altered by the MCO without notice and/or prior consent.
The contract has no provisions for appealing adverse decisions concerning Utilization Review, Quality Assurance, or Medical Management Decision.
Reimbursement will be less than the overhead.
The reduction in compensation is greater than acceptable.
Exclusivity—you must be able to provide to others.
The contract allows ability to assign without notice/approval or the ability to retroactively deny payment.
Billing limits are too short. Seek a 60-day period that begins with the end of the month in which service is rendered and be sure you can do this.
Presence of a "gag clause."
Reimbursement period > 60 days.
The MCO has the right to lower its schedule to match a lower contract that you sign; it may be retroactive.
You cannot terminate "with cause" such as:
Failure to make timely payments
Any changes by the plan in subscriber agreements, operational protocols, or administrative requirements affected by physician duties.
Material breach of contract by the plan.

Negotiate

- Increased payment for some of your most common procedures.

- A maximum amount that can be owed to the practice, by the plan, at any given time. If the plan exceeds that amount, have a remedy.
- Obtain the right to terminate the agreement immediately if not corrected in 5 business days.
- Continue to reorder services to covered patients at your usual customary rates.
- If you save the plan money, negotiate a share of the savings.
- A "without clause" termination. Try for a short period, settle on 90 to 120 days.
- Learn to negotiate. See Chapter 4 in this book.

ASSESSING THE EFFECTS OF AN MCO ON THE PRACTICE

- Perform a Plan Performance Comparison (Fig. 14–19).
- Determine the weighted average of the plan (% of total charges for a group of certain CPTs for which you are reimbursed by a managed care plan) (Fig. 14–20).
- Monitor the plan's AR separately.
- Create a statement for the plan's withholds and bill them when the payment is due.
- ALWAYS BE SURE THAT YOUR PATIENTS AND YOUR STAFF KNOW THE DIFFERENCE BETWEEN *PREAUTHORIZATION* AND *BENEFITS.* Many MCOs will preauthorize a procedure for a patient without knowing the patient's benefits. The patient should call to be sure that they have the benefit to pay for the authorized procedure.

Do More Homework

- Who is the Medical Director?
- Who is on the Board of Directors?
- Has it returned withholds?
- Where is it licensed? Who owns it? Check with the Secretary of State.
- What complaints have been filed? What is the malpractice history, operational or clinical?
- Does it pass on premium increases to physician reimbursement?
- If it is a capitated plan, do payments arrive on time and is there a current enrollees with the capitation check each month?
- Accreditation? NCQA? Dunn & Bradstreet? Moody's?
- Medical Loss Ratio—if high, maybe plan has limited financial flexibility; if low, maybe they don't pay providers.
- What are physician accreditation requirements? Board certification? CME's?

Deciding Whether to Join: Do I Need to Join?

- Average number of patients seen per week in the office?
- Can you absorb more patients?
- Average number of additional hospital visits/consults?
- Do your top referring physicians belong? Your competitors?
- Which employers offer the plan? Growth, history, average age?
- Is it financially responsible to join?

  Investigate the plan:

1. Department of Insurance or other state agencies
2. List of the doctors in the area; payment history; problems; denials. Has the plan added revenues to the practice?
3. National Council of Quality Assurance (NCQA 202-955-3500).
4. What is the average age of the Plan's A/R?
5. Market share
6. Number of insured lives
7. Recent annual report
8. Know the plan, not just the MCO
9. Patient and provider disenrollment figures
10. Hospitals in the plan?
11. Do they have a 1-800 number?

Special Problems

- The plan denies approval of what I think is appropriate.
  1. Inform the patient of the risks of not following my recommendation.
  2. Follow appeals process as outlined in the contract.
  3. Inform the patient, in writing, that they may purchase the recommended service at their own cost.

- Authorizations for service
  1. Remind the patient of the need for this with appointment confirmation call. (This is also a good time to review enrollment, remind the patient of co-pays and outstanding balances).
  2. If they forgot, remind them of your contract to provide service only with authorization.
  3. Call referring office and ask for a faxed authorization between two familiar contacts.

The Contract: Other Issues

- The plan should have access to the patient's records only as permitted by law and should pay for copying.
- Insist on written notice and preapproval before the plan uses your name in marketing materials.
- Include a statement in the contract that you are an independent contractor and will render all medical and surgical judgments without interference or control.
- The contract should be governed by your state law; disputes should be settled in your state.

PLAN	CHARGES	PAYMENTS (AVERAGE)	ADJUSTMENTS	GROSS COLLECTION %	NET COLLECTION %	NUMBER OF PATIENTS

MOST FREQUENTLY BILLED (BY UNITS) SURGICAL PROCEDURES AND PAYER PAYMENTS

FIGURE 14–19. PLAN PERFORMANCE COMPARISON TABLE

WEIGHTED AVERAGE OF THE PLAN

CPT Code	Frequency	Your charge	Gross charges	Plan Payment	Gross Payments
99211					
99212					
99213					
99203					
99204					
TOTAL					

Weighted Average Reimbursement (Total Payments) / (Total Charges)

Discount=100 minus weighted average

FIGURE 14–20.

- What is the plan's policy for dual insurance—i.e., both parents have insurance. "Birthday rule"? i.e., primary policy, closest to January or "male–female" rule, i.e., male primary; or "longevity" rule, oldest policy in effect is the primary?
- How are members identified?
- Make sure that authorizations and benefits coordinate.

Quality

Review the checklist below. "Quality" is very difficult to define.

1. Do you perform patient satisfaction surveys; compare them with peers; do you periodically institute plans to improve them?
2. Do you perform clinical outcomes surveys? Design your own or use a validated survey. Plan for a method to analyze the data. Institute a value compass for a frequently performed procedure.
3. Maintain patients' confidentiality as much as possible. If confidentiality is breached, make sure that you or your office are not responsible.
4. Be good to your staff so that your staff is good to your patients.
5. Give your patients a diagnosis or tell them why you can't. Don't be vague or evasive. Listen to what the patient is saying.
6. Whenever possible publish, speak, obtain CMEs and let your patients, the payers, your hospital, and your patients' employers know.
7. Follow practice guidelines established by your Specialty Academy.
8. Practice good business:
   - Create a patient information brochure (include hours, telephone calls).
   - Keep your patients informed of their lab or radiography results.
   - Keep your referring doctors informed.
   - Be available.
   - Know who your referral sources are, establish "VIPs," get the right name, address, phone and fax number. Use your patient information sheet to track referrals.
   - Know how you are paid (i.e., which payers pay how much?).
   - Schedule openings for "quick and easy" referrals.
   - Periodically randomly audit your own charts. Are allergies labeled? Have reports been called? Has your referring doctor been informed?
   - Learn about managed care contracts.
   - Insure appropriate coding.
   - Establish referral guidelines for your referring docs.
   - Send thank you notes when appropriate.
   - Charge reasonable fees.
   - Add new equipment and new services to your business.
   - Research any software that you buy.
   - Perform referring physician surveys.
   - Develop a practice prospectus.
9. *To thine own self be true.* Do everything you are capable of doing, refer the others. Be your patient's advocate and remind your patient that you are their advocate.
10. Establish a continuous quality improvement plan in your office for both the clinical and business aspects of your practice.

Getting Some Help From Others

When I designed this book I had the pleasure of meeting several experts who kindly provided me with their knowledge about several specific issues. These experts are listed in the sources at the end of this chapter.

Physician Assistants

Lynn A. Hughes, M.D., is a member of the AAO-HNS. Based in North Carolina, Lynn has utilized at least one physicians' assistant for the past 15 years. They:

- Do the physical exams for surgical patients.
- See patients on the initial post operative visit.
- remove packs, sutures.
- cover the office in the absence of the physician with ENT backup.

Each state has its own regulations. In North Carolina, two PAs is the maximum number. Both PAs and nurse practitioners require written protocols and cannot bill Medicare unless a physician is present. The physician must be available for immediate consultation and must review and sign and all dictated and written chart information within one week. PAs can write prescriptions but they cannot write refills for narcotics.

PAs require a degree plus two years in a medical school setting where they study side by side with medical students. They are generally paid between $60,000 and $90,000 per year.

The decision to use a physician extender(PA or nurse practitioner) is a personal choice. It is also dependent on local regulations and practice needs.

Revenue Tracking

Tracking revenues is essential in a managed care market. Several software products permit this. Physicians need to assess the software's ability to perform this function prior to purchasing (see Chapter 15). Our own fee schedules are overshadowed by insurers' "allowable" reimbursement. Reduced fee-for-service plans constitute a large percentage of revenue in many practices. Dr. Stephen Levinson has designed a method for analyzing the relative value of existing and future insurance contracts that pay by reduced fee for service. His analysis considers the volume of each CPT service performed in the practice. Utilizing this method, you can analyize how each plan would reimburse the practice if it were paying for all the services performed by the physician on an annual basis. This methodology compares more than fees and can establish a level playing field for analyzing current and future insurance contracts.

Keeping your finger on the pulse of your practice requires some quick methods to assess the vital signs of your business. May Schwartz, a physician reimbursement expert, recommends that two measurements are crucial. First, total your outstanding receivables 90 days or greater overdue and calculate this number as a percentage of overall receivables. If it is greater than 20%, there is evidence of exceptionally high financial losses. Second, divide your total charges by the number of months they represent giving your average charges per month. Your average months outstanding should range between .9 and 1.8. If it is higher than 2.0, you should proceed with an accounts receivable analysis.

Merging, acquiring, and selling your practice are individually specific issues. Please see Chapter 21 concerning this issue. Another excellent opinion can be obtained from C. Kay Freeman who is listed in the sources at the end of this chapter.

REFERENCES

1. Donabedian A: *Explorations in quality assessment and monitoring: The definition of quality and approaches to Its assessment.* Ann Arbor, MI: Health Administration Press: 1980.
2. Davies AR, Ware JE Jr: Involving consumers in quality of care assessment. *Health Aff* 1988; 7:33–48.
3. Moloney TW, Paul B: The consumer movement takes hold in medical care. *Health Aff* 1991; 10:268–279.
4. Rubin HR, Wu AW: Patient satisfaction: Its importance and how to measure it. In: Gitnick G., ed.: *The business of medicine: A physician's guide.* New York: Elsivier Science Publishing Co. Inc., 1991:397–409.
5. Rubin HR: Can patients evaluate the quality of hospital care? *Med Care Rev* 1990; 47:267–326.
6. Cleary PD, McNeil BJ: Patient satisfaction as an indicator of quality care. *Inquiry* 1988; 25:25–36.
7. Ware JE Jr, Hays RD: Methods for measuring patient satisfaction with specific medical encounters. *Med Care* 1988; 25:393.
8. Kertsz L: Patient is king. *Modern Healthcare.* April 29, 1996. 108.
9. Rubin HR, Gandek B, Rogers WH, Kosinji M, McHorney CA, Ware JE Jr: Patients' ratings of outpatient visits in different practice settings: results from the Medical Outcomes Study. *JAMA* 1993; 270:835–840.
10. Piccirillo, JE: The use of patient satisfaction data to assess the impact of continuous quality improvement efforts. *Arch Otolaryngol Head Neck Surg.* 1996; 122:1045–1048.
11. Isenberg, SF, Davis C, Keaton S: Project Solo: an independent practitioners initiative for confidential self-assessment of quality. *Am J Med Qual* 1996; 11(4).
12. Berwick D, Godfrey AB, Roessner J, eds: *Curing health care: New strategies for quality improvement.* San Francisco. Jossey-Bass, 1990, 55.
13. Radosevich D. Health Outcomes Institute, Bloomington, MN, personal communication.
14. Nguyen TD, Attkinsson CC, Stegner BL: Assessment of patient satisfaction: Development and refinement of a service evaluation questionnaire. *Eval Prog Plann* 1983; 6(3–4): 299–313.
15. Isenberg SF, Rosenfeld R: Problems and pitfalls in community based outcomes research. *Otolaryngology-Head and Neck Surgery,* 1997;662–665.
16. Berwick DM: Continuous improvement as an ideal in health care. *N Engl Med* 1989;320(1):53–56.
17. Imai M: *Kaizen: The key to Japanese competitive success.* New York: Random House, 1986.
18. Kano N, Seraku N, Takahashi F, Tsuji S: Attractive and must be quality. *Quality* 1984; 14(2):39–48.
19. Healthcare Marketing Trends, Nashville, TN. January 12, 1987, p. 4.
20. Segal ES: Maintaining communication in a time of uncertainty. *Arch Fam Med* 1995; 4:1066–1067.

SOURCES

Relative Values for Physicians
McGraw Hill Healthcare Management Group
1221 Venue of the Americas
41st Floor
New York, NY 10020
(800)-621-8168

Medicare RBRVU'S: Physician Payment Guide, 3rd edition.
AMA Order Dept.
(800)-621-8385

May Schwartz
Physician Reimbursement Issues
30 Tyler Road
PO Box 87
Waterville, NY 13480-0087
(800)-533-0860

Arte Maren
Employee Motivation
23647 Draco Way
West Hills, CA 91307
(818)-887-4416

C. Kay Freeman
Health Systems Strategies
500 Northpark Town Ctr. Suite 625
1100 Abernathy Road
Atlanta, GA 30328

Stephen R. Levinson, MD
Managed Care Payment Analysis
ASA, LLC
P.O. Box 308
Easton, CT 06612
203-371-4797

PAHCOM
Office Management, Employee Manual
Richard Blanchette
461 E. Ten Mile Road
Pensacola, FL 32552

Association of Otolaryngology Administrators
Office Management, Employee Manual
PO Box 3150
Iowa City, IA 52244
319-356-2371

Medical Management Monographs:
Financial Management; Managing Managed Care; Managing Medical Practice; Employment Management.
AMA
(800)-621-8385

Lynn Hughes, MD
Medical Assistants
11 Ardsley Ave. NE
Concord, NC 28025
704-788-1103

To contact Dr.. Isenberg:
Steven F. Isenberg, MD
1400 North Ritten Ave.
Suite 221
Indianapolis, IN 46219-3046
Phone: 317-355-1010
Fax: 317-355-1992, 317-355-1993
Email: projsolo@iquest.net
Voice mail: 317-596-0415

15

Information Management in Managed Care and Capitation

VINSON J. HUDSON

"If you don't measure it, you can't manage it." This was a key quote of Mark H. Spohr, MD, founder of MedSoft. He describes basic functions of managed care contract management:

- Allow the entry and definition of the terms of each contract.
- Calculate reimbursement based on the terms of the patient's insurance contract.
- Adjust accounts receivable to reflect expected reimbursement.
- Provide management reporting to show profit and loss under each contract.
- Provide for contract modeling using actual patient data to determine contract profitability during contract negotiations.

It requires knowledge to obtain the best information system solution for medical practice management in a managed care and capitation environment. Without knowledge, physicians will waste time, endure frustration, and add needless cost to their purchase. As a practice manager, you will monitor several managed care contracts over the next few years. Therefore, it's important to know the costs to manage patients and members or enrollees under multiple contracts in a fixed rate per patient system. With this in mind, we will select a managed care contract management application that is suitable for your practice.

■ Capitation and Measurement

Remember the "good old days" when a physician could compensate for lower income by increasing the fees charged for some services? This was the fee-for-service era where total financial risk fell on payers. The managed care generation of providers will face various structures of managed care plans where financial risk is shared. Managed care plans fix fees through capitation arrangements, motivating medical providers to use management tools to deliver cost-effective care.

Facing the Managed Care Market

The most difficult part of this capitation process is to track costs, especially when you've never had to do it. Traditional computer-based physician officemanagement/medical information system (POMIS™) could develop the numbers. Physicians can win under capitation if they understand what it costs to keep a practice running and plan physician compensation. This includes taking a closer look at fee schedules and current fee discount levels, specific services and facilities covered by the contract, practice patient visit levels, trends and capacity, and referral requirements.

Since the difference between the amount charged for services and the contractual adjustments in those charges continues to widen, physicians must protect their income and preserve the financial viability of their practice. Interviews with practice managers indicate that the current cost of providing services is becoming greater than the amount that the managed care payer market will bear. Thus, providers must redo their care delivery processes and reduce costs while simultaneously promoting the value of their care.

It is probable that managed care contracting will continue to grow as a foundation business strategy in medical office practices. Medical practice management should focus on information systems that support negotiation and management of managed care contracts.

A managed care contract is a formal or informal agreement between a payer (HMO, PPO, insurance company, employer, or employer group) and provider organization to reimburse patient claims on other than a total charge basis. Through managed care contracting, a medical practice assumes some share of financial risk by agreeing to per diem, discounted from fee schedule, per patient, or other reimbursement methodologies. In exchange, the medical practice expects financial gain.

Capitation as the Method of Payment

Capitation is a method of paying health care providers a periodic (typically monthly) per capita payment for the services delivered to the members' managed care plan who have selected the plan's provider. Physicians who have entered into or will inevitably enter into these managed care contract arrangements should understand how the payment system operates, how a capitated plan will work for them, and what automation tools are available to determine how to make a profit.

Capitation represents a fixed amount paid to providers for each enrollee assigned to them. The capitated patient is called a "member," "enrollee," "beneficiary," or "subscriber." The physician's payment is usually paid on a per-member-per-month basis, or based on a fixed percentage of the managed care plan's premium charged to the enrollee. These capitation payments do not increase for members who become seriously ill and require extensive care, nor do they decrease for members who do not seek medical care.

Capitation arrangements are based on group and individual membership. In a group arrangement, an HMO contracts with an independent practice association (IPA) or medical group composed of a group of primary care physicians, single specialty, or multispecialty. It pays them a capitated rate for all members. The group is responsible for internal and external compensation for all services. This is referred to as "full-risk" contract for outpatient services. This same group might negotiate a "shared-risk" contract between the managed care plan and the physician group.

For an individual capitation arrangement, an IPA is generally the capitating agent. The individual physician does not pay the specialist or other outpatient or inpatient providers directly; insted the capitating agent pays them.

Physician's Office Managed Care Contract Management Functions

Knowing the costs of managing patients under a fixed rate per patient system is crucial. Practice management consultants and billing services vendors describe the following functions for a computer system: (see Table 15–1)

1. *Calculate the number of encounters per month.* From the computer patient database, determine the *average patient base* and the *average number of visits per patient per year* and divide by the number of *months per year.*
2. *Calculate the overhead per encounter.* The financial application of the computer system solution provides the practice *overhead per month.* Divide this by the previously calculated *encounter per month.*

TABLE 15–1. Cost of Managing Patients

CALCULATION EXAMPLE FOR 2-PHYSICIAN PRACTICE	
Average Annual Patient Base of Practice (APB)	5,000
Average Visits per Patient per Year (AVPB)	2.4
Total number of Patient Encounters = 5,000 × 2.4	12,000
Number of Encounters per Month = (5,000 × 2.4) ÷ 12	**1,000**
Practice Overhead per Month (OHPM)	$32,000.00
Overhead per Encounter = ($32,000) ÷ [(5000 × 2.4) ÷ 12]	**$32.00**
Average Capitation per Patient per Month (ACPPPM)	$9.50
Practice Capitation Revenue per Month = 5000 × $9.50	$47,500.00
Capitation Revenue per Encounter = (5000 × $9.50) ÷ [(5000 × 2.4) ÷ 12]	**$47.50**
Copayment per Encounter (CPE)	$12.00
Copayment Revenue per Month = [(5000 × 2.4) ÷ 12] × $12.00	**$12,000.00**
Total Revenue per Encounter = (5000 × $9.50) ÷ [(5000 × 2.4) ÷ 12] + $12	**$59.50**
Profit (Loss) per Encounter = {(5000 × $9.50) ÷ [(5000 × 2.4) + 12] + 12} − (32,000) ÷ [(5000 × 2.4) ÷ 12]	**$27.50**

3. *Calculate the capitation Revenue per encounter.* Use the *average patient base* determined in step 1 and multiply it by the *average capitation per patient per month,* which results in a *capitation revenue per month.* Divide this result by the *encounter per month* calculated in step 1.
4. *Calculate the copayment revenue per month.* Multiply the *encounter per month* by the allowable *copayment per encounter* from each the member.
5. *Calculate profit (Loss) per encounter.* From the above data, the total revenue per encounter is determined by adding the *capitation revenue per encounter* and the *copayment per encounter.* Subtract the *overhead per encounter* from the latter result to arrive at the *profit (loss) per encounter.*

Although this is a simplified illustration, it shows the data elements that a managed care tracking computer application must monitor to minimize risk and maximize practice opportunity. Computers can automate these manual tasks better than people. The best managed care contract management application software should combine a member level database with effective software application tools for planning, population and member management, quality and value assessment, capitation management, contract negotiation, budgeting, management control, and process modification.

■ Information System Solution Selection Guidelines

Before selecting an information system solution with integrated managed care contract management functionality, do some basic planning.

1. *Create a selection team leader/selection committee.* Someone in the practice should lead the process of a group of responsible users of an ISS (Information Systems Solution) who will assist in defining the specifications for their particular functional areas. This is the first step in selecting the best ISS for your practice after your initial strategic practice assessment. Your efforts here will make later vendor responses more reliable.
2. *Develop a vendor/software shopping list.* Your practice needs a comprehensive, acccurate, and unbiased database of vendor profiles, including hundreds who have undergone a "satisfaction rating" from their customers. You should also utilize a Search and Match Service that uses provider specifications to search for a viable list of vendors. There are other sources with different information slants: Medical Group Management Association in Denver, Colorado, state medical associations, several trade publications, and consultants. From the initial list, eliminate those vendors who cannot meet your fundamental needs of application functionality, computer system platform, regional presence, product maturity, price, and so on.
3. *Contact five to ten vendors on the shopping list.* Develop a request for information (RFI) letter to each vendor. The vendors on your initial shopping list can generally meet your specifications, but you should go through a second round of vendor filtering.
4. *Conduct due diligence on the shopping list.* You should evaluate ISS vendors. Is it a stable organization? Obtaining accurate information about privately held vendors is difficult. You can begin with a Dun & Bradstreet report on the business for less than $100, which tells if the vendor pays its bills on time. Contact existing users to get their concerns.
5. *Ask questions; ask more questions; and/or negotiate.* Keep a running list of concerns and questions about how the purchase process works. When will the implementation and operation begin? Is there an installation/implementation schedule developed for you? Is training included in the price or is it purchased separately? If you decide to change business direction, how is your investment protected and continued support assured? If your questions have been satisfactory addressed except for a few low priority points, begin to negotiate. Some vendors won't change a policy. For instance, some vendors insist on a service contract for the first year of operation. Others will not release their software source code, but will agree on some escrow protection. Analyze what your practice needs and its position in the managed care environment.
6. *Analyze the terms of purchase and service contract.* Get legal advice to be sure that the language of the agreement is written for your organization. Obtain a typical customer agreement to examine what the vendor promises. This will help you determine your responsibilities and risks.

Developing a plan around these guidelines should increase the likelihood of selecting the best integrated managed care contract management application for your practice.

After you have analyzed your medical practice with your office staff or a practice management consultant and think you are ready for the selection process, you must take one fundamental step—selecting the core applications for your practice. Whether your practice is small or large, the following features differ only in complexity of system configuration and application functionality:

- *Eligibility, Benefits, and Electronic Data Interchange (EDI) Services.* Includes tracking a plan's members as they enter and leave the plan; determining which members are covered for what services along with any special payment arrangements; identifying out-of-scope services as outliers on the member's electronic file along with corresponding billing and payment provisions (e.g., discounts against the fee schedule); and tracking any coinsurance, deductibles, copayments, or maximum annual limits on treatment and developing a total for each encounter.

- *Referals and Utilization Management.* Permits the practice to efficiently manage referrals by automatically referring, tracking, and verifying several factors associated with participating specialists and other subcontractors. The system should maintain an updated medical-surgical database of the approved provider network.
- *Capitation Fund Pool.* Creates and groups fund pools according to the types of functions and activities needed to track.
- *Stop-Loss Insurance Tracking.* Capitated providers buy stop-loss insurance to limit their financial risk if a member develops a catastrophic condition. This feature should track individual members encounters, hospital stays, and referrals to other physicians over time so that claims are properly filed within the stop-loss threshold term of the policy. The application should also group and link individual member records, then automatically send out a notice when the stop-loss threshold is about to be crossed.
- *Charge Posting.* Posts payments and bills to the correct fund pool as received.
- *Audit Trail.* Permits retracing, retrieving, recreating, and manipulating old information. It then presents it in an appropriate format.
- *Maintenance of Risk Sharing Arrangement.* Tracks the contractual responsibilities for each member encounter.
- *Separating Fee Schedules for Different Providers.* Provides multiple fee schedules for each physician in the managed care contract.
- *Comprehensive Relational Database Management Report Generation.* Allows all database files and data fields to be manipulated for specific knowledge.
- *Tracking Number of Visits Allowed and Number of Visits Used.* Tracks the member's encounter activity.
- *Payer Authorizations.* Ensures proper authorization of members from the payer.
- *Contract Management.* Provides software tools for managing the managed care contract.
- *Claims Adjudication.* Determines whether the provider's claim of medical services performed satisfies all contractual obligations.
- *Write-off of Capitated Services.* Allows a write-off of capitated services that are part of the managed care contract.
- *Billing Carrier for non capitated Services.* Allows billing of payer for noncaptitated services required on the member.
- *Billing Member for noncovered Services.* Allows billing of member for noncaptitated services required on the member.
- *Billing Member for Copayment.* Identifies the copayment responsibility of each member and bills the member.
- *Tracking Write-offs by Doctor and Managed Care Plan.* Tracks managed care contract write-offs.
- *Handling PPO Members with a Fixed Amount Copay.* Differentiates capitated from discounted compensation.
- *Case Management.* Captures data for Healthcare Employees Data Information Set (HEDIS) reporting and other user-defined data requirements.
- *Clinical Outcomes Management.* Allows physicians to track their practice outcomes, such as complications, length of stay for members by procedure, number of procedures performed, postop readmission to hospital, and development of a measurement system to evaluate the effectiveness of specific treatments and the quality of the delivery system.
- *Integrating the Management of Fee-For-Service and Capitated Payment Accounting.* Allows capitated accounting to work with fee-for-service accounting systems.
- *Financial Management Systems.* Identifies those managed care plan members who may be receiving benefits outside of the capitation arrangements.
- *Operate on industry standard, open-architecture hardware and software.*

Systems or Turnkey Vendors

Systems or turnkey vendors provide practice management ISS on personal computer (PCs), workstations, midrange computers, and mainframes to various market segments. Most systems vendors have reseller arrangements with computer manufacturers for computers, system software, peripheral equipment, and even software from other companies (often the same companies used by their competitors). They then integrate these components into a practice management system of applications for the POMIS industry. Many of these vendors are also involved in other delivery approaches such as billing services and outsourcing services.

Most personal computer systems vendors service the solo through 10-physicians market. Workstation-based systems, consisting of Pentium computers, Digital workstations, IBM RISC System/6000, HP9000, and so on primarily service the 11-to 49-physicians market. These systems are typically UNIX-based operating systems running as servers to a number of distributed stations. Finally, the midrange/mainframe-based systems, consisting of

IBM AS/400, Digital VAX, HP 3000, and other larger systems, are characterized as high-volume, multiuser, multitasking, and multitreading transaction processing systems in group practices of 50 physicians and greater.

Billing Services Vendors

Billing services provide financial and accounting functions to medical office practices, typically off-site. They are an evolution of the past service bureau, using personal computers in the medical practice or other device to collect processing data rather than courier. Their services consists of bookkeeping, accounting, patient and insurance billing, accounts receivable management, and computer data personnel. Also included are insurance billing programs that include analysis and design of paper flow systems, design of charge document and implementation of billing control systems, insurance billing form preparation, financial and management reports preparation, and several office management service functions. This definition of billing services does not include the growing number of insurance claims billing services that *only* collect claims billing data from medical offices to format and forward to insurers or claims clearinghouses.

Some billing services may be defined as on-line computer services vendors who offer medical offices access to computer applications and data base storage at a central location. The vendors' host computer system is accessed by the physician's office via a terminal or personal computer over communications lines. This approach is a basic medical distributed processing business where personal computers are networked and tied to the host computer system.

Outsourcing Services Vendors

Some medical offices contract with outsourcing services vendors who provide consulting services, medical business office management, *and* billing/data processing services. They provide expertise in the financial and administrative management needs of the medical office. These services are similar to facilities management services or management services organizations marketed to the ambulatory care setting sector of the health care industry.

The outsourcing services vendor takes full responsibility for office setup, supervision of personnel, and accountability to practice operations. Expertise includes personnel management, billing procedures, fee structure, collections, office management, practice growth and control, and operation of an in-house computer systems if it exists. Compensation is typically received as a percent of collected revenues.

Pricing Descriptions

Table 15–2 summarizes the typical pricing of typical computer configurations by size and managed care plan. The solo and 2-physician ISS configuration system is primarily placed in primary care practices, urgent care centers, and active referral practices where the office handles about 30 patient visits per day. The 3- to 10-physician ISS configuration is primarily placed in small group practices of any type where patient visits range from 60 to 400 patients visits per day. The system serves a single or multispecialty environment. The 11- to 25-physician ISS configuration is primarily implemented in medium-sized group practices of any type where patient visits range from 300 to 1000 per day. The 26-to 99-physician ISS configuration is primarily implemented in large group practices of any type where patient visits range from 700 to 3500 per day. The 100 physicians and Greater ISS configuration is placed in large enterprise and integrated delivery system where the complexity of the applications and the computer systems hardware are needed.

Tables 15–3 and 15–4 summarize the pricing and configurations of billing services and outsourcing services vendors.

Physicians in any practice setting are increasingly depending on computer system solutions to assist in managed care office management. Because of their more complex financial aspects, managed care contract management, and scheduling needs, group practices are

TABLE 15–2. Typical Pricing Description of Full Computer ISS Configurations

Products/Services	*Solo & 2*	*3–10*	*11–25*	*26–99*	*100 +*	*MCP*
System hardware/software	$5,800	$25,840	$62,640	$253,000	$368,200	$54K–$435K
Applications software	$6,200	$25,500	$69,300	$225,000	$410,700	$240K–$1.2M
Maintenance and support	$2,200	$13,160	$26,500	$71,700	$132,413	$50K–$216K
Total	$14,200	$64,500	$158,440	$549,700	$911,313	$344K–1.9M

MCP = Managed Care Plan; 100 + = 100 physicians and greater; other items refer to practice sizes.
Source: Jewson Enterprises' POMIS Knowledge Base.

TABLE 15–3. Typical Pricing Configurations of Full Billing Services

Billing Services Medical Office Interface	*Cost and BudgetRequirements*
Dumb terminal or personal computer (PC) connected to host computer of billing services' processor. Depending on requirements, the in-office PC system may do some limited processing such as demand billing, statement printing, labels, appointment lists, etc. Modem communication is provided.	Pay an upfront fee for software and consulting Pay a charge on a per member per month basis or Pay a percent of collections (6–10% typical) Port charges and telephone line fees are extra Solo & 2-physicians range from $4000 to $7000 per year. A 10-physicians practice could pay $30,000 to $54,000 per year. Price depends on the in-office hardware/software and applications and services selected.

Source: Jewson Enterprises' POMIS Knowledge Base.

TABLE 15–4. Typical Pricing Configurations of Full Billing Services

Outsourced Medical Information System Interface	*Cost and Budget Requirements*
Managed care expertise Integrated delivery system expertise GUI interface	Pay an upfront fee for software and consulting Pay a charge on a per member per month basis or Pay a percent of collections (8–12% typical) Port charges and telephone line fees are extra

Source: Jewson Enterprises' POMIS Knowledge Base.

more likely to use sophisticated computer applications than solo practitioners. Computer systems in integrated delivery networks and large group practices are also more expensive than those in solo practices. Physicians are using computers beyond billing: health maintenance reminders, medical records, and other patient care tasks. Good managed care contract applications require research and development budgets that most small vendors can't afford. Even some larger vendors must look to external partners to deliver needs. Physicians are challenged not only to select the best functionality but the best vendor for the long term.

Vinson J. Hudson is president and industry analyst of Jewson Enterprises, an independent market research and analysis firm that has specialized in the medical office information system solutions field for more than 25 years. He offers a clearinghouse of "just-in-time" market intelligence in his field. His breadth of knowledge crosses several medical electronics and biomedical areas. He also develops personalized market surveys and reports, as well as presentations, to various audiences. He writes and contributes to several publications, and personally publishes the *Jewson Enterprises POMIS IQ Report,* a quarterly snapshot of industry intelligence. His telephone is always open to discuss this industry. Jewson Enterprises was formed in 1973 to specialize in market research and analysis in the Physician's Office Management/Medical Information Systems (POMIS™) industry. Clients include vendors, private physicians, group practices, applications software innovators, corporate acquisition seekers, investment bankers, practice management consultants, and publishers. The POMIS Knowledge Base is maintained through research and constant verification through regionally dispersed intelligence-gathering professionals.

Vinson Hudson holds a Master's of Science in Electrical Engineering and Medical Electronics from Stanford University. His industry analysis expertise includes claims/transaction clearinghouse services, hospital information systems. laboratory information systems, analytical instruments, operating room industry, patient monitoring systems, and others.

16

Malpractice Issues

THOMAS M. KIDDER

Medical and surgical practice has historically involved risk taking and hard work, usually balanced by great personal satisfaction and monetary rewards. Some physicians view managed care simply as a gentleman's agreement with a third party payer to provide a ready supply of patients in exchange for a discount on professional fees. The reality is that participation in managed care is much more complicated. The advent and rapid growth of managed care have, from the physician's standpoint, increased the risks and diminished some of the rewards. Just the opposite has been the case for MCOs and other third party payers. Risk has been shifted to the physician and the patient, while rewards—namely, profitability and reduced liability—have been eagerly garnered by MCOs. Total dollars spent on health care have not been reduced, only redistributed, with an estimated one-third of the managed care premium dollar going for administrative costs, such as overhead, executive bonuses, and building construction.

In this chapter, some risks unique to or accentuated by managed health care will be discussed from the perspective of a practicing physician. This chapter is not intended to be a source of legal or financial advice in navigating the unpredictable seas of managed care. Before becoming contractually involved, it is prudent to seek counsel from a qualified attorney, financial adviser, or risk management expert.

A comprehensive review of physician liability under managed care is also not the objective of this chapter. Rather, it presents the viewpoint of one physician relative to some issues germane to medical liability in this arena. I am grateful to the authors of the references cited at the conclusion of this chapter for highlighting and analyzing, in their writings, those areas of medical liability that are of special concern in managed care medicine. Any errors in interpretation are my own and not those whose ideas have helped me to synthesize a composite, pragmatic overview of this topic. For a more detailed discussion of any specific items contained in this chapter, the reader will find helpful information in these references.

In today's politically correct climate, it is truly a challenge to write anything that does not run the risk of offending somebody, not necessarily because of content but because of the author's choice of words. I have tried to write this chapter in a manner that is sensitive to the feelings of all potential readers. To keep this chapter reader friendly, the use of "he" or "she" should be regarded as interchangeable. Similarly, while I also disdain use of the term "provider" in reference to physicians and other health care professionals, for simplicity, and because managed health care plans include other entities (laboratories, imaging centers, hospitals, nursing homes, pharmacies, medical equipment suppliers, etc.) as providers of service to our patients, I will use the term provider to refer to any professional or entity that provides health care services to patients.

■ Why *Increased* Liability Under Managed Care?

In today's litigation-minded society, the specter of malpractice claims is ever present and has not really diminished over the past thirty-five years, despite various tort reform efforts. Managed care has, if anything, *increased* physicians' liability exposure. In an era when the doctor-patient relationship is already under siege—resulting from unrealistic expectations, our cultural reliance on litigation to resolve conflicts, the lure of unconscionable windfall monetary awards, less time available for unhurried communication between doctor and patient, weakening of the trust that patients have traditionally had in physicians by sensationalism in the print and audiovisual media—we now see introduced a variety of gatekeepers, physician-extenders, and other intruders into what was once, and still is in many cases, a very personal and sacred covenant between the patient and his or her doctor.

The presence of these interlopers has further distanced the physician from the patient; the risk of failure to diagnose and/or treat in a timely fashion is becoming an increasing source of medical liability claims and parallels the rise in office- or clinic-origin liability claims in contrast to those that arise in a hospital or operating room. The need to circumvent numerous administrative obstacles by a patient who is sick and anxious to obtain diagnosis and treatment engenders frustration and anger on the part of the patient and family members. The stage is thus set for a malpractice claim should anything go wrong. As specialty physicians, we can all recall cases where, had the patient been referred for definitive diagnosis and treatment more promptly instead of being repeatedly seen and misdiagnosed and improperly treated by "middle-men," the clinical problem could have been resolved more satisfactorily.

■ Managed Care *Is* Contract Medicine

The Contract Says It All (at Least, It Should)

Managed care medicine is essentially contract medicine. The totality of the relationship between you and the MCO—your mutual obligations, the financial and legal risks you incur, and the reimbursement formula—is (or should be) contained solely in the written contract you sign, including all exhibits, attachments, schedules, tables, and appendices referenced in the contract itself. It is of utmost importance that you thoroughly read, understand, and realize the ramifications, both explicit and implicit, of the document you sign, often referred to as the Provider Agreement, which establishes you as a participating physician.

■ Common Sense and Sound Business Principles

Getting along in the managed care environment will entail changes in the way physicians are accustomed to practicing. But doctors, by the very nature of their long training and the clinical problems they confront daily, are used to adjusting to changing conditions, even though many of us do so reluctantly because by nature we tend to be organized, compulsive, and more comfortable with a fixed routine. Applying ***common sense*** and ***sound business principles*** when dealing with MCOs is much like applying objectivity, experience, and continuing education to our daily clinical practice. Most of us have not received formal training in the business of medicine, and certainly very few physicians have had formal training in being able to understand, critically evaluate, and negotiate contracts.

Importance of Contract Language

Without going into detail about the structure and contents of a typical managed care provider contract—this subject is covered expertly elsewhere in this book—it has been my experience that, with a little effort, the majority of these contracts are actually intelligible to the nonattorney. It takes a little practice, but after reading through a few contracts, most of them follow the same pattern. Keep in mind, however, that *contract language is crucial*, and what appears to be a minor change in wording can make an enormous change in the way a court or arbitrator might interpret a contract clause. These contracts tend not to be too lengthy and are not usually written in arcane legalese, which used to characterize many older insurance policies, for example. The tide of consumerism has ushered in more easily understandable legal documents, at least in theory. However, the language is still critical to the interpretation and enforcement of a contract, so don't let your guard down because of reader-friendly, seemingly benign contract language.

Review of Contract by a Qualified Attorney

Since dangers may lurk in subtleties of language in provider agreements, most risk management experts advise physicians to have a qualified attorney review managed care contracts before signing. The physician himself or herself should always read and attempt to understand the contract, since attorneys and physicians have different perspectives on medical-legal issues. What is of concern to you from a medical standpoint may not be of great concern to your attorney from a legal standpoint. It is prudent to discuss with your legal consultant any problems you have with the contract and ask him or her to explain any terms or clauses you don't fully understand. Contract review by a qualified attorney can usually be obtained at reasonable cost and is money well spent if it helps to prevent more costly misadventures once you have affixed your signature.

Health Plan's Referral Network: Is It Adequate?

If an MCO has a number of "holes" in its physician panel—whether it is absence of certain specialties altogether, or lack of consultants whom you feel comfortable having your patients referred to, you should give careful thought to whether or not you want to become a participant.

Managed health care is medical care by contract. While the patient–physician relationship has always been recognized as a contract, under managed care the MCO also contracts with patients, physicians, facilities (clinical laboratories, imaging centers, hospitals, etc.), and suppliers of medical goods and services, often complicating your relationship with your patients. While the contract you sign with the MCO spells out *your* obligations, responsibilities, and liabilities as a participating physician, the contracts the MCO has with patients and other health care professionals and entities may significantly affect the way you are able to practice. For example, a pharmacy might, under terms of its contract with the MCO, not be able to supply a medication that you feel is essential and for which there is no equivalent for your patient.

Contract Negotiability

A contract is, in essence, an agreement between two parties, delineating the obligations, duties, and financial considerations governing their relationship. The fact that it is an agreement would imply that both sides have had the opportunity to negotiate into or out of the contract provisions that each party finds desirable or objectionable, respectively. Managed care contracts tend to be standardized, "one-size-fits-all" documents. While, in theory, contracts are negotiable, you may find that MCOs are either reluctant to or adamantly refuse to modify their boilerplate agreement, demanding that you sign it as is.

Just such an incident happened to me recently. A couple of weeks ago I received my biennial reappointment application form and a physician's agreement (contract) from a local MCO, for which I have been a participating physician for the past two years. I completed the application form, read the contract, and made some modifications in ink on the contract before signing it and returning it. The clause to which I most strongly objected required me to agree to accept *any* changes in policy or procedure that the MCO might, "from time to time," make in the contract. There was no statement that the MCO was required to notify me that any such changes had been made or what recourse I had, short of formally resigning as a participating physician, if I did not agree to accept the unilateral modification.

Shortly thereafter, I received a reply from the MCO informing me that the contract was nonnegotiable, that they would not accept the few changes I had made in the contract language, and that, essentially, I could take it or leave it. In my case, the number of patients I care for under that managed care plan does not constitute a significant portion of my patient population. I can understand their extreme reluctance to entertain modifications to their contract—especially if a number of their participating doctors make various changes before signing; it's much easier for the MCO to have one, uniform, standard "provider" agreement signed by all physicians, either primary care or specialist.

Acquiescing to their demand, however, goes counter to the two general principles of surviving in the managed care environment: use common sense and apply sound business principles in your dealings with managed care entities. Signing a contract that allows one party to unilaterally change the contract during its term, without any obligation to seek agreement or even notify the other signatory of the change, is tantamount to signing a blank check—it doesn't make sense! This scenario could pose a dilemma for a participating physician who has a significant proportion of his or her patient population enrolled in one particular managed care plan, which refuses to negotiate a modification to its contract.

Indemnification ("Hold-Harmless") Clauses

Most personal medical liability insurance policies will not cover, and may specifically exclude, additional liability assumed by the policyholder in entering into a managed care contract. The most obvious example of this assumed liability is the indemnification clause, commonly referred to as the "hold-harmless" clause, contained in many managed care contracts. These clauses, on cursory reading, often seem benign and innocuous. However, an indemnification clause may, either explicitly or implicitly, burden the participating physician with liability and damages for torts not under his or her control, potentially leaving him or her uninsured for legal costs associated with defense and/or with payment of damages. This liability may also arise out of, not direct patient care activities, but utilization review (UR), quality assurance, or credentialling functions that the participating physician may have agreed to perform under terms of the contract. It is imperative that written assurance be obtained, either from the MCO or your own personal liability carrier, that coverage is in force for claims arising out of your performance of these duties.

Are You Protected as a Utilization Reviewer?

Your contract may require you to serve in a utilization review capacity. Utilization review, while ostensibly employed to guarantee that "quality" patient care is being provided by participating physicians and other providers (and, in truth, it does in many instances, detect and remedy inappropriate or ineffective use of diagnostic or therapeutic measures), serves to control costs for the MCO, reviewing prospectively and/or retrospectively, services that are proposed or have already been provided. Utilization review, therefore, has a powerful function in determining whether to authorize or deny payment for requested or recommended services—all, of course, without ever having laid eyes on the patient! If a patient suffers harm because authorization for a service, determined retrospectively to have been medically necessary, was denied, those serving as utilization reviewers may be held liable for damages. Since your own personal medical liability policy will probably not cover the risk you assume by serving in this capacity, it is imperative that you obtain proof of coverage, either from the MCO or its carrier, or from your own liability insurer. Never accept a verbal "OK"—get it in writing!

Are You Protected as a Credentialler?

With regard to serving as a member of the credentials committee for an MCO, penalties arising out of antitrust or anticompetition lawsuits can be particularly severe. On one hand, you may be found liable for recommending membership and privileges for a physician who is later judged to have been medically negligent. On the other hand, you might be sued by a physician for restraint of trade or antitrust violation if you deny privileges or reappointment. While admittedly, evaluating physician performance, determining competence and skill, and deciding whether to reappoint a physician to the panel of participating physicians is a task that demands integrity and wisdom on the part of the credentiallers and carries with it a heavy responsibility, it is not without substantial liability exposure. The prudent physician will make certain that he or she is adequately insured before agreeing to participate in this function.

"Gag" Clauses

Currently, much attention is focused, both at the state and national legislative levels, on so-called "gag" clauses in some managed care contracts. There are various types of gag clauses, which may be included in provider agreements.

One type of clause bars the participating physician from criticizing the plan in any way. For example, the contract might require the participating physician to refer to a consultant on the MCO's physician referral panel even if the former did not truly believe that the panel provided a consultant competent to handle the patient's problem. The gag clause could prohibit the referring doctor from telling the patient that it would be necessary to go outside the plan to obtain the necessary medical services. Even an appeal by the participating physician of a UR decision to deny authorization might be construed as a violation of the contract, since it would, in a way, be a criticism of the decision rendered by the UR process.

A second way in which the gag clause might work is that it could prevent a participating physician from discussing the advantages and disadvantages of a given managed care plan with a plan subscriber or benefits manager when the contract between the employer/subscriber and the MCO was up for renewal. A physician may have, from experience in dealing with a particular MCO, an opinion as to the desirability of that MCO as a health benefits insurer. Yet the language in the provider agreement may constrain the doctor from discussing this important choice with the patient.

Perhaps most seriously, a gag clause may interfere with the physician's statutory obligation to obtain full informed consent from a patient by discussing diagnosis and treatment recommendations, options, and risks. For example, contract language may require the doctor to offer *only* those treatment options covered under the plan, even though the doctor may believe that a noncovered treatment would be more efficacious in a particular situation. Or, it might require prescription of a medication of inferior efficacy because the most effective drug is not listed on the MCO's formulary. Some gag clauses are so restrictive that they require the participating doctor to avoid mention of other options, even if the patient would be willing to pay out of pocket for them. Remember that signing a contract with such a gag clause does not relieve the physician of the statutory mandate to provide *full* disclosure.

Several states, including Massachusetts, Illinois, and New York, have either enacted or are now in the process of enacting legislation to restrict or prohibit the inclusion of gag clause language in MCO provider agreements. Federal legislation is also being drafted to address these issues on a national level.

A rather extreme, hard-to-believe form of contract gag clause actually prohibits the physician from showing the contract to or discussing it with *anyone*, including his or her attorney, financial adviser, business manager, or risk management adviser!

■ Basic Practice Principles Don't Change

Just as no two physicians really think alike (contrary to popular belief!), no two physicians are affected the same by the managed care environment. Nonetheless, some principles of medical/surgical practice and some issues pertaining to managed care and medical liability are common to many practicing clinicians. It is the intent here to examine several liability issues related to managed care that could have significant impact on the professional and personal life of a participating "specialty" physician.

Safeguarding the Patient's Best Interests

Some fundamental principles of delivering medical or surgical care to patients—some of which have their origins in antiquity—do not and should not change under managed care. The ***best interests of the patient*** should always be the physician's overriding concern, and his or her actions must be predicated on and driven by that concern. This principle is no less important or different than it is with traditional health care delivery. Your ethical obligations to your patient, regardless of third party payer arrangements, remain the same; nothing in your provider agreement with the MCO will abrogate these duties in the eyes of the law. Courts in various jurisdictions have consistently rejected the argument that considerations of cost justify substandard medical care. The interests of the MCO—minimizing spending and maximizing profits—are at odds with the interests of the patient and doctor, receiving and providing, respectively, the best quality medical care available.

Physician as Patient Advocate

It is imperative that the physician advocate vigorously for a patient if an MCO denies authorization for a medical service that he or she truly feels is medically necessary. This requires the physician to be familiar with the appeals mechanism, to file an appeal in timely fashion and in writing, and to follow through in protecting the best interests of the patient. If the appeals mechanism is cumbersome or ambiguous, direct contact with the medical director of the MCO should be made and the situation explained, both verbally and with a written follow-up letter or memorandum. If the MCO still denies authorization for a service that you deem medically necessary to prevent harm to the patient, you should either go ahead and provide the service yourself if possible, irrespective of reimbursement, or seek an alternative way of obtaining it. If you, as a participating physician, do not do all in your power to have the patient's medical problem appropriately managed, you may be held liable if the patient suffers harm or injury as a consequence.

In *Wickline v. the State of California*, the California Court of Appeals affirmed the responsibility of the physician to do all in his or her power to advocate for the patient when an adverse ruling is rendered by the MCO's utilization review process. In this particular case, a patient's lower extremity was amputated following complications of vascular surgery. The plaintiff asserted, and the appeals court affirmed, that premature discharge from the hospital materially contributed to the loss of her limb. Though the physician argued for additional hospitalization and was not, in fact, sued by the plaintiff, the utilization reviewer refused to grant an extension of hospitalization, and the patient was discharged after four days, sooner than either the physician or the patient thought was appropriate. However, the Court of Appeals was not satisfied that the physician had protested vigorously enough and reprimanded him. The court declared:

> The physician who complies without protest with limitations imposed by a third-party payer, when his medical judgement dictates otherwise, cannot avoid his ultimate responsibility for his patient's care. He cannot point to the health care payer as the liability scapegoat when the consequences of his own determinative medical decisions go sour.[13]

Standard of Care

Another principle that holds both for managed care and for traditional medical care is that you are required to meet the same ***standard of care*** as any physician of similar training and specialty, practicing under similar circumstances, and faced with a similar clinical problem. In this regard, it is important to read carefully the portion of your MCO contract having to do with standard of care. If the MCO prescribes the standard of care, you will still be held to the standard of care for your jurisdiction, even if the MCO's standards are *lower*. If, on the other hand, the standard of care prescribed by the MCO is *higher* than that of your jurisdiction, the law may find you liable if you do not adhere to the higher level of practice.

Advertising and Marketing

An issue related to and potentially affecting the principle of the standard of care has to do with the ***advertising and marketing*** of an MCO's health care system. You should request and examine all brochures, advertisements, and marketing materials distributed to benefits managers and subscribers. Satisfy yourself that the MCO is not making promises that they can't keep: for example, promising, implicitly or explicitly, services or levels of care that are unrealistic. Base your judgment on the MCO's fiscal strength, participating physician network, and the facilities (clinics, hospitals, outpatient surgery centers, rehabilitation or convalescent hospitals) with whom they have contracts. Any limitations on the services an MCO can provide, and what additional costs subscribers might incur if they must go outside the plan for care, should be clearly spelled out in the promotional literature.

Protecting Your Patient and Yourself from Adverse UR Decisions

As a participating specialist in a managed care plan, your clinical recommendations for diagnostic studies and treatment will be subject to review and either approval or denial by the utilization review committee of the MCO. There are some measures you can take to minimize your liability exposure with regard to utilization review decisions affecting the care you render to your patients:

1. *Provide full informed consent information* to your patient. Explain your assessment of the problem, options as to diagnosis and treatment (including your specific recommendation as to what you think would be the best option in this case), benefits, risks, and the consequences of no treatment. Document in the medical record that the informed consent process did indeed take place and the substance of your dialogue with the patient.
2. If UR denies authorization for your recommended course of treatment, and if you truly think the treatment is medically necessary, *don't fail to treat* and *don't abandon* the patient because of the UR decision. While the "medically necessary" issue may be debatable, your obligation under the law to recommend and provide, if the patient consents, treatment that you feel is in the patient's best interest is not abrogated just because the patient–physician relationship occurs in a managed care situation.
3. You must *vigorously appeal adverse UR decisions* on behalf of your patient. Depending on the urgency of the clinical problem and the expediency of the MCO's appeals process, register your objection promptly, in writing, keep copies of all correspondence with the MCO, and communicate directly with the MCO's medical director if necessary. A timely and persistent challenge to an adverse ruling by the MCO's UR process is essential. You may need to go beyond the appeals process provided for in your contract and in the bylaws of the MCO to absolve yourself from liability if the adverse decision results in harm to the patient.
4. *Confidentiality* of medical information is regulated by the statutes of your jurisdiction, not by the MCO's provider agreements or bylaws. State law supersedes contract language, and your actions with respect to preserving the confidentiality of medical information of your patients will be based on your compliance with statutory provisions in your own jurisdiction. In other words, you should protect, transfer, and release individual patient medical information the same way you do for your non-MCO patients.

Medical Records and Written Documentation

Good medical records are *as* important, if not *more* important, in managed care as they are in traditional health delivery systems. An *accurate, complete, objective, legible,* and *timely* medical record is frequently the most important defense a physician has in a liability lawsuit. It serves as the most permanent and credible repository of factual information in a medical negligence lawsuit. Years after an incident has occurred, memories fade, recollections differ, witnesses may or may not be available to testify, but the written medical record remains a constant.

Benefits of a Good Medical Record

A medical record meeting the criteria in the above paragraph provides protection to the patient and physician alike. Risk of error is reduced when essential clinical information is faithfully included in the chart. Patient care is generally improved when medical information is complete, easily readable, and accessible to all those involved in providing care. For the physician, the medical record frequently serves as the mainstay of legal defense in a liability lawsuit. Finally, it has fiscal importance in documenting the level of care provided, should a retrospective audit by government or other third party payer take place. This documentation may obviate the need to refund payments and/or pay heavy monetary penalties.

Care and diligence in the preparation and completion of medical charts and records, whether in the physician's office or in the hospital, are, admittedly, tiresome, laborious, and never-ending tasks. With the endless and varied demands on a physician's time, it is no wonder that chart entries are often illegible and lacking in sufficient detail to reconstruct the facts of a case several years later when an action is filed in court. However, most physicians who have been involved in medical liability litigation, either as defendants or as expert witnesses or consultants, will at least grudgingly admit to the supreme importance and effectiveness of a "good" medical record. Several defense attorneys have remarked to me that they have never been involved in a case where the medical record could not have been even *better* than it was—even if it was a good medical record—in terms of detail, objectivity, comprehensiveness, and explanation of rationale for a particular course of action having been taken. Of course, the temptation to "improve" the medical record ex post facto, for example, alteration of the medical record when litigation is likely or has already commenced should be rejected outright. It is possible to defend a poor or deficient medical record; it is virtually *never* possible to defend a case in which the medical record is known to have been altered.

Advice Regarding Medical Records

With regard to medical records or charts, some universal advice is worth repeating, whether regarding managed care or traditional care:

- Dictated, transcribed notes are legible and tend to be more complete than handwritten notes. Dictation and transcription, though adding to operating costs, will pay dividends in a more efficient, productive practice as well as enhance your risk management effectiveness.
- A good medical record does not have to be verbose or long-winded. Complete sentences and literary style are not as important as the information contained in the record: observations, meaningful

clinical data, documentation of findings, and interactions with patients, either in person or by telephone. Remember that level of service should be discernible from the medical record, so that the reimbursement you are requesting can be established from review of the chart.

- Only objective, relevant notations should be entered in the chart. Pertinent historical information and physical findings, lab and imaging data, documentation of informed consent, as well as some narrative reflecting your medical decision-making—for example, give your entries substance, reflecting your thought processes and your rationale for pursuing a particular clinical course—are all appropriate items to include in your chart notes. Assiduously avoid making any entries that could be construed as judgmental, insulting, or deprecating, or that reflect anger on your part toward the patient, a family member, or another caregiver. A good rule of thumb is to prepare the medical record as if you were expecting it to be read aloud in court several years hence. Would the reading of your chart entries help or hinder your case? Would you be embarrassed if your notes were read by a jury? The temptation is often great to play one-upsmanship or vent anger or frustration in the notes we jot in medical charts. Far better to suppress such an urge, remembering that the medical record is, first and foremost, a ***legal document***, and that indiscretion in its preparation may prove to be a millstone around your neck years later.
- An immutable rule that merits repetition is to *never*, for any reason, alter the medical record. If you wish to correct a typographical error, misspelling, or inaccuracy, do so in such a way that the original error is not erased. Put a single line through the error, note the change, and initial, date, and time the alteration. If the error is detected in a chart that is likely to be subpoenaed for litigation, make *no alterations whatsoever*, even with the precautions noted above. It is easier to explain an erroneous chart entry, than a chart alteration, to a jury.
- One last issue with regard to medical records involves patient confidentiality. The safeguards related to accessibility, transfer, security, and disclosure of confidential medical information are not nullified just because a patient is covered under a managed care plan. As mentioned elsewhere in this chapter, statutory provisions regarding confidentiality of medical information in a given jurisdiction supersede any MCO-provider agreement.

Questions about Plan Benefits or Coverage

You might be asked by patients whether certain services or benefits are covered by their managed care plan. Unless you are certain, you should not attempt to interpret the terms of their health plan for them. All questions related to plan coverage are best directed to the MCO administrator. For large group plans, these questions can sometimes be answered by the employer's benefits manager.

Financial Risks Under Managed Care

Perverse Incentives

A physician not only incurs unique and additional legal liabilities under managed care contracts; potentially major financial risk is also involved. One liability, which is a mixture of both legal and financial risk, arises out of ***perverse incentives***, for example, monetary withholds, penalties, or bonuses, that are used by MCOs to encourage cost containment, sometimes at the expense of appropriate medical care for the patient. The inverse relationship between the cost of services provided to the patient and the financial risk or loss assumed or incurred by the physician sets the stage for the unwary physician to cut corners in delivering medical care and fail to meet the standard of care in a given situation. Legislation to limit or eliminate these incentives in MCO contracts is presently under consideration.

Your Contractual Financial Responsibilities

In considering a managed care contract, pay attention to the portions that deal with your ***financial responsibility***: (1) What if the contract is terminated, by you or by the MCO, prematurely (disposition of withholds; unpaid balances on services already provided by you)?; (2) What if the MCO becomes insolvent?; (3) What if you are required to continue to provide services to plan subscribers for a period of time after termination of the contract? Other areas of financial liability, which are dealt with in other sections of this book, relate to indemnification of the plan by you for claims that may or may not have anything to do with negligence on your part, and compensation for time you spend on credentialling, utilization review or quality assurance functions.

Capitation Risks

Capitation contracts pose special financial risks for the participating physician. Depending on your patient population, costs for services could significantly exceed your capitation allotment. The contract should either specify a limit on cost overruns for which you are responsible, or some provision should be made for stop-loss insurance coverage.

ERISA Shifts Liability to the Physician

The indemnification ("hold-harmless") clause poses one of the greatest legal and financial risks to the physician signatory to an MCO contract. One major aspect of this problem has to do with ERISA, the federal Employee Retirement Income Security Act of 1974. Approximately 90% of MCO health plans are organized under the ERISA umbrella. What this does, in essence, is to shield the MCO from liability for medical negligence arising out of utilization review decisions to deny coverage. The courts have consistently upheld the immunity of ERISA-qualified MCO's from negligence claims. Therefore, in a medical negligence lawsuit arising out of an action taken by the MCO, if the MCO health plan is ERISA qualified, the only deep pocket the plaintiff can go after may well be yours!

REFERENCES

1. American College of Surgeons. Statement of recommendations to ensure quality of surgical services in managed care environments. *Bull Amer Coll Surg* 1994 ;79(12):30–31.
2. Barratt K: Reviewing gag clauses *Wis Med J* 1996;95(4): 249–250.
3. Benda CG, Rozovsky FA: *Managed care and the law: Liability and risk management: A practical guide.* Boston: Little Brown & Co., 1996.
4. Document #1043. Malpractice liability and managed care. California Medical Association Legal Counsel, September 1995.
5. Fischer JE: Ethical dilemmas in managed care. *Bull Amer Coll Surg.* 1995; 80(11):21–25.
6. Hirsch BD, Wilcox DP: Caution required when contracting with MCO's. *Texas Medicine* 1991; 89(12):40–42.
7. Karp D: Managed care will require adjustments in medical practice. In *Loss Minimizer.* Cloverdale, CA: David Karp Associates, March 1996.
8. Klein DG: Exploring snares in indemnity contracts. *Bull Amer Coll Surg* 1996; 81(4):30–33.
9. Larkin H: Lurking liabilities. *Amer Med News* June 26, 1995; 9–10.
10. Lobe TE: *Medical malpractice: A physician's guide.* New York: McGraw-Hill, Inc., 1995:367–384.
11. Manuel BM: Physician liability: New areas of concern under managed care. *Bull Amer Coll Surg* 1995; 80(2):23-26.
12. Palmisano DJ: Legal tips for the managed care age. *Bull Amer Coll Surg* 1996; 81(5):36–39.
13. *Wickline v. State of Cal.*, 228 Cal. Rptr. 661 (Cal. App. 1986), appeal dismissed (741 P.2d 613 Cal. 1987).
14. Younger P, Conner C, Cartwright KK, Kole SM: *Legal answer book for managed care.* Gaithersburg, MD: Aspen Publishers, Inc., 1995:143–171.

Thomas M. Kidder is an Associate Professor of Surgery at the Medical College of Wisconsin. He is the author of several book chapters and scientific presentations. Dr. Kidder has served as the Chairman of the Commission on Medical Liability and Risk Management for the State Medical Society of Wisconsin and the Risk Management Steering Committee of the Office of Commissioner of Insurance, State of Wisconsin. He is well known for his *Risk Management* Tip-of-the Month editorials. He has written extensively on such issues as the expert witness, managing the risks in situations of shared liability, and a physician's perspective on informed consent.

■ SECTION FOUR ■

The Physician's Response to Managed Care

17

Network Mergers and IPAs: The Legal Issues

MATTHEW L. HOWARD

The legal issues surrounding the creation of physician-owned networks, their mergers, and the formation and merger of independent physician associations (networks) are both complex and fluid. Lawmaking affecting these issues is proceeding a rapid pace. Theorizing that whatever the future holds will be colored by the past, the reader will therefore understand the rationale for emphasizing certain historical aspects of this subject.

Antitrust Law: The Background

Is There a Bias in Public Policy against Physician Organizations?

Physicians contemplating either establishing or participating in physician-owned networks must consider the legal implications of their decisions. The legal issues surrounding such networks and network mergers include issues of:

- federal antitrust law
- personal and professional liability
- unstated public policy to limit physician incomes and political power.

Bias Expressed by Policies Intended to Increase Physician Numbers

Physicians contemplating the recent controversy surrounding the Clinton administration's proposed national health insurance scheme sometimes forget the long history behind such efforts. National health insurance was first proposed by Socialist candidates for president shortly after the turn of the twentieth century. Active physician opposition dates to 1935, when the Roosevelt administration was rumored to be considering inclusion of national health insurance in the new Social Security system. Proposals were actually introduced during the Truman and Kennedy administrations. Each time, vigorous physician opposition led by the AMA helped defeat it. When the 89th Congress passed the Medicare legislation, physician opposition had become an affront to Lyndon Johnson and his successors. Johnson and other politicians were quoted as favoring reduction of the power of organized medicine to influence legislation. The Johnson administration sponsored legislation to increase the number of physicians, hopeful that increased numbers of physicians would lead to reduced costs for consumers and lack of physician unity through increased physician competition.[1] When costs spiraled upwards, the proponents of this policy feared they had made a grievous error.[2] It seemed that the wider availability of physicians, coupled with improved ability of a significant segment of the population to pay for care, was leading to increased supply fulfilling pent-up demand. Currently, that thirty-year-old policy is having its intended effect. The government intends for that effect to continue, and antitrust law is the likely vehicle to preserve reduced consumer costs and the lack of physician unity. The Federal Trade Commission (FTC) has been quoted as saying that any efforts to reduce resident physicians would be prosecuted as an anticompetitive measure.[3] This has not deterred younger physicians from recognizing the oversupply and proposing to reduce it.[4] Physicians, who have seen their incomes dropping in real terms for the first time in 50 years, are finding themselves forced to organize to protect their economic interests. In so doing, they are running up against the other bias embedded in public policy.

Bias Expressed by Interference with Physician Organization: Antitrust

Before discussing antitrust law, we should take a moment to recall the origins of the Sherman and Clayton Acts. This discussion will focus on federal antitrust law because the various state laws generally follow the federal lead. To avoid violations of local law, however, a physician engaged in network mergers or formation should always consult an attorney familiar with his or her state's antitrust law.

The United States underwent vigorous territorial expansion beginning in the 1840s, and continuing after the American Civil War, vigorous industrial expansion occurred concurrently. "Manifest destiny," a term coined in 1845 by newspaper editor John O'Sullivan, was the popular phrase expressing the burgeoning financial and industrial power of a nation discovering itself in possession of the power to implement its ambitions. He wrote, in justifying annexation of the Republic of Texas, that it was "the fulfillment of our manifest destiny to overspread the continent allotted by Providence for the free development of our yearly expanding millions." In short, "manifest destiny" was a philosophical or ideological rationale for imperialist adventuring as the nation expanded from the original 13 colonies.

During the latter part of this same period (1880 to 1910), industrial expansion in the United States led to formation of the first large corporations. It is reasonable to regard the spread of the trusts as a form of business imperialism, or the "capitalist's manifest destiny." John D. Rockefeller founded Standard Oil. Andrew Carnegie created U.S. Steel in 1901 by merger of multiple smaller steel companies. U.S. Steel controlled about 75% of the country's steel output in 785 plants with a total of about $1.4 billion in assets. Similar changes occurred in other industries.

The Birth of the Sherman Anti-Trust Act

Although the "Trusts" of that period do not seem so formidable to us in retrospect, they were regarded as a source of power separate from and threatening to the government. The politicians of the day found the "Giant Trusts" a wonderful target. Just as the modern politician campaigns against transnational corporations that "downsize" by heartlessly firing workers, the politicians of McKinley's and Teddy Roosevelt's day campaigned against the Trusts. In a manner strikingly similar to the imperialist foreign policy of the day, they developed an imperialistic domestic policy. This brought the power of the state to bear against business. The economic theorists of the day, and there is no shortage of their supporters today, felt that "monopoly" was harmful in and of itself. A monopoly could be used ruthlessly to raise prices for the profit of the "monopolists." Even where not complete, sufficient market share provided a power to destroy competition by price undercutting and then, after the competition went under, recouping lost profits by price gouging. To defeat this menace, the Sherman Anti-Trust Act was passed in 1890. It was designed to prevent another U.S. Steel, but it had other consequences. The occasional entrepreneur whose luck, inventive genius, or business skill leads to the creation of a dominant company in any field today must eventually face a charge of monopoly ("anticompetitive practices"). Physicians interested in countering the growing power of MCOs by organizing themselves into IPAs and physician owned networks must deal with Section One of the Sherman Act. It reads: "Every contract, combination in the form of trust or otherwise, or conspiracy, in restraint of trade or commerce among the several states, or with foreign nations, is declared to be illegal."

Claiming at least to support competition and the free market, Congress has placed stiff penalties on violations of the Sherman Act.[5] These laws clearly apply to healthcare enterprises in the same manner as to any other business activity.[6] Criminal violations are felonies. For physicians, this means the loss of one's license to practice medicine, prison terms of up to three years, and fines of up to $350,000 for individuals and $10 million for corporations.[7] Civil suits brought by parties claiming to have been harmed by monopolistic practices can lead to judgments in the millions of dollars, especially given attorneys' fees, court costs, and treble damages as allowed by the law.

Through the provisions of the Sherman Act, Standard Oil, American Tobacco and Du Pont Chemical were all partially disbanded and broken down into smaller companies. More recently, American Telephone and Telegraph was broken down into its components. Despite this, the modern multinational corporation dwarfs the trusts that precipitated passage of the Sherman Act. For example, in 1991 the two largest U.S. industrial corporations, General Motors and Exxon, had combined sales of about $227 billion.[8] This figure was greater (after adjustment for inflation) than America's estimated gross national product at the time of the Civil War, and more than the estimated combined sales of the over 200,000 U.S. manufacturing establishments in 1900.[9] It was larger than the gross national output of all but 13 of the almost 200 nations of the world.[10] The so-called "Baby Bells" that were left after dismantling of "Ma Bell" are beginning to merge into larger companies. In comparison, forming a network of otolaryngologists to negotiate with an HMO seems a minor matter. Physician activities are, however, granted little leeway under antitrust law.

This background is provided to remind readers that applying antitrust law to physician networks results from a perception that each physician's practice is a miniature U.S. Steel. Permitting collaboration between practices, it is presumed, will result in higher prices to consumers through monopoly power. Twenty-five years ago an argument could have been made that this was a valid view. At that time Medicare did not exist, and private insurance companies basically paid a flat fee or a fixed percentage of physician's charges. The patient was left to pay the balance in either case. An agreement between physicians to raise fees would have left patients with no choice but to pay the increased fee. Physician reimbursement, however, has changed faster than antitrust law.

New Applications for Old Laws

Demand for lower healthcare costs is leading to the rapid expansion of managed care organizations (MCOs). Physicians forced to accept the fees offered by the MCOs are seeking an equality of bargaining strength through the creation of provider networks. Under current law, the mere assertion that a network is being organized for that purpose will precipitate antitrust prosecution. By definition, a network of physicians is a group effort of physicians to establish pricing for a service. Thus, networks may violate antitrust law regardless of the stated motivation. Fortunately, such networks offer the possibility of efficiencies that can provide cost benefits to consumers. Physicians may argue that the benefits of competition to the consumer are outweighed by the savings obtained from anticompetitive combinations. This argument, however, carries little weight in the courts.[11] Unless specifically authorized by statute or regulation, anticompetitive actions will always be illegal. The rapid transformation of the American medical scene in the 1990s led the Federal Trade Commission (FTC) and the Department of Justice to issue a document: *Statements of Enforcement Policy and Analytical Principles Relating to Health Care and Anti-Trust.*[12] These "statements" pertain to various aspects of health care as a business while providing guidelines to avoid illegal activity.

"Per se" Violations in Antitrust

Interpretation of the Sherman Act, Section 1, has led to the assumption that certain activities are anticompetitive and in violation of the law.[13] These agreements are considered to be such that they would always, or almost always, lead to an increase in prices, a restriction in production or output, and harm competitors. These three activities are called "per se" violations. Once an entity is shown to have committed a *per se* violation, no justification or defense can be raised. One will note that each provision requires an "agreement". It naturally follows that a single person cannot commit an anti-trust violation.[14] The three per se violations are:

1. *Price fixing.* Example: agreeing to minimum or maximum prices; agreeing on common terms for installment payments such as the amount of down payment; or, agreeing to an interest rate. Physician created relative value scales were outlawed on this basis.[15]
2. *Group boycott.* Example: a group of physicians agreeing that none would sign a contract with Bleeding Heart Health Plan until more favorable terms were offered. Even if the refusal to sign resulted from judgments reached independently, the appearance of group action might well lead to an expensive legal dispute.
3. *Market Allocation Schemes.* Example: an agreement between two group practices of physicians in neighboring cities that each would refrain from placing advertisements in the Yellow Pages of the other's city.

By the terms of the act itself, two or more people are prohibited from engaging in unreasonable restraint of trade. Determining what is an unreasonable restraint of trade requires an analysis often referred to by the shorthand phrase, the "rule of reason."

Defining What Is Reasonable in Antitrust

Problems arise for physicians whose definition of reasonable conduct differs from the Justice Department's interpretation. Consider the following actual example. In a rural hospital with three anesthesiologists staffing the operating rooms, the workload was such that none of the three was working full time. Income was sufficient; the status quo was acceptable. A nurse anesthetist moved to town and applied for hospital staff privileges. One of the anesthesiologists addressed a staff meeting and made a strong case that if the nurse anesthetist began to practice, the resulting dilution of workload would harm the three anesthesiologists economically. He appealed to his colleagues to forbid the nurse anesthetist staff privileges: "We provide better care. We've stuck it out, taking call, being available on weekends and the like, because we want to remain in this town. If the nurse anesthetist gets much business, one of us will have to leave." What happens then in such a situation if the credentials committee legitimately wishes to reject the nurse anesthetist over concerns for his skills or his record of difficult interpersonal relations at his previous employment? The entire transaction is now poisoned by the anesthesiologist's speech to the staff meeting because a "contract, combination, or conspiracy" need not be the result of a formal written agreement.[16] An implied understanding is sufficient, and circumstantial evidence may lead a jury, which has a right to exercise considerable discretion in interpreting the facts, to infer criminal intent where none was intended.[17,18] Mere informal conversations which result in an appearance of a common fee schedule, a common action such as a boycott, or refusing to admit a nurse anesthetist to a staff may be sufficient to establish a "conspiracy in restraint of trade." Thus, if the nurse anesthetist sues on antitrust grounds, he may prevail. The anesthesiologist thought it quite reasonable to ask his colleagues for their assistance. The Justice Department would undoubtedly differ.

For most physicians in private practice, the major impediment created by antitrust law is its effect on collective bargaining. A group of unhappy otolaryngologists, negotiating as a consortium about the proposed reimbursement rate offered by an MCO, may find that they have engaged in forbidden concerted activity.

Restraint of Trade

A major restraint of trade, such the per se violations described above, is not judged by the "rule of reason." By their very existence, they are assumed to be anticompetitive and often lead to criminal prosecution.

The hospital staff previously described, especially the anesthesiologists, would more likely be sued in a civil action. Where a per se violation is not present, a court will balance the restraint factors against the arguments in favor of the challenged action. The restraint may be deemed reasonable if a reasonable argument can be made that benefits to society, such as improved quality of care, the provision of new services, and several other factors outweigh the effect of the restraining actions on market conditions and prices.

Fully Integrated Medical Groups

Medical groups that are fully integrated are generally exempt from antitrust challenge. This is a manifestation of a bias favoring HMOs built into antitrust law.[19] Fully integrated is defined with the existence of centralized marketing, billing and collections, claims processing, quality assurance, and utilization review. Thus, large group practices and HMOs such as Kaiser Permanente routinely bargain for pricing or deal collectively with third-party payers. Of course, a sufficiently large group would be open to challenge as a monopoly. In order to prove monopoly, the relevant market, defined either by product or geography, must be defined.[20] The existence of monopoly power in that market must be demonstrated, and it must be proven that the monopoly power was obtained, maintained, or enlarged by anticompetitive practices such as "predatory" pricing.[21,22] Since an accusation of monopoly generally requires a 65% market share, it seemed unlikely that this could occur in the U.S. healthcare market. The rapid consolidation of MCOs, corporately held hospitals, HMO mergers, and similar organizations in some aspects of healthcare suggest that monopoly power may soon be achieved.[23] An "attempt to monopolize" is also criminal conduct under the Sherman Act if intent to obtain a monopoly is accompanied by a "dangerous" probability of success. That speculative affect is sufficient for conviction.[24] Recently, the Department of Justice refused approval of Children's Healthcare P.A., a nonexclusive network of 65 pediatricians. The *Business Review Letter* stated, "Even a non-exclusive network can be anticompetitive when the network includes a large portion of the available providers in a relevant market. When a network has a large percentage of available providers, these providers face significant incentives to change their contracting patterns so that the network becomes *de facto* exclusive or to contract outside the network only on noncompetitive terms." This appears to represent rigid antiphysician enforcement. The proposed plan, however, risked rejection because it did not provide clear evidence of risk-sharing. A recent court case suggests that a more realistic view may be developing. Blue Cross and Blue Shield United of Wisconsin and its HMO sued the Marshfield Clinic, complaining of monopolization and anticompetitive pricing. The trial court found in favor of the Blues, but the Federal Appeals court reversed in a decision very important to physicians because of the grounds for their action.[25] The Court refused to consider the Marshfield Clinic's high rate of return, their high prices, or their success in signing up physician participants or customers as grounds for applying antitrust law. The Court noted that the clinic's success could result from higher quality, the greater cost of obtaining higher quality, and the natural monopoly which results from a rural location. The Supreme Court declined to further review the decision.

Section 7 of the Clayton Act forbids mergers if the result will be decreased competition.[26] The Department of Justice and the FTC have provided Horizontal Merger Guidelines to assist attorneys and physicians interested in whether their network merger will stand scrutiny.[27] Even where reasonable review suggests that a proposed merger is not anticompetitive, Section 5 of the FTC Act may forbid anticompetitive conduct, which violates the spirit of the Sherman and Clayton Act. While a constitutional scholar might find that too vague for enforcement, the Supreme Court has found otherwise.[28]

Physician Exclusion as a Manifestation of Restraint of Trade

Physicians excluded from a network may well be tempted to seek inclusion through a suit claiming illegal restraint of trade. Because there is a bias against large physician networks, as well as a propensity for courts to accept reasonable claims of concern for quality control, such suits are likely to be unsuccessful. The anesthesiologist described earlier defeated his intent by poisoning the credentials committee's chances to utilize legitimate quality issues as grounds for refusing staff privileges. Where a network is physician controlled, and therefore could be regarded by the regulating authorities as being composed of individually competing physician practices, exclusion of an otherwise qualified physician may lead to evaluation of the network as a "conspiracy or combination" in restraint of trade or a group boycott against the excluded physician. Therefore, it is important for networks to carefully define essential, job-related qualifications, and to investigate each physician applicant so as to defend attempts to exclude. It goes without saying that attempts to exclude on purely economic grounds are indefensible under the law. Where radiologists have challenged exclusive contracts for radiologic services on antitrust grounds, they have been generally unsuccessful.[29] In the *Capital Imaging* case, the appeals court found that even though there was a conspiracy in restraint of trade, it was not unreasonable. Even though the individual radiologists might have been harmed, the court ruled, the HMO in question contracted with fewer than 7% of the area's physicians, and served only 2.3% of the patients. Thus, antitrust concerns for society were not invoked. In *Hassan,* two allergists were terminated by a network allegedly due to failure to adhere to cost containment policies.[30] The physicians sued, alleging a group boycott. The trial court upheld the principle of economic credentialing, allowing termination for cost containment reasons related to competitive advantage and economic efficiency. In addition, the court found that the network in question controlled only 20% of the relevant market, and thus was not sufficiently large to come within the purview of the antitrust laws. For those physicians interested in establishing single-specialty networks, the court found that even an enrollment of 75% of physicians in the market was not sufficient to establish a per se violation of antitrust law. Thus, good-faith cost containment and quality control reasons for excluding a physician may survive an antitrust challenge, especially where there is little independent evidence of anticompetitive behavior.

■ Network Mergers

The antitrust implications of mergers between business entities are fairly constant.[31] Any merger that may "affect" interstate commerce comes under the jurisdiction of antitrust law. A merger of two networks of physicians, some of whose patients come from out of state, or where one has a contract with an HMO with a multistate presence, would clearly qualify.[32] Where the merger is in the form of an acquisition, merely sufficient representation on the board of directors to influence the business decisions of the acquired entity may trigger antitrust regulators.[33] There are special rules in effect for mergers and acquisitions of nonprofit organizations that are not considered here. As noted in Marshfield, special rules applicable to for-profit networks of physicians or other healthcare providers, as opposed to industrial or other businesses, are only just beginning to develop.

The Requirement for Notifying Regulators

A proposed merger must be reported to the FTC and the Department of Justice, on forms available from them, if it meets three requirements:[34]

- if either party to the merger is "engaged in commerce or in any activity affecting commerce."
- if the transaction involves the acquisition of assets or securities with voting rights where, for nonmanufacturing businesses, either the acquired or acquiring firm has assets or net sales of $10 million or more, and the other firm assets or net sales of $100 million or more.
- if the resulting transaction would leave the acquiring entity with securities possessing 15% or more of the voting rights or assets of the acquired party, or would obtain securities with voting rights or assets exceeding fifteen million dollars in value.

The filed forms are accompanied by a filing fee, currently $40,000, and a 30-day waiting period then ensues during which the regulators examine the reporting forms. The agencies issue a request for further information if they believe an anticompetitive result may ensue. If this is not issued, the parties can proceed with their transaction. If the request is issued, the parties must provide the information requested following which the regulators have an additional 20 days to evaluate. The 20 days only begin when the regulating agencies agree that they have received the information they requested. A review of trade law in the United States reveals that the Department of Justice and FTC pursue violators of the reporting law even where the ultimate conclusion is that the proposed merger has no antitrust implications. Noncompliance, or evasion of the reporting rules by creative structuring of deals, leads to civil penalties of up to $10,000 per day.[35]

Evaluating a Proposed Merger

Economic theory presupposes that businesspeople are "rational actors," who make business decisions after determining that proposed actions will lead to increased profits. Antitrust law is invoked only if increased profits may result from market power which will allow increased prices, reduced quality, or elimination of competitors without some overriding contrary consideration. Therefore, the regulators are interested in mergers that result in a controlling single entity that can raise prices higher than would prevail in a competitive market solely because competition has been eliminated. They are also interested in mergers that reduce the number of entities to the point that a de facto coordination between a few principal firms yields the same result. Because most mergers achieve profit through improved efficiency, and because benefits may outweigh the anticompetitive aspects of certain mergers, few mergers actually lead to antitrust enforcement. The regulating agencies have wide discretion whether to oppose any particular merger. If the expected efficiency is more than the harmful effect and the expected savings cannot be as easily obtained through some other means, an anticompetitive merger may be allowed.[36] This applies, however, only to the regulatory agency decisions. If a merger is challenged in court, the court is likely to take the position that if a merger reduces competition the benefits will not likely be passed on to the consumer.[37]

Evaluation of the merger will involve the same four steps referred to above. The relevant geographic market is delineated and the relevant product market is determined. From these two factors, the relevant competitors are identified and their market shares are calculated. This allows evaluation of the merger's impact on market share. If the market share of the merged entity is small, the merger is allowable. If it is sufficiently large, the merger is presumed to be unlawful. The fourth step is to determine if the presumption is correct after evaluating the proposed merger's anticompetitive effects, efficiencies to be expected, and whether mitigating measures might make the merger acceptable. The whole purpose of establishing a physician network, or merging two such networks, is to increase the appeal of contracting MCOs in contracting with the network. Since this would improve the network's bargaining position, the merger is anticompetitive by definition.

Antitrust Law: Safe Zones

Recognition of a new reality is gradually leading to changes in antitrust law. Where the anticompetitive practice involves sharing of financial risk among the participants, greater leeway has been permitted. "Safe zones" have been established by rule that provide exemption from antitrust challenge where certain criteria are met.[38,39] For exclusive networks, such as IPAs, no more than 20% of the physicians in each specialty participating in the relevant geographic market are permitted. For nonexclusive PPOs, or physician network joint ventures, the figure is 30% or less of physicians in each specialty with active hospital privileges. In either case, the physicians must share financial risk. Nonexclusivity is defined by showing that there are other competing networks, that members of the challenged network also participate in other networks and plans, that they earn income from outside the network, and that they are competing with other providers outside the network.

A single-specialty network interested in capturing a capitation contract with a major MCO may well include the majority of relevant specialists in the geographic area. The network's attractiveness to the MCO depends partially on the completeness of the coverage provided. This is of little concern to the MCO, whose costs are defined in advance through the negotiated capitation price. It should therefore be of little concern to the government. The rationale for antitrust action is protection of consumers from price manipulation. Price protection exists through the negotiated capitation price. Under current rules, however, an antitrust challenge would be likely.

■ Aspects of Physician Liability

The physician who is a member of one network, about to merge with or be acquired by another, may find that his or her careful decision to join based on rational evaluation of the networks rules and regulations, has been overridden by the merger. The rules of the new organization may differ from those of the old. The physician will need to ask: Does my original contract bind me to the new entity? Am I under contract to the new organization unwillingly? How do the rules differ? If there are differences, are they more favorable to me or less favorable? Is there a gag rule? Are the physician members of this merged network people with whom I would have voluntarily chosen to associate myself? What will be the effect on my referral pattern? What are the procedures for appealing unfavorable utilization decisions? Are the procedures equally protective of my patient's rights as the procedures in the original network or MCO were? What are the procedures for appealing unfavorable payment decisions? Are the procedures equally protective of my rights as the procedures of the original network or MCO were? Does the new entity have provisions in their contract to which I object? What recourse do I have? Other concerns will suggest themselves. In addition to the general comments above, there are some specific areas of concern.

Professional and Contractual Liability

The prudent physician will have evaluated a network's provisions for appeal of unfavorable utilization and payment decisions, whether they originate with an MCO with which the network has a contract, or from the network itself. Because liability may arise if physicians fail to act as their patient's advocate, the physician who is now a member of a new network must verify his or her right to appeal and the procedures for necessary to appeal.[40]

Similar considerations apply to gag rules, "hold harmless" agreements, restrictions on referrals for treatments or to physicians outside the network or MCO, practice restrictions, and other components of network and MCO contracts. The merger of two organizations into one creates a new entity. The physician neither contracted with nor joined this entity. If the surviving organization has the same rules as the network the physician originally joined, he or she can be comfortable with the result. If not, he or she must determine whether the rules now in effect are acceptable. If they are not acceptable, the physician must consider withdrawal.

Antitrust Liability

Section 8 of the Clayton Anti-Trust Act forbids the same individual from serving as a director of an officer of competing corporations, providing each corporation has capital, surplus, or undivided profits of more than $10 million, and that certain other requirements are met.[41] A physician participating in three networks could inadvertently violate these rules if one already met the threshold requirements and merger of the other two created a new entity that crossed the threshold.

The Changing World of Antitrust

The above discussion is based on current law. An FTC report has advised that a two-step analysis be applied to physician network creation and mergers.[42] The first step is to answer the question of whether the merger is "likely to result in credible efficiencies." The second is to ask whether those efficiencies are likely to deter the merged entity from engaging in anticompetitive practices or, on the contrary, to increase competition in a relevant market. Where these conditions are present, a merger would be approved unless the resulting market power concentration clearly outweighs expected efficiencies. It would seem likely that if such rules were implemented, some violations currently considered per se violations would be permissible. A speech by FTC Chairman Robert Pitofsky at a health care antitrust forum announcing an FTC intention to ease the rules on physician networks, implies that these suggestions may be incorporated into proposed new rules.[43] His proposal would allow application of "rule of reason" analysis to fee-for-service physician networks if significant quality or cost containment gains can be demonstrated, allowing per se analysis to be set aside. Nonexclusive arrangements would also receive lesser scrutiny.

Congress also has been taking an interest. The Judiciary Committee of the House of Representatives voted to recommend approval of 104 HR 2925, which would require "rule-of-reason" analysis for fee-for-service physician networks. The bill currently awaits full House action.[44] Clark Havighurst, a professor at Duke University School of Law, makes an illuminating comment on the proposed FTC regulations and HR 2925. He implies that bias exists against physician networks, saying that enforcement policy is based on "value judgments," and the "[y]ou should get away from the notion that rule-of-reason treatment is something you grant to people you like."[45] The formation of discounted fee-for-service networks, both multispecialty and single specialty, are essential if physicians are to have any collective bargaining power in the face of expanding MCOs. Revised FTC guidelines, whether compelled by statute or not, are essential if market-driven physician networks, free to benefit physicians through the availability of collective bargaining, and free to benefit patients through included quality control mechanisms, are to survive in a competitive world.

REFERENCES

1. Health Professions Manpower Act, 1968: Health Manpower Act, 1971.
2. Unger I: *The best of intentions,* New York: 1996, p. 363.
3. *Bull Am Col Surg* June 1996; 56(6): 81.
4. Young physicians press for solutions to doctor glut, *Amer Med News* July 8, 1996.
5. "Competition is our fundamental national policy," *United States v. Philadelphia National Bank,* 374 U.S. 321 (1963) [Citations to court cases in the format, ***nn*** U.S. ***nn*** where the letters "U.S." are bracketed by numbers (*nn*) are citations to opinions of the U.S. Supreme Court)].
6. "Anti-trust laws apply to hospitals in the same manner that they apply to all other sectors of the economy," *Boulware v. Nevada,* 960 F. 2d 793 (9th Cir. 1992), *Arizona v. Maricopa County Medical Society,* 457 U.S. 332 (1982).
7. And for dentists also. *See: United States v. Alston, D.M.D.,* P.C., 974 F.2d 1206 (9th Cir. 1992).
8. *World Almanac,* 1993, calculated.
9. *Grolier's Encyclopedia,* 1994 ed.
10. *World Almanac,* 1991.
11. *National Society of Professional Engineers v. United States,* 435 U.S. 679 (1978).
12. *Health L. Rep.* (BNA) 1376–1401 (September 29, 1994).
13. Codified in 15 USC § 1.
14. *Fisher v. City of Berkley,* 475 U.S. 260 (1986).
15. *Arizona v. Maricopa County Medical Society, supra.*
16. *American Tobacco Co. v. United States,* 328 U.S. 781 (1946).
17. *Theatre Enters. v. Paramount Film Distribution Corp.,* 346 U.S. 537 (1954).
18. *Esco Corp. v. United States,* 340 F. 2d 1000 (9th Cir. 1965).
19. The "new national health strategy" announced by President Nixon, February 18, 1971, quoted in *New York Times,* February 19, 1971.
20. *Consolidated Rail Corp. v. Delaware & Hudson Ry.,* 902 F. 2d 174 (2nd Cir. 1990), cert. denied, 498 U.S. 936 (1991).
21. "Monopoly power" is defined as the power to control price or exclude competition, *United States v. E. I. DuPont de Nemours & Co.,* 366 U.S. 316 (1961).
22. *Berkey Photo, Inc. v. Eastman Kodak Co.,* 603 F. 2d 263 (2d. Cir. 1979), cert. denied, 444 U.S. 1093 (1980).
23. For example, Columbia/HCA has increased its ownership of U.S. hospitals from 195 in 1994 to 347 at present, Hot issue: Dealing With Hospital Mergers. *Amer Med News,* July 8, 1996.

24. *Spectrum Sport Ltd. v. McQuillan,* 506 U.S. 447 (1993).
25. *Blue Cross and Blue Shield United of Wisconsin v. Marshfield Clinic,* 65 F. 3d 1406 (7th Cir. 1995).
26. *Brown Shoe Co. v. United States,* 370 U.S. 294 (1962).
27. 56 Frd. Reg. 41552 (September 10, 1992). Available also in *Trade Regulation Reporter,* Vol. 4.
28. *FTC. v. Motion Picture Advertising Serv. Co.,* 344 U.S. 392 (1953); *FTC v. Sperry & Hutchison Co.,* 405 U.S. 233 (1993).
29. *Capital Imaging Associates v. Mohawk Valley Medical Assoc.* (N.D.N.Y. 1992) 791 F. Supp. 956 aff'd, 996 F. 2d 537 (2d Cir. 1993).
30. *Hassan v. IPA* (E.D. Mich. 1988) 698 F. Supp. 679.
31. Section 7 of the Clayton Act, 15 USC §18, prohibits mergers and acquisitions "in any line of commerce or in any activity affecting commerce in any section of the country, [if] the effect of such acquisition may be substantially to lessen competition, or to tend to create a monopoly."
32. For example, see *Hospital Bldg. Co. v. Trustees of Rex Hospital,* 425 U.S. 738 (1976).
33. *American Crystal Sugar Co. v. Cuban-American Sugar Co.,* 152 F. Supp. 387 (1957), aff'd 259 F.2d 524 (2d Cir. 1973).
34. 15 USC § 18(a)(1)–(3), 16 C.P.R. §§ 801–803.
35. For example, *United States v. Cox Enterprises,* 1991–2 Trade Cas. (CCH) ¶ 69,450 (D.D.C. 1991) $1.75 million penalty paid after consent decree.
36. Merger Guidelines §4, "Physician Network Joint Ventures," U.S. Department of Justice and the FTC, Statements of Enforced Policy and Analyticial Principles Relating to Health Care and Antitrust, September 27, 1994, reprinted in 3 *Health Law Reporter 1391* (1994).
37. *United States v. Philadelphia Nat'l. Bank,* 374 U.S. 321 (1963).
38. There is a provision for a "messenger model" also, not discussed here. The essence of this exception to the rules is that a broker be engaged to negotiate price between insurer or HMO and the physician network.
39. Statement 8, "Physician Network Joint Ventures," supra.
40. *Wickline v. State of California* (1986) 192 Cal. App. 3d 1630, 239 Cal Rptr. 810.
41. 15 U.S.C. §19.
42. Cited *Am Med News.* June 24, 1996: 28.
43. May 13, 1996 in Chicago, quoted in *Amer Med News* May 27, 1996; 39(20):1.
44. Id. at 27.

Matthew L. Howard, M.D., J.D., currently practices medicine two days per week at the Kaiser Permanente Medical Center in Santa Rosa, California, and practices law four days per week in Ukiah, California. He provides consultation for physicians and attorneys on matters of staffing, credentialing, and professional liability matters. He represents claimants at administrative hearings before the Social Security Administration and, where necessary, pursues their claims in federal court. He holds Bachelor's (Chemistry) and M.D. degrees from UCLA, and completed an Otolaryngology residency at the Los Angeles County/USC Medical Center. He served two years with the U.S. Air Force. During nearly 20 years of private practice of ENT in Ukiah, he served terms as President of the medical society and Chief of Staff of Ukiah General Hospital. He has also served nearly 20 years on the volunteer faculty of University of California Schools of Medicine, and is currently Assistant Clinical Professor of Otolaryngology at UCSF. He has taught Business Law at Mendocino College in Ukiah, and presents a course in preventing malpractice suits at the American Academy of Otolaryngology/Head and Neck Surgery annual meeting.

18

Physician Organizations

JAMES UNLAND

■ Early Policy Decisions by the Founders

Once the decision to create a physician organization (PO) has been made and an initial founding group of physicians has been assembled, early policy decisions about the scope and nature of the organization must be made. The most important early policy decisions are:

- Defining the geographic scope and population catchment area. For antitrust purposes, most POs should seek to serve no more than 20% of the market.
- Defining the specialty mix; will the PO be single specialty or multispecialty, and if multispecialty, how broad will the range of specialist membership be?
- Determining the approximate number of physician members the PO ultimately wishes to have. The word "ultimately" is important here; planning should be based on a determination of the desired future size and market penetration of the PO, recognizing these goals may not be met in the first year.

Founding physicians are encouraged to make these decisions expeditiously and avoid months of discussion. It may be appropriate to bring in consultants or attorneys on a temporary basis to facilitate the "brainstorming" phase even if the PO chooses different experts to help form the organization.

■ Selecting Consultants and Attorneys

Physician organizations are relatively new entities and the number of individuals who have true expertise in creating them are limited. Therefore, it is vital to select consultants and attorneys with extensive experience in physician transactions and related issues.

Consultants are employed to provide business planning expertise and help guide the overall process of establishing and eventually operating a PO. It may be necessary to employ two sets of consultants—one firm for the planning and organizational work and a second for the operational work. Some consulting firms provide both types of experience. In any event, consultants should have the following qualities:

- Experience with physician transactions and, specifically, establishing POs.
- Sensitivity to the peculiarities of the specific project at hand and an appreciation of its special scope and purpose.
- Detailed knowledge of the step-by-step process of establishing a PO.
- The ability to differentiate the role consultants should play and the role the physicians should play. Often, consultants do work that the physicians should really do.
- The ability to make succinct, clear presentations that are result-oriented and that outline practical, action-oriented steps.

- Experience at negotiating transactions and collaborative arrangements among physicians. Evenhandedness in negotiations is critically necessary during the process of organizing a large number of physicians.
- Experience at working with health care attorneys and a thorough understanding of the legal issues so that recommendations made by the consultants can legally be implemented.
- Operational consultants must have extensive experience at managing medical practices and forming physician groups.
- Ability to cap consulting fees. Consultants should propose a "not-to-exceed" fee, although operational consulting fees are more difficult to cap than transactional/organizational fees. The process of integrating a PO operationally is less predictable simply because practices vary widely in their operational capabilities and in the relative sophistication of office staff.

Attorneys are utilized to provide overall legal and regulatory guidance, draft the necessary documents relating to formation of the PO, assist in certain negotiations, and review proposed managed care contracts. Attorneys should have the following qualifications:

- Prior experience at physician transactions, including PO formation. You want people who have been there before; educating lawyers is very expensive.
- Broad health care law experience, preferably including experience in hospital law and managed care law.
- Managed care contracting experience.
- A result-oriented, no-nonsense style. Endless discussion, lectures, and elaborations of legal fine points should be avoided. Physicians need attorneys to identify legal issues and propose workable solutions.
- All legal/organizational issues should be outlined in writing and systematically addressed in well-organized meetings. Don't let attorneys or the physicians "graze" from one nebulous topic to another. Every discussion should be oriented to making a decision or taking action.
- Commitment to a timetable and the willingness of attorneys to make the project a priority.
- A defined scope of work with benchmarks. Don't let attorneys run the whole organization; they are there to give legal advice and perform specific legal work. An organization should be able to be incorporated and totally organized from a legal perspective within a few weeks—not months!
- Ability to cap their fees. Good attorneys who have "been there" and know what they're doing also know how much work is involved in creating a PO; they should be able to quote a "not-to-exceed" price.

Incorporating the Entity

Even though a PO does not represent a merger of medical practices, a formal organizational entity must be created for the following reasons:

1. The PO concept involves permitting a large number of physicians to "master contract" under one umbrella. Therefore, it is necessary to create a single legal entity for that purpose.
2. A PO of any significant size will require at least a few employees to conduct important contracting and operational functions; the organization will also likely require a paid medical director. The creation of a single entity gives the organization a centralized structure enabling this to happen.
3. In addition to entering into master contracts with payers, the PO will need to enter into contracts with hospitals and other providers so that more integrated "joint contracting" can be offered to payers. In addition, a single-specialty PO will want to contract or subcontract with other physician networks; formal entity must be created for this type of contracting.
4. To provide the information systems, claims processing capabilities, and other operational infrastructure, there should be a central organizational entity that can contract with vendors and consultants.

Even though a central organizational entity is created, each of the individual practices or groups that is a member of the PO retains its existing corporate or organizational structure, its existing pension plan, its existing employees, and other characteristics defining it as a discrete legal/organizational entity. A PO is *not* a merger of medical practices; it is a managed care *confederation* with common managed care contracts, common information systems, and certain other shared capabilities.

Very early in the process, the PO founders, working with their attorneys and consultants, select the appropriate form of organizational entity. There are essentially three categories from which to select:

1. Corporation or variation thereof (professional corporation or limited liability corporation.
2. Partnership or limited partnership.
3. Tax-exempt foundation.

The most common form of organization of a PO is a the corporation or professional corporation, for the following reasons:

- A corporation can have stockholders, evidencing ownership in the entity or membership in the entity.
- A corporation can pay dividends based on the amount of stock owned. This may permit the founding members of the PO to receive somewhat higher dividends than subsequent members.

- A corporation can limit certain types of general liability and, under the proper corporate structure, malpractice liability can remain with the respective individual practicing physicians or groups that are members of the PO.
- If it becomes appropriate to merge the PO's medical practices into a fully integrated group, the initial PO corporate structure can serve as the entity into which the member medical practices become fully merged.

Some POs are formed as tax-exempt foundations. A tax-exempt foundation is usually exempt from federal and state income taxes, real estate taxes, and other taxes. If the foundation is established as a 501(C)(3), it can receive charitable donations and certain types of grants for research. In addition, if the member organizations of the PO ever merge into a fully integrated group, the tax-exempt foundation can, under certain circumstances, issue tax-exempt bonds and debt. However, there are certain disadvantages to tax-exempt foundations—they are subject to certain regulatory constraints, do not have stockholders, and cannot pay dividends.

Whatever form of organization is identified, it is important to have the attorneys form the organization expeditiously. For the purposes of continuing this discussion, we will assume that the form of organization of a PO is going to be a corporation or professional corporation.

Determining Officers, By-laws, and Governance

Assuming that the PO is going to be a corporation or professional corporation, it will be necessary to elect a president, vice president, treasurer, and secretary. This election should take place among the founders, with the understanding that after an initial period of time representing the start-up phase—usually one year—another election of officers can take place among the full membership.

Several policy decisions need to be made at this point:

- *Ownership and distribution of stock:* The founding members will need to decide whether all members of the PO will own stock or whether a selected number of members—usually restricted to the founding members—will be the stockholders. In some POs, the founding members are the sole stockholders because they contribute all the initial start-up capital. Other participants in the PO simply become "members" without owning stock. Under this scenario, the distribution of funds from managed care contracts and other earnings can (and should) be structured as an entirely separate matter unrelated to stock ownership. In other POs there are two classes of stock: Class A and Class B. Class A stock is usually held by the founding members and contains voting rights and certain other privileges that Class B stockholders do not have.
- *Membership rights and voting rights:* Regardless of the stock ownership and distribution structure, it is important early in the process to determine who will have voting rights on key issues. Normally, certain types of issues are voted on and approved by the Board of Directors or the Executive Committee. Other types of issues should probably be voted on by the entire membership. Some policy matters are so important that the entire membership should participate in the decision. PO founders must keep in mind that one of the anxieties independent physicians face in joining any organization is relinquishing control; hence, a PO should tend to be democratic and participatory irrespective of stock ownership.
- *Governance superstructure:* Most POs have a Board of Directors, an Executive Committee, and certain other committees. The Board of Directors should initially contain all the founding members. Later, the Board can be reconstituted to represent a cross section of membership in terms of specialty and geographic distribution. Physicians who are not on the Board of Directors can and should be involved in various committees, once again conforming to the philosophy of inclusion and participation.
- *By-laws:* Attorneys for the PO should review the various options relating to by-laws for the organization, including voting rights, attendance at meetings, membership, termination of membership, contracting rights, procedure for income distribution, and so on. Selecting the right attorneys and consultants who are experienced at forming POs can greatly expedite this decision-making process.

Establishing the Committee Structure

The founding members should establish four standing committees essential to operation of a PO, and one of the founding members should chair each committee:

- *Executive Committee:* This is the overall governing committee of the PO. This committee has the authority to make certain decisions as defined in the by-laws, and has the authority to hire individuals and enter into certain contracts, subject to the approval of the full Board of Directors or, as may be necessary, the full membership.
- *Contracting Committee:* This committee is responsible for negotiating managed care contracts subject

to approval by the Executive Committee and/or the Board of Directors.

- *Membership and Credentialing Committee:* All applications for PO membership are reviewed by this committee, which is also responsible for identifying and recruiting potential new physician or group practice members. This committee is responsible for establishing the ground rules of credentialing and membership subject to the Board's approval.
- *Operations Committee:* This committee is responsible for ensuring that the information systems and operational infrastructure are in place. It is also responsible for selecting and hiring an operations manager and selecting vendors for information systems, accounting, banking, and other types of technical support.

Although one of the founding members should chair each of the four standing committees—with the Executive Committee consisting in the early stages only of founding members—it is important that other committees eventually contain physicians who are not founding members and who may not even be stockholders. In addition, as the organization grows, it may be necessary to establish subcommittees or task forces. For example, the Contracting Committee may have a subcommittee that deals with HMOs and insurance payers, a subcommittee that deals with employers, and a subcommittee that negotiates subcontracts and joint venture contracts with other physician networks or hospitals.

Recruiting Membership and Credentialing

The single most important aspect of establishing a PO is identification and recruitment of the physician membership. The founding members must make some initial policy decisions in this regard that will greatly affect both the short-term and long-range viability of the PO:

- An identification of the specialty mix and specialty distribution. Will the PO consist of a single specialty, closely related specialties, or multiple specialties?
- What is the geographic area that the PO intends to serve, and what are the general population characteristics of this area?
- Does the PO intend to restrict its membership to board-certified or board-eligible physicians?

These three major policy decisions will influence all subsequent activities of the PO. It is vital that the founders decide as early as possible the types of physician specialties, how many physicians from each specialty, and the geographic/population target size.

Once these decisions are made, it is necessary to identify target goals for potential physician members. There must be a balance between PCPs and specialists; most of the sophisticated managed care plans have approximately a 50/50 split between PCPs and specialists.

To determine the approximate number of physicians within each specialty or subspecialty, the founders should analyze the ultimate population to be served by the PO—recognizing that it may take time to achieve that goal—and then target numbers of physicians by specialty based on widely accepted physician-to-population ratios. It is important that the geographic area as well as the population is adequately covered; it is not helpful to concentrate the physicians in a small geographic area if, in fact, the overall area to be served is quite large. Therefore, in major metropolitan areas it will be necessary to define "sectors" so that in each geographic sector the appropriate mix of specialists and PCPs is represented.

The issue of board certification can be emotionally changed and involve difficult decisions. In fairly sophisticated metropolitan areas, most large managed care plans have 80% or more board-certified physicians, and some require that more than 90% of the physicians be board certified. Many experts believe that large metropolitan managed care plans will soon require 100% of the participating physicians to be board certified or board eligible.

In outlying and rural areas, however, it is often difficult to find a high percentage of board-certified physicians. In fact, many outlying areas are fortunate to have any physicians at all. Thus, if the PO expects to cover these areas, the founders may decide to include physicians who are not board certified or board eligible to be members.

Once the initial policy decisions have been made, it is time to target specific physicians and begin recruitment. The key steps are as follows:

1. Identify the specific number of target physicians by specialty within each geographic "sector."
2. Prepare a brief written document describing the PO, its organizational structure, and objectives.
3. Ideally, the founding physicians represent enough of a cross section of the geography and the various specialties to be able to know and identify many of the physician recruits in each "sector." The founders should be in a position to know who is board certified, who is receptive to managed care, who is providing high quality care, and who is well connected with hospitals that eventually may become affiliated with the PO.
4. Information is distributed to physicians targeted for membership in the PO. Telephone conversations take place and faxes are transmitted.
5. One or more meetings of groups of potential physicians are held—the number of meetings depends

on the size of the PO—at which some of the key founders plus representatives of the consultants and attorneys make presentations about the PO and answer questions. Any physician or group practice contemplating membership in the PO will have a great number of questions. It is likely that two or three meetings will be held with potential physician members before they make a commitment.

6. Although it takes time to explain the PO to potential members and answer their questions, the overall recruitment process should have a timetable and a deadline for decision making. When physicians are initially approached about membership in the PO, the founders should indicate they are approaching a select group of physicians, but those individuals must decide whether to join within a defined amount of time. The exact amount of time for the recruitment process depends on the size of the PO and the geographic area covered, but typically ranges from 60 to 120 days.
7. When physicians indicate interest in the organization, they should be given an application form that requests relatively routine credentialing information. If board certification is a prerequisite to membership, and if the founders know the physicians whom they wish to recruit, credentialing should not be a major problem.
8. Formal acceptance of physicians into the PO should be as expeditious as possible, and physicians should be required to pay the membership fee on acceptance. Membership fees in most POs range from $500 to $2000 per member, with the average being around $1000 per member. These fees can be used to help defray some of the initial organizational expenses that the founders paid, plus create additional reserves for start-up expenses. As members are being recruited, the founders should begin identifying members who could serve on one of the four committees described previously.
9. After the committees are formed and individuals appointed, a major meeting of all PO members should be held. This meeting should be a combination social and business gathering. Members of the Executive Committee and the chairpersons of the other committees should speak briefly. If a manager has been hired, he or she should make a brief presentation, and the medical director of the PO should also present. The consultants and attorneys should be available to answer questions and speak briefly on technical topics. If vendors for information systems, operations management or technical services have been selected during the recruitment process, they should be introduced and available to answer questions as well.
10. Since most of the major policy decisions will have been made prior to or during recruitment, these decisions should be conveyed to the membership. Practical and logistical issues should be discussed, and a report given of any contracts that have been negotiated or are in process. Individual physician and group members should be briefed about what to expect in the next major phase, which is the operational integration of the group.

Policy Decisions Regarding Contracting, Claims Processing, Q/A, and Other Activities

Perhaps the most significant decision affecting the operations of a PO is whether the PO will initially contract on a discounted fee-for-service basis, a capitated basis, or both. This policy decision will have a significant impact on the degree of operational sophistication necessary to operate as a unified provider. For example, it is generally much less complicated to start a PO on a discounted fee-for-service basis because the physicians will be entering into contracts that basically involve an agreed-on fee schedule. On the other hand, capitation is certainly a much more advanced form of managed care, and the object of a PO should be to enter into capitated contracts as soon as practical.

Some POs begin with discounted fee-for-service contracts for the first year of operation. This gives the physicians an opportunity to get to know one another and allows time for certain utilization and Q/A procedures to be put into effect and for information systems to be integrated. Other POs are more aggressive and enter into capitated contracts immediately. When a PO enters into a capitated contract, it must have an integrated information system and a sophisticated utilization monitoring and Q/A program in place because capitation, by definition, means that the PO physicians are assuming financial risk.

A PO that enters into capitated contracts should also be prepared to perform claims processing and other administrative functions so that the organization can truly become "self-regulating." Some POs are able to enter into capitated contracts that are renegotiable within certain time parameters. If managed care is new to a geographic area or if a particular type of specialty managed care is new, payers are often willing to enter into capitated contracts with the understanding that the capitation fee can be renegotiated based on actual experience, so long as the PO is able to demonstrate that it is rigorously policing its members with respect to utilization and Q/A.

■ Determining the Physician Compensation System

The physician compensation system in a PO that enters into discounted fee-for-service contracts is relatively easy to establish. Generally speaking, each medical practice simply submits data regarding specific patient visits and procedures attributable to contracts that the PO has entered into, and the PO reimburses physicians based on the fee schedule, while subtracting some modest percentage of dollars for administrative overhead. In other words, in discounted fee-for-service organizations compensation is largely production based.

With respect to PO contracts that are capitated, however, the compensation system becomes somewhat more complicated.

■ Determining the Degree of Hospital Interaction and/or Collaboration

There is no question that effective POs involve hospitals in the contracting process in one way or another. However, it is important to establish a strategy regarding when and how to involve hospitals. Several factors are relevant here.

- A PO covering a large geographic area may ultimately need to involve several hospitals simultaneously. Attempting to do this in the early stages of PO formation may be impractical because of the logistical challenges of coordinating negotiations with several hospitals while simultaneously forming the PO. Therefore, with respect to a PO that covers an area involving more than one hospital, it may be wise to make the initial contracts only for physician services.
- If the PO wishes to contract with multiple hospitals, it should use the most efficient hospital as the starting point to establishing fee and cost structures. Later, these fees and cost structures would be presented to other participating hospitals.
- Asking hospitals for money or other organizational support should be undertaken with great caution. Under certain circumstances a hospital can provide useful technical support, but in accepting such support the physician founders must ensure that the lines of demarcation in terms of control are clearly delineated. Otherwise, there is a danger that the PO may not end up being a *physician* organization.
- If the PO is a regional entity composed of procedure-based specialists who work primarily in hospitals (e.g., cardiologists), it might be wise to work with a local hospital that has a high number of procedure rate but also is an efficient and cost-effective provider. This usually means working with a community hospital as opposed to a teaching hospital.

Three issues are especially important when considering hospital affiliations:

1. *The geographic location of the hospital or hospitals:* It is important that hospitals be located conveniently to physicians and patients within the geographic catchment area contemplated by the PO.
2. *Efficiency, quality, and cost:* These characteristics need to be in balance. Clearly, the best hospitals from the managed care perspective are those that are high quality and have the ability to provide efficient patient care at a relatively low cost. Automatically going to the lowest cost hospital without considering that institution's quality characteristics is not necessarily the best idea.
3. *The hospital's long term viability:* Managed care will force many hospitals out of business. Others will have to downsize significantly. Smart institutions are already downsizing and becoming much more efficient in anticipation of managed care. POs are advised to gravitate toward hospitals that are already consolidating operations, becoming more efficient, measuring and controlling costs, installing sophisticated information systems, and forming appropriate alliances with other hospitals.

It is not essential that a PO link with a hospital initially. A PO can contract only for physician services and professional fees and, later on, bring in the hospital component. Above all, physicians want to avoid carrying an inefficient hospital "on their backs."

■ Determining the Management Support Staff and Budget, Identifying Operational Infrastructure Requirements, and Developing a Master Timetable

The management and operational activities of a PO can be quite significant, especially if the PO intends to enter capitated contracts in which it handles credentialing, claims processing, Q/A, and utilization management. Each of these functions is specialized, and some require significant information systems and support staff. For a PO to develop the staff capabilities as well as hardware and software capabilities to perform all these functions in a totally self-sufficient manner can be cost prohibitive and impractical, especially in the early stages of the organization. Therefore, most POs are well advised to contract with qualified outside vendors to perform many of these functions, especially functions relating to expensive information systems.

The advantages of utilizing outside vendors for certain services are twofold:

1. Vendors with state-of-the-art systems provide a level of knowledge, experience, and focus that can be a great benefit to the PO both in its formative stages and when subsequently updating capabilities.
2. Most vendors can arrange contracts that pay the vendors out of incoming receipts, usually as a flat percentage of total receipts. This has the significant advantage of reducing the up front investment of the PO.

For the purposes of this discussion, therefore, we will assume that the PO is not going to develop all of its operational capabilities internally, at least not initially. Given that outside vendors will be utilized but that internal management staff will also be needed to some extent, a recommended division of functional responsibility between outside vendors and internal staff follows:

- *Medical office, clinical, financial, and management information systems:* These systems can be installed by qualified outside vendors who can place all the member medical offices on compatible information systems. With the proper information systems and the proper training of office personnel, it is not necessary to retain an outside practice management company, but it may be necessary to retain short-term practice management and information systems assistance.
- *Human resources training/retraining:* The PO should have an internal or external person dedicated to practice operations who can interface with the information systems vendor and coordinate the training and retraining of physician office personnel in the use of such systems.
- *Claims processing:* This is an area where the PO should consider contracting with an outside vendor, especially in the initial stages of the organization and particularly if the organization is entering into capitated contracts. The claims processing vendor can aggregate information provided by the information system. State-of-the-art claims processing organizations are also able to install "automated claims processing" and other paperless technologies.
- *Utilization management and Q/A:* Utilizing management information provided by the internal systems and by the claims processing vendor, the PO physicians and staff should perform their own utilization and management and Q/A functions. The ability to self-regulate in these areas is one of the main advantages of POs. As mentioned earlier, the PO should have a physician committee dedicated to these functions. It is also advisable eventually to have a full-time staff support person who manages and coordinates these functions; all the decision making and reviews, however, should be performed by physicians themselves. Large POs will need a dedicated physician employee (full or part-time) for this function.
- *Aggregation and formatting of information:* To secure managed care contracts and keep payers informed, it will be necessary to have the internal capability to aggregate information from various sources and format it into presentations to payers. The PO will need a manager of contracting. In the early stages of operations, this person can also handle aggregation and "packaging" of information pursuant to marketing and contracting. Eventually, however, the two functions of contract negotiations and marketing will need to be separated into two different individuals.
- *Contracting:* The PO should handle all contracting internally on a coordinated basis with a medical director and the manager of contracting. In the early stages of PO formation, a physician can probably handle both functions depending on the initial size of the organization. However, very soon after formation, the PO will require a full-time contracting staff person who should report to the medical director and also to the contracting committee.
- *Financial operations:* In the early stages of PO formation, an operations manager can direct both practice operations and financial operations. Eventually, however, the organization will need to have a chief financial officer.
- *Clinical operations:* The PO will need a physician medical director. Initially, this individual can assist with contracting and development of clinical protocols, utilization management, quality assurance, and credentialing. However, the PO will eventually require staff support to assist the medical director in carrying out these functions.

Selecting Outside Vendors/Products for the Operational Infrastructure

Selecting the right vendors and other outside experts is critical; these individuals can greatly assist with both start-up activities and ongoing PO operations. Some of the key start-up functions that can be performed by outside vendors are described below:

- Assistance with respect to initial PO formation and policy-making activities can be provided by attorneys and consultants. The consultants should also assist in budgeting, planning, and initial contract negotiations.
- Medical practice operational consultants can assist in assessing the member medical practices with respect

to information systems capabilities, relative sophistication of office staff, patient demographics, utilization characteristics, and financial characteristics.

- Information systems vendors can evaluate information systems requirements and, in the initial stages, develop a plan and budget to interface consistent information systems with other aspects of operations.
- The founding members of the PO should select an accounting firm to provide basic accounting services with respect to establishing the financial management functions of the PO.
- The founders of the PO should select a bank to provide specific services, including cash management and depository services. The right bank can also be a good resource for working capital loans, capital equipment loans, expansion loans, and other credit services.

As the PO emerges beyond the formative stage and into full-scale operations, it will be necessary to form relationships with vendors in certain critical areas. Some of the vendors who are conducting activities mentioned above should be able to easily transition into the full implementation stage. These operational areas of activity are as follows:

- Installing information systems and training practice staffs to operate those systems is perhaps the most significant operational challenge facing a PO. A PO cannot enter into capitation contracts without consistent information systems, and the organization is unable to market itself effectively to payers without the ability to aggregate relatively sophisticated types of utilization and quality data. All competition and managed care in the future will be based on information; therefore, these systems are essential if a PO is to mature into advanced managed care.
- With the capability to link into the PO's own information system, a claims-processing company can be helpful in handling all claims processing activity and in installing state-of-the-art automated and telemetric claims processing capabilities. The right outside vendor can also assist in bringing some or all of these functions in-house as the PO reaches the point where it can undertake its own claims processing.
- Practice management and human resource consultants may be needed to assist in training and retraining medical office staff, especially if the PO intends to enter into capitation contracts. This usually involves a relatively short-term engagement, with the consultants subsequently available "as needed" for troubleshooting and specific follow-up projects.
- It is possible that consultants and/or actuaries may be required to assist with analysis and negotiations pursuant to contracting. This is particularly true if the PO is involved in negotiations for capitation contracts. After the PO matures, however, this capability should be handled by the contracting manager who, from that point, should only need periodic technical support from outside sources.

Several principles apply to the selection of outside vendors:

1. They should have specific experience with physician networks in their respective field of expertise.
2. They should be able to demonstrate the ability to provide state-of-the-art services and products. This is particularly true of information systems vendors. Organizers of POs are advised to be cautious and methodical in selecting vendors with respect to information systems hardware, software, and support services. Vendors in the area of information systems are notorious for overpromising what their systems can do, for representing advances that are not yet implemented, and for not providing adequate follow-up services, training, and systems support.
3. Claims processing vendors should have specific experience in that field as well as the capability for automation and advanced forms of telemetry. They should also demonstrate a willingness to transition at least part of the claims-processing functions to the internal operations of the PO after the PO matures.
4. Bankers must be sensitive to and understand the medical practice business. They must have a demonstrated track record of making loans to physicians and POs, an understanding of the credit characteristics of such organizations and, above all, a willingness to lend money with a minimum of red tape. Be forewarned: relatively few banks possess these qualities.
5. Practice management consultants should have hands-on practice management experience, have worked in or with medical practices, and be able to understand all aspects of medical practice operations. They should also be individuals who can relate well to and be empathetic with the involved office staffs.
6. Accountants should have experience in handling the accounting and tax work for medical practices, including group practices. Accountants should be able to work collaboratively with information systems vendors to install effective financial reporting systems, payable systems, payroll systems, and other necessary accounting and financial systems.
7. Fees for all vendors retained to perform specific, short-term projects should be capped. Vendors who are providing ongoing services (i.e., claims management) should be willing take their fees as a reasonable percentage of collected receipts. Such arrangements minimize the upfront expenditures on the part of the PO.

8. Any vendor should be willing to transition the services being provided into the internal operations of the PO where appropriate. This is especially true in areas like information systems management, managed care contracting, practice management support, and—when the PO becomes large enough—claims processing. All these functions need not necessarily be performed internally; some vendors will continue to make it more attractive for the PO to contract with them than to bring a function inside. However, vendors should be willing to cooperate in transitioning these capabilities, if the PO desires to become operationally self-sufficient.
9. Vendors involved in developing state-of-the-art systems should be willing to bring those systems into the PO as new ideas and products come "on line." In addition, information systems vendors should be willing to customize system features that are appropriate for the specific PO.

Packaging Information for Marketing to Payers and Employers

Once the PO has been formed and has accumulated enough information from its member practices, the organization is in a position to present a comprehensive profile to payors and employers. This is the PO's first major marketing effort and represents the first opportunity to negotiate managed care contracts.

In the early formative stages, POs cannot be expected to have installed the kinds of sophisticated information systems and data retrieval systems that will eventually be present in the fully mature organization. However, this should not stop the PO from accumulating data available from participating medical practices and presenting a comprehensive profile to payers and employers. Practice management consultants and contracting consultants can greatly assist here in identifying the minimum required levels of information to present to potential purchasers of the PO's services. The initial "PO Profile" package, for example, might include the following information:

- A complete listing of the PO's medical practice members, their specialties, and their geographic locations. For group practice members, this should include a list of the individual physicians and their specialties within the group practice.
- For each physician listed, the hospital affiliation or affiliations.
- A map of the region showing the locations of medical practices and delineating primary care practices from specialty practices.
- A description of the PO's credentialing criteria.
- A description of the PO's organizational structure, its management, and operational plan.
- A description of the PO's contracting goals, both in terms of the types of contracts the PO wishes to enter into and the numbers, demographics, and geographic coverage of the populations the PO wishes to serve.
- Commentary regarding the PO's willingness and capabilities to enter into capitation and discounted fee-for-service contracts.
- Although it may be difficult to assemble such information for the first round of managed care contracting, information profiling aspects of the medical practices relating to utilization and quality would be helpful. Any special information about advanced procedures capabilities, research, or other advanced medical treatment activities would also be helpful. In addition, activities and programs relating to ambulatory care and preventive medicine should be described. These two areas are of special interest to payers—especially to self-insured employers.

In the first round of contract negotiations (which will involve contracting for the first full year of PO operations), most payers and employers will be sympathetic to the fact that a PO is not going to be able to present sophisticated quality and utilization information and may not be able to conduct full-scale claims processing activities. The important factor to convey to payers and employers is that the PO is committed to value, managed care, advanced information systems and quality monitoring, and, above all, to *physician-directed* self-regulation. Payers and employers will be especially impressed if a PO is willing to enter into capitated contracts even if those contracts may need to be renegotiable or otherwise adjusted at some point during the first year.

The structure of the PO itself will be a significant issue in the eyes of purchasers of health care services. Multispecialty membership is preferable to single-specialty POs, although some types of single-specialty organizations can be quite attractive if constructed properly (e.g., cardiology).

Even though multispecialty structures are more attractive to payers, POs that are top-heavy with specialists will be viewed less favorably than organizations with a balance of PCPs and specialists. Organizations that can reach a wide geographic area and provide relatively comprehensive services to various geographic sectors will also impress payors and employers. Finally, POs that are in the process of forming collaborative alliances with the more efficient hospitals in an area will be viewed positively by the payor community even if the first round of contracting does not involve joint-physician hospital contracts; at the same time, PO alliances with the wrong hospitals can be a significant hindrance to managed care contracting.

Contracting Negotiations

The nature of negotiations with payers will depend on the type of payor and the type of contract being negotiated—a discounted fee-for-service contract or a capitated contract. In general, discounted fee-for-service contracts are somewhat easier to negotiate and may create less of an administrative burden than capitated contracts. However, if structured properly, capitated contracts can give the PO much more control and can be more profitable.

Some relevant points with respect to contracting negotiations follows:

- Discounted fee-for-service contracts will most likely be predrafted "form" contracts prepared by the payers themselves, especially if the PO is contracting with HMOs, PPOs, or insurance companies. In such circumstances, it is important to have qualified people read the contracts in detail, focusing on (1) the fee schedules, (2) ensuring that the services to be provided are clearly described and that there is a delineation between covered and noncovered services, (3) ensuring the PO members understand and accept procedures with respect to preauthorizations and utilization review, and (4) ensuring that the PO clearly understands and accepts the billing and financial reporting procedures.
- Some discounted fee-for-service contracts can be negotiated directly with employers or other organizations. These situations may provide more flexibility for the PO to negotiate better terms in two areas. First, employers and organizations who do not have existing utilization and claims administration capabilities may be receptive to the PO handling these areas, including "self-regulation" of the U/R and Q/A processes. Second, the PO may be able to enter into an arrangement that begins as a discounted fee-for-service program, but later evolves into a capitated program. This has the significant advantage of permitting the parties to gather experience data on the covered population prior to entering into capitated arrangements. It also permits the PO to gravitate in a prudent manner toward capitation, which is the desirable end result.
- When capitated contracts are being considered either in the short or long term, it will be necessary to assemble enough information about the covered population and that population's claim experience to develop a capitation fee schedule. The capitation fee can be either a set per-member-per-month dollar amount covering all services or a combined arrangement in which the capitation fee covers only specific services, with a discounted fee schedule covering certain other procedures and services that are not as easily capitated. There are numerous ways to arrive at capitation fees; the most expeditious to study the actual claims experience of the population to be covered. This requires that the payer or employer share claims experience and cost information with the PO so that the parties can cooperatively analyze the information and arrive at a fair capitation fee.
- In new capitated contracts where the population has not been capitated previously, it is advisable to structure the contract so that the fee can be adjusted based on actual experience, especially during the first year of the new arrangement.
- Single-specialty POs will only be able to enter into discounted fee-for-service or capitated contracts with respect to the specialty services they provide, whereas multispecialty POs can enter into contracts for a much broader range of physician services. Although the scope of services of a single specialty PO is more limited, such organizations can "joint contract" with other POs and approach payers or employers on a unified basis.
- If a PO intends to team up with a hospital or hospitals for purposes of joint contracting, negotiations will be required between the PO and the hospital to ensure that the PO returns administrative control of its operations and that the PO's financial interests are protected. In addition, when a hospital is brought into the process, it is vital that the hospital's costs and fee structure be competitive and that there be a mechanism for controlling cost and fee increases. POs with a significant market presence can exert bargaining influence over hospitals to make their costs competitive.
- Managed care contracts should be flexible enough so that if new services and products are added to the PO's capabilities there is a mechanism for pricing and incorporating them into the master managed care contract. This is true both with respect to new medical services (or specialties added) and to enhancement of existing services—for example, moving certain procedures and tests from the inpatient to the outpatient setting and/or introducing enhanced diagnostic equipment, drugs, or other enhanced capabilities.

Adding New Members and/or New Affiliations

A PO can grow in several ways:

- Through the expansion of its geographical catchment area.

- Through the expansion of its population catchment area.
- By increasing the numbers of physicians within the PO's existing specialty complement.
- By expanding the PO's medical service capabilities through inclusion of new types of specialists not in the original organization.
- By forming "contracting alliances" with other POs or group practices.
- By forming "contracting alliances" with hospitals, medical centers, or hospital networks.
- By forming "contracting alliances" with home health agencies, networks of psychiatrists and psychologists, physical therapists, and rehabilitation specialties or other similar and logical vertical or horizontal relationships.

When new physician members or group practice members are added to the PO, it is important that they add appropriate and efficient capabilities to those of the existing PO. If a PO is successful, many additional physicians will want to join, but that does not mean the organization needs them. Additional physicians should be permitted into a PO *only* if:

- They conform to the credentialing criteria established by the PO's Credentialing Committee.
- They add a new service capability that is truly needed by the covered population, or they provide an existing service capability to a newly covered population or geographic catchment area.
- They are willing to conform to the PO's policies and procedures with respect to utilization management, quality assurance, office operations, and information systems.

If other types of providers such as hospitals and home health agencies are going to be included in or affiliated with the PO, it is important that the PO protect its own short and long-term interests and that the PO structure such arrangements to minimize the probability that the incoming or affiliated organization would detract from the organization in any way.

Simply because a PO has a capitated arrangement with payers does not mean that affiliated organizations must also be capitated, at least not initially. It is entirely possible to have a contract that combines capitation and discounted fee-for-service arrangements with respect to various component services. The essential ingredients for any organizations affiliated with a PO and entering into joint contracts are quality and cost effectiveness.

Above all, when affiliating with other organizations—especially hospitals—the PO must ensure that its control over both the master contracting process and its operations is not subrogated or otherwise compromised.

Marketing and Contracting

Contracting Policy Decisions and Goals

The contracting process for most physician networks—whether a PO or a fully integrated regional group practice—is likely to be an evolutionary process. There are several reasons for this:

1. Most newly formed physician networks may not have the management information systems and claims processing infrastructures necessary to enter into full risk-capitated contracting immediately. Many of these networks will choose to contract largely on a discounted fee-for-service basis during their first full calendar year of operation.
2. When physician networks do decide enter into capitated contracts, it may be advisable to capitate services gradually, beginning with office-based physician services. Under such combined arrangements, capitated contracts would be in place for certain defined office-based services and other professional services, and discounted fee-for-service contracts would continue in effect for hospital services and certain procedures and services that would remain expressly outside the capitation contract.
3. The inclusion of hospital services and other more intensive procedure-based services in capitated contracts can markedly increase overall risk as well as the administrative complexity of the program. Thus, in the early stages, many physician networks will choose to delay capitation of hospital and other advanced services.
4. The state-of-the-art of capitation, managed care contracting, claims administration, quality assurance, and other components of managed care will continue to change and evolve, bringing along technical enhancements that ideally can be used to the benefit of physician networks.

Some of the most important decisions that a physician network makes will need to be made in the early stages of network formation and will involve the issues of contracting policies and goals. These decisions—some of which have been referred to earlier but are worth repeating here—are as follows:

- Defining the specialties to be included in the network and the scope of services to be provided by the network.
- Defining the geographical and population catchment areas to be served by the network, both in the short term and the long term.
- Evaluating the payer markets; for example, insurance companies, HMOs, PPOs, self-insured employers, governmental entities, and other payers.

- Determining whether and how soon the network will be prepared to enter into capitated contracts.
- Making a realistic assessment of operational infrastructure capabilities and determining how soon those capabilities can be put in place given the relative stages of the network's formation.

Most new physician networks will need to transition gradually into more advanced forms of managed care contracting. However, the ultimate goals of all physician networks should be threefold:

1. To be become truly multispecialty in nature, either directly or through alliances.
2. To cover as wide a geographical and population catchment area as the market and antitrust regulations will permit.
3. To enter in to full-risk capitated contracts.

Above all, physicians forming a network should keep in mind that the most significant benefits of network formation will only be realized when the network itself is capable of assuming risk for a defined population. This occurs when physicians receive an appropriate pool of dollars and allocate resource utilization appropriately, thus "managing" patient care themselves.

Information Systems Infrastructure: The Critical Linchpin

In the future managed care era, all competition among health care providers will occur on the basis of information. Under widespread managed care—especially under capitation—the effectiveness and desirability of providers who serve or attempt to serve a defined population will be measured on the basis of the following factors:

- Geographical and population coverage.
- Relative utilization rates and resource consumption.
- Cost and cost effectiveness.
- Clinical outcomes measurements for the population being served.
- Credentialing criteria, scope of services, and ability to deliver noninstitutional care.

These key indicators will be evaluated by all payers, who will make a determination as to the *value* of the provider network relative to other options payers may have. Thus, to be able to compete in this kind of environment, a provider network—especially a physician-directed network—must be able to assimilate the kinds of information that can address these evaluative factors.

In fact, a national coalition of employers, HMOs, PPOs, and other payers has already developed the first generation of some of this required information. These reporting requirements are known as the Health Plan Employer Data and Information Set (HEDIS). HEDIS is the first generation of "core performance measures" designed to reflect health plan or provider performance through a common set of reporting standards that will enable payers throughout the United States to conduct comparative performance evaluations. It is beyond the scope of this book to present the HEDIS requirements in detail, but some of the items that HEDIS seeks to measure with respect to providers include:

- Measures of preventive care and health promotion including childhood immunization rates, cholesterol screening, mammography screening, other health screening tests, and health promotion/education programs.
- Measures of the effectiveness of prenatal care such as low birth-weight rate, the number of pregnant women for whom prenatal care began in the first trimester, and other measures of obstetrics effectiveness such as the percent of Cesarean sections.
- Measures of admission and readmission rates for acute and chronic illnesses.
- Outcomes measurements for treatment of cardiovascular diseases, cancer, and other high-profile health problems.
- Measures of admission and readmission rates for mental health and substance abuse problems.
- Measures of access to physician providers and urgent care providers.
- Measures of patient satisfaction with providers in a provider network.
- Detailed data on gender and age breakdowns for the covered population and the utilization rates for each subcategory.
- Utilization rates and costs for specific services such as hospitalization, inpatient surgery, outpatient surgery, chemotherapy, and other high-profile services or institutional settings.
- An analysis of the number of encounters, the number of procedures, the number of institutionalizations, average costs, and other parameters for high occurrence or high-cost DRGs in categories such as cardiovascular care, respiratory care/asthma, gynecological/obstetrics care, and cancer treatment.
- Global breakdowns and analyses of physician office encounters, other ambulatory care encounters and procedures, hospital inpatient utilization, maternity services, pediatric and newborn services, treatment of mental health and chemical dependency services, and other non-acute care.
- Financial breakdowns including costs by type of service and setting and including overall indicators of financial stability of the provider network.
- Information relating to quality assessment and improvement activities including detailed information about the quality assurance studies that have been

conducted, what areas of the provider network experience problems and identify need for improvement, what were the most important performance improvements the plan addressed during the most recent year, how did the plan improve the care of the population it serves, and what advances are planned in terms of expanding the delivery of services, scope of services, access, preventive care, case management, utilization, and risk management?

As comprehensive as this list seems, it is important to keep in mind that this is only the first generation of HEDIS reporting requirements.

In addition to the requirements relating to HEDIS and similar efforts, any provider network faces significant challenges with respect to its own internal administration and financial management. Therefore, most physician networks will probably need to contract with outside vendors to be able to "jump start" these capabilities in the early stages of network operation. Over time, the network can begin to develop its own internal information management system capabilities and transition those capabilities from outside vendors to in-house functions (although outside vendors may continue to remain competitive and efficient with respect to certain services).

Preparation of a Marketing "Package"

Even though a newly formed physician network is unlikely to be able to present the kinds of detailed information required under HEDIS in preparation for the first round of managed-care negotiations, the network should strive to prepare as comprehensive a profile as possible. Some of the kinds of information that can be presented in such a profile are found under "Contracting."

It is important for physicians to keep in mind that very few truly sophisticated physician networks exist in the United States. Most payers and employers realize that it takes time to assemble the physician members of a provider network and to install the necessary administrative and information systems infrastructures. Therefore, physicians should not be bashful or defensive about approaching payers and employers and opening negotiations with them even though many elements of the network may not be in place in time for the first contracts. If the physician network is constituted properly and has enough market presence, most payers will be willing to work with the network to develop contracts for the first year with the understanding that more sophisticated contracts will be developed later.

Contracting Issues to be Aware of

This part of the discussion will deal with major contracting issues that physician networks must consider prior to entering into negotiations with payors. The discussion covers both discounted fee-for-service contracts and capitated contracts. However, this discussion is not exhaustive; the reader is encouraged to work with local managed care experts, including qualified local health care legal counsel, and to consult other, more detailed sources of literature on managed care contracting.

One of the first major issues to address is who is doing the contracting? Is the physician network doing the contracting as a sole provider entity, is the physician network joining with other POs or fully integrated groups to engage in joint contracting, or is the physician network joining with a hospital or hospital network to negotiate a joint contract? The following points are relevant:

- If a physician network is the sole contractor in its own right, the nature of the contract to be negotiated will depend on whether the network in question is single specialty or multispecialty. Single-specialty networks will obviously be negotiating with respect to a more restrictive scope of services. In addition, the physicians in a single-specialty network may need to significantly alter their patterns of referral to other physicians, hospitals, and other providers especially if the contract in question is being negotiated with a PPO or HMO that has its own "approved list" of providers.
- If two physician networks are teaming up to negotiate jointly (or if a physician network is teaming with large group practices or other disparate physician providers), it will be important to: (1) select individuals who are authorized to negotiate officially on behalf of both networks and (2) prepare an information "profile" describing characteristics of each of the entities as well as the benefits that the combined entities bring to the table. In addition, the member entities of such a combined contracting confederation will need to conduct at least some negotiations with one another even before approaching payers so that the physicians themselves reach conceptual agreement concerning such issues as division of revenues, sharing organizational expenses, sharing information systems expenses, determining who will control management, and a number of other issues. The worst approach POs can take is to team up with one another, approach a payer and then begin bickering among themselves when contract negotiations get serious.
- If a physician network is going to be contracting jointly with a hospital or hospital network, it is vital that the parties reach agreement on several issues:
  Determine the exact type of structure through which the entities will negotiate.
  Determine who is going to do the negotiating on behalf of the parties (including the possibility that a

physician network representative and a hospital network representative will each attend all meetings and have equal representation in the negotiations).

Determine whether the "master contract" will flow through and be administered by the physician network, the hospital, or some new joint entity that the parties create (e.g., a PHO). Any physician will immediately recognize the critical importance of this issue.

Determine what kind of general contract the physician network is interested in as opposed to the hospital. For example, a physician network may be prepared for a capitated contract with respect to office-based physician services and professional fees, whereas a hospital may not be prepared for capitation and may prefer to start with discounted fee-for-service contract. If this is the case, the physician network must make absolutely certain that the hospital's discounted fee structure is competitive and that the physician network itself has veto power over unreasonable future hospital fee increases.

If the "master contract" to both the physician network and the hospital is going to be a capitated contract, the parties will need to have their own negotiations with respect to: (1) the administrative control of the contract and (2) the division of capitated dollars at the present time and in the future.

When a physician network is involved with a hospital in a joint "full-risk" capitated contract, the issues of risk and reward come in to play. Normally, the term "full-risk" means that the physician network and the hospital must work out an equitable division of risk sharing that is proportionate to the services being provided, the relative attributable costs of such services, and other factors.

Likewise, if the capitation contract results in the generation of savings and excess distributable funds, the physician network and hospital need to reach an accommodation about the relative distribution of such funds. The prevalent view of most experts is that since physicians themselves are the individuals most responsible (and in some cases solely responsible) for determining patient utilization patterns and resource consumption, then the physician network should reap most of the financial benefits of excess cash flow resulting from the master joint contract. At the same time, the physicians should bear in mind that even though the hospital may need to downsize and become much more efficient, it still has to replace vital equipment and maintain a competent clinical support staff as well as other support services. It is in the interest of the physicians in a network that is joint contracting with a hospital to keep the hospital as efficient as possible, but the covered population also must be well served by the hospital and satisfied by such services.

Once the issues of: (a) who is doing the managed care negotiating and (b) the relationship of the parties have been determined, numerous other issues arise with respect to the proposed managed care contract itself. As an initial matter, it is important to point out that physicians negotiating with payers may be handed a preprinted "standard" contract. Such a document should be regarded by physicians as a point of departure, not as a "take or leave it" ultimatum. Assuming that the physician network has established a reasonable critical mass that can be translated into a significant market presence, most items in a managed care contract can and should be negotiated. In this regard, it is vital that key executives of the physician network as well as key outside experts participate in reviewing the contract in detail and making recommendations concerning the negotiations.

With this in mind, some of the major managed care contracting issues that a physician network is likely to face follow. (The reader should again be reminded that this list is not exhaustive and that additional sources and experts should be consulted).

- If the physician network is contracting with an HMO, PPO, or insurance company, the entity with whom the physicians are negotiating should be asked to demonstrate its overall financial viability and experience. Managed care plans in this country have gone bankrupt, leaving participating physicians with thousands of dollars in uncollected bills and other liabilities. Consequently, the issue of the payer's financial soundness is not something to be taken lightly or glossed over.
- The physician network should assess the administrative capabilities of the payer if, in fact, the payer is going to perform administrative functions. This involves determining the payer's experience at conducting claims processing, the kind of information systems and management infrastructure the payer has, the kinds of reports and information the payer provides to participating physicians, and how the payer conducts utilization analyses and preauthorizations and a number of other issues.
- The physician network should evaluate the overall market presence of the payer in terms of the number of covered lives the payer will bring to the network and compare this with the network's number and composition of physicians to ensure that the physician network can, in fact, service the covered population.
- If the physician network is entering into a discounted fee-for-service contract with a payer, the network will usually perform patient care services and invoice the payer for the specific services provided based on the predetermined fee schedule. This raises the issue of the "collectibility" of funds

from the payer. Physicians should be forewarned that many managed care payers are agonizingly slow in paying claims and that many medical practices carry long overdue accounts receivable from such payers on their books. Some states have even enacted laws requiring insurance companies and managed care payers to pay within a certain time frame or otherwise suffer penalties. The entire issue of billing and collections is a critical one for physician networks entering into discounted fee-for-service contracts. Although this is not as much of an issue regarding capitated contracts, the issue of the timing of capitated payments, the basis for capitated payments, and related matters should also be addressed.

- The area of competition must be addressed regarding the activities of both the physician network and the payer. The physicians want to make certain that the payer is restricted in making contracts with directly competing physician networks or, at the very least, that the physician network in question is treated on a parity basis with other providers with whom the payer may contract in the given market area. In addition, the physician network wants to have the ability to market itself to other payers and to enter into other contracts without hinderance.
- The draft contract submitted by a payer to a physician network may include references to other documents, including fee schedules. It is important to review all documents that are referenced in any managed care contract. Furthermore, physicians should be forewarned of language in managed care contracts referring to "fee schedules prevailing at the time" or "the right to alter fee schedules at any time." It is important that a physician network has the ability to preapprove any changes in fee schedules or capitation rates; otherwise, the network is leaving itself open to potentially serious financial difficulties.
- The term of a managed care contract is usually one year, but some contracts have "evergreen" provisions permitting the parties to automatically renew the contract at the end of each year unless one of the parties exercises its termination rights. In addition to having the capability to terminate a managed care contract at the end of the contract year, a physician network should retain the right to terminate the contract during the year if the payer does not meet certain obligations.
- If capitation arrangements are contemplated in a managed care contract, the physician network should not accept capitated rates at face value but, instead, should analyze those rates to ensure that they are fair. As mentioned previously, newly formed physician networks are advised to enter into capitated arrangements in which the cap rate can be modified during the course of the first year, if necessary. The entire issue of capitation is one that must to be approached with caution and, if necessary, with outside experts, perhaps even actuaries.
- The "covered services" of any managed care contract should be listed as specifically as possible, delineating exactly the physician services that are covered and those that are not. It is customary sound contracting practice to exclude certain high-cost services—especially experimental or quasi-experimental services—from capitated contracts or discounted fee-for-service schedules. A related issue is whether a physician network is entering into a joint managed care contract along with a hospital; if so, certain hospital services may need to be excluded from the managed care contract as well.
- The profile of the members of the covered population should be studied and assessed for health risk. In addition, the payer should provide the physician network with detailed information regarding its underwriting criteria if, in fact, the payer conducts differential underwriting. Many managed care payers at the present time cover all families and individuals of an employed population, regardless of the incoming health status of those individuals. If the physician network intends to assume capitated risk, the exact nature of the health risk of the covered population in question needs to be determined.
- Capitated contracts can have any number of payment methods, including payment by virtue of percentage of premium, number of families, age/sex distribution, and other formulae. In addition, insurance companies and managed care payers all have various levels of copayments from patients at the time of service. These arrangements need to be examined carefully, both in terms of the initial payment arrangements and the ability to adjust payments at some future time. One arrangement that has been satisfactory to physician networks entering into capitation contracts is the payment of a flat rate per person per month based on a detailed analysis of a composition of the covered lives.
- Insurance and reinsurance coverage secured by the payer—and, if necessary, the physician network—needs to be determined. Most insurance companies, HMOs, and PPOs have reinsurance to protect their organizations against catastrophic losses. It is necessary to determine whether such reinsurance is adequate. In addition, with respect to full-risk capitated contracts entered into by the physician network, the network may need to acquire reinsurance in its own right.
- Malpractice liability and indemnification issues must be examined concerning both the physician network and the payer. If at all possible, a physician network should avoid indemnifying a payer against

malpractice claims or any other lawsuits. At the same time, the physician network wants to make certain that a lawsuit against the payer for irresponsible utilization review or preauthorization service denials are the sole responsibility of the payer. A physician should not be held liable if the physician recommends care for a patient and that care is denied by utilization review nurse or some other employee of the payer. Indemnification against this kind of liability should also be extended to protect the physician network from lawsuits against third party administrators (TPAs) who may be in the business of administering claims, conducting utilization review, and preauthorizing services on behalf of the payer.

- A physician network that is entering into a capitated contract with a payer should reserve the right to "self-administer" and "self-regulate." This means that the physician network should retain the option to bring claims processing, utilization review, preauthorization functions, quality assurance, outcomes measurement and all other administrative and management functions in-house, in return for which the capitated rate is adjusted significantly upward in recognition of the fact that the payer is no longer performing these functions and no longer incurs the overhead or the liabilities associated with these functions. Although it may be impractical to assume these functions during the first year of the contract, it should definitely be the longer term objective of any physician network to become self-regulating with respect to all capitated contracts.

Because of the high overhead and increasingly significant legal liabilities associated with administering managed care plans, most payers should welcome the opportunity to transfer these functions to a physician network. In fact, most enlightened payers have come to realize the facts of life of managed care: that the most highly evolved form of managed care from everybody's perspective is the physician-directed network that simultaneously assumes risk, self-regulates, and "manages" patient care.

Antitrust and Other Federal and State Regulatory Issues

The reader needs to be aware of three important qualifying factors in any discussion of antitrust and other regulatory issues:

1. The discussion that follows is intended to provide an overview of selected legal/regulatory issues and is not meant to be comprehensive. Furthermore, this information does not constitute legal advice and should not be construed as such.
2. This book is being written at a time when national health care legislation is pending in Congress. Legislation developed and passed by Congress is expected to make changes in antitrust laws and other laws and regulations governing medical practices, group practices, physician organizations, and integrated health care networks. The discussion in this section, therefore, takes into account only current laws and regulations, and the reader is encouraged to closely follow new developments in this rapidly changing field.
3. Adding to the transitional nature of federal laws and regulations in many areas, are state laws/regulations also in transition that may be subject to significant modification.

With these points in mind, it is the strong advice of this author that physicians contemplating forming a network of one type or another consult a qualified health care counsel in their state who has a familiarity with both federal and state laws/regulations as well as with pending changes affecting the activities and arrangements described in this book.

Antitrust Regulatory Activity

Let us first turn to a discussion of antitrust laws and regulations. The entire area of health care antitrust has been one of increased focus at both a federal and state level during the past several years, especially at the federal level. It should be noted that most state laws mirror federal laws in this area. Therefore, what is said about the antitrust area in this discussion from a federal standpoint will generally apply to individual states as well.

Selected antitrust issues with respect to physician network formation are as follows:

- The general purpose of most antitrust laws and regulations is to prohibit "anticompetitive" arrangements and activities. Three categories normally of interest to regulators are: (1) arrangements that because of their sheer size have the effect of dominating or monopolizing a market or of engendering a structure that has the potential for price fixing or locking out competitors, (2) arrangements wherein a number of independent competitors get together to fix prices and engage in other anticompetitive behavior, and (3) arrangements in which a monopoly or a "cartel" controls the supply, distribution, and pricing of products or services.
- Nonetheless, the U.S. Justice Department and the Federal Trade Commission have each recognized that managed care plans and integrated health systems possess characteristics that are of benefit to society. Therefore, laws and regulations applying to

other industries have been (and are being) modified to permit some flexibility in recognition of the fact that managed care providers need to aggregate services and apply consistent pricing to increase access to health services, make the provision of health services more efficient, and render health services more cost effective.

- At the same time, regulatory agencies do not want health care providers, including managed care providers, to create anticompetitive monopolies and cartels or to engage in price-fixing.
- In recognition of the need to balance antitrust regulations with the need for the consolidation and modernization of the health care industry, the Justice Department and the Federal Trade Commission have taken two important steps: (1) the establishment of certain "safety zones" for physician networks that include 20% or less of the physicians in each specialty within a geographical market who also "share substantial financial risk" and (2) to subject arrangements among health care providers and insurers to a "rule-of-reason" doctrine permitting some flexibility in the interpretation and scrutiny of specific arrangements.
- From a practical standpoint, a physician network that comprises 20% or less of the physicians in each specialty within a "defined geographic market area" will most likely not be susceptible to the allegation of creating a monopoly. In addition, just because the 20% safety zone has been established does not mean that networks comprising over 20% are automatically vulnerable to regulatory attack; it just means that those with over 20% market share may be scrutinized more carefully for anticompetitive behavior.
- The regulatory agencies make distinctions between independent health care providers who are coming together for the purposes of joint contracting as opposed to more integrated provider networks. Providers who otherwise compete against one another but are coming together for the purposes of joint contracting can, under certain circumstances, be accused of price fixing. To avoid exposure in this area, Physician Organizations, IPAs, and other loose affiliations of physicians or affiliations of physicians and hospitals need to be structured carefully and with the assistance of experienced health care attorneys.
- It is widely accepted that arrangements that are the least vulnerable to regulatory attack in the antitrust area are fully integrated arrangements in which physicians have true co-ownership. In addition, the regulatory agencies are favorably impressed by capitated arrangements in which the physicians share financial risk. In fact, the concept of "shared financial risk" is an important concept used by regulatory bodies when they apply the "rule-of-reason" doctrine to the examination of concerted contracting or other collaborative arrangements among health care providers.

Many physicians and hospitals clearly feel that the present antitrust laws and regulations are counterproductive when it comes to the need of the health care industry to consolidate and enter into collaborative arrangements. Many experts believe that these laws and regulations will be significantly changed and liberalized in the future and that the three tests of future arrangements will be:

1. Does the collaboration among providers increase access to health care services by consumers in the market being served?
2. Does the collaboration result in efficiencies that can be demonstrated to lower costs?
3. Does the collaboration preserve or even enhance the quality of the health care being provided?

It remains to be seen whether these guidelines will eventually supersede existing approaches for scrutinizing physician networks and other provider affiliations. Once again, the author recommends that in this period of transition the founders of any type of physician network consult qualified health care attorneys.

"Anti-Referral" Regulations

Another growing area of legislation and regulation can be described as "anti-referral" regulatory activity. At the federal level, the Stark bill initially dealt with this area, and a number of individual states have also enacted anti-referral legislation. Such legislation, broadly speaking, seeks to prohibit physicians from referring patients to laboratories and diagnostic centers in which the physician or a family member has an investment interest or other financial relationship. However, certain types of entities are exempted in most cases from this type of anti-referral legislation, including fully integrated group practices, prepaid health plans, and certain defined types of integrated health networks.

Like the area of antitrust, the area of anti-referral legislation is inevitably bound to undergo numerous changes in the next several years. Thus, qualified health care attorneys should be consulted in this area with respect to any type of physician network being formed.

It can be said that the fully integrated regional group practice as defined in this book is the kind of entity most likely to be exempted from anti-referral legislation—or at least less likely to be affected by such legislation than PO. This is because a PO is not a fully integrated entity with common ownership by and employment of physicians. The reader will recall that although management and information systems functions may be shared in a PO, the member practices remain as discrete legal and operating entities, and the member physicians of a PO can still enter into other contracts and arrangements independent of the PO. In fact, one of the reasons why successful POs are well advised to evolve into a fully integrated regional group practice is because the fully-evolved organization is more likely to be able to own and operate its own laboratory, diagnostic centers, home health agencies, and even hospitals.

Malpractice

A third major area of legislation and regulatory activity is the area of malpractice. An entire book could be written about this subject alone, and it is far beyond the scope of this chapter to enter a detailed discussion. Physicians are advised to be attentive to three areas relating to the overall issue of malpractice:

1. State "reforms."
2. Federal malpractice tort "reforms."
3. The definition of malpractice and related liabilities as they relate to managed care plans, including both payers and provider networks, and the potential liability interrelationships between providers and payers.

It is this last area where a remarkable amount of legal activity is taking place. A notable example is the growing tendency of patients to file suit against prepaid health plans or PPOs which deny care that physicians have recommended. Although the denial of patient care cannot technically be described as "malpractice," in such circumstances it is sometimes the case that physicians are sued simultaneously with the managed care plan.

The growing exposure to liability on the part of HMOs, PPOs, insurance companies, and other payers relating to aggressive utilization review, denials of service, and denials of claims dictate that physician networks and their attorneys pay special attention to the potential exposure to liabilities through contractual arrangements with such payers. As mentioned earlier in this section regarding contracting, it is essential that physician networks not take on unnecessary liabilities that should be borne solely by payers.

Insurance Regulations

Another area where regulatory scrutiny and legislative activity is expected to accelerate is the general area of federal and state insurance regulations. This area bears on the subject of physician networks because physician networks that become large enough may, in fact, wish to become full-service insurors as well. Although some states do permit provider networks to capitalize themselves and register as insurance providers, at the present time most states do not allow this per se. In states that do not permit the formation of provider-directed insurance entities, provider networks may find ways to establish a joint venture or another collaborative arrangement with an existing licensed insuror.

In any event, the most fully evolved form of managed care is the provider-insuror, and there is little question that legislation will be drafted permitting the establishment of such entities. Physicians interested in this area should keep in close touch with their state medical societies, either directly or through qualified health care attorneys.

Hospital–Physician Transactions

Hospital–physician transactions and relationships constitute another area of legislative and regulatory activity. This area potentially applies to physician networks in two ways:

1. Physician–hospital joint contracting may need to be examined from the perspective of antitrust laws and regulations.
2. Arrangements in which hospitals invest in physician networks, provide services to such networks, or otherwise support physician networks need to be carefully examined from the point of view of both the physicians and the hospital pursuant to "fraud and abuse" and "anti-referral." In general, these categories of statutes and regulations are intended to discourage arrangements in which physicians have a direct or indirect financial incentive to refer patients to a specific hospital. On the federal level, this entire area is scrutinized by both the Office of the Inspector General of the Health Care Financing Administration as well as the Internal Revenue Service. Certain "safe harbors" govern specific types of arrangements between physicians and hospitals, but, as with the other regulatory areas mentioned above, if the members of a physician network are contemplating the involvement by or with a hospital, qualified health care attorneys should be consulted.

In addition, the author stresses that the physicians in any kind of physician network who are having discussions with a hospital or hospital system should not rely solely on the hospital's attorneys for guidance about arrangements and regulatory issues. Any such discussions require that the physicians involved have their own qualified health care attorneys who have the exclusive purpose of looking after the physicians' interests.

James J. Unland graduated cum laude from Harvard College (BA, 1972). He received his MBA from the University of Chicago Graduate School of Business Administration in 1975. Jim has authored numerous books and video programs on the subject of physician-directed organizations. He is the managing editor of *The Journal of Healthcare Finance* and the editor of *First Illinois Speaks.*

As president of the Health Capital Group, Mr. Unland oversees a Chicago-based firm which has branch offices in Dallas and Pittsburgh. The firm provides a wide range of consulting and management services to medical practices, hospitals, and other types of health care providers. Their consulting services include: mergers and acquisitions of medical practices, medical practice valuation, group practice formation, formation of provider managed care networks, structuring and negotiating transactions, and assisting financially troubled organizations. Management services are oriented primarily toward medical practices, physician networks, and hospital-physician entitles through the firm's affiliate, The Health Systems Network Alliance, the firm provides comprehensive medical practice and provider network management services.

Although the Health Capital Group deals with all types of healthcare organizations, Mr. Unland spends most of his time dealing with physicians and hospitals. His activities include structuring and negotiating medical practice mergers and acquisitions, medical group practice formation, valuing medical practices, and formation of provider-based health care networks.

19

Single-Specialty Networks: The Mature Network

GARY STONE

Managed care companies (HMOs, PPOs, POSs, PHOs) are increasingly penetrating the medical marketplace and acquiring ever increasing numbers of subscribers to their health plans. They bring with them demands on physicians to sign capitated or discounted fee-for-service contracts, or the risk of losing a large portion of their patient population. With little or no expertise, management background, or database to assist them, these physicians commit to and sign contracts that include capitation or other commitments that place them at risk (see Fig. 19–1).

The author has served as founder and medical director of a large ENT single-specialty network in South Florida that currently consists of 80 providers serving a capitated population of 900,000. The following represents a summary of this 6-year experience. A plan of action is outlined to assist physicians in structuring a single-specialty network and negotiating a contract with payers to provide care to a large managed care population. This will include data processing requirements to provide the associated utilization analysis, measurement of quality and appropriateness of care, and deal in detail with the *equitable distribution* of funds.

■ Definition of a Single-Specialty Network (SSN)

A single-specialty network is an independent practice association (IPA) of specialists in one field offering comprehensive market coverage for the geographical area served. The network is a vehicle for marketing and implementing health insurance payer contracts and provides the physician leadership and provider participation necessary to carry out that implementation. And finally, the network should deliver practical and realistic cost reduction in health care delivery while providing effective management of utilization and quality measurement of services.

■ History of ENT Networking in South Florida

Prior to 1990 and the implementation of the first South Florida ENT single-specialty network, negotiating leverage resided solely in the hands of the health care companies. Proposals for reduction in fee schedules were offered to the community at large and only those who accepted were invited to remain as providers. Under pressure from the state and federal government as well as large employers, reduction in health care costs were carried out with cost reduction as the primary priority and measurement and maintenance of quality a secondary factor. Difficulties in implementing these cost-cutting changes were enhanced by the failure to form partnerships with providers. In 1990, the first SSN in otolaryngology was formed and obtained its initial contract with the Blue Shield HMO carrier, offering 54,000 capitated individuals to the newly formed IPA network of 28 providers. This represented a service area of three counties. In the ensuing 6 years, rapid growth occurred in both the number of insured lives and total number of contracts signed.

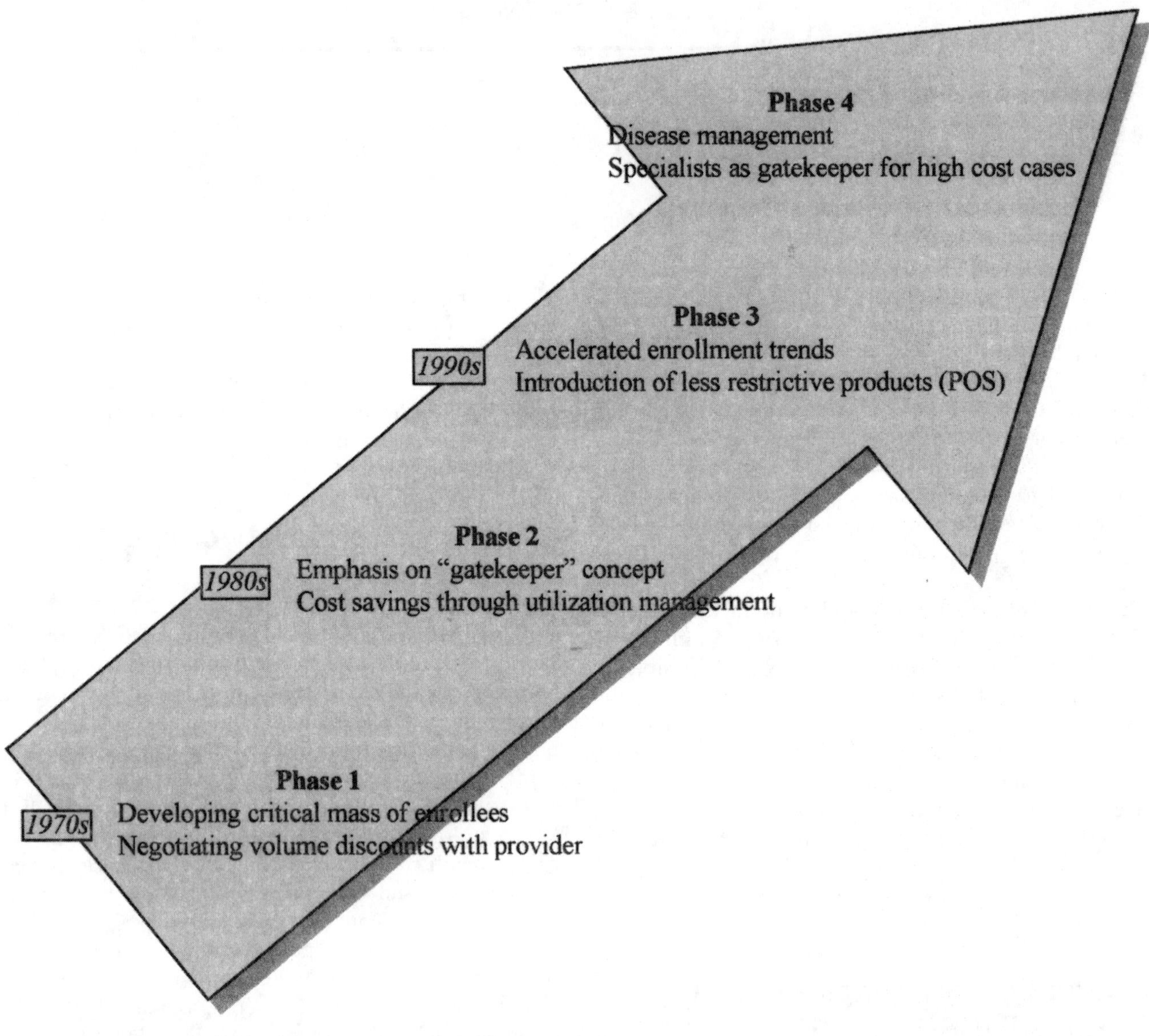

FIGURE 19–1. The Evolution of Managed Care—Moving Toward a Fourth Phase

E.N.T. HMO
MEMBERSHIP

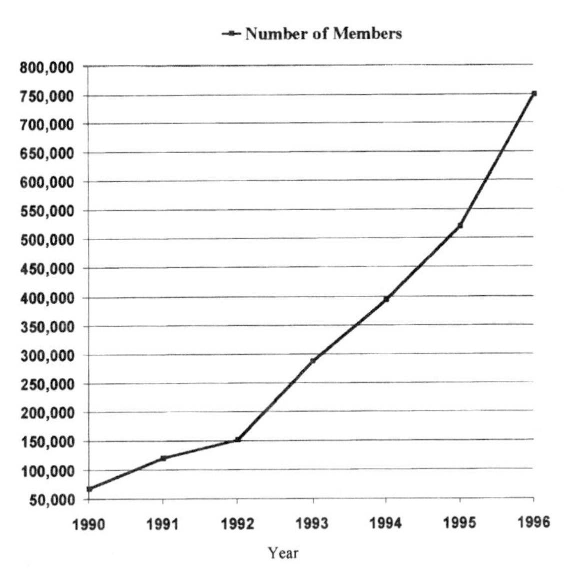

E.N.T. HMO
CONTRACT

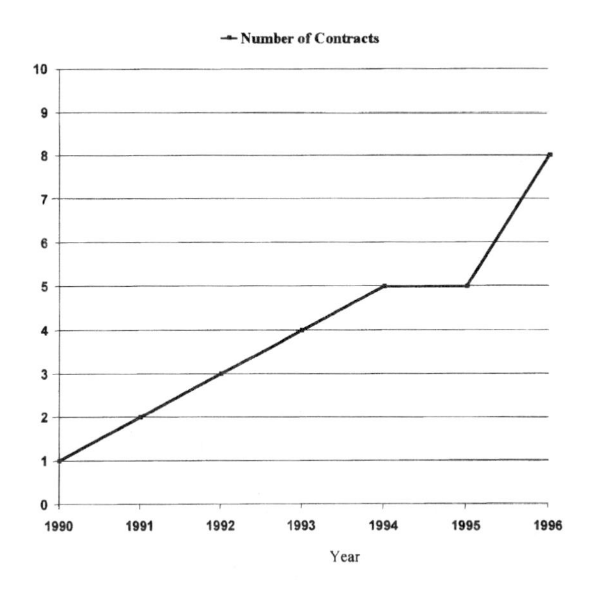

FIGURE 19–2. Rate of growth

Figure 19–2 outlines the rate of growth of both the capitated population and the number of managed care contracts obtained.

This success of the single-specialty networking experience in South Florida can be attributed to the following factors:

- A well-designed infrastructure and delivery system.
- Experienced management.
- Realistic pricing.
- Appreciation of payer needs.
- Physician involvement.
- Thoughtful economic incentives.
- Partnership formation between the network and the management of the managed care organization.

For 6 years, utilization management has been accomplished by *peer* physicians performing claims review with associated CPT code correction, adoption of practice and referral guidelines, and cooperation of participating specialists. While largely accomplished automatically through computer algorithms to correct for creativity in billing practices, a significant component of this is also achieved through peer physician review of all operative, pathology, and consultation reports occurring for the month being processed. Through peer physician management of the network, we have been able to attain an equitable distribution of funds allocated for otolaryngology care in our community.

Structuring a Single-Specialty Network

The SSN development has a logical evolution and should develop as shown in Table 19–1.

Lead Physician Selection

The lead physician or medical director of the SSN should have recognized clinical expertise and some background in managed patient care experience. Some level of management skills and expertise are helpful as well as computer literacy, at least to the extent of having familiarity and ease of interpreting statistical data reports. A degree of entrepreneurial motivation is also desirable to serve as a driving force for the efforts that will be required to bring the network to fruition.

A subset of minimum responsibilities for the lead physician for a network would consist of:

TABLE 19–1. Structuring a Network

Lead physician selection
Formation of the business entity
Contracting with providers
Formation of advisory committees
Marketing the network to payers
Establishing data processing capability

1. **Act as liaison between provider and payer.** Serving as liaison with the medical director of the managed care plan is a vital function at work here. A line of communication between medical directors of both organizations is usually established and contributes to the significant enhancement of quality of care delivered. Problems on either side are brought to the table for discussion and resolution without involving the patient, the employer, or other parties representing the recipients of care.
2. **Availability.** The lead physician or a designee will have to be available primarily by telephone for problems as they arise. These will usually consist of logistical problems regarding precertification, provider availability, patient's requesting referral to tertiary care or out of area facilities, and complaint resolution.
3. **Selection of the specialist provider panel.** The lead physician in conjunction with the medical director and network manager of the HCO will agree on the final list of specialist providers who will be under contract to deliver the care. These decisions will be based on geographical representation, perceived quality of care, subspecialty representation, and university or tertiary care referral services.
4. **Contract development.** The lead physician will, along with the appropriate advisory committee, be responsible for development of a provider contract prepared by the legal representative of the organization. Key points to consider in developing these contracts will be whether any restrictive language will be included to allow participating providers to join other competing networks as well as facilitate the joining of the network as a provider while at the same time allowing for a clearly stated clause for resigning or cancellation of the contract so as to accomplish what has been referred to as "easy in/easy out contracting."
5. **Payer contract negotiating.** The lead physician will be responsible for coordinating all marketing and payer negotiation activities with the goal of achieving an increasing market share for the network.
6. **Development of data processing capability.** The lead physician will coordinate the development and/or procuring of data processing services to fulfill the requirements of claims adjudication, utilization review, quality assessment and management, and implementation of shared savings programs.
7. **Establish relative value scales.** The lead physician, as chairman of the steering committee, will spearhead the establishing of the relative value system to be used in the claims adjudication process. This can be simply by the adoption of an existing relative value scale (e.g., Medicare, RBRVS, McGraw-Hill) or by devising a customized system based on usual and customary charges for providers in the network and the relativity that exists therein.
8. **Establishment of utilization review and payment criteria.** Here the lead physician will coordinate the development of algorithms and other guidelines to establish policies regarding rebundling of unbundled claims, CPT codes to be included or excluded in the claims processing, etc.
9. **Establish quality assurance programs.** The lead physician with the quality management and shared savings program will direct the establishing of all quality assurance programs required by contract and/or implemented to achieve the contracted shared savings programs. Additionally, these programs will be structured around NCQA and other regulatory agency guidelines.

Formation of Business Entity

Early in the evolution and development of the SSN, a decision will have to be made regarding the nature or type of business entity to be formed. Although this decision will largely be governed by legal advice and individual goals and objectives of the organizers of the network, Table 19–2 summarizes the usual choices available for accomplishing this goal.

Contracting with Providers

In the development of provider contracts, the following factors will have to be considered:

1. **Restrictive Language.** A decision will have to be made whether or not providers will be allowed to sign other network contracts in the area and thereby be allowed to serve as providers for a multitude of managed care plans. This author is a proponent of this policy since I have significant concerns about being asked to sign any managed care or network contract that restricts participation in other such plans. If the other competing network is more successful at marketing their product, this could have catastrophic consequences on the provider's market share and his or her medical practice income.
2. **Cancellation Clauses.** It is advisable in all provider contracting to allow for what has already been described as "easy-in/easy-out" cancellation clauses. These are usually accomplished by providing for so-called no cause cancellations by either party of the contract with a reasonable notification period usually consisting of 60 or 90 days. In this manner, the essential risk or "downside" is that the provider will be obligated to provide care for a number of patients over a 60 or 90-day period and agree to accept as full compensation the network payment for these patients.

TABLE 19–2. Organizational Sturctures

Type	Features
Joint venture by contract	Easy to establish Inflexible Useful only in initial stages of development
General partnership	No federal income tax imposed at partnership level Unlimited liability
Limited partnership	Creates general and limited partners Complex entity General Partner carries liability
Corporation (S or C)	Shareholders sheltered from business liability C—Corp or S—Corp S—Corp limited to 35 Shareholders
Not-for-Profit corporation	No taxes No earnings to shareholders except "arm's length fees"
Limited liability corporation (LLC)	Limits shareholders' liability Partnership status for tax purposes Most popular form for IPA

3. **Non-Compete Clauses.** Occasionally a provider contract will stipulate that anyone who leaves or terminates his or her relationship with a network may not proceed to engage in the formation of a competing network for a period of time such as one year. This has been devised to prevent participating providers from serving on advisory committees of one network and then using this information to form a competing entity. This may or may not be allowed by contract as is deemed appropriate by the organizers of the network.
4. **Antitrust Considerations.** Much has been written about pending and proposed changes to the anti-trust laws as they relate to IPAs and specialty networks. Indeed, much of this information has been conflicting and confusing. In the same week, one medical newsletter reports that the Feds will be tightening their enforcement of antitrust regulations while another periodical reports a trend toward slackening of enforcement. There have been few antitrust actions brought against IPAs to date, even though in many cases these IPAs exceed the "safe harbor" membership threshold of 30% of the licensed practitioners in the community. Whether this is the case because they have achieved safe harbor by virtue of the "rule-of-reason" principles or because the Justice Department in general has backed off in enforcement is a matter of conjecture. At a time when both government and market forces are encouraging the formation of managed care networks to facilitate the transfer of risk from the payer to the provider, it can be argued that the rigid interpretation and enforcement of antitrust regulations would be counterproductive.

Formation of Advisory Committees

Advisory committees serve as a vital tool in the management of the single specialty network. Committees are designated to serve in key areas to assist the governing body of the network in establishing all policies and procedures.

1. Steering (Utilization-Peer Review) Committee. The steering committee is concerned with all questions and issues relating to utilization management of the network. It will be concerned with claims adjudication issues whether they are relative value based or issues of creativity of billing. The committee structure should provide for geographical representation from each of the areas served by the provider network as well as additional representation from each of the subspecialties and the university or tertiary care facilities. The South Florida steering committee consists of 14 members with the following breakdown: Dade County—4 members, Broward County—3 members, Palm Beach County—3 members, Martin County—1 member, Pediatric Otolaryngology—1 member, Neurotology—1 member, University of Miami—1 member. The steering committee has concerned itself with guidelines for referrals from the network to the tertiary centers and establishing equitable reimbursement schedules for university participants in the network. A subset of this committee has recently engaged in establishing guidelines for reimbursement for disease and diagnosis management to neutralize the incentive to overutilize in a fee-for-service reimbursement environment. When the management of serous otitis media was examined, it was found that the utilization of audiometry and tympanometry varied from occasional to routine use at every office visit. In an attempt to achieve the goal of equitable reimbursement of the network funds each month, a policy is currently being devised to allow for global reimbursement for this diagnosis on a monthly basis. It is believed that this will allow for individual treatment styles and the utilization of office diagnostic modalities on an "as needed" basis. Similarly, a steering committee policy has been established for only one reimbursable endoscopic procedure at each office visit to obviate the problems of reimbursement when multiple office endoscopies are billed at the same setting.

2. Quality Management and Shared Savings Committee. The quality management committee may meet in conjunction with the steering committee as we usually have done in Florida. This committee has structured a comprehensive quality program each year to comply with contractual obligations to our payers as well as establish a value-added benefit for MCOs to contract with our networks. One such study has dealt with the procedure of bilateral myringotomy with tubes (CPT 69436-50). In a population of children under the age of 6, a study was conducted to track the percentage of children with documented pretreatment with antibiotics prior to surgery compared to the overall incidence of surgery. Over a period of time through network and steering committee educative processes, including the sharing of the data with network providers, we have been able to document a progressive increase in the number of pediatric patients receiving prophylactic antibiotic treatment prior to surgery as well as an overall decrease in the incidence of surgery in this population. This is an ongoing study that documents the effectiveness of physician management of the delivery of health care.

3. Marketing and Negotiating Committee. This committee is dedicated to the marketing and active negotiation of the SSN to payers in our community. This includes the development of graphic demonstration of the added benefits provided by the network to both our payers as well as our patient populations.

4. Provider Relations Committee. The provider relations committee usually serves as a subset of the steering committee. It is concerned with complaint resolution and promptly responds to all inquiries or complaints received from members (patients), PCPs, network providers, MCOs or the employer groups representing the subscribers. The committee investigates all such complaints, documents both sides of the issue and responds to the payer with written recommendations, conclusions, and/or corrective action recommendations.

5. Data Processing Committee. This committee is concerned with structuring the algorithms that are used to assist in claims adjudication. In addition, the committee, in conjunction with data processing personnel, structures the format of reports to be used to implement the quality assurance and shared savings programs.

Marketing the Network to Payers

To successfully negotiate a payer contract, certain general guidelines should prevail. First and foremost is to identify which payers in your community are the largest managed care providers and which ones are entertaining the development of an exclusive relationship with an SSN. This information is obtained by promoting an awareness that your network exists and is anxious to partner with the payer. Identifying the payers and the decision makers within each organization is critical and can be accomplished by direct telephone communication with the medical directors and directors of network development in each of these organizations. It is useful to consult with colleagues already under contract with these companies and solicit assistance from hospital administrators who have similar relationships in place.

To assist in this marketing effort, keep in mind the reasons why HMOs and other MCOs are increasingly turning to SSNs for the delivery of their specialty care and why SSNs are successful. Inherent in this is the understanding of the importance of forming the *partnership* with the payer. The majority of my professional career was spent in an era when most payer relationships were adversarial. The payers saw most specialists as greedy individuals who were insatiable and uncooperative; specialists saw most payers as profit centers dedicated to denying or delaying reimbursements and coverage of benefits for the sake of the bottom line rather than the subscriber/patient beneficiary. This relationship for so many years has in my opinion contributed to the problem we face today with patients and their employers unhappy with the health care system and demanding radical changes. Forming this partnership with payers (frequently fellow physicians serving as medical directors) is imperative if we are to return to a position of influence and/or control policy making and implementation.

Why are managed care companies contracting with single specialty networks?

- **Cost Reduction**
  - Professional fee discounts
  - Hospital utilization savings (shared or full risk)
  - Administrative cost savings (e.g., claims processing, UM, QA, etc.)
- **Provider Relations**
  - Attracting desired physicians to plan
  - Buffering plan from criticism
  - Managing provider issues
  - Providing specialty expertise conveniently
- **Utilization Management**
  - Practice profiling
  - Expert claims review
  - Concurrent review (within and outside service area)
  - Incentives

- **Quality Management**
  - Credentialing and Recredentialing
  - Peer review
  - Participation/liaison with plan's QM Committee
  - Establishing clinical guidelines
  - Disease state management programs
  - NCQA and HCFA
- **Marketing**
  - Premium reductions/ increasing market share
  - Differentiation of product
  - Prestigious local and national physician leadership
  - Quality enhancement/disease management
  - Direct access
- **Data Processing**
  - Electronic data transmission from providers
  - Electronic data transmission to payers
  - Sophisticated reporting capabilities (QM, UR)
  - HEDIS guideline management
  - Geographic access software

Why are single specialty networks successful?

- Physicians are active partners.
- Specialists understand their specialty best.
- Businesslike approach to MCOs.
- A value-added product is created.
- SSN serves as vehicle of dissemination of payer policies.
- Vehicle for QA program integration.
- Provide network contracting for HMO through single negotiation and single signature contracting.
- Shared leadership expertise and ideology in case of multispecialty MSO or through steering committee input.
- Vehicle for implementation and delivery of shared savings programs.
- "Peer" physician network management when "peer" is defined as same specialty and board certified.
- The SSN serves as the best example of the Group Without Walls, especially for the solo practitioner.

HMO contracts with SSNs usually include an exclusive relationship to facilitate the assumption of risk. This means that the network will be responsible for providing all of the care in that specialty and patients will be obliged to stay within the network to receive full benefits of their contract for care. Only in this way can the network safely assume the risk of caring for the contracted population at a fixed rate of reimbursement. This usually entails accepting a ***capitation rate.***

The capitation rate is a fixed monthly payment based on the size of the contracted population of insured lives that month and is expressed as a rate **per member per month (pmpm).** It transfers the risk of overall utilization to the network and delegates all or part of the claims adjudication, utilization review, and quality management activities.

The first mandate to successful negotiation of a capitation contract in otolaryngology is to clearly define the inclusions and exclusions in the proposed contract. Nothing will have as much impact on the adequacy of the capitation rate as this clear understanding of what the network is financially responsible for.

Capitation Rate Negotiation

Arriving at an equitable capitation rate can be a difficult, frustrating, and even catastrophic experience if all the services to be included in the contract are not clearly defined. The capitation rate must be based on *accurate* data reflecting the overall past cost experience for ENT. It is strongly advised that all such past experience be supplied in detailed CPT occurrence data for a period of one or two years. This data should then be compared with other ENT databases for capitated populations to establish correlation or differences that can be readily explained by demographics, level of service, or other obvious differences in the populations. Comparison databases are available for Medicare, Medicaid, and commercial capitated populations and should be sought out and used to assist in making informed decisions regarding the validity of proposed capitation rates.

With 14 years experience in capitating otolaryngology services at both the individual practice and large SSN levels, I recommend that all the following services be clearly identified as to whether they are *included* or *excluded* in the contract:

- Routine office audiometry (air, bone, speech)
- ABR (BSERA) and ENG testing
- Office X rays
- Allergy testing and treatment
- Hearing aid dispensing
- Surgical assistant/co-surgeon reimbursement
- Facility fees or tray fees
- Advanced head and neck surgery
- Skull base surgery
- Cochlear implants
- University (tertiary care) referrals

In addition, consider carefully and completely the following factors that will impact the adequacy of the capitation rate:

- **Point of Entry.** Will the point of entry into the system be by referral from the PCP (gatekeeper model) or by patient self-referral directly to the otolaryngology office. This will have significant impact on utilization and the capitation rate.
- **Population Mix.** What portion of the total population being offered for capitation will be Medicare, Medicaid, or commercial members? Traditionally, a separate capitation rate is negotiated for each of these populations in view of the significant variation

in utilization associated with each group. Avoid any offer of a "blended" or average single capitation rate. This carries the significant risk that the managed care company will more successfully market their Medicare product out of proportion to others (the Medicare cap rate is always higher than the commercial rate) and the blended contractual rate will adversely impact the network.

- **Out of Area and Out of Network Claims.** An out of area claim results from a patient seen by a physician in a remote geographical area while an out of network claim arises when a patient is treated at a nonparticipating hospital or by a noncontracted physician called in when no other is available..
- **Size of Contracted Population.** Finally, consider the total size of the population and what effect any "catastrophic" illnesses will have on the total cost of care. Obviously, the larger the population size, the more the occasional major, high-cost services rendered will be "buffered" by the large monthly budget.

As you can see, arriving at a capitation rate involves consideration of many variables that dramatically impact the cost of the ENT care you will be responsible for. For this reason, I urge you to avoid any quoted "average" capitation rates—or at least interpret them keeping the above information in mind. At best, any "average" capitation rate will have a range of at least plus or minus 50% until all the variables are defined.

Why Capitate Now?????

"Why should I capitate now if my waiting room is full and I don't have to?" "What's the harm in putting it off as long as possible?" These seemingly innocent questions almost demand the automatic conclusion that there is no harm in waiting. However, I would like to propose one possible alternative reasoning. There appears to be universal agreement in this country at the present time that physician fees and scheduled reimbursements are being slowly and progressively ratcheted down. In most capitation negotiations, the payer proposes to offer an **exclusive** population of members/patients for a pmpm rate that is a ***discounted*** rate based on the actual expense experience for ENT care for the previous one or two years. Therefore it becomes apparent that there is a significant potential downside risk to delay negotiating such a contract now. If you allow your community reimbursement levels to be ratcheted down until the payer's annual costs are reduced to their lowest historic levels and base the capitation rates on these lowered rates, there is much to be lost in the long run. On the other hand, rates based on high utilization rates and high expense histories tend to be higher and more favorable for negotiating shared cost savings programs.

Other factors to consider in payer contract negotiating include the term of the contract, automatic renew of contracts, annual capitation increases based on cost of living and/or merit, stop-loss clauses to protect for unexpected overutilization, exclusive rights of first refusal for geographic expansion of the payer market (e.g., statewide expansion), and so on. In general, the longer the term of the contract the better, as long as you can rely on the validity of the data that the capitation rate was derived from or adequate stop-loss protection is in place.

Network Implementation

The following guidelines should be used to ensure the smooth, timely implementation of your single specialty network:

Set a realistic timetable for implementation. Table 19–3 is a sample 120-day timetable for network implementation:

Network provider selection includes the following

- Quality providers
- Geographical coverage proportional to geographical distribution of insured population
- Hospital coverage
- Avoid churning of patient population
- Subspecialty coverage
- University (tertiary) coverage

Selection of the provider panel is a joint decision made by the network and the payer. Usually, the panel is constructed by the network management based on the above guidelines; final approval with or without mandated modifications comes from the payer. Geographical and hospital coverage should be adequate to allow for vacations and other contingencies to avoid being responsible for out-of-network charges. Previous large volume providers for the proposed population should not be excluded from the proposed panel without concern for the churning of the patient population that will occur if large numbers of patients under care have to change doctors as a

TABLE 19–3. 120-Day Implementation Timetable

Day	
1–30	Determine service area
	Determine desired network size
30	Sign letter of intent
30–60	Agree on cap rate
60	Sign contract
60	MSO mails termination of notice
90	Form steering (peer review) committee
120	Network operational
120	Implement network claims processing

result of the new contract. Finally, adequate subspecialty coverage should be contracted for (e.g., pediatric otolaryngology for pediatric ICU coverage).

Establish Data Processing Capability

Reimbursement Methodology

The first data processing design decision that must be made is whether reimbursement to providers will be fee-for-service or subcapitation to each provider. In the fee-for-service scenario, overutilization is incentivized and must be managed by careful data tracking and active involvement of the steering committee. The alternative, direct subcapitation obviously incentivizes underutilization, which is more difficult to monitor especially when in some cases only a telephone contact from the patient occurs and there is no written record to audit. Accordingly, each network will have to make this choice.

My network capitation experience has been with network reimbursement based on a modified, relative value, fee-for-service system. All clean claims received during the month are entered into a custom data processing system. Each procedure has been assigned a relative value from a custom-designed RVU scale. At the end of each month, the total number of RVU points generated are tabulated and reviewed by the lead physician. The capitation funds available for the month are entered into the data system and when divided by the total number of RVU points generated that month result in a point dollar value. Reimbursements are then tabulated by patient for each occurrence and a detailed explanation of benefits is generated to be sent to each physician with his or her check for that month.

It is imperative to understand that in this case the *overall network is capitated,* but all *providers are reimbursed on a fee-for-service basis.* Therefore, there remains an incentive to overutilize, which must be managed by detailed data analysis and peer management with adherence to network policy. Obviously the higher the total number of points, the lower the value of each point and vice versa. This explains why the actual dollar value of reimbursement experienced each month varies. ***Appropriate utilization*** maximizes reimbursement and can result in higher reimbursement than was experienced prior to capitation. This concept relies on each and every provider becoming a ***partner in utilization*** and, when universally adopted, can result in the highest quality health care delivery while maintaining adequate and equitable compensation.

■ Utilization Management

The steering committee under the direction of the lead physician reviews all utilization reports for the month and selectively reviews all operative, pathology and consultation reports. Custom computer algorithms are constructed to facilitate this task. A report detailing all PCP referrals for the month is generated and reviewed for changes in referral rates or patterns. While it is reasonable for the network to be responsible for follow-up care under its control, the rate of new referrals from PCPs is out of our control and if excessive ("dumping") can severely impact reimbursement. Accordingly, this is closely monitored and outliers are dealt with by the payer to whom the PCP is under contract.

In selected cases, precertification is performed by our network staff using guidelines established by the American Academy of Otolaryngology-Head & Neck Surgery. These activities have been concentrated in the areas of Bilateral Myringotomy with Tubes, T&A, and Endoscopic Sinus Surgery.

The Tragedy of the Commons

Perhaps the biggest challenge facing the peer utilization committee deals with the dilemma that the network as a whole is striving to achieve the lowest possible utilization compatible with delivery of high quality health care, while at the same time the individual provider is still best served by overutilizing in a fee-for-service reimbursement environment. This follows the economic doctrine of "The Tragedy of the Commons" as described by Garrett Hardin and relates to the individual incentive versus the shared incentive trade-off, or the fact that one's privatized gain exceeds one's share of the commonized loss. Everyone would be better off if the whole group consumed less (RVUs), but any one individual is better off by consuming more. And, since people are more motivated based on individual rewards rather than group rewards, all individuals end up consuming more. Herein lies the challenge for peer review!

The most effective tool for achieving utilization "parity" in the network has been through the development of global reimbursement. For instance, a single value is established for reimbursing an initial visit/consultation and includes any audiological, endoscopic, or other office diagnostic procedure associated with that visit. The same is true for return visits. This principle can be applied to disease state management wherein a single global fee is paid for the management of each case of serous otitis media whether it is treated conservatively, surgically, or a combination of the two.

"Peer" Review

Whenever I refer to peer review, I define "peer" as a physician in the same specialty who is board certified in that specialty. One of the many strengths of SSNs lies in the fact that only otolaryngologists are reviewing the work of otolaryngologists. It is imperative that we do this if we are to survive this health care revolution we are witnessing. We are also reminded historically that: "Peer review by physicians is remedial, while peer review by bureaucrats is punitive."

The lead physician and steering committee serve to gather and disseminate utilization review and quality improvement data with providers and to bring to the peer review table all issues for resolution. In view of the successes experienced by networks doing so across the country and the receptiveness of payers to have us perform this function, we remain successful. The biggest danger for failure remains by default because physicians fail to participate in these committees for the ill-conceived reason that this constitutes "conspiring" with the enemy. In my opinion, the biggest failure on the part of organized medicine has been our failure to sit at the table with payers and regulators who are designing the model of health care delivery for the twenty-first century. It is time to form this partnership that has been in large part responsible for our successes to date.

Quality Assurance

Although, the responsibility for providing quality assurance oversight of the network remains with the payer as an undelegated service, the design and implementation of these programs remain the primary function of the network's quality assurance committee. These programs are designed to ***impact*** the level of care, not just measure it. This involves incorporating quality outcomes measurements into these studies and can be achieved through records review or by patient satisfaction surveys. By sitting on the quality improvement committee of each of our payer companies, these activities are coordinated and integrated with those performed by payers to conform to HEDIS and NCQA requirements for certification and successful marketing.

To date, our quality assurance programs have involved the management of serous otitis media, septoplasty surgery, and T&A surgery (indications and outcomes). In the management of serous otitis media, we have docmented through successive studies the increasing incidence of prophylactic antibiotic treatment with concurrent decreasing incidence of surgical intervention.

Annual Report Card

An annual reevaluation of our network with the payer includes the receipt and evaluation of an annual report card. This four-part evaluation consists of:

1. **Patient Satisfaction Survey.** A large sampling of patients referred to a physician over the previous year are polled for overall satisfaction and perceived quality with questions involving accessibility, timeliness of appointment, courteousness of staff, whether provider answered questions willingly, etc.
2. **PCP Satisfaction Survey.** A sampling of PCPs are polled regarding availability of specialist to discuss the case, provision of written consultation report within five days of the day of service, etc.
3. **Log of Complaint Calls.** All telephone calls made involving complaints from members are logged and the incidence is compared from year to year. Our network has developed a computerized tracking mechanism for all complaints that documents both sides of the dispute and outcome of its discussion at the Steering Committee.
4. **Utilization Goals—Attained Cost Savings.** All networks are evaluated for attainment of utilization goals mutually agreed to by the network and the payer. In the case of shared savings programs, the attainment of these goals is associated with bonus reimbursement to the network providers.

Figure 19–3 depicts a sample of the satisfaction survey report regularly compiled by our largest payer.

Shared Savings Programs

The development of shared savings programs is an increasingly more essential and promising component of the partnership between the SSN and the MCO. All current negotiations for new or expanded contracts include these discussions and should be actively pursued. There can be no question that reduction in all health care expenditures is becoming a mandate and will occur whether we physicians are a part of its implementation or not. Hence the reduction in hospital length of stays, maternity care length of stays, shift of surgery from inpatient to outpatient setting, and so on continues even to the extent that some of these become state legislative issues. It is imperative that these remain professional issues rather than legislative ones and shared savings programs are one of the solutions to this problem.

The shared savings program establishes a baseline from past experience of the payer and establishes the percentage of sharing of any savings that subsequently occur through the efforts of the network management and participants. Thus, reductions in length of stay for head and neck surgery patients when compared with historical numbers results in revenue sharing just as the reduction in overall incidence of myringotomy with tubes surgery does.

The SSN is the vehicle for the delivery of the shared revenue program and has the added responsibility of establishing and maintaining a sophisticated data system to monitor these activities.

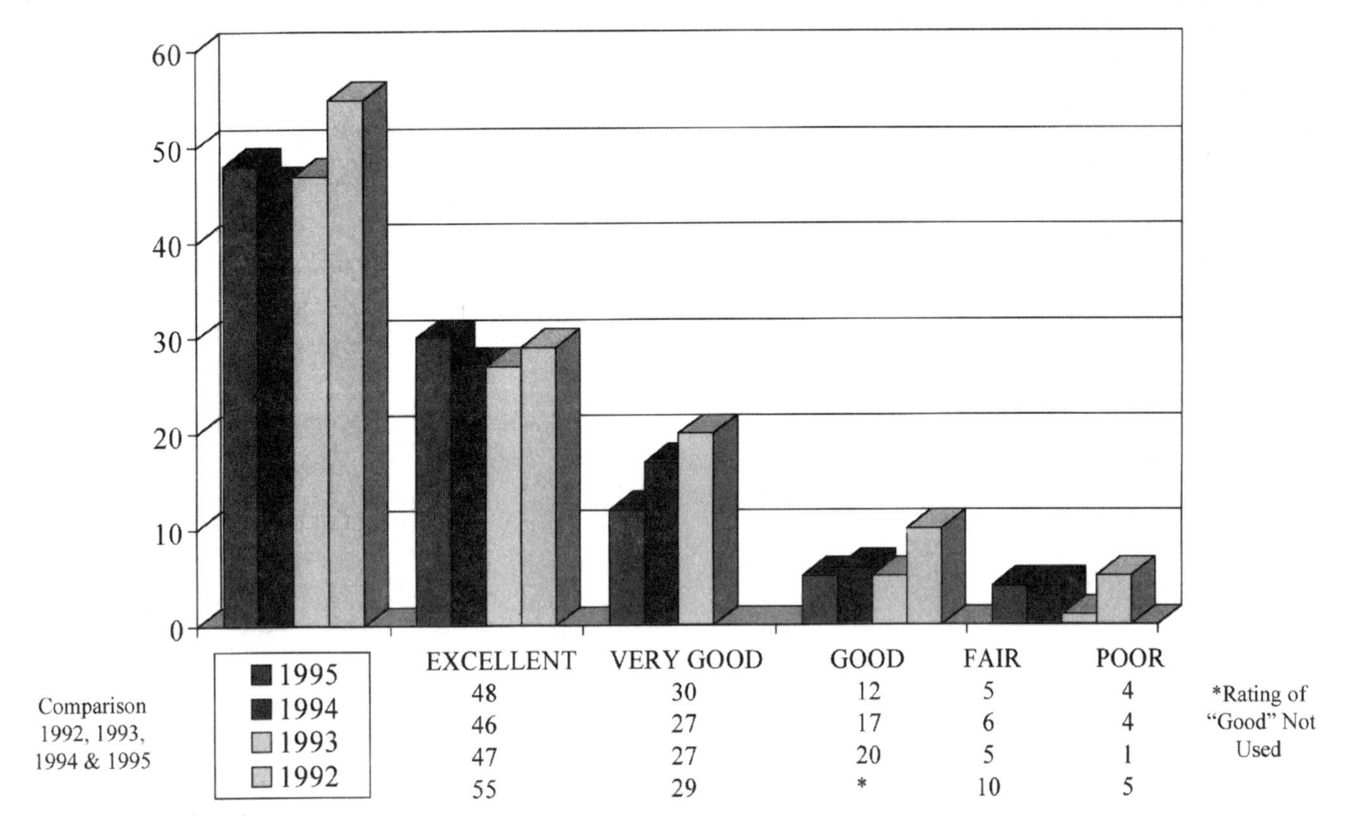

FIGURE 19–3. Overall member satisfaction with ENT network

■ Group Purchasing Benefits

As the SSNs increase in size and join to form a "portfolio" of networks, it becomes feasible to develop a group purchasing cooperative as an added value incentive for network participants. First and foremost in this regard is the development of a group professional malpractice insurance cooperative. Additional programs are planned to include the purchase of office supplies, medical disposable supplies, and preferred rates for electronic claims transmission clearing house rates.

■ Conclusion

The Golden Rule in medicine states: He Who Has The Gold, Rules. In the case of managed care, the gold is the number of insured lives, subscribers, members, potential patients, or whatever you prefer to call the exponentially increasing population switching to managed care and capitated plans. While the actual degree of market penetration by managed care varies from one area to another and state to state, it is apparent that all communities are following the same pathway. It is clear that integration of medical practices into larger, more cost-efficient entities is becoming a vehicle for survival. The single-specialty network model has met with success in meeting the demands of payers while simultaneously affording the specialist the most autonomy possible in this environment. It allows the formation of a partnership between the network and the MCO and elevates the physician manager to a vital role in this partnership. The ability to competitively bid for capitated and exclusive contracts for large populations is a further advantage. The bottom-line results of our network experience has been:

- Attainment of equitable fee schedules.
- Input from all participating specialists.
- Practice growth and expansion.
- Sharing a collective negotiating voice.
- Negotiation of shared risk savings programs.

Attaining these goals has been facilitated by the development of a custom data processing system to collect capitated funds into a pool and reimburse providers on a fee-for-service basis in an attempt to preserve the best features of fee-for-service health care delivery. At the same time, we have developed a model of peer physician review and management to establish the role of the physician manager and promulgate the continued physician management of health care.

REFERENCES

Fickenscher K, Buettner S: Lessons from the trenches in physician integration. *Physician Exec* June 1996; 22 (6) 14–18.

Hardin G: The fortune encyclopedia of economics. Henderson DR, ed. 1993:88–91.

Lazarovic J: Specialty capitation and effectiveness assessment. *Physician Exec* January 1993:19(1): 32–35.

Gary Stone, MD, FACS, is the founder and director of a large physician-operated single specialty network in South Florida. The network currently consists of 80 providers serving a capitated population of 900,000. Dr. Stone has lectured extensively on the initiation and development of physician directed networks. His seven years of experience have lead to the refinement of data processing requirements necessary for providing the associated utilization analysis, measurement of quality and appropriateness of care, and deal in detail with the equitable distribution of funds.

20

Single-Specialty Networks: Initial Stages

MICHAEL D. WEISS

The health care marketplace of today has changed drastically over the past several years, creating rapid shifts in the practice patterns of all physicians.

Control of patient referrals has also shifted out of the patients' hands and more directly to the PCP. With managed care, this also shifts control of reimbursement to the PCP, hospital, HMO, or third party administrator involved. Naturally, all these middlemen want their share of the total pot before it ever reaches the specialist, leaving only a portion of already reduced funds to eventually be distributed. One of the reasons PHOs have rarely worked is because of this very principle—that is, the hospital, and often the PCPs who are running the plan, have to get the first share. This is a two-tiered system with the specialists in the lower class.

Multispecialty groups and partnerships with hospitals are an attempt by doctors to avoid the control problems developed by the hospitals and HMOs and return more control directly into the hands of the physicians themselves. Although this is a step in the right direction, there is a sufficient amount of distrust on the part of specialists that they are still concerned about receiving their fair share. Specialists often see the same individuals running the multispecialty groups that they dealt with in the previous arrangements.

One method for circumventing this problem, and maintaining a level playing field, is to unite individual practices within a single specialty into their own bargaining network. The **single-specialty network** (SSN) is the best means for a particular specialty to control its interactions with all players in the health care arena, including other specialties, primary care groups, HMOs, hospitals, and third party payers. Most specialists feel that no one can be better trusted to look out for their own interests than themselves. Contract negotiations are performed by that specialty on behalf of that specialty. A comfort level is thereby achieved.

Clearly, a major goal of the SSN is to ***retain independence*** and ***control as much as possible its own destiny.*** There are other major factors to consider, including:

- Retaining independence. Each individual practice also remains independent, operating in a group-without-walls type of arrangement. Groups are unified into an independent contracting entity (IPA model) for those contracts they have negotiated together. Currently, the limited liability corporation (LLC) structure is popular for this purpose. Individual practices own the LLC and use it to contract for professional medical services. Other aspects of the individual practices may remain separate, if they so choose.
- Maintaining or increasing market share.
- Maintaining income in an environment where payment to physicians, especially specialists, is being significantly reduced.
- Providing a product attractive to payers to secure contracts for services.
- Developing economies of scale. If income levels are to be monitored with declining revenues, expenses must also decline. One way to achieve this is to combine services, in the LLC or other contracting entity

to reduce overhead. Possibilities for savings come from centralized billing, purchasing, personnel, or other support services.
- Creating a viable bargaining unit that can operate both independently and jointly with other similar groups to its best advantage.

Bearing in mind this last item, the door for a variety of other networking possibilities is opened:

- Networking with other single-specialty groups in other specialties to negotiate jointly for contracts.
- Networking with similar single-specialty groups in surrounding geographical areas to negotiate for larger contracts in a particular specialty.
- Networking with multispecialty groups for carve-out positions for those areas that cannot be handled adequately by the multispecialty-specialty group.
- Adding value to the capabilities of an SSN by contracting or networking with university centers, where needed, to provide tertiary care. In return, the single-specialty group may be able to enhance and expand geographical coverage for a university center by providing primary ENT care for the university center's contracts.

The SSN is an extremely attractive concept for insurers. When done properly, it can provide a turn-key approach by supplying for a ready-made single specialty referral coverage for an entire region. This SSN can offer a multitude of services in one package, including: administration, credentialling, quality assurance, utilization review, and outcomes tracking. Economies of scale are achieved by requiring the payer to negotiate only one contract. The cost savings are readily apparent and will strengthen the network's bargaining position.

Contracts can be made in a variety of fashions, but an ***exclusive*** panel, one in which the SSN is the only provider for that specialty, is the most desirable. These may be on a fee-for-service or capitated contract basis. Some proposals may include both.

Other issues such as organizational structure, governance, antitrust concerns, quality assurance, utilization review, disbursement of revenues, competition, and exclusivity all must be addressed by the group. Many of these issues are directly related to the local demographics and internal dynamics of the group.

For the sake of group survival, certain fundamentals must be kept in proper perspective. The single specialty network is strictly a business and does not replace the local medical society. It is *not* a union or instrument of social change. It should, however, be manageable, flexible, and adaptable to different proposals and requirements from various insurance companies. It must also be responsive to the constant changes in the health care industry.

The toughest challenges are actually getting the network started and formulating its ideal structure. For the purposes of this discussion, we will limit our focus to the single specialty IPA or LLC. These entities, other than actual mergers, are the basic form of practice networking.

Always keep in mind that an IPA is strictly a vehicle for negotiating contracts. There is no integration of services of any sort in the IPA model. In other forms of practice integration, ranging from the group-without-walls concept to total merger, there are varying levels of this type of integration. These include centralized billing, combinations of pension plans, and consolidation of offices. In the group-without-walls model there is a central administration, while the individual offices remain as separate profit centers. Each of these offices must stand alone in terms of profitability, but most of the management functions, such as billing, contract negotiation, and pension are centralized. A still higher level of integration is total integration of practices.

The greater the level of integration, the greater the need for doctors to sacrifice the individual aspects of their practice styles, and the greater the need to share information such as patients and revenue with their competitors. There is often a natural reluctance to enter into this sort of arrangement. The IPA structure, therefore, is often the best way for these practices to organize. As the IPA is solely a negotiating vehicle, it is often the most palatable solution to this problem.

When creating any type of network or IPA, there are naturally extensive prerequisites that need to be considered before the group can be a viable unit. Months of planning and preparation are usually required.

First, a high priority in the group's formation should include creating an outline of items necessary for the structure and operation of the group. These items then must be prioritized and analyzed as to expense. A typical outline should include:

- A statement of the goal or mission of the group.
- Development of an organizational team of doctors, each with a specific role. In particular, one doctor should be chosen to coordinate activities and act as a liaison between the doctors, lawyers, consultants, etc., in the early stages.
- Development of a task timetable.
- Determination of appropriate geographic area to be covered and how membership will be decided.
- Creation of committees for quality assurance, utilization review, credentialling, and fee structure (in appropriate sized groups).
- Legal assistance to formally structure group and assure no antitrust violations.
- An experienced administrator/negotiator for the group and a third party administrator (TPA) for the

disbursement of funds and tracking purposes. This latter item (TPA) may be researched, but isn't t really necessary until the first contract is obtained.

- Identification of value added services that set your group apart from individual practices or competing networks for marketing purposes.
- Other items as necessary.

The first goal in any project is to define your goal or mission, a major component is the identification of your target payers. By identifying your target, you can more easily determine the group's structure. A target market must be identified. If you are going after insurance contracts, you must put on a businessperson's hat and identify the payers to whom you can market your product.

The key in selling any product is to give the customer (third party payers) the product they want or need. An obvious need is low cost. ***Structuring your organization to meet the needs of the third party payers is another major factor.*** This creates an attractive product for the carriers and makes your group more desirable, a factor that implicitly enhances your group's value during contract negotiations.

Our IPA serves as a great example of how this works. In the Maryland area, several large insurance companies establish centers around the state for their HMO products, organizing themselves in strategically located health centers (i.e., staff model). For each of these centers a *separate* contract, specific for that center, is negotiated by a central administrative office with each participating ENT (or any other specialty) group. These contracts are usually exclusive and capitated and typically involve a specialty practice close to the primary care site.

It seemed obvious to a number of us in practice in the northern Baltimore suburbs that if we negotiated deals together we would become a much more attractive candidate to payers. We hoped to obtain a better deal when these contracts were being negotiated. We organized into a legal entity to avoid antitrust violations. Furthermore, by offering the HMOs several different group practices that would be participating jointly with all the different centers, patients would have a choice of practices to which they could be referred.

The response to our initial inquiries with the insurance companies came as a surprise, but it was the basis of the creation of our IPA. We were told that while the idea for the organization was attractive, it wasn't much of a benefit to them to combine negotiations for 3 or 4 centers when they still had 10 more around the state to negotiate. In other words, ***the benefit to the insurance company was having to negotiate only one contract in the region.*** An equally important lesson is: They told us what they needed, and we provided the product. The northern Baltimore IPA quickly became the Maryland IPA.

Not every group, of course, is faced with the same geographical needs and requirements. Those organizing the group must consider a number of items. The first is whom the contract will cover. Other questions are the number of patients and the distance required for these patients to visit your offices. Who is providing the patients? Are they from a neighborhood center, as described in the staff model above, or are they spread out in various individual practitioner's offices in the region? Are the offices conveniently located to make the group attractive? Don't forget: the identification of neighborhoods in some places may be equally as important as distance in miles.

Next consider with whom you will be negotiating. Obviously, if your practice is only negotiating directly with the HMO down the street, you do not need any type of network for bargaining purposes. In most medium to large communities, however, the actual negotiations may be through a central office that will cover a more regional area, rather than a more local one. Hence, the need for a well-defined geographical network.

Make sure that the group you form is of a size that is not only appropriate for your purposes, but also manageable. The smaller the group, the more cohesive and manageable it will be. As size increases, so do management problems, including problems with physicians' time, personnel, physician cooperation, and financing.

While all areas may be represented geographically, there may be significant differences in the numbers of covered patients for any region. Some contracts can potentially be more focused on some providers than others, or more concentrated in only certain areas of the region. For instance, a contract with an urban factory-based payer may have less penetration into the more distant suburbs. In our group, a small portion (2%) of the total payment each month to the IPA for capitated contracts is divided equally between all members regardless of the number of patients seen. While not a large sum of money, this offsets the feeling on the part of some members of a disparity of patients in a particular plan. It psychologically strengthens the group's cohesiveness. There are many ways that these problems can be addressed. With the addition of more contracts and patients, these differences will eventually be reduced or minimized.

Remember that size is an advantage and that *this is another bargaining point to utilize* during negotiations. Don't be afraid to remind the payer of the geographical representation that your group is offering. Payers will be more interested in a total deal than in negotiating numerous small ones. Use this fact to remind the payer of your group's attractiveness.

As physician networks, IPAs are taking on a wide variety of forms. One concern common to all when starting such a network is the actual costs involved. Depending on how this is done, expenditures can range from modest amounts to as much as $100,000. One reason for this disparity is fairly simple: costs are directly proportional to the organization of the game plan and the amount of work the doctors themselves are willing to put into the actual formation of the group. Certain costs s uch as legal fees are naturally unavoidable. These too can get out of control if not carefully analyzed during this process. Use of consultants can, in some cases, be helpful in enabling that group to organize its plans in an efficient manner and *save* money by avoiding unnecessary expenditures.

While the work of creating an IPA is considerable, no one but the doctors themselves can fully determine what is best for them. An active, participatory role is essential. Doctors are often overwhelmed when they finally understand the volume of work that is necessary, since organizing a network requires many of the same policy-making decisions that would go into making any type of health care organization. Not only do physicians need to be recruited, but credentialling, utilization review, and quality assurance policies must be determined and stated in writing if the IPA is of any substantial size. Legal issues need to be decided with the appropriate documents drawn. It is extremely tempting for physicians, busy in their own practices and having little expertise in these areas, to hire a third party to perform most of the work in the IPA's creation when the goal of the consultant should actually be to *assist* and *guide* the doctors. By proceeding in this fashion, fewer unnecessary expenditures result and the goal can be kept in focus. I will highlight several of the major points in your agenda, although this is not totally inclusive.

- Choose a development committee with a leader to coordinate tasks. Initial items should include membership, finance, fee schedule, legal issues, quality assurance, and utilization review. A individual or committee should be chosen to complete each task with a timetable. A group leader is important for coordinating efforts, making sure the timetables are met, and maintaining the group's momentum.
- Legal fees are necessary, but it is recommended that every proposal by any law firm for its services be scrutinized in advance. In the case of Maryland ENT Physicians, we opted for a flat fee, choosing not to contract on an hourly basis specifically spelling out what was to be provided in the contract. Much of this material may be provided to similar groups so that the necessary work can be quickly obtained. One aspect of the work that is highly recommended is an antitrust analysis for your group's geographical distribution. The cost of this can certainly be negotiated in advance. Proposals from several firms to do this work are also recommended.

The work required for organizing the group is extensive, yet much of it can be done in the doctors' offices. In the beginning, there is no need for a separate office or secretary. While the Maryland IPA has an administrator, he and the doctors creating the network worked out of their own offices initially. Our only early office expenditure was a central telephone line with voice mail that was utilized when the contracts were obtained. Thus the president, administrator, secretary, treasurer, and credentialling and quality assurance committees were all located in separate offices. This caused no problem for the membership but, more important, created *zero* overhead.

Consultants can be helpful, but the real substance of the organization is determined by the doctors and the organizational committee. Think of creating your IPA as if you were building a new home. You would certainly hire the services of an architect or builder. What these individuals cannot do, however, is build a house to suit your needs without a considerable amount of input from you. Otherwise, the house that is built will be *theirs*, not *yours*. Where doctors are not directly interacting with the consultant in development of the IPA, costs can escalate and the resulting product will be less than ideal for that particular group. If the organizing physicians assume the lion's share of creating the network, costs will be minimized and the momentum will be established to obtain contracts.

If a consultant is utilized for guidance, that person should be considered in a similar fashion to choosing an attorney, accountant, or other professional. Physicians are in a frenzy trying to form networks and opportunists also abound. While many so-called health care consultants are well intended, there are also good number whose expertise and experience is marginal. Some of these consultants may also have very little real experience in actually dealing with the third party payers with whom the contracts must be negotiated. Many physicians are also reluctant to join another group, having been burned in the past with multispecialty ventures that have failed for these reasons.

Nonetheless, while much of this work involving creation of IPAs and networking systems is new, experienced individuals are available who have started or are operating functional, successful groups. They can offer substantial help.

The most common question I am asked is management of the money, the method of distribution, and whether or not this is done in house or by a third party administrator (TPA). This issue is actually one of the *last* items that needs to be completed. After all, there is no money coming in until the first contract has been obtained. There is no reason to contract with any particular TPA group until such time as you actually *need* one. You certainly need to investigate to find a group to manage the disbursements in the manner you set up, as well as to track outcomes and identify outliers whose billing may deviate from the norm. There is no reason, however, to pay for their services prematurely. In certain cases, the carrier itself may provide this service although this may allow *them* to control the data, rather than you. Many groups may want to develop their own TPA at the outset. While this may be appropriate for some, the time and expense required might best be spent in organizing and getting the first contracts. It will probably cost less to pay for these TPA services at first, and develop your own as the IPA matures.

In summary, while organizing physicians may assume a variety of different forms, the IPA model is often not only the easiest to create, but often the most marketable form of network. It is geographically complete and offers physicians an opportunity to organize themselves as a group, yet maintain their independence. Unavoidable costs can be minimized by maximizing direct physician participation in the group's creation. Use of outside resources is helpful in initiating the development of any SSN, but must respond specifically to the needs of the organizing physicians. Creation of a procedural outline will enable the group to analyze and appropriately prioritize its efforts to maintain efficiency and control costs, while maintaining its primary focus. Direct and continuing physician involvement in the earliest and subsequent stages of the creation process will be one of the most important factors in ensuring success.

Michael D. Weiss, M.D., has been pivotal in the creation of Maryland ENT Physicians, Inc., an otolaryngologic specialty network in Maryland. It is an independent practice association model with approximately 50 members covering the entire state of Maryland, District of Columbia, and the northern Virginia suburbs. Maryland ENT IPA has been formally in existence for approximately two years and has four managed care contracts covering 250,000 lives, with ongoing negotiations with other carriers covering an additional 600,000 lives. These contracts contain both fee-for-service and capitated components. In addition, his IPA is a physician-directed initiative that has been able to keep start-up and administrative costs to a minimum by increasing direct physician involvement in its administration.

21

Mergers and Acquisitions

T. FORCHT DAGI AND JAY MAYES

The purpose of this chapter is to serve as a guide the recent wave of practice mergers and acquisitions in the health care industry. This phenomenon is virtually uncharted. We propose to examine why mergers and acquisitions are pursued, how they might add value, how they might best be implemented, the purposes they serve, and the problems likely to follow in their wake. The chapter is split between a macroeconomic view of the health care trends, a discussion of the role mergers and acquisitions have played in responding to market pressures, and a guide to evaluating, implementing, and planning practice mergers and acquisitions.

The chapter focuses on mergers of individual group practices. This narrow focus does not begin to exhaust the range of mergers and acquisitions that the health care industry has experienced. Nevertheless, we believe that many, if not most, of our observations also pertain equally well to mergers and acquisitions on a broader scale. These will not be our focus, nor do we intend our observations to address activities of publicly traded corporations conglomerating physician practices either uniquely or as part of a broader health care acquisition strategy.

The Impetus for Mergers and Acquisitions in Health Care

In the mid-1980s, Lee Iacocca proclaimed that the price of every Chrysler sold included $600 for health care. At about the same time, insurance companies began to tighten their traditional underwriting policies for health care, with the manifest effect of reducing coverage and the number of covered lives. The AIDS epidemic in cities like New York and San Francisco placed an enormous burden on public health institutions and public hospitals. By the late 1980s the idea that an inordinate and ever enlarging proportion of the GNP was devoted to health care had been firmly implanted in the American mind.

Health care reform was a centerpiece of the Clinton presidential agenda during Clinton's first campaign. The mandate was clear: reduce costs while maintaining quality and improving access. How this mandate was to be implemented was not so obvious. The debate over health care reform became increasingly ideologized during the first six months of the presidency. All sides—those seeking radical change, those recommending incremental change, and those desperately defending the status quo—contrived to influence the public through a combination of intimidation and self-righteousness.

By the summer of 1994, the impetus for change had attenuated. The 103rd Congress achieved no consensus on health care reform. In the wake of the Republican victory of November 1994, health care lost considerable importance as a political spark. Still, the debate has polarized stakeholders into two groups. One is ideologically sympathetic to the idea that health care ought to be treated as a regulated utility. The second concedes a need for change, but ascribes the need primarily, if not exclusively, to market considerations.

The industry still anticipates an unstable future. Even without the passage of major legislative initiatives, a series of cascading administrative regulations and unrelenting downward pressure on price by employers are likely to reduce quite measurably the options for returns on investment.

Given the political climate, nothing much may change in the political arena. The realities, however, matter less than the fears. The central question is not whether things will actually change, but whether they will be perceived as about to change. Irrespective of what the new control mechanisms might eventually be, market or government, physicians have increasingly lost control of the health care industry.

In an effort to maintain income levels in the face of imminent structural change, practitioners have begun seeking economies of scale and increased market presence, or power. Market power has also been the objective of physicians trying to move from the commoditized position to which they have been relegated by payers who have come to see them as one of many potential vendors in the health care arena. *Pari passu,* a number of corporate institutions and investor groups have discerned an opportunity for profit through the exchange of guaranteed patient flow for deeply discounted fees and restructured payment systems. *The proliferation of merger and acquisition activity among and between various sectors of the health care industry constitutes part of the attempt at a cogent response to these pressures on the theory that larger groups might exert a larger market influence or benefit in other ways by one or more of the following mechanisms:*

1. Negotiating power.
2. Undertaking risk and cutting out middlemen.
3. Establishing practice standards.
4. Controling the provision of care in all its ramifications.
5. Instituting economies of scale to reduce costs.
6. Controling patient flow.

Several of these mechanism serve the same goal and are, for all intents and purposes, functionally inseparable.

The phenomenon of mergers and acquisitions in medicine constitutes quite a bit more than the mere assemblage of practitioners and institutions of various sorts and sizes. This phenomenon represents, simultaneously, a manifestation of and a response to fundamental changes in the relationships of payers, practitioners, patients, and institutional providers. The relationships in question are best described in terms of control of four dimensions of medical practice: patient flow, payment, access to care, and quality.

Changing Models of Medical Practice

The traditional model of medical practice was centered around a contractual relationship between doctors and patients. The physician consulted in response to the patient's request. The patient was the client. It was widely understood that other stakeholders might wish to interfere with this relationship. For this reason, virtually every code of professional medical ethics and tort law canonized an aversion to such interferences in some way. Professional codes insisted on privileged communication, personal responsibility for continuity of care, liability for outcome, and other ethical obligations that fostered the model of individual physicians relating to individual patients.

Although the patient could leave the physician, the physician was limited in his or her liberty to leave the patient. A physician could, however, refer the patient. For this reason, to the extent that the control of patient flow dwelt elsewhere than the patients' hands, it dwelt in the hands of the physician. The relationship between physician and patient was contractual. The patient or the patient's surrogate—family or employer—was responsible for payment. Even if the patient didn't have adequate means to pay, the physician was obligated, at least in some ethical frameworks, to provide charity care.

In the traditional model, access to care was a function of ability to pay and of regional physician supply. Quality control was seen as an internal, professional matter for the colleges of medicine or their equivalents (e.g., specialty organizations, boards of licensure) to oversee.

Although it is highly likely that the traditional model did not ever exist in anything vaguely approaching a "pure form," it serves as a reasonable, if probably mythical model from which to indicate directions of change along the four dimensions we have noted. Tables 21–1 and 21–2 summarize the traditional, the current, and two probable future scenarios for health care, minus any significant structural change in the industry.

One possible scenario is payer domination. In this scenario, market power is achieved in relation to one's ability to purchase health care for a large number of patients. Federal approval of Provider Supported Networks (PSNs) may challenge the payer domination achieved by aggressive marketing of cost control to employers. These employers initially lacked the sophistication to purchase and evaluate managed care plans based on health outcomes.

Another scenario involves the evolution of linkages and strategic alliances among physicians, hospitals, and payers. In this situation, there is an opportunity, given the proper facilitating mechanisms, to create integrated health systems (IHS) utilizing horizontal (same specialty or service type) and vertical (cross specialty in the simplest form, but more likely combining the sources of funding, the venues for service, and the sources of patients in one organization—e.g., physicians, hospitals, nursing homes, home health care providers, and payers) mergers to achieve integration. The ascendance of IHSs may be limited, however, by continued price pressure from managed care organizations on hospital costs and permissible population bed days; by the slow pace of hospital dominated information systems to contend with outpatient information; and by unwieldy governance structures. IHSs seem to be plagued by an inability to marshal the resources and the will required to anticipate or respond to the marketplace as it changes.

TABLE 21–1. Roles of the Four Main Players in Health Care*

Scenarios	*Models*	*Physicians*	*Patient*	*Payor*	*Hospital*
Past	"Traditional Model"	All aspects of decision making	Compliance with physician recommendation Payment	N/A	Providing capital-intensive equipment for specialized procedures and nursing care
Present	Transitional Model 1980s	Delivery of HC within constraints defined by patient	Participation in decision-making process	Utilization management; reimbursement schedules	Credentialling, quality control, utilization review
Future Options	Payer Dominant Scenario	Delivery of HC within constraints defined by payer	Consent in formal (legal sense); little or no physician choice	All aspects of determining site, span, and intensity of service	Seconded to payer
	Integrated Health System Scenario	Delivery of HC within fixed allotted portion of premium dollar; physician controls quality, access; offers acute and preventive care	Active part of personal health prevention and decision making; decision made on basis of unbiased informed consent	Marketing based information re price, quality, and patient satisfaction; delivers fixed % of premium for provision of care	Part of HS; information linkage-hospital, physician; clinical/financial information
	Physician Dominated	Administrative responsibility: full risk for the premium dollar including both health care provision and administration	Physician patient partnership in the therapeutic relationship, only physician assumes financial risk	Middleman marginalized or actually unnecessary	A vendor to physician organization

*HC: healthcare HS: health system

TABLE 21–2. Dimensions of Control in Health Care

Scenarios	*Models*	*Patient Flow*	*Payment*	*Access*	*Quality*
Past	"Traditional Model"	Physician	Patient	Physician and patient	Physician
Present	Transitional Model 1980s	Payer and Physician	Payer	Payer and Physician	External quality monitors; hospitals, payers, regulators, licensing boards
Future Options	Payer Dominant Scenario	Payer	Payer	Payer	Payers, regulators, licensing boards via proxies
	Integrated Health System Scenario	Physician and integration of strategic allies	Integrated Health System (IHS)	Physician—caps on services determined by IHS and marketplace	Physicians/providers—outcome, cost, patient satisfaction
	Physician Dominated	Physician and physician organization	Physician organization under direct contract with employer	Employer decision; physician under accepted guidelines	Physician organization

For the physician, this is an era of rapid and frightening change. Job satisfaction is at an all-time low.[1] The factors affecting the way medicine is practiced and the way physicians must relate to one another, to hospitals, and to insurers are out of their control. The traditional doctor patient relationship has been besieged by employers, government agencies, and insurers.

Because physicians as a group lack experience in working with large organizations, they tend to focus on control issues rather than on the mission, the vision, and the purpose of new enterprises. As a group, physicians tend to dismiss the need to outline objectives clearly. The focus on control has also contributed to the inability of physicians to organize productively and assume positions of leadership as the health care market changes.

The Growth of Supplier Power

In this chapter, the term "supplier" will be used to refer to those institutions that control patient flow to providers or reimburse for care. Payors, insurers, employers and HMOs, therefore, all count as suppliers. The growth of supplier power has resulted in increasing infringement on physicians' professional prerogatives. The term "supplier" is contrasted with "provider." In the current economic environment, the most important suppliers are those who provide money, patients, or services on which physicians depend for their livelihood. The term is often used as a term of art to refer to payers and employers.

Payers increasingly insist on largely ceremonial, but time-consuming preauthorizations (approval) and second opinions before undertaking treatment. They have steadfastly resisted any claim for accountability for the results of delay or denial. Physicians are subject to the vagaries of complex criteria for what procedures and treatments will or will not be reimbursed as well as retrospective claims review in which payment to the physician is delayed and not infrequently reduced or denied after the fact. Employers have turned to self-insurance and quality determination systems to more clearly focus their power on meaningful but poorly defined outcomes.

On the government transfer side, regulations have established phased reductions in Medicare and Medicaid reimbursement and have eliminated many opportunities for cost shifting or increasing return on investment through referrals to physician owned, medical service-related businesses.

Professional education has also been affected. Physicians in the past were relatively autonomous and individualist. This trait was encouraged during training at both the undergraduate and postgraduate level. Cost effectiveness was not part of this training scheme. Medicare, in fact, conceded the need to reimburse some residency training-related expenses at a higher than usual rate so that specialty training might continue.

In response to supplier pressure, however, from both payers and employers, medicine has begun increasingly to focus on cost-related, as opposed to disease-related issues. Organized medicine has also responded by moving from a defensiveposture with respect to maintaining the vestiges of market power to a more aggressive posture intended to regain that power.

Another important factor is the growth in national organizations dedicated to the documentation of outcome quality (NCQA, FACCT, and others). There are quality-directed partnerships between employers and payers, and there has been increasing interest in public access to physician quality data (e.g., NCQA "Quality Compass" on the Internet). Quality outcome indexing has also been suggested as a meaningful gloss on unrelenting cost control.

Mergers, Managed Care, and Integrated Delivery Systems

How have these factors influenced the growth of health care mergers? Mergers in health care are driven by the need to compete in an environment in which concerns regarding the cost of care and access to care override almost all other considerations, *and come to be controlled by someone other than the physician.* Although the dimension of quality is never absent from the rhetoric of change, only in exceptional cases have considerations of quality driven payers to choose facilities or providers a priori.

To make sense of this phenomenon, it is helpful to explore the relationship between the goals of health care reform and the structural changes that have been proposed for the industry.[2] The nonfinancial goals of health reform stripped of the ideology are the achievement of universal access to care at a defined level of quality. There are several strategies through which these goals might be attained. The first issues that must be addressed is the relationship between the provision of care and its reimbursement. There is precedent (worldwide) for provision of care in government institutions; compulsory participation in prepaid "sick funds" that either own or source out the provisions of care on a competitive basis; and various hybrids. In the absence of ideology, the provision of care can be distinguished from the reimbursement for care. (The term "ideology" as used in this discussion is meant to be descriptive and not prejorative. It refers to the tendency to invest ideas with immunity against criticism because of beliefs about their inherent merit.)

The issue of ideology cannot be ignored, however. Three arguments drive health care reform in the United States: concerns regarding efficiency and effectiveness; concerns regarding quality and access; and ideological beliefs regarding the benefits of centrally planned, centrally regulated, and (in most cases) collectively owned health care delivery systems. The first two arguments do not necessarily require structural changes in the industry unless there were no other means of obtaining the desired outcome and, even then, there would not necessarily be any preconceived ideal form of health care system. The same cannot be said of the third argument. Here, central planning, government regulation, and collective ownership are perceived to be beneficial *on their merits*.[3] The same can be said for most single-payer concepts. This is why the specific ideology of reform has the potential to be so influential.

In the late 1970s, Alain Entoven, a liberal economist at Stanford, proposed to offer individual subscribers enrollment options with differential pricing corresponding to different types of coverage. HMOs, for example, might carry lower premiums. In this way, he reasoned, the selection process could be managed competitively. This concept came to be known as managed competition. In subsequent years, the concept was broadened to refer, more generally, to any system in which cost differentials would be used in an attempt to influence consumer or payer choice.

Many critics of the existing health care system have argued that managed competition will act to enhance the existing market system and direct it toward universal coverage and cost containment. It is not altogether clear, however, how the fact that differences in the cost of insurance options are borne by subscribers necessarily results either in universal coverage or in cost containment. In California, for example, even though 60% of state workers and retirees along with a very large percentage of other workers participate in managed care plans, universal access and universal coverage are not appreciably closer to being achieved. And with respect to cost control, recent legislative initiatives singled out fee-for-service plans for rate regulation, and exempted non-fee-for-service plans from legal strictures such as the corporate practice of medicine doctrine and referral free prohibitions.[4]

The concept of managed care *as originally articulated* did not necessarily lead to specific structural changes in the health care industry, although it did encourage cost reductions as one dimension of competitive advantage among insurers. The approach of President Clinton's proposed health plan,[5] in contrast, was to legislate the establishment of health plans (a specific type of insurance program) to be purchased through a process of competitive bidding, from which fee-for-service practices and small providers would be de facto excluded. This *did* requires structural changes in the industry. The changes that were required became, in fact, part of the administration's social agenda.

While forward looking merger of practices was one part of the response to managed competition, the wave of mergers preceded the Clinton administration. In the 1980s, declining hospital occupancies and the Medicare prospective payment system resulted in joint ventures and vertical integration among hospitals and practitioners. The purpose of these moves was to replace lost sources of income and guarantee patient flow. Physicians invested in diagnostic and outpatient surgery centers, while hospitals invested in physician groups. Some physician groups merged, but there was no immediate sense of urgency to restructure *practices* as opposed to *services*.

About 1991, however, mergers changed in character. They derived increasingly from single specialty groups and disease or condition management "carve-outs." They emphasized exclusivity and were willing to incorporate a shared insurance risk with the payer through a capitation mechanism.[6] They also represented a response to a threatened shift in the equilibrium of power involving physicians, hospitals, and payers, the three major components of the health care system. Thus, the locus of competition shifted. Practitioners and institutions merged, and practitioners and practitioners merged, with both groups intending to dominate the market and dictate terms should a takeover ensue.

There are ample opportunities for profit if an organization can provide an integrated network of PCPs, specialists, and inpatient and outpatient facilities. Contracts can be let to insurers or, in some instances, directly to employers. The physician base limits the size of the network, and the institutional base limits the capital intensive services that can be provided. Insurers, however, have claims experience and actuarial data that are critical to effective bidding.

As a result, there has been a rush on the part of physicians to consolidate and then sell practices while they still retain value. According to one survey, one-third of all hospitals have purchased physician practices, and an additional 40% plan to do so imminently.[7] Over 50% of hospitals and physician groups are thought to have joined or created networks. A major goal has become that of participating in, or forming, an integrated network subject to well-defined, and relatively controlled competition.

Hospitals traditionally utilized their market power and capital resources to bind physicians and assure a referral base. The competitive capability of debt-ridden hospital-dominated systems is altogether uncertain, however. Hospital consolidators have been reluctant to acquire either payers or physician groups, although this reluctance may be in the process of changing.

In most cases, horizontal integration precedes vertical integration. Groups of specialty compatible physicians merge. Pairs of hospitals enter into formal alliances. Large insurers acquire smaller ones. After the achievement of horizontal integration, networks of practitioners and institutions, practitioners and insurers, or hospitals and insurers are created. Finally, an integrated network is attempted.

Few groups have actually followed the full route of horizontal integration first and vertical integration second. Those that have are generally HMOs and very large intexgrated clinics like the Lahey Clinic, which moved from Boston to the suburbs after purchasing a hospital in Burlington, Massachusetts, or the Mayo

Clinic, which went so far as to form its own medical school. Allegheny General Hospital in Pittsburgh, another example, recently purchased two medical schools, while Kaiser Permanente, which owns a series of hospitals on the West Coast, has also endowed specialty chairs at medical schools with which the hospitals have become affiliated.

■ The Growth of Managed Care

The Nixon-supported HMO ACT of 1973[8] mandated that employers offer an HMO option for health care to all employees. During the ensuing 20 years, HMOs experienced tremendous growth in enrollment (see Table 21–3).

The HMO-based consolidation of covered lives[9] has created considerable market power for HMOs and other patient suppliers. The scope of the term "supplier" has already been noted, but merits further clarification. For purposes of this chapter, the term supplier will refer to HMOs, insurer, and payers who finance health care through collection of insurance premiums, and can control patient flow in various ways. They are suppliers because they supply patients to health care providers. Increasingly, large employers have achieved the scale, scope, and experience necessary to act as direct suppliers of patients to providers. However, most employers have continued to require payers to deliver physician networks and administrative services. Providers are physician groups, hospitals, skilled nursing facilities, and others who deliver direct health care services to patients.

HMOs have used their market power to drive down the cost of health care. Lower costs are translated into lower premiums to employers and further growth in HMO enrollment. Enrollment growth results in economies of scale that HMOs can apply to health care delivery services and administrative functions. Larger HMOs achieve additional dollar savings because increased patient numbers lower the actuarially determined economic risk from adverse patient outcome. Size spreads the risk across a larger pool of insurance premium dollars. Other patient suppliers such as insurance companies, employer coalitions, and health care purchasing cooperatives such as CALPERS (California Public Employees Retirement Services) have also experienced consolidation of covered lives and growth in market power.

Consolidation market power has allowed HMOs to competitively bid down the price of health care services. For the purposes of this chapter, the term HMO will be used as a proxy for all suppliers. Supplier market power permits reduction in HMO reimbursement for services provided by physicians, hospitals, and other suppliers. In exchange for accepting this "volume discount" in reimbursement, providers gain the opportunity to deliver care to the HMO's large population of patients. The alternative, for provider groups, is to be excluded.

From the physician's perspective, loss of control over patient flow affects market power, capacity utilization, professional pride, and, in the long run, professional skill. Thus, there is considerable risk to being excluded from the 50,000 to 200,000 HMO lives.

HMOs have exercised their market power to "change the rules of the game" for American physicians. As summarized in Table 21–4, a comparison of certain key features of physician practice in the early and late 1980s shows clear evidence for a structural shift and for significant rule changes. Three features were in large measure responsible for physicians' interest in practice mergers.

First, physicians were increasingly asked to respond to RFPs (requests for proposals, or contract bids) to provide care to very large populations of geographically dispersed patients. Scale efficiencies and market power tended to favor those who could provide large-scale geographical coverage. This was especially true for the primary care specialties of family practice, obstetrics and gynecology, and pediatrics.

A second factor favoring broad geographic representation was the emphasis on the so-called "wellness model" of care.* Proximity facilitates convenience, access, and

TABLE 21–3. HMO For-Profit Managed Care vs. Not-for-Profit Patient Enrollment for the United States According to an Employer Survey (*N* = number surveyed)

HMO and Not-for-Profit Enrollment		
	1988 (1665)	*1993 (1953)*
For-Profit Managed Care Enrollment (% of employees)	29	51
HMO For-Profit Enrollment (Millions of lives covered)	15.4	24.8
Not-for-Profit Enrollment (Millions of lives covered)	17.2	20.4

*The "wellness model" is distinguished from the "disease model" of earlier times. Historically, patients sought out physicians services as a result of specific illnesses or complaints. Physicians, in turn, construed their professional roles in terms of diagnosing and treating specific illnesses. There also existed another view of the physician. From Hippocratic times the physician was urged to encourage "health" through dietetics, salubrious environmental influences, and the like. This second role was emphasized when the primary function of Western physicians (but not, for example, Ayurvedic physicians) was limited to diagnostics, and was deemphasized when Western physicians found more active treatments in which they could engage. To some extent this role was adopted by the sanitarian and the primordial public health physician of the early nineteenth century, but they did not engage in patient care. The twentieth-century public health physician also did not engage in patient care. It remained for the latter part of the twentieth century to revisit the idea of involving physicians in *preventative* treatment and advice. The wellness model represents an articulation of the belief that preventative examinations and prophylactic interventions of asymptomatic populations improves their health and well-being, and is also cost effective.

TABLE 21–4. HMO (Supplier) Consolidation and the Rules of Play

	Prior to Early 1980s	*Since the Mid-1980s*
Supplier (insurer, employer, HMO) Purchasing Power	Low—many small HMOs employers lack consensus on solution to health care cost	Highly concentrated—lead HMOs and employer coalitions achieving critical mass of covered lives to consolidate market; knowledge of drivers of health care costs support contracting
Method of Physician Reimbursement	Fee-for-service, discounted fee-for-service	Fee-for-service, discounted fee-for-service, global, per diem, and increasingly capitation
Medical Group Size	Solo or small group practices	Large, growing single and multispecialty group practices
Focus of Care Provided	Care for individual patient or family unit	Care for a population of patients—"covered lives"
Physician Practice Objectives	Treatment of specific identified disease states or illnesses	Focus on the prevention of illness and early detection of illness to minimize the severity and cost of illness
Geographic Locus of Medical Care	Local community—"12 mile rule"[10]	Responsible for large numbers of covered lives—suppliers drive to physician providers who have geographical distribution and desired level of integration to serve their population; also suppliers centralized and localized some acute care services

compliance with respect to routine care and regular medical surveillance.

The third key feature driving the physician merger trend was the introduction of managed care and capitated payment for physician services. Managed care implies that either the HMO or a contracted physician group is actively monitoring utilization of health care services and promoting the delivery of the "appropriate" number and kinds of medical therapies prescribed to patients by physicians.

Under capitated payment, physicians agree to accept a fixed reimbursement from the HMO in exchange for providing all contractually agreed services to the HMO's patients. For physician groups to engage in intelligent and profitable capitated contracts, they must project the health service needs for the patient population and the medical group's expected cost to deliver the required services. Bidding to provide care under a capitated contract is more likely to be profitable for medical groups who start out on a strong clinical and financial basis, and who can provide geographical coverage sufficient to sustain enlarging populations with lower actuarially determined financial risk to the capitated group. (This is an important point. There is *no* good reason to grow a practice so it can accommodate an enlarging population base with a *higher* actuarially determined risk.)

Physicians practicing under capitated patient contracts must change the way they view the delivery of services to patients. Historically, financial incentives have encouraged physicians to view a patient as a profit center; for example, providing more services to the patient will generate more profit/revenue for the physician. In a capitated reimbursement system, patients are a cost center; for example, providing more services to the patient increases the cost to the capitated physician and reduces his or her profit/revenue.

HMOs believe that capitation provides appropriate and necessary incentives to physicians to manage care in accordance with implicit or explicit corporate priorities. They also believe that large, so-called Integrated Medical Groups (IMGs) can more successfully manage care in this manner because their capital structure affords them the ability to build the infrastructure support (information systems to track patient financial and clinical outcomes, utilization review, case management, patient satisfaction surveys, etc.) necessary to monitor and impact patient care. Independent of their potential ability to manage care more successfully, larger physicians groups have the opportunity to create market power and their own economies of scale, and perhaps the capital base to become a PSN. In the past, HMOs have worked with all willing physician providers (solo, small physician group, or large group) on an individually contracted basis because the supply of unmanaged patients who paid full freight for care met or exceeded the capacity of the physician. That is no longer the case. Physicians are now dependent on discounted reimbursement from HMOs to cover expenses. As a result, HMOs can choose whom they will.

HMOs prefer the administrative efficiency and reduction of overhead that comes through contracting with fewer and larger physician provider groups. In technical jargon, this process is called "trimming the provider panel." HMOs also prefer to work with groups that they feel have somehow "captured the idea" of working with managed care. This preference is related to the fact that most physicians, at least initially, actively resent the imposition of constraints on their practice habits and do not possess the mindset required for successful participation in managed care. Those that either understand the constraints of managed care a priori, and are well disposed toward them, or at least come to accept them, tend to gravitate toward larger groups, or, in the current environment, to create them in response to needs. And to the extent that mergers occur *in response* to the contracting requirements of managed care, a commitment to participate in the managed care process is implicitly articulated and generally recognized as such by HMOs.

Although this chapter will not focus on the subject as such, the idea that mergers in health care serve as a signaling mechanisms aimed at suppliers (as well as to competitors, though to a lesser extent) deserves at least passing mention. Just as corporations can follow the route of becoming a "virtual" corporation, integrated health networks can be "virtual" in the sense that while they may not possess exclusive call on *all* providers on whom they draw, they have obtained capacity commitments from enough of them to be able to offer, with confidence, the level of integrated service required. The larger provider group formed expressly for the purpose of participating in such networks signals, in virtue of its formation, a commitment to participate.

There is also a practical side to this commitment: having expanded capacity, the group is likely to dissolve unless patient flow to match capacity can be secured. Professionals in medicine tend to be unhappy unless they are utilized fairly fully, because their self-image is typically related on some level to production and demonstrations of competence. Thus, an expanded group becomes dependent on HMOs for patient flow. The shift of power that this dependence entails, if understood and not resented by the provider, smoothes the relationship between the two and may lead, in the ideal, to a strategic networking partnership. The vision of a strategic partnership is limited only by reimbursement. It will remain a practical possibility only so long as pressures from premium revenue, from payer administrative costs, and from diminishing profits do not result in too low a reimbursement to providers. When premium reductions are passed down to the providers to maintain stock market profits in the face of employer price pressures, strategic networks will collapse.

In summary, physicians have found it necessary to seek alternatives to their traditional practice mode (solo or small group, single-specialty practice) to respond to the market power that HMOs and other suppliers have achieved. Many physician mergers were in fact defensive. They were motivated by fear, by the desire to secure practice revenue streams, and by the belief that size could lead to a balance of power. These mergers lacked the vision and imagination to achieve true and sustained market power for physician groups. Medical practice groups can grow through acquiring new physicians (scope economies and enhanced revenue) or increasing the number of covered lives the group serves (scale economies and reduced costs). Either process, if correctly conceived and properly managed, produces additional capital and supports further growth, if called for.

Mergers and Networking amongst Physician Groups

Structural Frameworks: Physician Group Mergers and Networking Activity

The power conveyed by mergers tends to make groups competitive with other groups and attractive to integrated health systems. Networking, in comparison, tends to provide practice groups access to patient populations not otherwise attainable. The contrast between merger activity and networking activity is demonstrated in Table 21–5.

There is a spectrum of different types of physician networking activity that falls between the small group practice and a fully integrated medical group. Options vary from loose physician networks constructed to share resources (shared leasing arrangements not resulting in a new legal entity) to full and formal practice acquisitions in which the buyer purchases the assets and liabilities of the seller and the seller ceases to exist. All network models share the objective of sharing opportunities to contract with payers to provide care to the large populations of patients that payers have organized (supplier market power).

The most common models for physician networking are described in detail in Table 21–6. Models differ in the degree to which they require physicians to surrender

TABLE 21–5. Comparison of Merger and Networking Opportunities for Medical Groups

Type of Provider	*Advantages to Merging*	*Advantages to Networking*
Primary Care Providers	Economies of scale and control of patient flow make the group an attractive partner and takeover target. Larger groups of primary care specialists come to control large numbers of patients, and therefore patient flow. Control of patient flow allows primary care groups to control the cost of specialty care and other forms of tertiary referral care (including hospitalization) through most-favored referral strategies. Successful cost control also makes the group attractive to other providers and to payers, leading to increasing economies of scale, and increasing numbers of patients under control. In capitated systems, this leads to improved cash flow. In cases of practice liquidation, terminal value is generally arrived at as a combination of one year's cash flow and the net present value of future earnings from patients in the practice.	Empower primary care provider to control aspects of patient flow, quality of care, protocols for care for a larger organization. Provides for increased capacity, contracting abilities. Providers can compete for larger managed care contracts or use network to develop their own managed care network. Reciprocal commitments with networked partners result in stable relationships that can be broadened to include employers and government agencies.
Specialists	Capturing market segment with limits allowed by law (currently estimated at between 20 and 34%, pending clarification from Department of Justice). INcreasing monopoly power. Establishing barrier to competition. Refining practice to desired mix. Improving life style. Improving quality of care through participation in medium-scale clinical studies. Enhanced reputation factor.	Guaranteed patient and cash flow with predictable capacity utilization. Potential for subspecialization through exploitation of large patient base-market dominance.
Multispecialty groups	Mergers of multispecialty groups lead to potential for full vertical integration (e.g., Mayo Clinic-outpatient clinic, hospital, nursing home and rehabilitation facilities, public health unit, medical school, residency and fellowship training programs, ancillary, professional training programs), and with addition of its own HMO—status as a "fully integrated health system"	Market dominance and further growth. Forward and backward Integration with insurers and HMOs. Lowered risk through enlarged patient pool. Improved utilization of capital intensive facilities.

autonomy, whether in the form of independent clinics or practice routines. Four common practice relationships are encountered: (1) PPO (preferred provider organization), (2) IPA (independent practice association), (3) GPWW (group practice without walls), (4) IMG (integrated medical group).

Each step along the continuum from PPO to IPA to GPWW achieves more of the putative potential benefits of the fully integrated medical group. Each step also moves the individual physicians further along the path of escalating intra group cooperation and dependence. This move results in a gradual surrender of physician autonomy on some levels. As a practical matter, clinical decision-making autonomy is usually largely preserved except in IMGs, where protocols and other management tools (including physician incentives) are used to routinize patient care in ways that would not work in looser organizations.

This view of the market suggests that physicians must prepare to relinquish autonomy as an unavoidable consequence of ongoing market changes in health care. The merger process allows for some control over the process. Physician networking creates market power through contracting. Networking also offers the potential for economies of scale and some capital to support key practice support functions required for managed care.* The

The idea of *managing care* (as opposed to *managed care*) implies that *medical groups* rather than payers develop internalize processes that support active efforts to monitor and control patient flow. The ideologized view of the process emphasizes potential improvements in cost control without sacrificing quality. The idea is to establish simultaneous efficiency and effectiveness measures for the population under contract patients. Mechanisms that might be invoked include clinical case management, linking patients clinical and financial outcomes, and utilization review. The process is not very different from what is encountered in managed care. The distinction has to do with who is in control—the payer or the physician group.

TABLE 21–6. Merger and Networking Models for Physician Group Practices (*Note:* Key features of each model are in bold face)

Models for Physician Group Networking and Merger (Listed in increasing level of physician commitment to an integrated medical group)

Model	*Legal Structure*	*Physician Autonomy Office*	*Physician Entry Revenue Stream*	*Disadvantages of Model*
PPO—preferred provider organization	New legal entity created only as contracting vehicle; **no MD equity; Cannot accept capitation**	MDs retain autonomy; **retain existing independent office**	Open Panel—any willing MD can join; usually dominated by subspecialists; **MD independent revenue stream; does own billing**	**No common fee schedule; no change in MD expense side; open panel approach means no managed care strategies**
IPA—independent practice association	New legal entity created for contracting; **equity based (min. value); can accept capitated contracts**	MD retains practice autonomy except for IPA contracted patients; **retain existing independent office**	Invitation only; **IPA collects fees; MD otherwise independent revenue stream for other patients**	**Difficult to generate capital; no change MD expense side; weak incentive to manage care**
GPWW—group practice (clinic) without walls	**New legal entity to independently house entire back-office business functions for all MDs; greater equity base and profit sharing; accepts capitation**	**MDs retain existing independent office; GPWW establishes separate business office for common back-office functions**	Invitation; **shared expenses; revenue flows through GPWW but MDs retain separate profit center for each office**	**Limited scale economies multiple offices; lacks group discipline, culture, and financial incentives to manage care; diffuse governance**
IMG—integrated medical group practice	**creation of a single legal entity; significant MD equity**	**All MDs are employed by group; single main clinical office, possible satellite locations**	Invitation; **group compensation system; single or multispecialty group**	**Limited access to capital; single site may be unattractive to payers and raise**

group can actively manage care by creating physician incentives, developing internal case management, monitoring clinical and financial patient outcomes, and creating information feedback loops to group physicians.

Various networking models will appeal differently to individual physicians as a function of their understanding of and commitment to health care change and the degree to which they have completed the cultural transformation to a group practice mentality (the ability to change). The degree of managed care maturity in their local market (increasing maturity is defined as a higher percentage of covered live under managed care), and the presence of existing large medical groups also influence a physician's willingness to network.

The observation that physicians in a given market are moving closer to an IMG model implies either that the market is more mature and a higher level of physician integration is required to remain competitive, or that local physician leaders have the foresight and the entrepreneurial energy to become market leaders and move ahead of HMO penetration into the local market

When Do Practice Mergers Work?

Practice mergers do not suit every situation. Before engaging in a merger, the principals involved must ask some very fundamental questions about the purpose of the merger and the business they are trying to create. So fundamental is this point that it is useful to back away from the specific problems of practices contending with managed care to look at the theory of mergers in terms that are broader than medicine alone.

Businesses create value through any of the following four strategies:

1. Enhancing efficiency—innovating to lower costs.
2. Innovating new products or processes—improving the quality of the product relative to market requirements.
3. Establishing market power.
4. Rewriting the rules of the business to their advantage.

The consolidation of physicians into larger group practices has the potential to create value through each of the four strategies. But if there is any question about the ability of the larger group to capitalize on its size or on the opportunities that a larger group provides, the logic behind the merger must be rethought. The strongest promise for success of medical groups as groups—the one that best exploits the promise of enlarging scope—probably emanates from the full merger of physicians into IMGs. Since IMGs are arguably the most valuable, it is worth examining them in order to dissect out the components that might benefit smaller enterprises as well.

Enhancing Efficiency-Innovating to Lower Costs

Mergers create economies of scale. First, as the group grows, it employs additional physicians and achieves increasing economies of scale in administrative and clinical management support. The potential benefits include the ability to reduce the number of clinic sites and the elimination of redundant back-office support (billing, collections, transcription, medical records, etc.). There will also be opportunity to achieve economies of scale over staffing, capital equipment needs, human relations management, and management for the practice. Back-office overhead for small physician practices typically consumes 35 to 50% of the practice revenue. It is important to recognize that savings generated may not immediately result in lower overhead because of the need to divert these savings into the development and purchase of additional practice-support capabilities, especially information systems for purposes of record keeping and documentation, quality assurance, and utilization review. Also, the initial cost of merging, which is often considerable, must be amortized.

Additional economies of scale follow in relation to the types of physicians who make up both the original and the merged group. Primary care physicians have become the linchpin for patient care in most managed care models. Consequently, a strong PCP network creates market power. The specialist also requires a strong base of PCPs to assure an adequate supply of patients. Although we will not address the issue here, the new dependence of the specialist on PCPs represents a significant change in the physician power structure that must be managed effectively in growing integrated medical groups.

The second economy of scale derived from practice growth relates to a reduction in financial risk that accompanies the ability to care for larger and larger populations of patients. This concept is outside of the scope of this chapter except in a very theoretical way. Nonetheless, it is of great practical importance to groups who undertake financial risk for populations of patients under capitation or through some other arrangement. This factor should probably not be regarded as a major impetus for merger, even though it serves as a strong incentive for the continued growth of medical groups

Product Innovation—Quality Improvement

Quality control first became an issue external to the medical profession through hospital QA initiatives. Most of these initiatives were undertaken in response to outside regulatory pressures. Initially, these programs were designed to identify physicians who fell below a certain standard. The standard was generally set by the hospital staff. Later, payers began to address quality issues indirectly through their interest in controlling health care costs. They defined quality as the lack of significant variation from external norms. These norms were often based on extensive but inflexible data bases that could identify outcome standards but often failed to take into account sensitive and legitimate confounding influences such as patient age, acuity, and complexity. Physicians as a group rejected this model of external case management as inappropriately based on control and the primary desire to limit cost.

The economies of scale derived from physician merger present the opportunity for physicians to regain control over patient care quality. Medical groups at risk can establish clinical models of case management that differ from external control models in several respects:

1. It is based on a model of identifying best practices.
2. It is internally motivated.
3. It is supported by combined clinical and financial patient outcomes.
4. It arises from the ongoing relationship between the medical groups' physicians and the patient.
5. The physician group derives direct financial reward from limiting utilization of services.

Prior to capitated reimbursement, payers retained all the financial reward derived from physician efforts to be cost effective. The moral hazard for the patient is apparent. With capitation, there is both a moral hazard for the physician to the extent that reimbursement depends on cost savings, but there is also an element of financial and legal risk involved with providing too little care since inadequate or untimely care may be more expensive and give rise to malpractice suits.

The generally accepted, but as yet unproven premise suggests that quality costs less. A driver of value for physicians merging is the opportunity to prove this assumption and control the data. Whoever first amasses and controls this information in a given market will have significant, and quite possibly very long lasting first mover advantages.

Establishing Market Power

The issue of market power for the growing medical group has already been noted. Some data that illustrate the point are derived from the history of suppliers and providers in the Minneapolis/St. Paul medical market. In 1990, in Minneapolis, 65% of physicians were members of medical groups. This figure compares with a national average of 30%.[11] The chronological development of the Minneapolis medical market is presented in Table 21–7.

The evolution of the Minneapolis market demonstrated the rising market power of the medical groups. The rate of HMO growth slowed in 1987–1988. Several factors came to play in the Minneapolis market, but a dominant factor was the rise in market power of large medical groups that had gained sufficient market power and integration to bypass the HMOs and successfully contract directly with employers to provide health care to their employees.

Rewriting the Rules of the Business

Whoever establishes the standards to which an enterprise, a business, or an industry must adhere earns a distinct market advantage. The rules of the game continue to change rapidly in health care. Suppliers initiated changes in the rules of the game. To the extent that large groups control certain aspects of the economic and service components of the industry, they may exert significant influence on how the next iteration of modifications will appear. One example is antitrust regulation as it applies to health care. Medical groups forced a reconsideration of antitrust legislation as they responded to market changes through the merger process.[12]

Benefits Associated with Group Mergers

The reasons behind medical group mergers and the gains associated with multispecialty medical group formation are summarized in Tables 21–8 and 21–9. Many of the benefits associated with IMG formation do not pertain to horizontal merger models.

Trends

The rate of physician movement from traditional solo to group practices has accelerated over the last decade. This trend was only minimally apparent before the late 1970s and early 1980s. In 1960, only 11% of physicians were in group practices while in 1980 30% were. There were 10,762 physician groups in 1980 and by 1987 the number had increased to 17,516.[15]

Not only has the number of medical groups increased significantly, but the groups are increasing in size as measured by the number of physician members in the group. According to the American Medical Association Council on Long Range Planning, the number of group practices with greater than 100 physicians members is expected to continue to grow at 12% per year the 1990s.[16]

The Alliance Formation Process for Physician Group Practices

A formal guide to the formation of medical groups has not been described to date to the best of our knowledge.

TABLE 21–7. Minneapolis/St. Paul Market Evolution

Unstructured: Phase I 1972–1980	***Loose Framework Phase II 1980–1986***	***Consolidation Phase III 1986–1990***	***Integrated Health System-Phase IV 1990–present***
Independent hospitals, physicians	Hospitals and physicians under price pressure	Hospitals form systems (alliances)	Employers form coalitions to purchase health services
Slow growth of independent HMOs	Excess inpatient hospital capacity	Aggressively recruit PCPS	Systems manage patient populations
Employee benefit expansion Unsophisticated purchasers of health care	HMO, PPO enrollment balloons (supplier market power)	Gain leverage on HMOs	
		Become platform for integration	
		Development of large multispecialty, primary care, and IPA physician groups	
		Specialists practice underutilized; discounts increase	
		Lead HMOs achieve critical mass, begin to consolidate	
		Selective contracting by major purchasers	

TABLE 21–8. Why Physician Groups Will Seek Affiliations or Mergers

Access to managed care patients through hospital or health system's contracts
Access to capital to expand group
Compensation support
Physician recruitment incentives and practice guarantees
Systems support; top-flight management, information systems
Need to "cash-out" older, retiring partners
Desire to create equity in the practice by physician owners
Facilities and equipment
Seeking strong partner with "deep pockets" for risk-sharing managed care contracts
Relief from administrative hassles
Relief from financial losses experienced by the group
"Bandwagon" effect of other groups merging, affiliating, and being acquired

TABLE 21–9. Factors Driving the Success of Multispecialty Groups[14]

Comprehensive range of physician services and ancillary services
Patients have one familiar organization as their "Medical Home"
Well positioned for managed care—strong physician recruiting position
Payers believe multispecialty groups will be well positioned for managed care and that they can truly manage care and impact clinical decision making of physicians in primary care specialties
Subspecialty physicians need strong primary care base to maintain referral volume
Payers utilize PCPs

In this section, we offer a model for the merger of a small (3 to 5 physician) group into a larger one. We will address a series of issues, each one from the perspective of both the smaller and the larger group alone.

Initial Phase: Assessing Strategic Match

Question 1. How competitive is the existing practice of each partner?

- **Small Group Perspective:** Examine the reputation and governance structure of the larger partner. Determine the smaller group's potential role in the merged groups strategic plan and become familiar with the large group's current strategic plan. Explore the larger partner's access to capital for practice growth and for building and/or enhancing information systems required to support practice management tools (quality assurance, utilization review, linked clinical and financial data for patients, etc.). Identify the existing payer contracts that the larger partner holds and determine concordance with small group's current patients and contracts.

  Determine the potential of these contracts to add patient volume to the smaller group. Identify what geographic coverage would be achieved and what new payer contracting options might become available following the merger.
- **Large Group Perspective:** What is the smaller group's reputation for quality, patient satisfaction, ability to work on a team, commitment to measuring clinical outcomes, and learning from feedback about their clinical and financial performance. Clarify whether the smaller partner can handle any additional volume of patients that might come from existing or anticipated new payer contracts.

Question 2. Does the merger create a win-win environment?

- **Small Group Perspective:** Physicians in the small group must feel that the loss of personal and practice autonomy is offset by the income security and ability to participate in capitated contracts expected from the association with the larger group. The larger group is better positioned to deal with managed care and capitated contracts and is expected to have more secure and greater current and future access to patients. Physicians in the smaller group can also win by realizing a reduction in the administrative hassles of running the day-to-day practice, and by gaining scale advantages that allow greater capitalization of practice growth and practice support tools for such a superior information systems. Physicians in the small group can also regain some control over clinical practice through capitated contracts that support an internal, clinical model of case management rather than an external, payer-driven control model of case management. The external model is frequently viewed as "sledgehammer."
- **Large Group Perspective:** The large medical group will experience benefits through growth in the size and breadth of its physician network (economies of scope). Size and geographical distribution enhance the group's coverage and builds its market power. Increased market power supports more balanced negotiations with the powerful suppliers. In addition, the larger practice creates a larger revenue base and multiplies the larger group's economies of scale. Scale economies provide capital to further expand the physician base and acquire the practice support tools necessary to efficiently compete for capitated contracts.

Question 3. Are the existing group cultures compatible?

- **Choosing partners:**
  1. Professional and personal compatibility
  2. Commitment to group as well as individual success
  3. Criteria to explore:
     a. Standards for clinical care—equal or preferably exceeds community standards
     b. Physician longevity—desire for continuing practice and targeted retirement age

c. Practice attitude—attitude towards work (hours, days, call, etc.), practice style, utilization of referral to specialists and/or out-of-practice physicians (ease of referral, limitations on referral), and utilization patterns for ancillary services such as laboratories and radiology.
d. Attitudes about charity care and community service
e. Attitudes and time allotted for community medical governance roles
f. Respect for personal time off

- **Barriers to physicians achieving success through merger:**
  1. Control issues
  2. Autonomy
  3. Politics
  4. Ego

Physicians who are unable to accommodate to changes in these domains after initial discussions and analysis of the potential governance structure of the new group will not support successful completion of the merger. The cultural change required may be more significant if there is substantial size discrepancy between the two groups.

Physicians must look beyond the past: The current evolution of health care suggests that physicians will be required to move from autonomous practices to organized groups. For most physicians, the ability to successfully make this transition dependents on their achieving a clear and complete picture of the patterns of change in health care and the potential impact that these changes will have on practice options and patient volume. Consequently, much of the cultural evaluation occurs during the educational process as each group assesses the partners' abilities to perceive and respond to the cultural transformation required to adapt to structural changes in health care.

Finally, cultural fit must be evaluated from the perspective of each partner's ability to internalize the global structural elements of a successful merger (Table 21–10).[17] At the stage of implementation, mergers require cooperation based on trust and the embedded cultural ability to internalize growth through team work.

Initial Phase Evaluation: Stakeholder Blessing. Both external and internal stakeholders must be able to see substantive benefits to gain their support and sponsorship for the alliance.

Internal Stakeholders

Question 1. Who are the internal stakeholders?

The potential stakeholders with respect to privately held medical group mergers include the following:

1. Majority shareowners, generally physicians
2. Minority shareowners, e.g., COO or office manager
3. Employees of the medical group

Question 2. What are the concerns of the physician stakeholders?

Physician owners of small medical groups are accustomed to having explicit unfettered authority over their practice, their business, and their employees. The key issues for gaining physician blessing are listed in Table 21–11.

Question 3. What are the minority owners' concerns':

Minority stakeholders are usually long-standing valued employees within the physician group. Their concerns will focus on the value of their investment (exchange value of shares in existing group) and job security. The merger process must balance the job security of these managers and the need for the new group to build and protect itself for the future. This is particularly important if the merged group is considering downsizing back-office support to enhance scale economies and/or closing some office sites.

Question 4. What are employees' concerns?

Employees must be kept fully informed and educated about the importance of the proposed merger to the groups' future success and their own job security. They will have concerns regarding job security and benefits under the new group. Retention of retirement benefits is especially important to long-standing employees. All concerns should be addressed openly and honestly.

Employees also need to be educated about future directions and changes in health care so that they can

TABLE 21–10. Successful Merger—Cooperation Is the Dominant Objective

(Factors Favoring Competition or Cooperation in Strategic Alliances)

	Favor Cooperation	*Favor Competition*
Strategic Intent	Maximize joint competitive advantage	Maximize firms competitive advantage
Proprietary Resources	Manage shared resources	Protect and develop
Organizational Control	Through control systems and cooperation process	Through hierarchy and control systems

TABLE 21–11. Gaining Merger Blessing from Physician Stakeholders

Issue	*Concern*	*Recommendation*
Physician compensation	Frequently crucial issue to MD proceeding; must be short-term winners and losers	Clarify proposed impact on compensation; Emphasize long-term benefits to merger, and MD income security
Structure—corporation or partnership	MDs sacrificing control in merging; ego, autonomy, and politics play a role; Opportunity to remain full (equal) partner in new group	Equal partner with limited additional financial buy-in is best received; structure should be thoroughly thought out and presented to all physicians
Governance structure	MDs sacrificing authority and control; differential partner size raises issue of balance of power	Ideal proposed governance board of 5–7 members; represents a transition involving decentralized decision making, and shareholder delegation of authority-building trust
Officers of merged group	Loss of authority and voice in group decisions	Blended slate—significant leadership and administrative skills; requires a medical director who reports to the Board of Director; shareholders must approve the slate
Pension plan	Concern regards preservation of benefits and control of investment decisions	Negotiated structure designed to preserve as many benefits as feasible considering the cost structure delivered to the merged group; be supportive of desires and remain flexible and creative
Clinic name	Loss of long-standing personal and professional identity	Minimize effects of competition over name; MD referrals are made to the MD; only the public (self) refers based on the practice name; Name is to convey message to general public—*marketing* is predominant real issue
Physician employment agreement	Loss of autonomy; salary, benefits, retirement, departure outside of retirement, vesting period for partnership	Frequently seals the foregoing issues; considers the good of the group as well as the needs of the individuals; effective agreements give the group the power to govern its members—**protecting the group protects the individuals**

understand the reasons for merger. It is important to stress that protecting the group protects the employees.

External Stakeholders:

Question 1. Who are the external stakeholders?

- **Patients**—Patients should be informed after the merger and reassured that the merger will not eliminate their relationship with their physician. Patients should also be informed about the benefits to be expected from the merger; for example, expanded patient service benefits that might be offered because of the enhanced geographical reach merger group and the economies of scale apparent in the larger group.
- **Marketing**—Patients who direct or self-refer and physicians who refer to physicians in the group will need to know about the changes. Appropriate marketing strategies should be part of the strategic plan for implementation, but reassurance will be important as soon as the merger intent is made public whether by intention or not. Ideally the new group should invest a percentage of its revenue for marketing, planning, and new patient acquisition. The merger itself may generate additional specific patient benefits that offer marketing opportunities.
- **Government**—Government becomes an external stakeholder through the regulatory process. First, antitrust questions must be considered. Efficiencies created by the merger may become an important issue in antitrust defense. These efficiencies are equally important in gaining the support of internal stakeholders and should be acknowledged during initial stakeholder blessing. Second, the government is an external stakeholder to the extent that the merged group either holds or plans to hold Medicare or Medicaid contracts. Frequently, these programs are administered through suppliers who have specific programmatic and health care needs in mind when they request contract bids from

providers. This issues should be considered in the strategic vision that evolves during the stakeholder blessing phase.

Intensive Phase Evaluation: Winning Internal Stakeholder Support

Question 1. How do we anticipate and deal with coalition behavior?

The proposed merger will initially be threatening to physician owners, managers, and employees. Winning support requires open and honest communication and stakeholder education about structural changes in health care and the need to position the medical group for the future. Group leadership must assume a very active role in this process. General objectives are outlined as follows:

1. Line up support for the merger as early as feasible. Understand who the stakeholders are and which members may form coalitions against the merger.
2. Know the nature of stakeholders demands; *for example,* are employees' jobs secure, will salaries change, what are the new reporting relationships; what degree of business or practice autonomy must be sacrificed by physicians, who controls the pension plan, what equity will be obtained in the new company, will personal salaries change?
3. Understand the political behavior and the process by which potentially dissenting coalitions will form and evolve; for example, understand who the employees trust and listen to; which physician factions within the group may see the future differently (*e.g.,* young physicians or older physicians).
4. Individuals and groups can achieve the power to restructure conditions so that organizations pursue goals that better suit their own agendas; therefore, listening to them, educating them, and winning their support is worth the time and energy required.
5. These individuals tend to use manipulation, bargaining, and coalition formation with interest groups to achieve their purposes; know who these group will be and involve them early in the planning and especially in the solutions.
6. Coalitions tend to build around issues. Opportunities for success may be maximized as follows:
   Make all different issues visible—let them be aired.
   Create a clear sense of the purpose intended through the merger.
   Gain commitment by anticipating and managing coalition behavior.
   Gaining commitment should take the form of finding the right way to accomplish a goal rather than winning.
7. For these reasons, the following strategy should be pursued
   Listen and understand internal stakeholders.
   Know how to handle internal coalitions.

Be prepared to address all the issues identified as concerns of the physician stakeholder

Question 2. Who are the formal and informal physician leaders in the group?

Many small medical groups do not have clearly established leadership. Leadership tends to occur through a committee of the whole. Concordant with the hierarchical organization of their medical training, physicians have a strong tendency to accept seniority as an appropriate requisite for leadership. The proxy of experience offered by this model may or may not coincide with the leadership and administrative skills necessary to successfully lead a practice group through a merger. The merger process requires talented and trusted leadership and may result in alternative leaders stepping forward.

A second confounding problem of leadership in small physician groups is the perception that the receiving of the medical degree makes the physician equivalent to any other physician colleagues in all aspects of medical group governance. This notion is quite independent of experience or administrative training and conveys a strong sense of personal authority about group decisions. The natural play on this posture is that decisions are made by a majority of all physicians in the group. Consequently, the objective must be set to educate and seek buy-in from all group physicians.

Intensive Phase Evaluation: IV Development of a Strategic Plan

Once the blessing and matching phase is complete, it is necessary to develop a comprehensive strategic plan that takes the two medical groups through an in-depth analysis. Prior to this intensive sharing and analysis phase, it is appropriate to enter into a confidentiality agreement to protect both parties in the event that the alliance is not concluded.

1. The process of strategic planning is well defined. We will not attempt to duplicate a description of the process, but will focus instead on several key issues. The potential partners must identify synergism to be obtained in the creation of the joint entity.
2. Physicians have very demanding schedules. It therefore may be appropriate to consider a strategic planning retreat to identify an agreed on strategic vision, common goals, and opportunities;
3. A formal analysis of strengths, weakness, opportunities, and threats associated with the merger may assist participants in focusing beyond immediate problems associated with planning the merger.

4. Unless one of the groups contains leadership experienced in strategic planning and merger activity, it may be appropriate to utilize a consultant facilitator to lead the discussion at the strategic planning retreat. The characteristics of physician group leadership identified above suggest that a facilitator may be valuable in this process. Mutually agreed on non-physician leadership from both groups may represent an equally acceptable option. Few physician leaders in small medical groups have the necessary experience to lead groups through this strategic planning process.

Conclusion

There are several reasons to consider practice mergers or acquisitions:[18]

- Increasing geographical coverage
- Contracting efficiencies
- Economies of scale
- Access to improved information systems
- Access to sources of capital for further growth
- Access to improved management
- Market power.

Physicians are generally inexperienced about working in organizations. The three-way interchange of security, control, and autonomy is particularly problematic. To avoid conflict later on, it is advisable, in a very formal manner, to:

- Articulate the perceived advantages accruing from a merger.
- Reach consensus regarding the nature of the business that will be developed *and how this business will be different from that pursued by each party to the negotiation separately before the merger.*
- Articulate the reasons for merger with the specific parties involved.
- Probe and articulate the core competencies of each party.
- Articulate the strengths, weaknesses, opportunities, and threats accompanying each party to the merger.

After this step has been completed, a feasibility plan should be initiated, together with the development of a formal business plan. The business plan should include:

- Clearly articulated objectives for the merger
- Structure and control issues
- Distribution of equity
- Control of clinical (as opposed to administrative) decision-making
- Management and governance
- Compensation formulae.

Although it may not necessarily have to be included within the business plan, serious consideration should be given to articulating a scheme for *dissolution and liquidation* of the merger, and whether a formal merger, rather than a looser networking alliance, is necessary to achieve the stated objectives.

After the merger has been formalized, but before it has been implemented, the merger should be informally, but pointedly discussed in the physician community. Physician leaders who have been supportive up until this point may now waver. If the merger has been arrived at by a process of increasing and inclusive consensus, however, wavering is less likely. Implementation, the last step in the process, assumes acceptance of the roll-out model and continued consensus on the part of the physicians involved.

There are no magic formulas to determining whether a merger will work, or whether it is even advisable to try. *Unless the specific objectives of a merger can be fully articulated, and unless alternatives can be explored and demonstrated to be wanting, and unless the objectives can be demonstrated to hold the* ***reasonable*** *promise of increased advantage to all stakeholders, the merger is likely to fail.* There is a whole portfolio of approaches to physician alliances. The merger and acquisition process is the most definitive and the most difficult to undo. The advantages of flexibility achieved through other linkage vehicles may outweigh the advantages of a merger, particularly in view of the expense involved, the relatively difficult dissolution process, and the fact that most mergers involve the relatively intimate alliance of former competitors.

The importance of developing efficient communications must not be underestimated. A formal communication process must be established, one that highlights the vision of the merger and combines small group discussions with the full and efficient dissemination of information. Multiple avenues of communication are best.

Mergers typically involve a shift in leadership as they evolve from planning to implementation and from implementation toward maturity. This may brook resentment, particularly insofar as more senior physicians, who have traditionally been accorded leadership roles in the culture of medicine, become eclipsed by younger physicians or by administrators, whose familiarity with managed care surpasses their own. The resentment that frequently interposes can be somewhat restrained through a process of education aimed at bringing all members of the merging groups to a similar level of theoretical expertise and affording those with special interest the opportunity to take on more prominent roles. The key for individual physicians is a willingness to commit personal time and energy, and, for the group, a willingness to enlarge the circle of governors. Leaders of a group will usually require focused education, which the group should support.

Information needs in merged groups encompass the traditional domains of practice administration, patient demographics, compensation, scheduling, patient records, utilization, and qualifying physicians and assistant staff. In addition, consideration should be given to the specific needs associated with the development of clinical protocols, outcome measures, patient satisfaction surveys, provider satisfaction surveys, case management, risk management, and contracting needs. It is critical to plan for an information system capable of supplying the infrastructure for the complexities of true integrated health systems.

The function known as "human resources" in large corporations—employee management and benefits, hiring, firing, investment in education, holidays, and the like—is typically handled relatively informally in small groups. As groups merge, this function may require more formal attention. As groups engage in integrated systems of care, it will also be necessary to develop a coterie of employees with specific managerial experience in the fields of ambulatory care, managed care, home health, and pharmacy.

ACKNOWLEDGMENTS

We wish to acknowledge the contribution of Professor Harbir Singh of the Wharton School of the University of Pennsylvania. Professor Singh offered invaluable guidance and teaching, and helped us conceptualize the models for mergers in health care that have been set forth.

REFERENCES

1. Beckham JD: Integrated health care delivery systems: A guide to successful strategies for hospital and physician collaboration. *Quorum Health Resources* Tab 200:p 5. Thompson Publishing Group. December 1993.
2. This discussion draws on a number of sources including: Hall MA: *Managed competition and integrated health care delivery systems.* 29 *Wake Forest Law Review* 1 (1994); Hitcher CH, Richardson C, Solomon JE, Oppenheim CB: *Integrated delivery systems: A survey of organizational models.* 29 *Wake Forest Law Review* 273 (1994); Iglehart JK: *Health policy report: Managed competition.* 328 *N Engl J Med* 1208 (1993); Kissick WL: *Medicine's dilemmas. Infinite needs versus finite resources.* New Haven: Yale University Press, 1994; Enthoven A: Consumer-choice health plan: A national health insurance proposal based on regulated competition in the private sector. 298 *N Engl J Med* 650, 709 (1978); Enthoven A: The history and principles of managed competition. 12 *Health Affairs Supplement* 1993, 20 ff.; Baker N: Health care reform: Summary of the Clinton administration's health reform plan. 26 *J Health and Hospital Law* 289 (1993); Frankford DM: Neoclassical health economics and the debate over national health insurance: The power of abstraction. 18 *Law and Social Inquiry* 351 (1993); Johnson LB: Playing doctor: Who controls the practice of medicine? 66 *St. John's Law Review* 425 (1992); Kohler MR: When the whole exceeds the sum of its parts: Why existing utilization management practices don't measure up. 53 *University of Pittsburgh Law Review* 106 (1992); Sanders SJ: Regulating managed care plans under current law: A radical reversion to established doctrine. 20 *Hofstra Law Review* 73 (1991); Nguyen NX Derrick FW: Hospital markets and competition: Implications for antitrust policy. 19 *Health Care Management Rev.* 34 (1994); Brewbaker WS III: Health care price controls and the takings clause. 21 *Hastings Constitutional Law Quarterly* 669 (1994); Relman A: The new medical-industrial complex. 303 *N Engl J Med* 963 (1980); Chase-Lubitz JF: The corporate practice of medicine doctrine: An anachronism in the modern health care industry. 40 *Vanderbilt Law Review* 445 (1987).
3. See, e.g., Navarro V: Medicine under capitalism. New York: Prodist (1976) pp. vii–x; xii–xiii; 135–169; Bennet A: U.S. marxists thrive despite communism's demise. *The Wall Street Journal,* September 6, 1994, page B1, continued B4; Relman AS: The new medical-industrial complex. *N Engl J Med* 265:963–970, 1980; Harris R: A sacred trust. New York: Penguin Books (1966).
4. Hall, *op. cit.* at 4; H.R. 3600, 103 rd Congress, 1st Session, §§ 1322, 1407 (1993).
5. H.R. 3600, 103rd Congress, 1st Session.
6. In capitated systems, the insurer or payer pays a *per capita* fee to the health care provider in anticipation of need. No additional utilization fee is ever paid. The provider shares insurance risk with the payer in the sense that the capitation fee is intended to cover all services provided. It is to the explicit advantage of the provider to calculate the exposure with utmost care, because the costs of any services provided above the level or quantity anticipated must be furnished free of marginal reimbursement.
7. Hall at 7, notes 11–14.
8. Iglehart JK: Health policy report: The struggle between managed care and fee-for-service practice. *N Engl J Med* 1994; 331:63–67.
9. Covered lives is the number of persons that an HMO, other payer, or provider has agreed to provide health care services for under contract (usually expressed in thousands).
10. Holdren RC: Competing in a merger and acquisition era: How much is a medical practice worth? *Healthspan* 1994; 11(4):37–39. Holdren articulates the 12-mile rule: people won't travel more than 12 miles without extraordinary effort from the medical practice, but once they are in a feeder network, they will travel long distances for procedures.
11. Report of the AMA Department of Professional Activities. American Medical Association (1990).
12. This particular aspect of health care reform has not yet been decided. At the time of this writing, the U.S. Department of Justice insists that no more than 20 to 34% of specialists in any one market, for example, merge. In practice, however, networks have been granted a relative immunity from adhering to this finding, which has yet to be fully tested in the courts.
13. Hospital Strategy Report. 1992. 4(9):5–7. Buy or build physician organizations as a magnet for referrals and a partner in managed care contracting.
14. *Integrated Health Care Delivery Systems.* 1993; Tab 200:p. 40.
15. Report of AMA Council on Long Range Planning, *Am Med News* 1994;32(29):12–13.
16. Ibid.
17. From lecture notes, Professor Harbir Singh, Wharton Executive MBA Program, Corporate Development: M&A (Management 721, fall semester, 1994).
18. Fickenscher K, Buentner S: Lessons from the trenches in physician integration. *Physician Executive* 1996; 22:14–18.

Jay Mayes, M.D., is a board-certified neonatologist who is co-founder of an innovative 15-physician neonatal-perinatal group practice that delivers coordinated, single-source care to high-risk pregnant mothers and their babies in Phoenix, Arizona. He graduated from Indiana University Medical School in 1974, and then moved to Phoenix to complete his Pediatric Residency and his Neonatal-Perinatal Fellowship. Dr. Mayes was a director of the Arizona State Newborn Transport Program and the director of the Newborn Intensive Care Unit at Phoenix Children's Hospital.

Dr. Mayes left his medical practice in 1993 to attend the Wharton School at the University of Pennsylvania. While completing his business degree, Dr. Mayes formed Integra Consultants, Inc., a provider of home care services to newborn and pediatric intensive care patients; and Samaritan Health Plan, a 150,000 member HMO in Phoenix, Arizona.

Dr. Mayes received his M.B.A. from the Wharton School in 1995. He is currently the Vice President of Medical Affairs for HealthPartners Health Plans, Inc., the second largest HMO in Arizona. HealthPartners Health Plans is a 400,000 member, provider-owned HMO that resulted from the merger in July 1996 of Samaritan Health Plan in Phoenix, Arizona and Arizona and Partner's Health Plan in Tucson, Arizona.

22

Evolving a Single Specialty Into a Multispecialty Network

RAMIE A. TRITT

When Dr. Steven F. Isenberg asked me to write a chapter in this text, I willingly accepted the opportunity since Atlanta has allowed me the opportunity to develop significant experience in managed care. Having said that, I must caution that "all health care is local." Therefore, whatever you read in the following pages may not apply directly to what is happening in your local community today yet it may be very apropos in the future.

As soon as this chapter's topic was finalized, I began a Medline search to see what else has been written about single-specialty networks evolving into a multispecialty network. I quickly found out that much has been written about multispecialty networks that started from a primary care base and multispecialty networks that are part of a integrated health care delivery system.[1,2,3] However, I could not find anything written about a multispecialty network that had evolved from single-specialty networks. The reader's community may or may not allow development of a model similar to what has happened in Atlanta. However, certain principles are true guiding lights that should stay constant as managed care organizations develop throughout the nation. I hope to leave you with those principles and with some comfort that managed care can be successfully integrated into your practice.

It is said that "good judgment comes from experience, and experience comes from bad judgment." With that in mind, I will start our Atlanta story by letting you know that I trained at McGill University in Montreal, Canada. While living in Montreal, I experienced the Canadian medicare system. When I first arrived in Atlanta in 1978, there was just talk about HMOs coming to the city. By 1980, the first HMO—HealthAmerica—had arrived and within a few months I had become the first otolaryngologist to contract with an HMO. By 1982, our group had increased to three physicians and we were now on a capitated contract and providing otolaryngic services to 25,000 HealthAmerica members. HealthAmerica went through its own growth and consolidation, eventually being bought by HealthCare and subsequently MaxiCare. By 1985, the plan had 50,000 lives and we were still the only group providing otolaryngic services. MaxiCare, however, had lost control of utilization and we suffered the consequences. We found ourselves providing otolaryngic services for nominal dollars since we were committed to our capitated fee. MaxiCare was bought by Kaiser and still the bleeding did not stop. At that point we tried to reach a new agreement with Kaiser. They had a different agenda, however, and we went our separate ways.

By 1990 the local health care market had started to change and HMOs were becoming more numerous. United HealthCare, which at that time was not well known, had come into Atlanta by buying a HMO known as Health First. I was contacted by the local representatives of Health First and asked to look at a new concept. The concept was to group together otolaryngologists from the greater Atlanta area into a single-specialty network that would provide otolaryngic services to 45,000 Health First members. Shortly afterwards, our group of four, along with fifteen additional otolaryngologists, embarked on the first otolaryngology specialty network in the greater Atlanta area. Two years later, Cigna HealthCare of Georgia decided to capitate otolaryngologists. Our group, which by then numbered eight physicians, was awarded the greater Atlanta Otolaryngology contract. One year later, we were chosen by Aetna Health Plans of Georgia to administer their otolaryngology network. Currently, our group of sixteen otolaryngologists, in conjunction with other otolaryngologists throughout the greater Atlanta area, provide otolaryngic care to 350,000 lives through our capitated contracts. As president and medical director, I have been involved in all aspects of the development and management of these networks.

"Change is the only constant thing" is a saying that rings true when it comes to health care in the 1990s. The same events that are happening in Atlanta are also occurring in many areas of the country. I realized approximately a year and a half ago that the single-specialty network is an excellent model, but one that will not accommodate the needs of all payers as they look for "their best model." For various reasons, the payers in Atlanta have strongly encouraged and supported the growth and development of single-specialty networks. All these networks have had years of experience in administering capitated contracts. Accompanied by peers from other specialities, we formed a multispecialty network in 1995 that now consists of approximately 650 physicians in fifteen specialities. GMG (Georgia MultiSpecialty Group) is committed to accept capitated contracts from payers and has now finalized its first contract with a national HMO while continuing negotiations with other payers. In addition, both our single-specialty network and GMG are having in-depth discussions with vertically integrated systems in the hope of achieving a relationship that allows the horizontally integrated single-specialty network and the integrated multi-specialty network (GMG) to work with and provide otolaryngic care and multispecialty care in vertically integrated health care systems.

Now let me try to detail the principles that we followed at our inception and how we have evolved those principles. The initial concept was to determine how to capture market share. Obviously that is still important, but the reality of the situation is that a new paradigm has evolved. The new and critical paradigm is "quality of care, quality of service and cost." We now focus our energies and initiative on these three overriding themes. Understanding the new paradigm and expanding on each of these themes will be the thrust of this chapter.

■ Forming a Single Specialty Network: Why Do It?

I remember going to an AAO-HNS meeting a few years ago and discussing what we were doing in Atlanta with our single-specialty networks. Most of the physicians were either not interested or were saying that there was no need for that type of product in their market. Last year, at the Academy meeting, our group, Atlanta Ear, Nose & Throat Associates, P.C., had a booth where we demonstrated to our colleagues how to develop a network. We also presented our new software product that handles the data processing and claims administration functions of the networks. At last year's meeting, more physicians were interested in the concept of a single-specialty network and the evolution into a multispecialty network. However, many still asked the question: "Why should we do it when there is no present demand for this in our community?" In the next few paragraphs, I hope to answer everyone's doubts about the need, either present or future, to develop single-specialty and multispecialty networks in their geographic areas.[4,5]

More and more throughout the country we are seeing patients move into HMO, Point of Service (POS), and PPO networks. When patients move to managed care networks there is a 15 to 25% cost advantage compared with indemnity insurance products. When patients move to capitated systems there is up to a 40% cost advantage. You can therefore easily understand why insurance companies strongly encourage the employer community to enroll their employees into a managed care network.[6]

For many years, payers have been looking at the physician cost-quality matrix. In simple terms it means that there is a huge cost to the payers, which is passed on to employers. Even if certain physicians provide quality care, they may be eliminated. What payers are looking for is an environment in which providers provide high quality care and low utilization (see Fig. 22–1)

Payers have realized that they can achieve high-quality care and low utilization by having physicians manage care in a capitated environment. This has lead to a fertile environment for physicians to gain back some of their lost control. This also has allowed the development of single-specialty and multispecialty networks in which specialists are able to control care at a very reasonable cost.

For physicians, single-specialty and multispecialty networks give us a chance to maintain or even gain market share depending on our local and regional health care environment.[4] It allows us a fair chance of getting our portion of the premium dollar. It enables specialists to be at the negotiation table with hospitals and PCPs with a united and strong voice to argue and get our share of the health care dollar. Properly formed and controlled, specialty networks can equal the balance of power with PCPs. United HealthCare is a leading example of a major payer that not only strongly supports but encourages the development of specialty networks.[4] Atlanta has been at the cutting edge of this specialty network development that is now reaching the California coast.

With a multispecialty network, the specialists can share in full risk contracts and get their portion of the savings when utilization is controlled. Part of the hospital savings and savings earned by achieving medical expense goals are passed on to the specialists. For years, the American consumer has desired access to a specialist whenever the

Physician Cost-Quality Matrix

HIGH QUALITY

High Utilization	High Quality	**Ideal** Low Utilization	High Quality
Good, but too pricey		Good all around	
High Utilization	Low Quality	Low Utilization	Low Quality
Bad all around		Bad but improving	

LOW UTILIZATION

Payers have realized that they can achieve high quality care and low utilization by having physicians manage care in a capitated environment. This has lead to a fertile environment for physicians to gain back some of their lost control. This also has allowed the development of single specialty and multispecialty networks in which specialists are able to control care at a very reasonable cost.

FIGURE 22–1. Physician Cost-Quality Matrix

need or want has arisen. By having a cost-effective specialty network in place, you will be able to answer the call of the payer when the American consumer starts clamoring for improved access or direct access to specialists. For example, in Georgia laws have been passed allowing direct access to dermatologists and gynecologists. At the same time, the insurance carriers desire to control costs. That is why specialty networks are very advantageous to the payer.

From a very practical day-to-day and style-of-practice viewpoint, there are great advantages to having a specialty network in place (see Table 22–1). We all are faced with the need to have our surgical cases approved. Usually this is done by a nurse or nonmedically trained person. In specialty networks our own colleagues review the difficult and questionable cases. As the physicians, we get to talk to our colleagues to explain the rationale and the need for a particular procedure.

TABLE 22–1. Why Do It—Summary

Maintain and increase market share
Major market shift to managed care products
Participate in hospital and other risk-sharing programs
Input into QA/UM and surgical criteria protocols
Develop advanced information systems
Gain opportunity to participate in network administrative role
Participate with colleagues in a specialty network
Position yourself for future changes in health care

Single-specialty networks allow the physician to develop quality assurance and utilization review protocols that govern the care of the network. This is advantageous when compared to working within the confines of non-otolaryngic friendly quality assurance protocols such as Milliman and Robertson. In our networks, physicians sit together on a quality assurance committee and oversee our own utilization and set our own protocols. The payers delegate (but do not relinquish) the quality assurance and utilization review functions to the single-specialty network. Again this allows us the luxury of "communicating with our own colleagues" and working together on a collaborative basis without necessarily having to merge member practices. By developing networks, you will also be forced to develop information systems that allow for accumulation of data. This data will allow you to be prepared to function in the new era of medicine. Another advantage of being involved and actually running a specialty network is that some physicians who are business minded can assume administrative functions. This will allow some physicians to earn funds that are presently being spent on nonmedical administrative personnel.

Finally, I see the day (as it is happening in certain markets today) when most of us will have an opportunity to contract directly with employers.[7] Those entities that have the longest track record will obviously have the upper hand. This takes us full circle back to the beginning when I mentioned that maintaining market share is a significant advantage of being involved in single-specialty and multispecialty networks.

■ Forces That Will Stop You

By now I hope you have gotten the urge to start to set up your own single-specialty or multispecialty network. Human nature being what it is, you are going to be thinking about all the hassles and difficulties that you will be facing as you set out to achieve your goal of establishing a premier network. To try to help you through the quagmire I will now list some of the typical concerns that I hear from physicians who are in the early stages of setting up a network.

One of the first concerns is the amount of work and effort, which includes many, many hours after the regular clinical workday, involved in setting up the network. It will obviously take months to achieve the goal of a fully operational network. We are all accustomed to hard work and we should not forget our residency days. We did it then and we can do it now. A more realistic concern is the natural frustration that sometimes develops when we have to deal with our colleagues in a business environment. Some individuals do not appreciate or recognize the effort and leadership skills that are needed to start and implement a specialty network. You may have to deal with negative comments spoken directly to you or more likely behind your back. There will also be the natural resistance of your colleagues to compensate you financially. Try to remember that being fair is reasonable but "business is business." In other words, if you or your colleague puts in the effort and hours to organize and implement a network, they should be financially compensated. Sometimes everyone else is looking for the next person to start the ball rolling. There will have to be a person or group of people willing to step up to the plate and lead the charge. Let the leaders step up.

Every community and every region has different market forces. Your market may be heavily dominated by PCPs controlling the delivery of health care. Do not let that stop you from developing specialty and multispecialty networks. It is important to realize that specialists can get on a more equal footing with the PCPs. The trend is starting to occur throughout the country, and we are seeing IPAs in California requesting proposals from specialists and asking them to form specialty networks. PCPs realize that they do not know all the ins and outs of every specialty. They can shift risk to the specialists and still do well financially.

Like any new business, there will be costs to start the network. Invest in your own future and you will succeed. Look at Wall Street where every company invests in itself. As physicians, we have been reluctant to invest in our own businesses. Some of us are now waking up and realizing that now is the time to put money back into our own businesses. We should not drain our businesses each year by taking all income as ordinary income. Everyone needs to realize that there are costs to setting up an organization.

Some colleagues are concerned about the need to set up sophisticated information systems and develop quality assurance committees with clinical guidelines. A need to follow the NCQA (National Committee for Quality Assurance) guidelines is a standard in the market place.[8] If your community does not have people who are able to do it, you can obtain it from outside your community by contacting organizations such as ours. Payers will frequently help you in establishing the protocols. When you are just starting out, you will not have all the data available to feel comfortable in knowing how and what to bid on a capitated contract. Once again, there are books and articles written on this subject and many individuals with experience are now available to help you through this process.

Some physicians are just worried about giving up their autonomy in the practice of medicine because of having to accept network guidelines and protocols. The reality of the situation is that we all work within accepted guidelines. In a network, however, the guidelines are more structured or at least more visible. The caveat is that in the specialty networks we are usually the ones able to develop and administer those guidelines.

Some communities still have essentially little or no managed care penetration. Physicians constantly say that they are concerned that if they set up a network and go to a payer that they will be driving the prices downward in their market place. My view is the opposite. I believe that you will have the upper hand, can exert significant impact in your market place, and will be able to achieve significant market share for the future.

In summary, the forces that will tend to stop you are the forces of uncertainty and the unknown. If you analyze these forces, however, you will realize that most are business concerns that we are all smart enough to grasp. As I keep saying to my colleagues, there is the practice of medicine and the business of medicine. Let us not fool ourselves—managed care is the business of medicine. The other concerns about working together as a team within the network should be something that we easily overcome as soon as we realize the benefits.[9]

How to Build a Multispecialty Network

I will tell you how we developed our multispecialty group in Atlanta. Every market is different, but you can pick up ideas from each market that will apply to yours. In Atlanta, the payers have encouraged and supported the development of single-specialty networks. We therefore started with a base of very strong specialty networks. Taking the *best* specialty networks (*best* meaning those that had the most managed care experience and most contracts), we merged these networks into a "specialty" multispecialty network using the legal entity known as a limited liability company (see Table 22–2 of GMG's specialities—primary members and affiliate members). Currently, we are partnering with different PCP panels to form a "specialty–primary care" multispecialty network. This allows us the flexibility of affiliating with numerous primary care panels. It permits us to contract with payers or MCOs that already have a primary care panel. Thus, our multispecialty organization (GMG) is not tied down to one particular model or locked into any specific payer model. The goal of any multispecialty network should be an ability to contract with as many managed care organizations and payers as possible.

TABLE 22–2. GMG Member Networks

Primary Members
Allergy
Cardiology
Dermatology
Gastroenterology
Neurology
Neurosurgery
Oncology
Ophthalmology and Optometry
Orthopedics
Otolaryngology
Plastic Surgery
Podiatry
Radiology
Surgery (General, Colo-rectal and Vascular)
Urology

Affiliate Members
Endocrinology
Infectious Disease
Nephrology
Obstetrics/Gynecology
Pulmonology
Rheumatology
Sleep Medicine

In our model, we first started with the single-specialty network. Obviously, the otolaryngology network is best known to me, but what I am about to tell you applies to single specialty and multispecialty network formation in general. To develop a network you must do the following: Establish a group of physicians who will be the core group and the physician leaders. This group will be making some early critical decisions such as:

- Defining whether the group will be a single-specialty network or a multispecialty network.
- Determining the geographical scope of the network.
- Deciding on the number of physicians to be admitted into the network.

Generally, several physicians will comprise the Executive Committee of the network. This is crucial when dealing as a multispecialty network. For a single-specialty network, situations arise when one individual may be the leader and sole organizer of the entity. In that case the physician leader must have the support of all the physicians from the onset.

- Very early on in the process a governing board is formed and a legal entity is organized. This entity can be a regular corporation, limited liability corporation, or partnership. Legal counsel is always obtained and preferably you will find an attorney with experience in medical transactions including physician organization formation, health care law, and regulatory experience.

- The board will chose a president, and the president will serve on the executive committee with the other physician leaders. A medical director will be selected from one of the physician leaders, as well as a physician whose responsibility is to supervise and preferably be actively involved in contracting functions between the MCOs and the network. In addition to the financial/contract committee, there will be credentials, quality assurance/utilization management, and marketing/business development committees. The organization chart of GMG is shown in Figure 22–2 as a representative model for a multispecialty group formed by single specialties.
- Early on in the process the executive committee must select other specialities to participate in the network. If it is a single-specialty network, all the

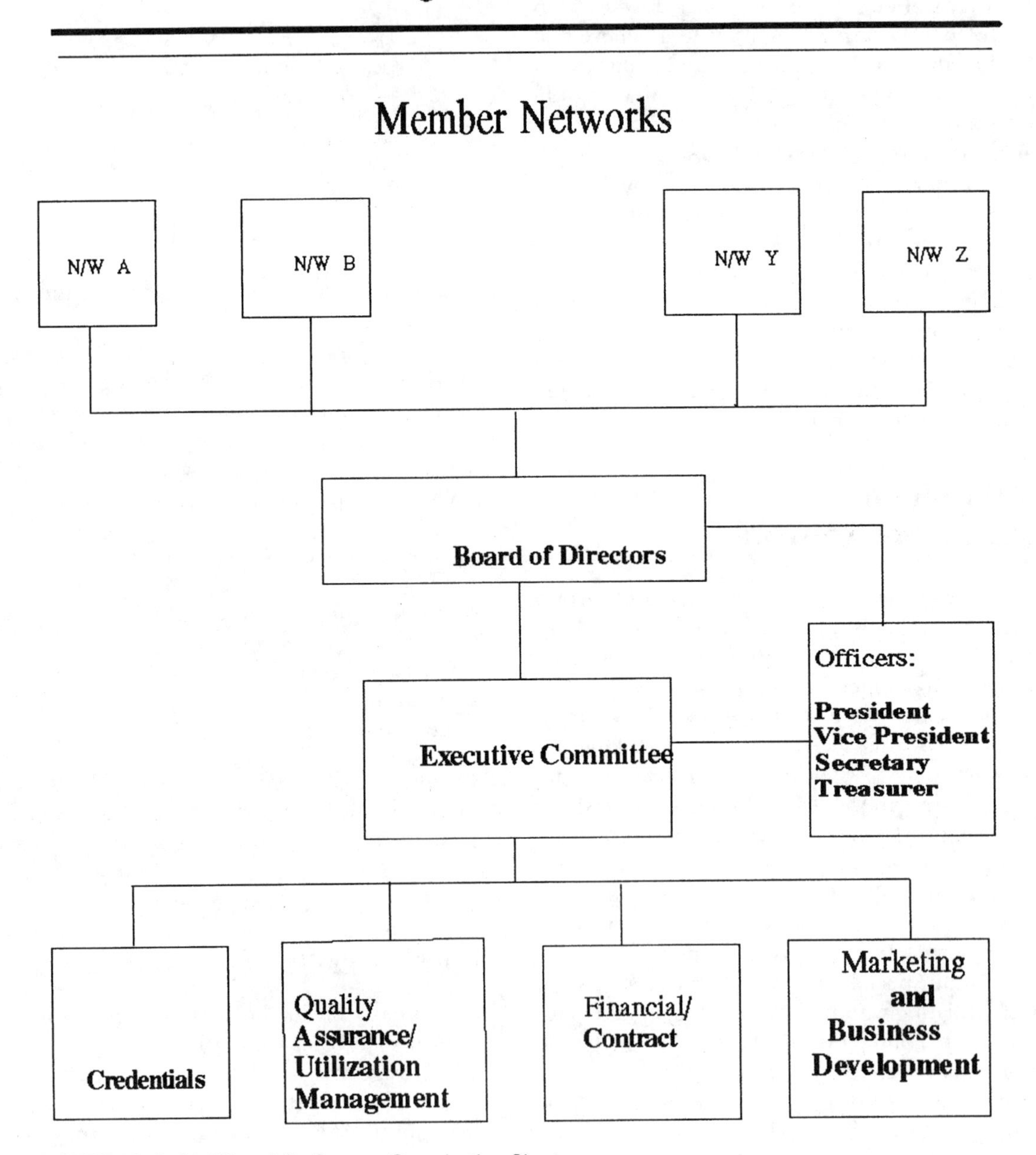

FIGURE 22–2. MultiSpecialty Group—Organization Chart

physicians will be limited to that specialty. In the multispecialty organization, each network has the responsibility of determining its own individual members. However, the credentials committee has the authority to add members to a particular network if there is a lack either in geographic access or specialty/subspecialty care that is required by the payers and is not being met by the individual network. Managed care organizations in your community will provide you with data about which physicians are cost-effective utilizers. Usually physicians will have their own reputation that precedes them. Networks should try to obtain the physicians who are well respected in the community since it will strengthen the organization.

- During the process of choosing physicians it is important to be able to "interact" with your member physicians. Therefore, the personality of a physician may preclude his or her admission into the network even though from a quality standpoint the person provides cost-effective care. Likewise, all physicians in the network, including those on the executive committee, must be open to constructive criticism about following network guidelines and protocols.
- Board certification is usually a criteria for choosing physicians and MCOs. Look for a network to have at least 90 to 95% of its physicians board certified.
- Network leaders must determine the compensation method for the physicians. Options are:
  - Capitation fee (per member per month or per member per year)
  - Discounted fee for service
  - Utilization of relative value units—RVUs or utilization of Medicare RBRVS payment system.
  - Any combination of the above
- One of the most critical parts of the utilization management program in a specialty organization is the very strong precertification system for all surgeries. Before any surgery is done, it is precertified by a nonphysician reviewer who utilizes the previously agreed on surgical criteria guidelines that have been developed by the QA/UM committee. If a case is not approved by the nonphysician reviewer, it is immediately brought to the attention of the physician reviewer. Only a physician reviewer can deny a case. Communication is achieved with the requesting physician to let him/her know why the case has been denied. Frequently it is a matter of inadequate documentation and, with the appropriate documentation, the case is approved. The surgical guidelines we use in our networks are those approved by the American Academy of Otolaryngology Quality Assurance Committee with modification for the following procedures—septoplasty, endoscopic sinus surgery, ventilation tube insertion, tonsillectomy and adenoidectomy, and uvulopalatopharyngoplasty.
- At time of payment, all claims are initially reviewed by the nonphysician network administrator or delegated personnel. Once again, final review by the physician reviewer is done to make sure that all network guidelines have been met. For example, multiple procedures are paid at a percentage of the regular fee, as done by MCOs.
- Strong information systems are needed to handle all types of reports that the payers request. More and more reports are required since the payers have to meet NCQA guidelines. The best information systems have an open architecture so that data can be retrieved and analyzed in many ways. An example of such an information system is CAPSYSTEMS, our own propietary system.
- Every organization needs strong advisers whose motivation is to see the network thrive. For a network to thrive it must have covered lives and continue to grow in its number of covered lives. These advisers need experience in managed care with emphasis on network development, contacts in the payer community, experience with requests for proposals from MCOs, and the ability to bring in experts if the advisers do not have all the knowledge or experience. Advisers can be paid on either a fixed monthly fee or a percentage of the capitation dollars coming into the specialty organization monthly.
- When bidding on a payer contract, it is important to analyze the payer's past utilization history for both the number of procedures and the dollar amount paid on the procedures. Procedures are analyzed for both office and outpatient/inpatient surgical procedures. Office procedures should be further subdivided into evaluation management (E/M) codes, audiology, and so on. Surgical procedures should be analyzed for the number of endoscopic sinus surgery, septoplasty, tonsillectomy and adenoidectomy, ventilation tube, and other procedures that have been done. All this information will allow you to determine the best capitation rate for your proposal.
- Carve-outs need to be negotiated. An example of a carve-out in a specialty contract is otoneurologic procedures.
- If a payer does not provide you the needed information to bid on a contract because it is a new product (such as a new point of service product) being developed by the payer, use national historic data as a guideline. It is also important to find out which age group the payer is trying to sign up and if the payer

is using any other criteria to try to narrow or expand its scope of potential patient enrollees.[10]

- Day-to-day operations of the network need to be performed by the network administrator or other assigned personnel. This is obviously critical since the majority of the networks will have physicians who actively practice medicine (such as myself) and who are not full-time physician administrators.

Specifics of a Multispeciality Organization

Once developed and organized, the multispecialty network will need a business plan. This is usually done by a business consultant and the plan will include a mission statement, business activities, and financial projections for the organization.

Your mission statement should include the following critical points:

- Provide cost-effective, high-quality professional services through a comprehensive network of qualified specialists in the metro area and throughout the regional area.
- Promote integration in the organization and delivery of specialty care, creating cost efficiency in both administration and health care delivery.
- Facilitate, market, and promote direct negotiation between various payers and the entire network; provide legally allowable advantages to the group, while minimizing administrative costs.
- Provide meaningful utilization data for payers and participating specialty networks, and develop proactive managed care strategies, including capitated care.
- Promote the development of appropriate clinical guidelines and other quality improvement standards for the use of specialty care and enhance the quality of patient care through these standards.
- Enhance the growth and success of member specialty networks, by expanding marketing opportunities and offering services to improve network administration.

Business activities should be very focused to market and administer contracts between the network and payers. Specific business activities should include:

- Soliciting and negotiating agreements to provide specialty physician services on behalf of payers, either on a fee-for-service or capitation basis.
- Accepting a global capitation payment for the entire network, and appropriately distributing it to the individual member networks.
- Providing contract administration services for member networks, including claims payment, withhold administration, utilization review, and data collection, analysis, and reporting.
- Providing consolidated data collection and reporting on behalf of all member networks to payers.
- Monitoring experience of each member network under the multispecialty contracts.
- Establishing guidelines to be followed by all member networks on such issues as provider credentialing and contracting, quality assurance programs, and practice protocols. It will be the responsibility of each member network to develop and administer standards specific to their network that are consistent with the overall guidelines established by the multispecialty network.
- Offering a more integrated approach to delivery of specialty care, coordinating protocols among specialties to avoid duplication of services, and insuring the highest quality of care developed in the most cost effective manner.
- Recruiting and contracting with new specialty networks to ensure comprehensive coverage by the multi-specialty group.
- Contracting with nonmultispecialty networks or provider groups as necessary to allow the multispecialty organization to meet its obligations under managed care contracts.

The above list of business activities may be undertaken directly by your organization or through contracts with other consultants. The scope of activities may also be expanded as needed to promote the organization's mission.

In addition, very detailed information should be developed for the marketing plan, operations of the organization and the financial projections should be as conservative as possible to avoid future disappointment.

Conclusion

I hope I have been able to stimulate you to start a multispecialty organization in your local health care market. If you are already involved in such organizations, then perhaps the above information will be useful. Finally, I am more than happy to receive telephone calls and help my colleagues with their questions, thoughts, or concerns about single-specialty and multispecialty networks.

REFERENCES

1. Terry D: Integrated health care in California's managed care capital. *Managed Care Q* 1994; 2(4):24–34.
2. Risk R, Francis P: Transforming a hospital facility company into an integrated medical care organization. *Managed Care Q* 1994; 2(4) 12–23.
3. Colie C: Guiding the integrated delivery network. *Healthcare Forum J* November/December 1994: 16–23.

4. Pope, T: New program gives specialists control. *Managed Healthcare News* November 1995: 26B–26M.
5. Dial, WF: Trend toward specialty capitation growing. Managed Healthcare News. 1995 December 28B–28K.
6. Menefee PH: Managed care—Still a growth industry. The Robinson-Humphrey Company, Inc. July 15, 1996: 9–10.
7. McCally JF, Nauert RC: Direct contracting: The future is now. *MGM Journal.* March/April 1993: 23–29.
8. Standards for Accrediation. National Committee for Quality Assurance, 1995 edition.
9. Unland JJ: Physician-directed managed care efforts in the United States. *Medical Practice Management.* January/February, 1996: 163–173.
10. Inspecting a new plan: You're due diligence. *Physician's Managed Care Report.* May 1996: 52–53.

Ramie A. Tritt, M.D., graduated with honors from medical school, McGill University, Montreal, Canada, in 1973. He completed his otolaryngology residency at McGill and then followed, in 1978, with a fellowship in otology and head and neck surgery at Upstate Medical Center in Syracuse, New York. Since then, he has been in private practice in Atlanta, Georgia.

Dr. Tritt has been involved in managed care since the early 1980s. He administered the capitated otolaryngology program for Health America, the first HMO in Atlanta. Currently, he is President, Medical Director, and Administrator of three otolaryngology capitated networks in Atlanta (United HealthCare of Georgia, Cigna Health Plan of Georgia, and Aetna Health Plans of Georgia). These networks have approximately 350,000 covered lives.

In 1995, Dr. Tritt spearheaded the formation of GMG (Georgia MultiSpecialty Group) and has served as president since its inception. This organization is a limited liability company consisting of 15 specialty networks with 650 physicians. GMG has now finalized its first contract with HealthSource of Georgia and is in negotiation with numerous other payers.

Dr. Tritt is on the advisory board of American Health Consultants, their Physician's Managed Care Report, and is also on the advisory board of Columbia's Ambulatory Surgery Division–ENT Section, and Health Source of Georgia. In July 1996, Dr. Tritt cofounded Physicians' Speciality Corp., a physician practice management company focused on the ear, nose, throat, head and neck, and related specialities. Dr. Tritt is chairman and president of Physicians' Speciality Corp., which became a publicly traded company on the Nasdaq National Market System (NASDAQ) in March, 1997.

23

Will Doctors Take Back Health Care?

UWE E. REINHARDT

Two distinct shifts of control over the nation's health system threaten to erode the medical profession's traditional dominance over American health care. First, there is a rapid shift of control from the supply side of the health sector to its demand side. Physicians sit on the supply side of the sector. Second, there is a gradual but inexorable shift of control away from government toward private regulators—the managed care industry. Because organized medicine traditionally has held much sway over government, the latter has actually been a very timid regulator. By contrast, the modus operandi of private regulators can resemble the rough tactics of bounty hunters who are less easily manipulated than is government.[1] The bounty, of course, is the difference between the premiums collected up front by the bounty hunters and the cost at which they procure health care from doctors, hospitals, and pharmacies.

Both shifts are facilitated by pervasive excess capacity in the health system that has developed over the past two decades. As Jonathan Weiner has projected in a recent study on the physician workforce, for example, if 60% of the American population were enrolled in carefully managed private health plans, such as HMOs, then about 140,000 specialists and 25,000 generalists in the pool of 571,000 physicians now estimated to be available in the year 2000 actually would not be needed in that year.[2] Whenever the supply side of any market exhibits that much latent excess capacity, it is easy to bring it to its heels simply through the ancient principle of *divide et impera*. We are witnessing the onset of that process now.

It is possible that, in the next millennium, the typical American physician will resemble the typical American engineer who is employed in a large corporation that is managed by non-engineers—often by experts in finance. The question is whether this trend toward greater dependence of physicians on nonphysicians is inevitable, or whether the medical profession can retain (and, in part, regain) its hitherto powerful position in the health system. The central thesis of this chapter is that the profession may be able to retain its hold on the health system, although probably only with the help of government. The question is whether physicians will have the vision to grasp that opportunity and the staying power to maintain that position. On that question the jury is still out.

Why Physicians Lost Professional Autonomy

Until about the late 1980s, American physicians and their allies, hospitals and the health care manufacturing industries, dominated all facets of the health system—the clinical, the economic, and the political.

The bulk of these providers' revenue flowed to them from a highly fragmented private and public insurance system, whose governing principle was to provide each insured patient completely free choice of doctor, hospital, and pharmacy at the time of illness. Although large third-party payers, notably Medicare, Medicaid, and some of the larger Blue Cross/Blue Shield plans did enjoy enough market power to exercise varying degrees of control over the prices of health services, the principle of free choice robbed all third party payers of the leverage to control the volume of services going into the treatment of patients.

Furthermore, few politicians, private-sector executives, or policy analysts then dared to question the clinical autonomy of physicians. That reluctance reflected in good part its awesome political power. But it also rested on the naive notion that modern medicine is a reasonably exact science and that physicians could be trusted to apply that exact science to human suffering without caving in to the financial conflict of interest inherent in fee-for-service medicine. As long as physicians were in taut supply and, therefore, assured of comfortable incomes, the latter assumption seemed plausible.

Under these circumstances it is not surprising that eventually the size, the configuration, and the total cost of the American health system was driven largely by its supply side, and that the annual growth of health spending eventually rose to double-digit rates, far in excess of the annual growth of the nation's gross national product.[3] Nor is it surprising that this loosely structured system generated startling interregional variations in clinical practice patterns, in prices of health services, and, hence, in per-capita spending on health care—a fact illustrated graphically in the recently published *Dartmouth Atlas of Health Care*.[4] In an earlier study of payments made in 1989 by Medicare to physicians treating elderly patients in various cities of the United States, for example, it was found that, after adjusting the expenditure data for intercity differences in the demographical composition of the elderly population and even for intercity differences in the fees paid physicians in that year, the adjusted per-capita spending per Medicare beneficiary ranged from a low of $ 822 in Minneapolis, Minnesota, to a high of $1,847 in Miami, Florida.[5] These intra-U.S. variations in per-capita health spending exceed the comparable international variations within the industrialized world. Data of this sort, which first became available in the early 1980s, have become a nettlesome challenge to the medical profession, which has never been able to explain these variations with appeal either to the health status of the populations being served or health outcomes.

It was, of course, only a matter of time before those who write most of the final checks* for health care—government (accounting for close to all health spending) and private employers (accounting for another 35%)—reacted sharply to the rapid annual growth in health spending and the growing research literature on geographical practice variations. The profession's inability to explain these variations gradually eroded its authority and unfettered clinical autonomy.

The first volley in this reaction actually came not from the private sector, but the federal Medicare program. In 1983, that program replaced the traditional retrospective full-cost *reimbursement* of individual hospitals—a method that actively encouraged regional variations in costs—with a more uniform, nationwide schedule of prospectively set global payments for some 500 distinct medical cases. That was the first large-scale attempt to shift at least part of the financial risk of a patient's illness directly onto the shoulders of those responsible for managing the treatments of patients. Medicare followed that move, in 1992, with the imposition of a federally set, uniform fee schedule covering all Medicare patients nationwide. That move ended the individual physician's long-standing prerogative to determine, within fairly broad limits, his or her fees under the Medicare program.

Both measures, however, still left control over the volume of hospital admissions and physician services largely in the hands of physicians, as did virtually all private insurance contracts. In the end, that control could be wrested from physicians only when anxious private employers were able to persuade their equally anxious employees to give up their long cherished freedom of choice of providers at time of illness in return for continued provision of employer-provided health insurance. That crucial concession enabled employers to enroll their employees in selected health plans, each empowered to procure health care only from a select set of preferred physicians, hospitals, and pharmacists.

Selective contracting, in the face of pervasive excess capacity in the health system, has been the vehicle on which control over health care has moved from the supply side to the demand side of the health sector. A health plan's power to limit the insured to a set of preferred providers ipso facto endows that plan with the power to exclude from its roster any provider it finds wanting, either because that provider's prices are too high or, in the case of physicians, because the volume going into the treatment of particular illnesses exceeds clinical practice guidelines. Selective contracting is the foundation of what is has come to be known in the United States by the generic label "managed care."

■ Forms of Control over Physicians: Prudent Purchasing a la Carte versus Capitation

Health plans can exercise their newfound control over the providers of health care by means of two distinct contractual models. The first can be described as the *prudent purchasing model* and the second as *capitation* or the *incentive alignment model*.

*Actually, all health spending originates in the budgets of private households. Government and business are merely conduits for that flow of funds from private households to the providers of health care.

Under the *prudent purchasing model*, the health plan shoulders the financial risk for the insured's illness in return for an annual premium. It then procures needed health services prudently, and a la carte, from a selected set of providers, largely on a fee-for-service basis. The essential feature of the model is that the providers of health care do not assume the financial risk of the patient's illness. That risk remains on the shoulder of the health plan. Using the economic leverage of selective contracting, however, and pitting individual providers of health care against one another under the *divide-et-impera* principle, the health plan can extract steep price discounts from physicians, hospitals, and other providers of health care. Using the same leverage, the health plan also gains the ability to proctor the providers' practice patterns and, if necessary, to micromanage the treatment of patients through the application of practice guidelines.

Together, the ability to extract price discounts from providers and impose micromanaging on the physician–patient relationship tend to be lumped together under the generic label "managed care," although there remains some confusion around the precise meaning of that term. Some authors confine the term "managed care" strictly to the proctoring and, if necessary, the micro-managing of the volume of services going into the treatment of patients. Others include in the term the practice of health plans to extract price discounts from the providers of health care. Still others dilute the definition further by including in it virtually any attempt by third party payers to influence the price and utilization of health services, even if it is merely the imposition of deductibles and coinsurance on patients.

Under the second model of control over physicians, the *capitation* or *incentive alignment* model, the health plan absorbs the financial risk of illness from patients against payment of a premium, but then shifts that risk partly or wholly onto the shoulders of the providers of health care who are paid a flat capitation payment for that role. This shifting of risk to the providers of care is the quintessential ingredient of "capitation." Strictly speaking, the premium an insured pays to an insurance carrier could be viewed as a capitation payment as well, but that is not common usage of the term. Capitation in health care always implies that those who make the decisions concerning the treatment of patients (or those who control the delivery of health care within a health care facility, such as a hospital) are made to bear the financial risk inherent in their own decisions.

Although the *capitation model* spares the health-insurance plan proper the need to manage care, the network of providers who do assume full risk for the cost of treating patients must control its members through some form of managed-care techniques. That may be the reason why the concept of "capitation" is so often confused with "managed care." Managed care may be a natural consequence of capitation; but managed care does not necessarily imply capitation. It can go perfectly hand in hand with fee-for-service compensation of providers. Probably because "managed care" is so often (and erroneously) taken as a synonym for "capitation," one frequently encounters in the literature one of the oddest of dichotomies: that between "fee-for-service compensation" (a method of paying providers) and "managed care" (a method of controlling volume). The proper dichotomy is between fee-for-service compensation versus capitation, and between managed care versus the complete, unfettered clinical autonomy over medical treatments that *individual* physicians enjoyed under the classic indemnity insurance.

Full-fledged *capitation* models under which providers take full risk for all of the insureds' medical needs are still relatively rare in the United States. Aside from the long established group or staff model Health Maintenance Organizations—such as the Kaiser Foundation Health Plan or the Health Insurance Plan of New York—which effectively integrate the insurance and the health-care delivery function within one organization, full-fledged *capitation* arrangements between independent health plans and independent provider groups (such as multispecialty group practices and their subcontractors) have emerged mainly in California. But there are many hybrid models in between the *prudent purchasing model* relying strictly on fee-for-service compensation and the pure *capitation model*. Under some arrangements between insurers and providers, PCPs may be capitated for their own services and share in the residuals of budgeted risk pools for the services of specialists and hospitals.

From the viewpoint of physicians, the pure *capitation model* is a mixed blessing. On the downside, the model does saddle physicians (and other providers of health care) with the unaccustomed task of managing the financial risk of their own patients' illnesses. Furthermore, any arrangement that effectively rewards physicians financially for withholding health services from patients is apt to strain the physician–patient relationship, if patients are at all aware of that incentive. On the other hand, however, the capitation model does shift the task of micromanaging health care out of the offices of a distant health plan and into the hands of a presumably collegial community of physicians whose techniques of controlling the individual member within that collegium might be more mindful of the physician's professional sentiments and, therefore, less nettlesome to the individual physician.

It is reasonable to expect that, once the task of managing the full financial risk for their patients' illnesses has been fully mastered by physicians, they will be tempted to form what is now known as Provider Service Networks (PSNs) capable of contracting directly with either government, large private employers or associations of small employers and individual families. That approach would eliminate the insurance industry as middleman between payer and provider and capture for providers the profits now earned by that middleman. It is for precisely that reason that the insurance industry is unlikely to push capitation onto the providers of health care, if it can at all avoid it. From the insurer's perspective, the preferred model remains the prudent purchasing model, based as it is on the *divide-et-impera* principle. The coming decade will show which of the two models will carry the day in American health care.

■ The Nature of Provider Service Networks (PSNs)

Provider Service Networks (PSNs) are an integrated network of physicians, hospitals, pharmacies, and other allied health care facilities that are capable of assuming full financial risk for the cost of a group of insured patients. The integration of the PSN may be physical, in the form of a large campus linked to a set of satellite facilities that are owned by the PSN or under exclusive contract with it. Alternatively, the integration of the PSN may be merely virtual, by means of a set of contracts and information systems that bind together a dispersed set of freestanding parties.

A PSN may be organized by a group of physicians who control the capitation payment per insured life and, with it, the allocation of financial resources within the PSN. Alternatively, the PSN may be centered on a hospital that controls the capitation and its allocation among members of the PSN. Finally, the PSN may take the form of joint ventures between hospitals and physicians with shared control over the capitation, although the stability of such models can easily be jeopardized by a power struggle between physicians and the hospital.

The concept of PSNs gained prominence during the budget battle of 1995, which included a highly partisan debate over proposed reductions from the projected growth paths of Medicare and Medicaid spending. Traditionally, any such "cuts"—which, in truth, have always been mere reduction from future growth—have been vehemently protested by organized medicine and the hospital industry, with dark hints of rationing and a general deterioration of the quality of American health care. In return for graceful acquiescence to the very sharp reductions proposed by the 104th Congress in 1995, physicians and hospitals were promised legislation that would greatly facilitate the formation of PSNs capable of competing head on with health plans organized around insurance companies. This legislative relief is of two kinds.

First, the American Medical Association has long sought removal of certain antitrust strictures that currently hinder the formation of physician-run PSNs. In particular, organized medicine wants to see a replacement of the current *per se* rule (which holds that certain behavior is ipso facto or *"per se"* a violation of competition, even if that is actually the case) with rules that force the antitrust authorities FTC and the Justice Department) to prove that a particular behavior by health care providers in a particular instance actually is harmful to competition.[6] Given the thin staffing of the two antitrust agencies and the cumbersome methods of proof in such matters, the proposed switch in rules would literally give the providers of health care effectively a free hand in organizing PSNs.

A second form of legislative relief sought by the providers of health care is exemption from the strict rules that state governments impose on commercial insurers. In particular, physicians and hospitals would like to be excused from the costly monetary reserve requirements that must be met by commercial insurers. The providers argue that, unlike commercial insurers who must purchase from outsiders all the care they promised the insured, the members of a PSN themselves constitute the needed reserve, for they provide much or all of the promised care. Just how willing a group of physicians would actually be to absorb the cost of an unexpectedly large run on this hidden reserve (by unexpectedly high morbidity) is an open question. In any event, apparently persuaded by the logic put forth by organized medicine, the 104th Congress was prepared to grant PSNs exemption from the otherwise onerous monetary reserve requirements.

In the meantime, the FTC has revamped the antitrust guidelines under existing law with an eye to facilitating the easier formation of PSNs, thereby removing the pressure by organized medicine for more formal and sweeping legislative relief that might eviscerate the FTC.[7]

Current legal restriction probably have not been the only reason why PSNs have found it difficult to get off the ground. For their part, private employers have not been accustomed to contracting directly with providers of health care and, so far, have preferred to contract with their long-standing partner in health care, the insurance industry. By contrast, the federal and state governments are likely to be much more open to the idea of signing full-risk contracts directly with the providers of health care. Although the legislation to that end is likely to remain hostage to partisan bickering in the 105th Congress, there actually is widespread sentiment in both parties to let the managed care industry control both the cost and the quality of health care financed by the Medicare and Medicaid programs and to give providers a prominent role in this process. In other words, if the medical profession will soon regain its erstwhile dominance over American health care, it may well have to thank its traditional nemesis: the government. Ironies are one of our health system's major by-products.*

*One of these ironies is that, if cost and quality control for the Medicare and Medicaid programs are to be turned over to competing, private regulators (managed-care companies), the government must put in place an regulatory infrastructure that makes that competition fair and efficient. Such an infrastructure is otherwise known as "managed

■ The Prospect of Provider Service Networks

The prospect of PSNs in the future of American health care remains a hotly debated topic. Some observers believe that physicians and hospital executives lack the culture and skills to manage large, vertically integrated health systems that combine the insurance function with health care delivery. There is, for one, the fundamental question whether physicians can perform the traditional functions of commercial insurers—marketing, underwriting, and risk management—more cheaply than the commercial insurers. Furthermore, there is the question of how easily eagles can be made to fly in formation—that is, what organizational structures it will take to make physicians cooperate clinically and economically. Will physicians be able to resist the perennial temptation to sell the cash flows they control to the highest bidder on Wall Street? It is an intriguing question, to be revisited below.

Other observers, however, believe that PSNs can and probably will play a significant role in American health care and may even come to dominate the managed care industry. Paul Ellwood,[8] widely regarded as a pioneer in the development of "managed care," made that point in a recent interview with the editor of *Medical Economics*, as did the present author in an earlier issue.[9] In the Institute of Medicine's 25th Anniversary Symposium held in early 1996, Jeff Goldsmith deplored that

> Many cost management activities taking place in our health care system today are superimposed upon the doctor/patient relationship. Physicians find it necessary to have phone conversations with a far-distant nurse about what they can or cannot do to patients they have known all of their lives for any clinical decision that involves more than a few hundred dollars.[10]

He went on to conjecture that

> As health plans shift risk to physician organizations, responsibility for effective clinical decision making is going to devolve from a bank of nurses talking over 800 numbers to the communities of physicians who are at-risk. . . . As risk devolves onto these physician enterprises, so will responsibility for setting clinical standards and for policing them.[11]

From the viewpoint of physicians, this is an optimistic vision. It implies that physicians will be able to achieve two related objectives. First, it is assumed that physicians will be able to develop for their "enterprises" *stable* organizational structures capable of preserving the clinical autonomy of physicians. Second, it is assumed that physicians will nurture the general public's trust in the ethic driving these organizational structures. That will not at all be easy under capitation.

Both objectives probably are easiest reached with a purely collegial organizational structure that resembles the structure of a private university. A university is nothing other than a not-for-profit, capitated, vertically integrated, multispecialty, pedagogic group practice. There is, of course, some hierarchy among professionals in the university. There is a president, there are deans, and there are chairs of academic departments. Well-run universities, however, take care that the perquisites accorded different levels within that hierarchy are not too visibly different. As a general rule, for example, the salary of the president does not exceed that of ordinary full professors by more than a factor of 2 to 3, and the salaries of full professors, in turn, tend to be only about twice the salary of newly hired assistant professors. Great care is taken in most universities not to set the appearance of the "corporate office" apart too much from that of the rest of the campus. Finally, and most important, neither the faculty nor any other staff have ownership rights in the university; they are all mere employees.

Although the top managers of a university do, on occasion, move the levers of power available to them, for the most part the governance of the institution proceeds on open, collegial debate and consensus. Most important, individual faculty members enjoy a high degree of autonomy over their teaching and research activities. To be sure, the content and quality of their teaching is monitored by the department chairs (and by students) through questionnaires completed by students at the end of each course, through formal, published reviews of the professor's style and course content by students, and through behind-the-scenes monitoring of his or her syllabi and final examinations by the department's chair. Furthermore, the products of the faculty's research are routinely subjected to strict and often brutal outside peer review and monitored internally by means of regular reports to the dean of the faculty. Even so, in their day-to-day activities, most professionals in a well-run university enjoy a high measure of what physicians would call "clinical autonomy."

Although he does not say so explicitly, the "community of physicians" Jeff Goldsmith has in mind probably resembles more the collegiate setting of a university than an investor-owned corporation. Some prominent physician enterprises—for example, the Mayo Clinic, the Marshfield Clinic, and the Oxner Clinic—probably come close to this campus atmosphere. These organizations have been stable over time and have gained the trust of the

---

[regulated] competition." The required infrastructure for managed competition will resemble nothing so much as the Health Insurance Purchasing Cooperatives (HIPCs) that were the centerpiece of the Clinton Plan and drew so much opposition, especially from the insurance industry. Some large, progressive private employers aside, managed competition is not now operative in the private sector.

general public, meeting the two objectives set forth above. Although these clinics have traditionally rendered their services to patients on a fee-for-service basis, they probably will be able to preserve the patient's trust in them even under full-fledged capitation.

At the other extreme of the organizational spectrum, however, one could imagine purely capitalist organizational structures in which physicians own shares that can be traded for cash, at least under certain circumstances. Such structures might approximate employee-owned business firms, such as the Avis car rental company which has been owned in the last nine years by its 13,500 employees, but is now in the process of selling itself to the highest bidder, a hotel franchiser. In a recent editorial on that transaction, *The New York Times* pointedly observed:

> Worker-owned firms—even those that are profitable like Avis—have a tough time surviving from one generation to the next . . . Apparently the financial gain [to the workers, from the sale of the firm to outsiders] outweighs for Avis workers the psychic value of owning the firm.[12]

For similar reasons, physician-run PSNs based on the raw capitalist model are not likely to remain collegial for long. One can conjecture that, over time, they will be likely to develop rigid hierarchies with corporate offices whose inhabitants may have M.D. degrees, but march to different financial drummers than the rank and file in the trenches and, for all intents and purposes, differ from ordinary executives with M.B.A degrees mainly in that, once upon a time, they knew what makes the human body tick and how to repair it. Salary differentials in these capitalist structures would be likely to vary much more than in a truly collegiate structure, and so would the distribution of ownership rights.

The rank and file in a purely capitalist PSNs are likely to be removed even further from the corporate M.D. officers, if the latter decide to enhance the entity's financial capital through joint ventures with outsiders—for example, with an insurance carrier.* One would imagine that the corporate M.D. officers in such a joint venture will, sooner or later, begin to shop all of the entity's future cash flow to outside investors, to cash out their presumably sizeable own stakes when a good deal comes along—M.D.s in the rank and file be damned.

Like the Avis deal remarked on by *The New York Times,* such a deal may look sweet enough even to physicians in the trenches. For enough cash up front, they may be willing to trade in their profession's autonomy. The rank and file would be the more likely to be disposed that way, the more their corporate officers in their daily work resemble nonphysician executives in ordinary business firms and the less the rank and file have to lose.

In between the purely collegiate and the purely capitalist model lie other forms of organization suitable for PSNs—for example, the partnership structure typical of law firms and some investment banks. These organizations group their professionals into two distinct categories with different rights and duties: partners, who have non-tradeable ownership rights in the firm, and associates who are willing to undergo years of quasi-indentured labor in the hope of becoming partners one day. New partners are elected to that rank by the existing partners, presumably on the basis of their ability to bring revenue to the firm. Partners enjoy the privilege of garnering not only profits generated strictly by them, but also a good part of the profits generated by the quasi-indentured associates who are employees.

Would such partnerships be more stable, over time, than the purely capitalist model based on tradeable equity shares? If investment banks serve as a guide, they might not be all that stable. Two decades ago most investment banks were partnerships of this sort. In the meantime, the senior partners of most of them have cashed in their stakes through conversion of the partnerships into publicly traded companies. On the other hand, most law firms and many accounting forms have retained their partnership structure, at least so far.

Would such medical partnerships as easily gain the trust of patients and the media as the truly collegial structure on the model of, say, the Mayo Clinic? It probably would depend on the extent to which the partnership *appears,* to outsiders, to be profit driven. If the senior partners in M.D. partnerships were known to take home incomes coming anywhere close to those routinely enjoyed by senior partners in law firms or investment banks, these incomes might trigger ire among patients and the media and nurture ever deeper suspicion about "capitation" and "managed care." Indeed, the media might be busily fed with derogatory information by "deep throats" from the ranks of hardworking, underpaid, and disillusioned junior associates within these partnerships.

■ Conclusion

When the managed care industry has reached maturity sometime early in the next millennium, will the medical profession once again dominate the American health system, as it has for so long in the past? The concise answer to that question is "It depends."

*Joint ventures between clinical enterprises and outsiders—for example, an insurance carrier—would make sense if the clinical enterprise is an academic health center solidly anchored in a wider academic structure or solidly committed to the not-for-profit status. In such joint ventures, *individual* physicians—even those in the corporate office—do not hold ownership rights that can be sold to outsiders.

It is clear that the complete professional autonomy that the *individual* American physician has traditionally enjoyed in health care will, before long, be a thing of the past. In his or her daily work, an *individual* physician's clinical decisions are likely to be monitored and constrained by some organization, whether run by physicians or nonphysicians. Debates over that form of autonomy are moot by now. The question is merely whether physicians as a group will be ruled by the insurance industry under the *divide-et-impera* principle, as is increasingly the case today, or whether physicians can topple that industry from its current pinnacle of power and make it subservient to the dictates of physician-run PSNs, just as that industry had been subservient for so long to the medical profession's dicta, until about the mid-1980s. The central thrust of this chapter is that the answer to the latter question hinges in no small part on the organizational structure physicians choose for their PSNs, for two reasons.

First, the structure itself may be inherently unstable over time. A purely capitalist structure for PSNs may lead individual physicians to sell their professional autonomy in the long run for high, onetime monetary profits in the short run. If a sellout is what it turns out to be, history will say that in the late 1990s American physicians had a short moment of glory where they could cash in on the networks they had formed—and then they went back into permanent servitude to Wall Street.[13]

Second, the organizational structure of PSNs will also determine their acceptance by patients who, through their choices as enrollees in competing health plans, will determine the future shape of the managed-care industry. It is reasonable to suppose that, in this respect, the purely collegiate model would be an easier sell than are models that, by their very structure, highlight the profit motive driving modern medicine. That will be doubly so under full-risk capitation of PSNs, a method of payment that inevitably arouses suspicion among patients and in the media.

It appears that the U.S. Congress is open to the idea of letting physicians play a more dominant role in the managed-care industry—perhaps *the* dominant role. Whether or not the medical profession will be able to rise to that challenge remains to be seen.

REFERENCES

1. In this connection, see Reinhardt UE: The new social contract in American health care: Three-tier medicine, with bounty hunting. Forthcoming in *Health Economics*, October 1996.
2. Weiner JP: Forecasting the effects of health reform on U.S. physician requirements: Evidence from HMO staffing patterns. *JAMA* July 20, 1994; 272(3):333–50.
3. Congressional Budget Office: *Trends in health spending: An update.* Washington, DC: US Government Printing Office, June 1993.
4. The Center for the Evaluative clinical Sciences: *The Dartmouth Atlas of Health Care.* Chicago: American Hospital Publishing Company, 1996.
5. Welch WP, Miller ME, Welch HG, Fisher ES, and Wennberg JH: Geographic variation in expenditures for physicians' services in the United States. *Engl J Med* March 4, 1993; 328(9):621–627.
6. Burda D: FTC previews doc network antitrust rules, *Modern Healthcare,* June 24, 1996; 8.
7. *Ibid.*
8. Why doctors will take back health care. Interview with Uwe E. Reinhardt, *Medical Economics* December 26, 1995; 72(24):72–87.
9. How doctors can regain control of health care. Interview with Paul M. Ellwood Jr., M.D., in *Medical Economics.* May 13, 1996; 73(9):178–91.
10. Goldsmith J: Risk and responsibility: The evolution of health care payment, in Institute of Medicine: *2020 VISION: Health in the 21st Century,* Washington, DC: National Academy Press, 1996; 55.
11. *Ibid.*
12. Why worker owners sell out, *New York Times,* July 7, 1996, p.8.
13. Why doctors will take back health care, *op. cit.,* p. 87.

Uwe E. Reinhardt, a native of Germany, has taught at Princeton University since 1968, rising through the ranks from assistant professor of economics to his current position. He has taught courses in micro- and macroeconomic theory and policy; accounting for commercial, nonprofit, and governmental enterprises; financial management for commercial and nonprofit enterprises, and health economics and policy.

Professor Reinhardt received his Bachelor of Commerce degree from the University of Saskatchewan, Canada, in 1964. He was also awarded the Governor General's Gold Medal as the Most Distinguished Graduate of his graduating class. He received his Ph.D. in economics from Yale University in 1970. His doctoral dissertation was entitled "Physician Productivity and the Demand for Health Manpower." He has received honorary degrees of Dr. Sci. from the Medical College of Pennsylvania and Mount Sinai School of Medicine, City University of New York.

Although Professor Reinhardt's research interests since that time have centered mainly on health economics and policy, his work has also included topics in corporation finance, including benefit-cost analyses of the Lockheed L-1011 Tri Star and the Space Shuttle.

In 1978, Professor Reinhardt was elected to the Institute of Medicine of the National Academy of Sciences. He served on the Governing Council from 1979 to 1982. He also served on a number of study panels at the Institute, such as the Committee on the Implications of For-Profit Medicine. Currently, he serves on the Institute's Committee on Technical Innovation in Medicine and the Committee the Implications of a Physician Surplus.

From 1987 to 1990, Professor Reinhardt was a member of the National Leadership Commission on Healthcare, a private-sector initiative established to develop options for healthcare reform. He continues to serve on that organization's successor, the National Leadership Coalition on Health Care, cochaired by former Presidents Carter and Ford. He is past president of the Association of Health Services Research, and is still a member of the board. From 1978 to 1993, he served on the Board of

Trustees of the Teachers Insurance and Annuity Insurance Association and was a member of its Mortgage Finance Committee.

Professor Reinhardt has served on a number of government committees and commissions, among them the National Council on Health Care Technology of the then US Department of Health and Welfare from 1979 to 1982, and the Special Medical Advisory Group of the Veterans Administration from 1981 to 1985. From 1986 to 1995, he served three consecutive three-year terms as a commissioner on the Physician Payment Review Commission (PPRC), established in 1986 by Congress to advise it on issues related to the payment of physicians. In 1996, he served as a member of the Committee on the U.S. Physician Supply of the Institute of Medicine (IOM) of the National Academy of Sciences. He is currently a member of the Council on the Economic Impact of Health Reform, a privately funded group of health experts established to track the economic impact of the current revolution in healthcare deliver-and-cost control. In 1996, he was appointed to the Board of Health Care Services of the Institute of Medicine, National Academy of Sciences.

Professor Reinhardt has also served on editorial review boards for numerous journals, such as the *Journal of Health Economics,* the *Milbank Memorial Bank Quarterly, Health Affairs, The New England Journal of Medicine,* and the *Journal of the American Medical Association.*

Index

Academic Medical Center Consortium, 150
"Accept assignment" method, 14
Accessible population, 105
Accountability, of health care providers, 68, 78–79
Accountant services, 264
Accounting
  automated, 236
  by independent practitioners, 22
Accounts payable, 224
Accounts receivable, 221, 224
  efficiency improvement of, 189
  outstanding, 230, 271
Accreditation
  of hospitals, 79
  of managed care organizations, 227
Accreditation standards, for managed care providers, 60, 227. *See also* Board certification; Credentialing
Acquired immunodeficiency syndrome (AIDS) epidemic, 295
Acquisitions. *See also* Mergers and acquisitions
  as mergers, 253
Actuarial cost method, of capitation rate estimation, 5–7
Addiction, health care expenditures for, 167
Adenoidectomy
  outcomes study of, 106
  surgical guidelines for, 321
Adenotonsillar disease, quality of life assessment in, 106–107
Administrative costs, of managed care, 239
  as managed care contract issue, 59–60
Administrative personnel, in health care system, 167, 169
Administrative services, flow charting of, 185
Adverse drug reactions, 118
Advertising
  by managed care organizations, 243
  for staff, 199–200
Advocacy, for patients, 78, 177, 243
  professional liability and, 254
Aetna Health Plans, 315–316
Age factors, use in capitation payment estimation, 6
Agency for Health Care Policy and Research, Patient Outcomes Research Teams, 100
Allegheny General Hospital, Pittsburgh, 301
Allergy immunotherapy, outcomes study of, 207
Allocation bias, 102, 103
Ambulatory surgery, increased use of, 3
American Academy of Otolaryngology, Quality Assurance Committee, surgical guidelines of, 321
American Academy of Otolaryngology-Head and Neck Surgery
  obstructive sleep apnea syndrome clinical severity staging system, 88
  Outcomes Research Small Project Grant, 100–101
  precertification guidelines, 285
  referral guidelines, 26–27
American Academy of Pediatrics, 27, 94
American Academy of Physician Executives, 176, 205
American College of Physicians, 3–4, 27
American Group Practice Association, 138
American Health Care Policy and Research, 26–27
American Journal of Medical Quality, 177
American Medical Association
  antitrust position of, 328
  Ethical Issues in Managed Care, 78, 79
  opposition to national health insurance, 249
American Society of Anesthesiologists, 88
American Telephone and Telegraph (AT&T), 143, 250
American Tobacco, 250
Analysis of existing practice, 63–64
Analysis of existing practice costs, 64
Antibiotics, as otitis media with effusion treatment, 88
Anticompetition law, 242
Antireferral regulations, 273–274
Antitrust law, 55, 307
  credentialing and, 242
  historical background, 250–251
  penalties on violations of, 250
  per se violations of, 251, 252, 255
  physician organizations and, 257, 273–274
  provider service networks and, 328
  reform of, 254, 328
  "restraint of trade" determinations of, 251–253
  "rule of reason" of, 251, 252, 255
  "safe zones" of, 254
  single-specialty networks and, 281
APGAR score, 88
Appointment scheduling, 218, 221
  common problems in, 188
  computerized, 186, 192
  emergency, 14
  physician time templates for, 186, 188
  of work-in patients, 188, 190
Appropriateness studies, 87–88, 108–109
Arbitration, of managed care contract disputes, 62
Archives of Otolaryngology-Head and Neck Surgery, 87
Atlanta, Georgia, otolaryngology networks in, 315–316
Atlanta Ear, Nose and Throat Associates, P.C., 316

AT&T. *See* American Telephone and Telegraph
Audits, 61, 236
Autonomy
of patients, 73–75, 78
of physicians, 73, 74–75
in group practice, 304
loss of, 325–326
in multispecialty networks, 319
in physician groups, 304, 309
during professional training, 299
Avis, 330

Back-office overhead, 306
Barach, Alvan, 114
Bartering, 221
Begin, Menachim, 37
Benchmarking
of capitation contracts, 9
for clinical improvement, 142–158
clinical value compass approach in, 144, 145, 146, 148, 150, 151, 152, 153, 154
process of, 143–147
worksheet for, 144, 145–146, 150–153
definition, 142–143
in outcomes assessment, 86
of patient satisfaction surveys, 204–207
of staff requirements, 198
in total quality management, 215–216
Beneficence, 77
Benign prostatic hypertrophy, effect on quality of life, 87
Berwick, Donald, 213
Bias, in outcomes research, 102, 103, 104, 192
Bier, August, 103
Billing
automated, 236
balance, 61
collection policies, 14, 224
off-site services for, 237
outsourcing of, 220
profile report use in, 67–71
Blue Cross/Blue Shield, 277
control over health care costs by, 325–326
electronic claims submission to, 16
Blue Cross/Blue Shield United of Wisconsin, 252
Board certification, 76, 227. *See also* Credentialing
of multispecialty network members, 321
Bowel surgery, clinical improvement benchmarking for, 147–158
Boycott, as antitrust violation, 251–252, 253
Brainstorming, in contract negotiations, 39, 40, 41
Brute force sample, 105, 105
Budget, annual, 219, 220

California, managed care in, 300
California Public Employees Retirement Services (CALPERS), 301
Camp, Robert, 142
Capital Imaging antitrust case, 253
Capitation, 3–10. *See also* Contracts, capitation (incentive) model
adverse effects on health care quality, 74–75
benchmarking in, 9
definition, 3–4, 234
differentiated from managed care, 327
full-physician, 5
full-risk, 5
as malpractice lawsuit risk, 306
physician's financial risks in, 245
for physician groups, 302
primary care, 4–5, 8–9
reinsurance and, 9–10
risk-shifting in, 327
types of, 4–5
Capitation rate
actuarially sound, 65
analysis of existing practice and, 63–64
analysis of exising practice costs and, 64
average, 284
calculation of, 64–65
actuarial method of, 5–7
physician productivity method of, 7–8
definition, 283
factors affecting, 283–284
as per member per month (pmpm) rate, 283, 284
for physician organizations, 271
for single-specialty networks, 283–284
CAPSYSTEMS, 321
Carnegie Corporation, 250
Carotid artery resection, 88
Carpal tunnel syndrome surgery, clinical quality improvement of, 129, 130, 133, 134–139
Carter, Jimmy, 32
Carve-outs, in specialty network contracts, 321
Case management, 77
automated, 236
Case rates, 3
Case series, 101
Cashier, job description of, 194
Causality, 101, 102
Certified medical assistants, 191
Chamberlain, Neville, 32
Chance, in outcome studies, 103
Change concepts, in clinical improvement, 158–163
Change management guidelines, for clinical improvement, 136, 138–139
Change scores, 110
Charity care, 296
Check-in protocol, for patients, 189, 190–191
Children's Healthcare P.A., 252
Chronic Sinusitis Survey, 89, 90–91
Cigna HealthCare, 315
CINAHL database, 150
Claims
automated adjudication of, 236
"clean," 56, 62
discounted fee-for-service, with risk-pool withholds, 57
electronic submission, 16, 192
processing of
by physician organizations, 262, 263
vendors for, 264
rejected, 20
follow-up of, 12–13
as malpractice liability, 274
unpaid, follow-up of, 12–13
Clayton Anti-Trust Act, 250, 252, 255
Clinical coordinator, job description of, 194
Clinical improvement, 117–165. *See also* Continuous quality improvement; Project Solo; Quality assurance and control
benchmarking in, 142–158
case example, 147–158
definition, 142–143
process of, 143–147
worksheet for, 144, 145–146, 150–153
change concepts of, 158–163
Clinical Improvement Worksheet for, 128–142, 163–164
carpal tunnel syndrome surgery case example, 129, 130, 133, 134–139
change management guidelines for, 136, 138–139
core clinical process and, 128–129
fundamentals of, 163–164
hip replacement case example, 160–163
users' manual for, 139–142
clinical value compass approach, 117–128
context of, 158
Plan-Do-Check-Act cycle in, 117, 130, 134–142, 153–154, 160, 163–164
Clinical practice guidelines, 327
patient and physician autonomy and, 75–76
models of, 75
Clinical severity staging system, 88
Clinical trials
comparison with outcomes research, 99–100
functional status assessment in, 94
quality of life assessment in, 94
Clinical value compass method, of health care value assessment, 117–128
benchmarking with, 143, 144, 145, 146, 147, 148, 150, 151, 152, 153, 154
case example, 122–125
value measures in, 122, 124–125
worksheet for, 119–122, 124, 125
Clinton administration, health care plan of, 249, 295, 300, 329n.
Cochlear implants
cost effectiveness of, 92
effect on quality of life, 90
Cohort studies, 101
"Collectibility," of payments, from managed care organizations, 270–271
Collection policies, 14, 224
Community-based outcomes research, 93, 207
Community-based practice, total quality management in, 213, 215–216

Comorbidity
  definition, 85
  as outcome studies factor, 102
Comorbidity survey, 207
Competition
  among physician organizations, 271
  among physicians, 249
Computed tomography staging systems, of chronic sinusitis, 91
Confidence intervals, 104
Confidentiality, of medical records, 61, 79, 227, 229
  physicians' failure to respect, 173
  in quality assessment, 167, 176–177, 205–206
  state laws and, 244, 245
Confidential Self Assessment of Quality, 205–207
Conflicts of interest, in managed care, 73, 74, 77
Confounding, 103
Congress, United States
  89th, 249
  104th, 255, 328
  105th, 328
Conjunctivitis, assessment instruments for, 89
Connell, Laurence O., 79
Consecutive sample, 105
Consultants. *See also* Vendors
  contracting, 265
  medical practice operational, 263–264
  practice management, 264, 265
Consultation charges, in-hospital, reimbursement for, 14
Continuous quality improvement (CQI), 167
  by independent practitioners
    in business management, 219–226
    checklist for, 229
    expected quality in, 215
    expert advice sources for, 229–230, 231
    in facility and operations management, 224–225
    effect of managed care organizations on, 227–230
    one-dimensional quality in, 213, 215
    with outcomes-based marketing, 207–213
    patient satisfaction surveys for, 204–207, 209, 210
    in practice management, 216–219
    practice prospectus and, 213, 214
    in referral services management, 219
    revenue tracking in, 230
    in staff management, 219
    total quality management in, 214, 215–216
    unexpected quality in, 215
  patient satisfaction and, 174
  Project Solo and, 176–177
Contracts
  automatic renewal, 271
  capitation (incentive) model, 326, 327
    full-risk, 327
    payment methods, 271
    of physician organizations, 261, 262, 265, 266, 267, 270
    self-administered/self-regulated, 272
  definition, 134
  discounted, fee schedules of, 56–57
  discounted fee-for-service, 56, 57, 261, 262, 266, 267, 270–271, 321
  full-risk
    definition, 234
    of physician organizations, 270, 271
  for independent practitioners, 225–226
  legal issues of, 51–65
    administrative costs, 59–60
    amendment provisions, 61–62, 63, 226
    authorized communications, 56
    authorized services, 56
    balance billing, 56
    capitation issues, 63–65
    "change in law" section, 63
    clean claims, 56, 62
    closing practice to new patients, 61
    continuing care after termination, 62–63
    coordination of benefits, 7, 61
    covered services, 56
    credentialing, 60
    demographic information, 58–59
    discount fee-for-service rates, 56
    disputes resolution, 56, 62, 226
    eligible enrollees, 56
    emergency services, 56
    excluded services, 56
    exclusivity terms, 63, 226
    fee schedules, 56–57
    gag rules, 77, 226, 242, 254–255
    "hold harmless" (indemnification) clauses, 226, 242, 246, 271–272
    incentive pools, 56
    in-network, 56
    key procedural sections, 61–62
    legislative regulation, 63, 242
    management issues, 59–60
    medically-necessary services, 56, 77, 244
    medically-unnecessary services, 59
    out-of-network, 56
    payment rates and schedules, 56
    point-of-service, 56
    precontracting issues, 54–55
    premimum creditation to risk pools, 57
    as Provider Agreement, 240
    provider manual, 60
    records requirements, 61, 227
    reimbursement periods, 226
    risk-bearing/risk-shifting payment schemes, 57
    risk pools' function and flow, 57–58
    shared-risk, 234
    specialist reimbursement, 58
    stop-loss insurance, 59
    termination clauses, 62–63, 76–77, 277, 280, 281
    "termination" of disruptive patients, 60
    term of contract, 62
    timely payment, 56
    utilization management, 56, 241–242
    withholds in discount schedules, 56
  localization of, 65
  multiple, 233
  negotiation of, 31–49, 54–55
    adverse emotions in, 37
    Best Alternative to a Negotiated Agreement in, 42–43, 45–46
    brainstorming in, 39, 40, 41
    checklists for, 47–49
    communication principles, 47
    concept of, 31–33
    deception in, 43
    definition of, 31
    disjointed interests in, 40–42
    escalating/extreme demands in, 44
    four-quadrant analysis in, 40, 49
    "hard bargaining" approach in, 34, 35, 43–46
    by independent practitioners, 226–227
    integrated, 31, 32
    interests versus positions in, 38–39
    lock-in positions in, 45
    misperception and misunderstanding in, 36–37
    model for, 32
    objective criteria for, 42
    partisan, 31–32
    by physician organizations, 266
    positional bargaining approach, 45–46
    positional pressure tactics in, 43–44
    "principled bargaining" approach in, 34, 35
    principles of, 48
    problem avoidance in, 38
    psychological warfare in, 43
    skills required for, 32, 33–34
    "soft bargaining" approach in, 34, 35
    substantiative versus nonsubstantiative issues in, 35–38
    terminology of, 39
    twelve commandments of, 46
  nonnegotiability of, 241
  of physician groups, 302–303
  prudent purchasing model, 326–328
  renegotiation, 61–62
  renewal dates, 187
  review by physicians' attorney, 240
  selective, 326, 327
  of single-specialty networks, 280–281
  termination of, 62–63, 76–77, 271, 280, 281
  terminology of, 55–56, 240
  types of, 51–54
Control groups, 101, 102, 105
Convenience (grab) sample, 105
Coordination of benefits (COB), 7, 61
Copayments
  automated billing for, 236
  in capitation contracts, 6–7
  collection of, 224
  as patients' responsibility, 61
  as practice cost analysis factor, 64
Core values, 79–80
Coronary artery bypass grafting, mortality rate, 118, 126

Corporations
industrial, 250
limited liability, 281, 289–290
multinational, 250
multispecialty networks as, 319
not-for-profit, 281
physician organizations as, 258–259
Corticosteroids, as otitis media treatment, 107
Cosmetic surgery, 77
Cost analysis, patient, 221, 222
Cost containment, antitrust law and, 253
Cost-effectiveness research, 92, 94
Cost per service, in capitation contracts, 6
Covariates, 102–103
CPT-4. *See* Current Procedural Terminology codes
Credentialing, of managed care providers, 60, 76–77
economic, 76–77, 253
legal liability in, 242
in multispecialty networks, 321, 322
in physician organizations, 260, 267
as provider network value indicator, 268
Crosby, Philip, 213
Current Procedural Terminology codes
use in analysis of practice data, 63–64
use in capitation rate estimation, 5, 6, 64, 283
payment reductions on, 57
use in reimbursement process, 12, 17, 20–22, 189
use in revenues per relative value unit calculation, 221, 223
use in revenue tracking, 230

Dartmouth Atlas of Health Care, 326
Dartmouth COOP Project, 125–126
Dartmouth-Hitchcock Medical Center, 126
Accelerating Clinical Improvement Bowel Surgery Team clinical improvement quality study, 147–158
"Data dredging," in outcomes studies, 104
Data processing committees, 282
Decision analysis, 92
Decision making, medical, 79
Deductibles, as patients' responsibility, 61
Delphi Forecasts, 216
Deming, W. Edwards, 127, 203–204, 213
Demographic factors, use in capitation payment estimation, 6
Detection bias, 102, 103
Discounted fee-for-service contracts, 56, 261, 262, 266, 267, 270–271, 231
risk-pool withholds and, 57
Discounted fees, 3, 327
Disease-specific clinical outcomes, 100
assessment instruments for, 88–90, 110–113
Dizziness
assessment instruments for, 89, 90
cost-effective analysis of, 95
effect on quality of life, 90
Dizziness Handicap Inventory, 89, 90
DOCSHARE, 177, 205–207, 215
Du Pont Chemical, 250

Editorial peer review, 100–101
Electronic claims submission, 16, 192
Electronic payment submission, 16
Ellwood, Paul, 100, 329
Emanuel, Linda, 78–79
Emergency management, in independent practices, 224
Emergency room charges, reimbursement process for, 14
Employee Retirement Income Security Act of 1974, 246
Employees. *See* Staff
Employers
direct managed care contracts with, 53–54, 318
health care expenditures by, 326
Encounter data, 63–64
Encounter forms, 14, 15
computerized, 186, 192
Entoven, Alain, 300
Epidemiology, 101–103
Epworth Sleepiness Scale, 88
Estimates, statistical, 103
Ethical Considerations in the Business Aspects of Health Care (Woodstock Theological Center), 78, 79
Ethical Issues in Managed Care (American Medical Association), 78, 79
Ethics
of managed care, 73–81
conflicts of interests, 73, 74, 77
core values, 79–80
guidelines for, 74, 77–79
organizational ethics, 74, 79–80
physician-patient autonomy, 73, 74–77, 78, 304, 309, 319, 325–326
provider accountability, 78–79, 80
of medical practice
patient advocacy, 243
patients' best interest, 242–243
Ethics report cards, 78–79
Experimental studies, 102
Explanation of benefits (EOBs), 13–14, 17, 20
External study validity (generalizability), 104, 105
Exxon, 250

FACCT, 299
Facility management, in independent practices, 224
Family practice, geographical coverage of, 301
Federal Trade Commission, 249, 272–273, 328
antitrust law reform proposals, 255
Horizontal Merger Guidelines, 252
merger reporting requirement, 253
Statements of Enforcement Policy and Analytical Principles Relating to Health Care and Anti-Trust, 251
Fee-for-service compensation, 327
patient satisfaction with, 172
payer-related risk of, 233

Fee schedules, 13–14
of discounted managed care contracts, 56–57
managed care organizations' amendments to, 57
Feinstein, Alvan, 85
Florida Power and Light, 143
Flow charts
use in clinical improvement analysis, 134, 138, 139, 140–141, 160, 161, 162
use in office efficiency planning, 185–186
Formularies, restricted, 76
Foundation for Accountability, 68
Freeman, C. Kay, 230
Functional health status
as clinical improvement indicator
in benchmarking, 144, 145, 146, 147, 148, 150, 151, 152, 157
for carpal tunnel syndrome surgery, 134, 135, 137
with clinical value compass approach, 118, 119, 122, 124, 126–127
definition, 85

Galbraith, William Kenneth, 185
Gatekeeper concept, of managed care. *See* Primary care physicians, referrals by (gatekeeper role)
Gates, George, 93
Generalizability, 104, 105
General Motors, 250
Generic drugs, 76
Geographic variation, in health care utilization rates, 87
Georgia MultiSpecialty Group, 316, 319–322
Getting to Yes (Fisher and Ury), 31, 33, 37
Glasgow Coma Scale, 88
Goldsmith, Jeff, 329
Government. *See also* Antitrust law
health care expenditures by, 326
responsibility for health care costs, 171
Gross Domestic Product, health care expenditures as percentage of, 117
Gross National Product, health care expenditures as percentage of, 295
Group boycott, as antitrust violation, 251–252, 253
Group practice. *See also* Physician groups
without walls, 290, 304, 305
Gulf War syndrome, 77
Gynecology, geographical coverage of, 301

Halo effect, 101–102, 103
Harvard School of Public Health, Program for Health Care Negotiation and Conflict Resolution, 31
Hassan antitrust case, 253
Hawthorne effect, 206–207
Head and neck cancer
clinical severity staging of, 88
outcomes research in, 89, 93
quality of life assessments, 91–92, 94

Head and neck reconstruction, microvascular free tissue transfer technique in, 94
HealthAmerica, 315
HealthCare, 315
Health care
aim of, 118
delivery structure for, 85
disease model of, 301n
physicians' control of, 325–332
practice principles of, 242–245
primary care model of, 23
quality of
effect of capitation on, 4, 74–75
importance of, 167–175
indicators of, 68
managed care organizations' monitoring of, 77
patients' perception of, 167, 174
stakeholders in, 100
value of, 117–118
clinical value compass assessment of, 117–128
wellness model, 301–302, 301n.
Health care costs
annual rate increase, 3
as clinical improvement indicator
in benchmarking, 143, 145, 146, 147, 148, 150, 151, 152, 157
for carpal tunnel syndrome surgery, 134, 135, 136–137
in clinical value compass approach, 119, 122, 124, 125, 126–127
effect of HMOs on, 301
as percentage of Gross Domestic Product, 117
physicians' responsibility for, 167, 171
Health care expenditures
annual trends, 4, 326
per capita variations, 326
percentage received by physicians, 167, 168
Health Care Finance Administrators Common Procedure Coding System, 20
Health Care Financing Administration, 274
Health care purchasing cooperatives, 301
Health care reform, 117–118
Clinton administration plan for, 249, 295, 300, 329n.
for mergers and acquisitions, 295–296, 299–300
Health insurance
employer-provided, 3, 74
for medical office employees, 220
national, 249, 295, 300, 329n
Health insurance companies. *See also* Health insurance providers; *names of specific companies*
effect on health care costs, 171
percentage of health care expenditures received by, 167, 168
physician organizations' contracts with, 266, 270
underwriting policies restrictions of, 295
Health insurance plans, patients' questions about, 245
Health insurance providers
physician networks as, 274
provider service networks as, 328, 329
Health Insurance Purchasing cooperatives, 329n
Health Maintenance Organization (HMO) Act of 1973, 301
Health maintenance organizations (HMOs)
antitrust law and, 252
"any willing provider" laws for, 53
capitation payments by, 3–4
contracts, 51, 53
with physician groups, 302–303
with physican organizations, 266, 270
with single-specialty networks, 282–283
enrollment, 301
physician workforce and, 325
first otolaryngologist contracted with, 315
effect on health care costs, 301
horizontal and vertical intgegration by, 300
information sources about, 52
patient satisfaction with, 172
staff model of, 77
startup time, 52
state licensure, 52, 54
Health Outcomes Institute, patient satisfaction survey by, 204–205
Health Plan Employer Data and Information Set (HEDIS), 68, 236, 268–269
Health plans, 300
control over physicians by, 325–328
factors affecting patients' selection of, 172
Insurance Reference Guide to, 187
inventory of, 187
Plan Summary Sheet for, 187
Quick Reference Grid for, 187, 188
Health Services Resource Group, 174–175
Health status, definition, 99
Hearing aids
comparison with otologic procedures, 95
effect on quality of life, 90
patients' satisfaction with, 89, 207, 209
Hearing loss
assessment instruments for, 89
conductive, hearing aid use in, 95
Hearing screening, in infants, 95
HEDIS. *See* Health Plan Employer Data and Information Set
Hemorrhoidectomy rates, geographic variation in, 87
Henry Ford Hospital, referral guidelines, 26
Henry Ford Medical Group, 23, 27–28
Hippocrates, 74
History data, 63
Hitler, Adolf, 32
Hospital-based analysis, as outcomes measure, 67
Hospital consultation charges, reimbursement process for, 14
Hospitals. *See also names of specific hospitals*
health care role, 297
joint ventures, 300, 328
mergers and acquisitions, 55
percentage of health care expenditures received by, 168
physician network-affiliated, 274
premature discharge by, 243
specialists' partnerships with, 289
vertical and horizontal integration with practitioners, 300–301
Hospital staff privileges, exclusion of medical professionals from, 252–253
HSQ 12, 207
Hughes, Lynn A., 230
Human resources consultants, 264
Hungate, Robert, 117
Hypotheses, post hoc, 104
Hysterectomy rates, geographic variation in, 87

Iacocca, Lee, 295
ICD-9-CM. *See* International Classification of Diseases, Ninth Revision, Clinical Modification codes
Imaging technology guidelines, of capitation contracts, 8–9
Incentive pools, in discount schedules, 56
Incorporation. *See* Corporations
Independent practice associations (IPAs), 289, 304, 305. *See also* Single-specialty networks
antitrust law and, 254
contracting committees, 52
contract negotiation function, 290
managed care contracts, 234
Independent practitioners
challenges faced by, 203
continuous quality improvement by, 203–231
in business management, 219–226
checklist for, 229
expected quality in, 215
expert advice sources for, 229–230, 231
in facility and operations management, 224–225
effect of managed care organizations on, 227–230
one-dimensional quality in, 213, 215
with outcomes-based marketing, 207–213
patient satisfaction surveys for, 204–207, 209, 210
in practice management, 216–219
practice prospectus and, 213, 214
in referral services management, 219
revenue tracking in, 230
in staff management, 219
with total quality management, 214, 215–216
unexpected quality in, 215
contracts for, 225–226
Infants, hearing screening in, 95
Inference, clinical, 103–104
Infertility treatment, 77
Information management. *See* Management information systems
Informed consent, 78, 244
Inpatient review, concurrent, 3

Inpatient surgical procedures, capitation rate estimation for, 321
Integrated health systems, 296, 297, 298
Integrated medical groups, 302–303, 304, 305, 306
  model of, 307–312
Internal consistency, of surveys, 110
Internal medicine, referral process in, 24
Internal Revenue Service, 274
Internal validity, of outcomes studies, 104, 105
International Classification of Diseases, Ninth revision, Clinical Modification codes
  use in capitation rate estimation, 5
  use on encounter forms, 14
  use in reimbursement, 12, 20, 189
Internet, 216
Inventory control, 220
IPA. *See* Independent practice associations
Isenberg, Steven, 93

Japanese, industrial quality improvement techniques of, 143, 203, 213
Johnson administration, 249
Joint Commission on the Accreditation of Healthcare Organizations, *1996 Comprehensive Accreditation Manual for Hospitals*, 79
Joint ventures, 254, 281, 300, 328
Journal of the American Medical Association, 87
Juran, Joseph M., 213

Kaiser Permanente, 252, 301, 315
Kaizen, 213
Kelsch, John, 158
Kelvin, William, 113
Kennedy administration, 249

Laboratory results, patients' reports of, 216–217
Laboratory services, anti-referral legislation for, 273–274
Lahey Clinic, 300–301
Laryngeal cancer
  outcomes research in, 94
  quality of life assessment of, 91–92
  TNM tumor staging of, 88
Laryngeal diseases, outcomes research in, 94
Laryngectomy, quality of life assessment of, 91–92, 94
Legal fees, 221
Legal services, 258, 261–263
Levinson, Stephen, 230
Liability, in managed care, 226, 254–255. *See also* Malpractice liability
  contractual, 254–255
  for employees' negligence, 219
  financial risks, 245–246
Line item posting, of payments, 13

Malpractice insurance, 63, 220
Malpractice liability, 239–246
  advertising/marketing-related, 243
  capitation-related, 306
  effect on health care costs, 171
  failure to report laboratory results-related, 216
  gag clause-related, 242
  legislative reform of, 274
  physician networks' risk of, 271–272, 274
  utilization review-related, 241–242, 243–244, 246, 254, 272, 274
Managed care
  administrative costs of, 59–60, 239
  as contract medicine, 240, 241
  definitions, 327
  differentiated from capitation, 327
  financial risks of, 245–246
  new paradigm for, 117–118
  patient management costs in, 234
  phases, 278
  physicians' skill requirements in, 33
Managed care information sheet, 225
Managed care organizations
  accreditation/licensure, 227
  fraudulent payment discounts by, 13–14
  independent practices and, 227–230
  information sources about, 227
  legislative regulation of, 76–77
  Medical Loss Ratio of, 227
  physician credentialing by, 76–77, 242
  physicians' exclusion from, 76–77
  plan performance comparison of, 227, 228
  revenues from, tracking of, 221
Managed competition, 300, 328–329n
Management, as managed care contract issue, 59–60
Management information systems, 192, 233–238
  for multispecialty networks, 318
  for physican organizations, 262, 263, 264
  pricing descriptions, 237–238
  selection guidelines, 235–237
  vendors, 236–237, 264, 265
Managers, 198–199
Managing care concept, 304n
Manifest Destiny, 250
Marcus, Leonard J., 31
Maren, Arte, 219
Market allocation schemes, as antitrust violation, 251
Marketing
  by managed care organizations, 243
  outcomes research-based, 207–213
  by single-specialty networks, 282–283
Marketing and negotiating committees, 282
Marshfield Clinic, 252, 329–330
Matrix and reference manual, 14
MaxiCare, 315
Mayo Clinic, 300–301, 329–330
McGill University, 315
McGraw-Hill Relative Value Units, 6, 17
McKinley, William, 250
Medicaid
  as capitation population class, 6
  control over health care costs by, 325–326
  cost increase control of, 3
  electronic claims submission to, 16
  managed care organizations' control of, 328
  projected growth reductions, 328
Medical education, 299
Medical Group Management Association, 235
Medical Loss Ratio, 227
Medically necessary treatment, 56, 77
  malpractice liability implications of, 244
Medically-unnecessary treatment, 59
Medical office practices
  capitation rate estimation for, 64, 321
  cost analysis of, 64
  time estimation for, 218, 221
Medical Outcomes Study, 25, 93, 113, 204
Medical practice models, 296–299
Medical records. *See also* Management information systems
  alteration of, 245
  confidentiality of, 61, 79, 227, 229, 244, 245
  management guidelines for, 218, 244–245
    for efficiency improvement, 189, 191
  use in malpractice litigation, 244–245
  as outcomes research basis, 107–108, 114
  physician's failure to respect, 173
  state laws regarding, 244, 245
Medical schools, ownership by clinics and hospitals, 300–301
Medicare
  Canadian system, 315
  as capitation population class, 6
  control over health care costs by, 325–326
  cost increase control for, 3
  electronic claims submission to, 16, 192
  managed care organizations' control of, 328
  medical specialty training funding by, 299
  projected growth reductions, 328
  prospective payment system, 300, 326
  Resource-Based Relative Value Scale, 6, 17, 321
  uniform fee schedule, 326
Medicare beneficiaries, per-capita expenditures on, 326
Medications
  generic, 76
  health care expenditures for, 168
  preapproved lists of, 76
MEDLINE database, 150
MedSoft, 233
Menière's disease, outcomes research in, 93
Mergers and acquisitions, 295–314
  antitrust regulations regarding. *See* Antitrust law
  health care reform and, 295, 299–300
  HMO contracts and, 301–303
  by hospitals, 300–301
  impetus for, 295–296
  managed care growth and, 301–303
  networking versus, 303–305
  among physician groups, 303–312

dissolution and liquidation, 312
economies of scale, 306
external stakeholders, 310–311
human resources management, 313
information needs, 313
internal stakeholders, 309–310, 311
leadership, 312–313
market power, 306–307
model, 307–312
networking versus, 312
quality of care and, 306
trends, 307
supplier power and, 299, 301
Meta-analysis, 88, 107
MetLife, 17
Minneapolis/St. Paul, medical group mergers in, 306–307
Monopolies, 250, 252
Morbidity, factors affecting, 6
Multinational corporations, 250
Multispecialty networks, 265, 307, 308
contract negotiations by, 318–319
development from single-specialty networks, 315–323
business plan, 322
credentialing of members, 321, 322
incorporation, 319
organization chart, 319, 320
quality assessment programs, 322
full-risk contracts, 316
networking versus mergers by, 304
networking with single-specialty networks, 290
obstacles to, 318–319
physician organizations as, 268
rationale for, 316–318
as specialty-primary care network, 319
Multivariate analysis, 104
Myocardial infarction patients, health care quality improvement for, 122–125

Naisbitt, John, 100
National Committee for Quality Assurance, 217, 286, 299, 318, 321
Health Plan Employer Data and Information Set (HEDIS), 68, 236, 268–269
National health insurance
Clinton administration proposal for, 249, 295, 300, 329n.
historical background, 249
Natural history, of disease, 103
NCQA. *See* National Committee for Quality Assurance
Neurosurgeons, referrals to, 23–24
New Hampshire Hospital Association, 150
Newsletters, 216
Nixon, Richard M., 301
Not-for-profit corporation, 281
Nottingham Health Profile, 90
Nurses, 167, 169, 191
Nursing homes, 168

Observational research, 102, 105
Obstetrics, geographical coverage of, 301
Obstructive sleep apnea syndrome
clinical severity staging of, 88
outcomes assessment of, 94, 95–96
quality of life assessment of, 106–107
Office data, types of, 63–64
Office efficiency. *See* Operational management
Office insurance, 220
Office managers, 198, 199
Office visits
as physician productivity indicator, 7–8
scheduling of. *See* Appointment scheduling
Operational management
efficiency improvement techniques for, 185–192
automation use, 185, 191–192
flowcharting, 185–186
identification of problem areas, 185–186
process reengineering and process improvement, 192
updating of operations, 186–191
in independent practices, 224–225
Opthalmology, subspecialty fellowships in, 23
Optimally-managed care, 9
Ordering log, 220
O'Sullivan, John, 250
Otitis media, outcomes research in, 92, 95, 107
quality of life assessment in, 94, 106–107, 110–113
Otitis media with effusion
clinical practice guidelines for, 108–109
cost-effectiveness studies of, 94
outcomes research in, 88, 93, 94–95, 107
Otolaryngologists
outcomes research by, 207–213
peer review by, 285–286
profile reports by, 68–69, 70–71
referrals to, 24
Otolaryngology
outcomes research in, 106–109
appropriateness studies, 87–88, 108–109
clinical severity staging system, 88
community-based research, 93
disease-specific assessment instruments, 88–90
future directions, 93–96
patient-based research, 106–107
patient satisfaction assessment, 93
pediatric, 88, 93, 94–95, 107, 282
process assessment, 108–109
records-based research, 107–108
referral guidelines for, 25, 27–28
single-specialty networks of, 277–288
Otolaryngology-Head and Neck Surgery Conference, outcomes research recommendations of, 93–96
Otology, outcomes research in, 95
Otorrhea, posttympanostomy, 88
Outcome, definition of, 85
Outcome data, 67
Outcomes management, 100, 101
Outcomes measurement, 204
categories, 67–68
as clinical improvement indicator
in benchmarking, 143, 145, 146, 147, 148, 150, 151, 152, 157
in carpal tunnel syndrome surgery, 134, 135, 137
with clinical value compass method, 117–128
instruments for, 85–86
results data use in, 64
Outcomes research, 85–98, 99–115
American Academy of Otolaryngology-Head and Neck Surgery grant for, 100–101
appropriateness studies, 87–88, 108–109
bias in, 102, 103, 104, 192
clinical severity staging system, 88
community-based, 93, 207
comparison with clinical trials, 99–100
comparison with randomized controlled trials, 101–103
cost-effectiveness research, 92
cross-sectional studies, 90–92
definition, 67, 99–100
disease-specific instruments, 86, 88–90
epidemiological basis, 101–103
essentials of, 106
by independent practitioners, 207–213
meaningless, 101
differentiated from meaningful, 105–106
meta-analysis, 88, 107
methodologic requirements, 86–87
as observational research, 101, 105
patient-based, 100, 101, 106–107
process assessment, 100, 101
prospective studies, 90–92
records-based, 100, 101
retrospective studies, 90–92
statistics use in, 103–105
types of, 86–87
Outpatient surgical procedures, capitation rate estimation for, 321
Outsourcing, 219–220, 237
Oxner Clinic, 329–330

Park Ridge Center for the Study of Faith and Ethics, 79
Partnerships, 258, 281, 282, 330
Patient account specialist, job description, 194
Patient-based outcomes research, 100, 101, 106–107
Patient call back sheet, 216–217
Patient cost analysis, 221, 222
Patient incident reports, 217
Patient Outcomes Research Teams, 100
Patients
best interests of, 242–243
demographics of, as managed care contract issue, 59
direct payments by, 61
disruptive, 60, 218

Patients (*Continued*)
  dissatisfaction with physicians, 173, 174. *See also* Patient satisfaction; Patient satisfaction surveys
  new
    closing practice to, 61
    preregistration of, 12, 186, 188, 189, 190
    registration of, 185
Patient satisfaction
  as clinical improvement indicator
    in benchmarking, 144, 145, 147, 148, 150, 151, 152, 157
    in carpal tunnel syndrome surgery, 134, 135, 136
  clinical value compass approach, 119, 122, 124, 126–127
  in continuous quality improvement, 174
  with managed care cost, 172
  with managed care quality, 172
Patient satisfaction surveys. *See also* Project Solo
  form for, 178
  implementation and methods of, 174–175
  by independent practitioners, 209, 210
  as mail surveys, 113
  by single-specialty networks, 286, 287
  validity and reliability, 113
  Visit Rating Questionnaire for, 113, 175, 178, 204–205, 207
Patient services, flow charting of, 185
Patient Visit Rating Questionnaire, 113, 175, 177, 178, 204–205, 207
Payment discounts, fradulent, 13–14
Payment rates. *See also* Fee schedules
  as defined in managed care contracts, 56
Payments
  collection of, 270–271
  direct, by patients, 61
  line item posting of, 13
  retrospective denial of, 74
  schedules for, as defined in managed care contracts, 56
Payroll management, 224
Pediatrics
  geographical coverage, 301
  in otolaryngology, outcomes research in, 88, 93, 94–95, 107, 282
Peeno, Linda, 73
Peer review
  editorial, 100–101
  in single-specialty networks, 279
Petty cash, 221
Physician assistants, 191, 230
Physician cost-quality matrix, 316, 317
Physician groups
  capitation payments to, 5
  hospitals' investments in, 300
  increase of, 307
  managed care contracts, 234
  networking by, 303–305
Physician-hospital organizations
  capitation payments to, 5
  contracting committees, 52
Physician networks. *See also* Multiple-specialty networks; Physician organizations; Single-specialty networks
  antitrust law regarding, 249–254
  exclusion of physicians from, 252–253
  as health insurance providers, 274
Physician organizations, 257–275
  accountant services, 264
  banking services, 264
  by-laws, 259
  claims processing, 261, 264
  committee structure, 259–260
  consultants for, 257–258, 261, 263–264
  contracting by, 261, 262, 264, 269–272
    capitated contracts, 261, 262, 265, 267, 270
    negotiations, 266
    policies and goals in, 267–268
  contracting alliances of, 267
  credentaling of members, 260, 267
  early policy decision making by, 257
  expansion, 266–267
  governance superstructure, 259
  hospital affilitations, 262, 265, 266, 267, 269–270
  incorporation, 258–259
  information systems, 264, 268–269
  legal issues affecting, 256–259
    antitrust law, 249–254, 255, 257, 272–273
    physician liability, 254–255
  legal services for, 258, 261–263
  management and operational activities, 262–263
  market "package", 269
  membership rights, 259
  number of members, 257, 260
  physician compensation system, 262
  profiles, 265, 269
  public policy-related bias towards, 249–250
  recruiting of members, 260–261
  regulatory issues affecting, 272–274
  specialty mix of, 257, 265
  stock ownership distribution in, 259
  vendor services, 262, 263–265
  voting rights, 259
Physician-patient relationship
  autonomy in, 73–75, 78
  effect of capitation on, 327
  as contractual relationship, 296
  deterioration of, 239–240
  ethics of, 242–243
  in managed care, 240, 241
  patient advocacy in, 78
  patient dissatisfaction with, 173
  patient-perceived quality in, 175–176
  practice management guidelines for, 218–219
  quality improvement guidelines for, 229
Physician productivity method, of capitation rater estimation, 7–8
Physicians
  income decrease, 249–250
  job satisfaction, 299
  percentage of health care expenditures received by, 167, 168
Physicians' Information Exchange (PIE), 177, 180, 205–206, 215–216
Physician withholds. *See* Withholds
Physician workforce, 167, 169, 249, 325
Piccirillo, Jay, 94
Pitofsky, Robert, 255
Placebo effect, 101–102, 103
Pliny the Elder, 103
Plume, Stephen, 216
Point-of-service, 56, 316
Postage, cost management for, 220
Postoperative outcomes survey, 207, 210
PPO. *See* Preferred provider organizations
Practice administrators, 198, 199
Practice growth monitor, 221, 222
Practice guidelines. *See* Clinical practice guidelines
Practice management
  consultants for, 264, 265
  for the independent practitioners, 216–219
Practice managers, 198, 199
Practice pamphlets, 216
Practice principles, 242–245
Practice prospectus, 213, 214
Preadmission testing, 3
Preauthorization, 299
  differentiated from precertification, 14
  as malpractice liability risk, 272
  relationship to patient's benefits, 227
Preauthorized admissions, 74
Precertification, 3
  differentiated from preauthorization, 14
  for surgery, 74, 321
Precision, statistical, 104
Preferred provider organizations (PPO), 304, 305
  antitrust law and, 254
  "any willing provider" laws for, 53
  contracts, 52–53
  discounted services of, 51
  network broker model of, 53
  patient satisfaction with, 172
  physician organizations' contracts with, 266, 270
Pregnancy, adolescent, health care expenditures for, 167
Premiums, credited to risk pools, 57
Preregistration, of new patients, 12, 186, 188, 189, 190
Preregistration coordinator, 194, 195
Preventive medical services, 76, 168
Price fixing, as antitrust violation, 251, 254
Primary care capitation, 4–5, 8–9
Primary care model, of health care system, 23
Primary care physician groups, networking versus mergers by, 304
Primary care physicians
  capitation payments to, 4–5
  fees, comparison with specialists' fees, 24–25
  referrals by (gatekeeper role), 278
    economic incentives for, 53, 58
    guidelines for, 25–28
    profile reports, 69

rates, 24
to single-specialty networks, 285
referrals to, 23
satisfaction with single-specialty networks, 286
specialists' dependence on, 306
specialty network development and, 318
Problem solving, 122
Procedure codes. *See also* Current Procedural Terminology codes, International Classification of Diseases, Ninth Revision, Clinical Modification codes
profile reports and, 68, 70
Process assessment, 100, 101, 108–109, 114
Process improvement techniques, 192
Process reengineering, 192
Productivity, of physicians, 7–8
Product quality, 203–204
Profiling/profile reports, 67–71
definition, 67–68
of lifetime health care costs, 128–129
of physician organizations, 256, 269
of surgery costs, 207, 211, 212, 213
in total quality management, 216
Project Solo, 93, 167–182, 204–207
benchmarked measurement process of, 167, 175, 177
confidentiality in, 176–177, 205–206
Confidential Self Assessment of Quality method of, 167, 176–177
definition, 167
peer development and direction in, 177
Patient Visiting Questionnaire of, 113, 175, 177, 178, 204–205, 207
Physicians' Information Exchange of, 177, 180, 205–206, 215–216
quality as central vision of, 175–176
Proportional hazards regression, 104
Prostatectomy rates, geographic variation in, 87
Provider manual, 60
Provider relations committees, 282
Provider service networks, 327–330. *See also* Multispecialty networks; Single-specialty networks
care options outside, 76
definition, 328
legislative regulation of, 328
organizational structure
capitalist, 330, 331
collegial, 329–330, 331
physicians' exclusion from, 76–77
role in health care system, 328–330, 331
Provider Supported Networks (PSNs), 296
Proxies, in outcomes assessment, 86
Prudent purchasing model, of managed care contracts, 326–328
Purchasing costs, of independent practitioners, 219
P values, 104
Pyriform sinus carcinoma, quality of life assessment in, 92

Quality-adjusted life-year (QALY), 92
Quality assurance and control. *See also* National Committee for Quality Assurance
antitrust law and, 253
in multispecialty networks, 318, 322
in physician mergers, 306
prior to managed care, 296
as Project Solo goal, 176–177
in single-specialty networks, 280, 283, 286, 318
Quality management committees, 282
Quality of life
definition, 85, 99, 109
effect of sensory impairment on, 90
health-related, 109
Quality of life assessment
assessment instruments for, 86, 90, 105, 109–114
in otolaryngology patients, 106–107
retrospective, cross-sectional and prospective studies of, 90–92
Quality of Well-Being Scale, 86, 90
Quality outcome indexing, 299
Quarterly statistics form, for independent practitioners, 221, 223

Radiology services guidelines, of capitation contracts, 8–9
RAND, 25
Random error, 109–110
Randomization, in outcome studies, 102
Randomized controlled trials, comparison with outcome studies, 101–103, 114
Random sample, 104–105
Reception area, cleanliness and condition of, 224
Receptionist/registrar, job description, 191, 194
Reception protocol, 190, 191
in independent practices, 224–225
Record-based outcomes research, 114
Records. *See* Medical records
Records-based outcomes research, 107–108, 114
Referral coordinator, job description, 194
Referral network, adequacy of, 240–241
Referrals, 296. *See also* Primary care physicians, referrals by (gatekeeper role)
automated tracking of, 236
guidelines, 23–30
development of, 25–27
in otolaryngology, 27–28
legislative regulation of, 273, 274
medical report letters in, 109
by patients, 217
process of, 23–25
rates, 23–24
effect of referral guidelines on, 24–25, 28
reception staff's verification of, 12
scheduling for, 229
unauthorized, 20
Referral sources, management of, 219, 229
Reflux-type symptoms, description and classification of, 94

Registration, of new patients, 185
Regression to the mean, 101–102, 103
Reimbursement. *See also* Payments
percentage payment on, 17
Reimbursement specialist, job description, 194, 196
Reimbursement systems, 11–22
collection policies, 14, 224
"domino effect" in, 12
efficiency of, 189
electronic claims submission in, 16, 192
encounter forms for, 14, 15, 186, 192
flow charting of, 185
monitoring of, 17–20
staff's expertise in, 12–14
Verification of Eligibility and Benefits forms for, 16
written policies for, 14
Reinertsen, Jim, 138
Reinsurance, 9–10, 59, 271
Relative value scales, 285
resource-based, 6, 17, 321
of single-specialty networks, 280
Relative value units, 321
revenues per, 221, 223
Relman, Arnold, 79
Requests for proposals, 301
Rescheduling, of patients, 218
Resource-based relative value scale (RBRUS), 6, 17, 321
Responsiveness, of surveys, 110
Results data, 63
Revenue tracking, 230
Rhinitis, assessment instruments for, 89
Risk-bearing, 57
Risk pools, 57–58, 327
Risk-sharing, 3, 4, 233, 234
Risk-shifting, 57
Rockefeller, John D., 250
Rolodex file, 185
Roosevelt, Franklin D., 249
Roosevelt, Theodore, 250
Rosenfeld, Richard, 93
Royal College of Radiologists Working Party, referral guidelines, 24
Ruff, Howard, 101

Sadat, Anwar, 37
Sampling methods, 104, 105
Scheduling, of patients. *See* Apppointment scheduling
Schwartz, May, 230
Second opinions, 299
Selection bias, 104
Sensory impairment, effect on quality of life, 90
Septoplasty, surgical guidelines for, 321
Service contracts, 221
Sex factors, use in capitation payment estimation, 6
SF-36, 86, 90–91, 107, 207
Shared savings programs, for single-speciality networks, 286
Sherman Anti-Trust Act, 250
Sickness Impact Profile, 86

Single-specialty networks, 269, 277–288
antitrust law and, 292
consultants for, 292
contract negotiations by, 289, 290, 291
credentialing, 292
definition, 277
development committee, 292
development into multispecialty networks, 315–323
rationale for, 316–318
economies of scale, 289–290
implementation, 284–285
initial stages, 289–293
legal services for, cost of, 292
as limited liability corporation, 289–290
marketing of, to payers, 291
motivation for, 316
networking options for, 290
number of members, 291
obstacles to, 318–319
physician organizations as, 265, 266
preooperational planning and organization, 290–293
quality assurance in, 280, 286, 292
recruiting of members, 292
reimbursement systems, 285
revenue disbursement procedure, 292–293
shared savings programs, 286
structuring of, 279–284
advisory committees formation, 281–282
capitation rate negotiations, 283–284
contracting with providers, 280–281
marketing to payers, 282–283
organizational structure, 280, 281
selection of lead physician, 279–280, 290
third-party administration, 290–291, 292–293
utilization management by, 285–286, 292
Sinusitis/sinus surgery, outcomes research in, 93, 95, 107
appropriateness studies, 87–88
assessment instruments for, 89
quality of life assessment of, 90–91, 106
surgical guidelines for, 321
Smoking, health care expenditures for, 167
Social Security system, national health insurance inclusion in, 249
Software
for independent practices, 225
for managed care data management, 225
for revenue tracking, 230
Specialist physician groups, networking versus mergers by, 304
Specialists
fees, comparison with primary care physician's fees, 24–25
income reduction for, 289
patients' access to, 316–317
as percentage of all practicing physicians, 23
referrals to. *See* Primary care physicians, referrals by (gatekeeper role)
reimbursement, within capitated systems, 58
utilization review of, 243–244
Spohr, Mark H., 233
Staff
advertising for, 199–200
computer terminal access, 191
efficiency improvement, 185, 191
hiring, 199–200, 201
interaction with patients, 217–218
involvement in quality improvement, 213, 216, 219
job descriptions, 185, 191, 194–197, 199–200
management of, 193–201, 219, 221
operations checklist for, 193
reimbursement activities, 12–14
salaries, 200
skills, 199–200, 201
Standard of care, 243
Standard Oil, 250
Stark bill, 273
Statistics, in outcome research, 103–105
Steroids, as otitis media with effusion treatment, 88
Stop-loss insurance, 59, 245
automated tracking of, 236
Study sample, 104–105
Subspecialists, subcapitation, 58
Subspecialization, 23
Substance abuse, percentage of health care expenditures for, 167
Surgeons, referrals to, 23–24
Surgery
capitation rate estimation for, 321
cost profiling of, 207, 211, 212, 213
precertification for, 74, 321
urgent, scheduling of, 14
Surgery coordinator, job description, 194, 197
Surveys, 109–110
reliability of, 109
validity of, 110
Systematic sample, 105

Target population, 104–105
Tax-exempt foundations, physician organizations as, 258, 259
Tax regulations, managed care contract implications of, 55
Technical Assistance Research Project (TARP), 216
Telephone
use in patient management, 216–217
voice mail systems, 186
Termination
of care for disruptive patients, 60
of managed care contracts, 62–63, 76–77, 277, 280, 281
Third parties. *See also* Health insurance companies; Medicaid; Medicare
in health care relationships, 74
Tinnitus, assessment instruments for, 89
TNM tumor stage, 88
Tonsillectomy
effect on quality of life, 95
mandatory second opinions for, 107–108
rates, geographic variation in, 87, 107–108
surgical guidelines for, 321
Total quality management, 179, 204
benchmarking in, 215–216
in community-based practice, 213, 215–216
by independent practitioners, 221
Transfer bias, 102, 103
Transsexual surgery, 77
Treatment denial, as malpractice liability risk, 274
Treatment protocols, 60. *See also* Clinical practice guidelines
development by managed care providers, 65
physicians' liability for, 59
Truman administration, 249
Twain, Mark, 101, 109
Tympanostomy, as otorrhea cause, 88
Tympanostomy tubes, pediatric use of, 87, 94, 108–109
quality of life assessment of, 110–113

Uncertainty, statistical, 103
Unemployment insurance claims, 220
United HealthCare, 315, 316
U.S. Justice Department, 272–273, 281, 328
Horizontal Merger Guidelines, 252
merger reporting requirement, 253
Statements of Enforcement Policy and Analytical Principles Relating to Health Care and Anti-Trust, 251
U.S. Steel, 250–251
U.S. Supreme Court decisions, on antitrust violations, 252
University medical centers, networking with single-specialty organizations, 290
University of California, Los Angeles, 24
Unmanaged care, 9
Utility costs, 221
Utilization data, managed care organizations' monitoring of, 76
Utilization rates, in capitation rate estiamtion, 5–6
Utilization review, 74, 241–242, 262, 263
automated monitoring of, 236
legal liability associated with, 241–242, 243–244, 246, 254, 272, 274
in single-specialty networks, 280, 281–282, 285–286, 318
in specialty networks, 317
Uvulopalatopharyngoplasty, 88, 321

Value equation, for health care, 118
Vendors
of management information systems, 235
for physician organizations, 262, 263–265

Ventilation tube insertion, surgical guidelines for, 321
Verification of Eligibility and Benefits Form, 16
Vertigo
  cost-effective analysis of, 95
  effect on quality of life, 90
Veterans Administration Cooperative Study, for laryngeal preservation, 93
Violence, health care expenditures for, 167
Visit Rating Questionnaire. *See* Patient Visit Rating Questionnaire
Voice, assessment instruments for, 89

Wennberg, John, 87
Weymuller, Ernest, 93
Wickline v. the State of California, 243
Withholds, 3
  in discount schedules, 56
  reserved from risk pools, 57
  return by managed care organizaitons, 227
Word-of-mouth recommendations, by patients, 216
Working Group on Accountability, 78–79
Wound infection rate, postsurgical, 118

Xerox Corporation, 142, 143

Zip code grouping, for analysis of practice data, 64